THE KEY TO EATING WELL AND BEING HEALTHY IS IN YOUR HANDS!

Before you snack, shop, cook, or dine out again, get the scoop on all the foods you eat in this completely updated, revised, and expanded guide. With more than 6.5 million of their popular counter books in print, Annette B. Natow, Ph.D., and Jo-Ann Heslin, M.A., R.D., C.D.N.— nationally recognized professional nutrition educators— are the trusted source for the information you need to lose weight, prevent disease, increase your energy levels, and live a longer, healthier life. This easy-to-use, easy-to-carry reference offers essential up-to-date nutrition information for more than 17,000 foods, featuring reliable counts for:

- Calories
- Fat
- Cholesterol
- Protein
- Carbohydrates
- Fiber
- Sodium

THE COMPLETE FOOD COUNTER
3rd Edition

If you eat it, you'll find it here!

Books by Annette B. Natow and Jo-Ann Heslin

The Calorie Counter
(*Fourth Edition*)

The Cholesterol Counter
(*Seventh Edition*)

The Complete Food Counter
(*Third Edition*)

The Diabetes Carbohydrate and Calorie Counter
(*Third Edition*)

Eating Out Food Counter

The Fat Counter
(*Seventh Edition*)

The Healthy Heart Food Counter

The Healthy Wholefoods Counter

The Most Complete Food Counter
(*Second Edition*)

The Protein Counter
(*Second Edition*)

The Ultimate Carbohydrate Counter

The Vitamin and Mineral Food Counter

Published by POCKET BOOKS

THE
COMPLETE
FOOD
COUNTER

Third Edition

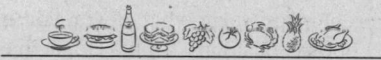

Annette B. Natow, Ph.D.
Jo-Ann Heslin, M.A., R.D.
With the Assistance of Karen J. Nolan, Ph.D.

POCKET BOOKS
New York   London   Toronto   Sydney

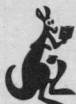

Pocket Books
A Division of Simon & Schuster, Inc.
1230 Avenue of the Americas
New York, NY 10020

Copyright © 1999, 2003, 2006, 2009 by Annette B. Natow and Jo-Ann Heslin

A previous edition of this work was published in 1999 by Pocket Books as *The Most Complete Food Counter*.

All rights reserved, including the right to reproduce this book or portions thereof in any form whatsoever. For information address Pocket Books Subsidiary Rights Department, 1230 Avenue of the Americas, New York, NY 10020

This Pocket Books paperback edition January 2009

POCKET and colophon are registered trademarks of Simon & Schuster, Inc.

For information about special discounts for bulk purchases, please contact Simon & Schuster Special Sales at 1-800-456-6798 or business@simonandschuster.com.

Manufactured in the United States of America

10   9   8   7   6   5   4   3

ISBN-13: 978-1-4165-6666-3
ISBN-10:   1-4165-6666-X

*To our families, who support us
through every project:*

*Harry, Allen, Irene, Sarah, Meryl, Marty, Laura, George,
Emily, Steven, Rebecca, Joseph, Kristen,
Brian, Karen, and John.*

ACKNOWLEDGMENTS

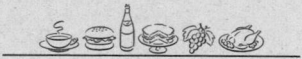

For graciously sharing her knowledge, Karen J. Nolan, Ph.D.

For all her continuous support and help, our agent, Nancy Trichter.

For her suggestions and editing skills, Sara Clemence.

Without the tireless cooperation of Stephen Llano and the production department at Pocket Books, *The Complete Food Counter,* Third Edition, would never have been completed.

A special thank you to our editor, Micki Nuding.

And, we would like to thank all of our readers for their suggestions and questions. Your input helps us to provide you with the most useful information.

"…foods though so numerous and varied in form, can be reduced to rather simple terms."

Mary Swartz Rose, Ph.D.
Feeding the Family
The MacMillan Company, 1919

CONTENTS

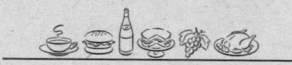

PART ONE

Brand Name, Nonbranded (Generic), and Take-Out Foods

PART TWO

Restaurant Chains

INTRODUCTION

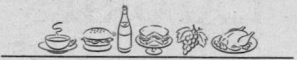

Listen to any group of people talking, and the conversation almost always turns to food—what's the best choice for lunch, the current popular diet, or the latest health report. Everyone loves to talk about food. And everyone has questions about their health.

We wrote *The Complete Food Counter* to give you answers. It is a handy, easy-to-use, *complete* food and nutrition resource, listing nutrient values for more than 17,000 foods, along with information on how to get enough of or limit each nutrient listed.

Let's talk about food—it's fun.
Let's talk about nutrition—it's important to your health.

1

UNDERSTANDING CALORIES

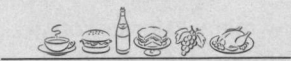

Calories are calories, whether they come from apples or chocolate fudge. Every time you eat, you take in calories. All foods, except water, have some.

Your body is a machine that uses food calories as fuel. When the amount of fuel you take in equals the amount of fuel you need to run your body, your weight remains constant. There is no extra fuel to store and no deficit to make up. Eat too many calories, and your body uses what it needs and stores the rest for future use—in places like your thighs, hips, and waist. Eat too few calories, and your body draws on its fuel reserves to meet demands. Your thighs, hips, and waist get slimmer as your fuel surplus is depleted.

Again and again, studies have shown that if you cut calories, you lose weight. It doesn't matter if those calories come from bread, meat, or salad dressing. When you eat too many calories, even from healthy foods, you gain weight. The key to long-term weight control is to burn as many calories as you eat.

AND THE NUMBERS ARE?

On average, we eat 300 more calories a day than we ate 35 years ago and we weigh 24 pounds more.

Women eat 1,880 calories a day; men eat 2,620.

To find out how many calories you need each day, you need to do two things. First decide, how much do you want to weigh? Not your current weight, but what is your target weight? Then select an activity factor that fits your current activity level.

1. Your target weight is: _____

2. Your activity factor is: _____

   20 = Very active men

   15 = Moderately active men or very active women

   13 = Inactive men, moderately active women, and people over 55

   10 = Inactive women, repeat dieters, seriously overweight people

3. Target Weight × Activity Factor = Calories needed each day.

   For example, if your target weight is 130 and you are a moderately active woman (factor 13), you need about 1,600 to 1,700 calories a day.

   130 pounds × 13 = 1,690 calories

Eating this amount of calories each day would guarantee weight loss, because you are getting only enough calories to support your target weight, not your current heavier weight. Add extra exercise to your regular routine, and the weight will come off even faster.

FAT FACTS

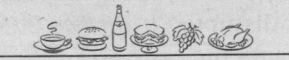

The simplistic view that all fats are bad and you should eat less fat is no longer accurate. The more accurate message is:

- Not all fats are bad for you.
- The type of fat you eat may be more important than how much you eat.
- A moderate fat intake can be healthy.

Don't head for the bacon grease just yet. Even though the current research suggests that a moderate fat intake may be healthier, no one is suggesting a *high* fat intake is good for you. Eating too much fat puts you at risk for:

- Heart disease
- Stroke
- High blood pressure
- High cholesterol
- Cancer
- Obesity
- Diabetes
- Arthritis
- Gout
- Age-related macular degeneration (ARMD), a leading cause of blindness
- Alzheimer's disease, a leading cause of dementia

A high fat diet may even disrupt your body's clock. We all operate on a 24-hour circadian cycle that regulates sleeping, waking, fluid balance, body temperature, heart output, oxygen use, and gland functions. When the body's clock is disrupted it throws off our internal signals, including appetite control. Researchers have found a misaligned body clock can increase the risk for obesity and diabetes. More recent research on animals confirmed that a high fat diet disrupts normal circadian rhythms— another good reason to eat a moderate amount of fat.

Total Fat— should be 20% to 35% of total calories

Americans have gotten the message that a high fat intake is not good for them. Current consumption studies show we eat about 33% of our daily calories as fat. That is close to the upper end of the recommended 20% to 35% of total calories each day.

The following table will help you set your own daily target fat intake. First, select the number of calories you eat each day. Next, select the percentage of fat calories you wish to eat, and the chart will give you the grams of fat to aim for daily. This means if you regularly eat 1800 calories a day, you should eat somewhere between 40 grams (20%) and 70 grams (35%) of fat each day.

If you aim to eat 20% to 25% for your daily calories as fat, you will be eating a low fat intake. Thirty to 35% is considered a moderate fat intake. Either can be part of a healthy eating plan.

DAILY TARGET FAT INTAKE			
CALORIES PER DAY	**PERCENTAGE OF FAT CALORIES EACH DAY IN GRAMS**		
	20%	25%	30%	35%
1,000	22	28	33	39
1,100	24	31	37	43
1,200	27	33	40	47
1,300	29	36	43	51
1,400	31	39	47	54
1,500	33	42	50	58
1,600	36	44	53	62
1,700	38	47	57	66
1,800	40	50	60	70
1,900	42	53	63	74
2,000	44	56	67	78
2,100	47	58	70	82
2,200	49	61	73	86
2,300	51	64	77	89
2,400	53	67	80	93
2,500	56	69	83	97
2,600	58	72	87	101
2,700	60	75	90	105
2,800	62	78	93	109
2,900	64	81	97	113
3,000	67	83	100	117

CONSIDER THIS

It's been shown over and over again that people have trouble sticking with a low fat eating plan.

Moderate fat intakes are more satisfying, and people find them easier to adopt for the long haul.

CONTROLLING CHOLESTEROL

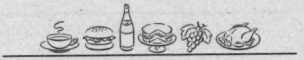

Total Cholesterol

Desirable: less than 200 mg/dl
Borderline high: 200 to 239 mg/dl
High: 240 mg/dl or higher

High cholesterol quietly does damage to your body, building up on the walls of your arteries. Over time, this buildup can cause the arteries to harden, a process called *atherosclerosis*. If arteries get narrowed, blood flow to the heart muscle is slowed down and may even be blocked. A blocked artery to the heart can cause a heart attack. A blocked artery to the brain can cause a stroke.

High cholesterol does not cause any symptoms, so the only way you know if your cholesterol levels are too high is through a blood test. It's important to know what the results mean.

Total cholesterol is just that—the amount of cholesterol in a given volume of blood. It is measured as the number of milligrams (mg) of cholesterol in 1 deciliter (dl) of blood, which is slightly less than a half cup. For example, 222 mg/dl = 222 milligrams of cholesterol per deciliter of blood. To make things simpler, your doctor may give you just the number, 222, rather than the more complete measurement. To reduce your risk for heart disease, you want your level to be below 200.

YOU SHOULD KNOW

It's wise to fast for at least 8 hours before getting your blood drawn.

Eating a high fat meal within 4 hours of a blood test can affect the results by raising blood fats.

If your number is good—total cholesterol is close to 200—you can eat a moderate cholesterol diet, which contains 300 milligrams or less cholesterol a day. If your cholesterol number is less than desirable, or if your doctor has prescribed a cholesterol-lowering medication, you should eat a low-cholesterol diet, with less than 200 milligrams a day.

Total cholesterol isn't the only number that matters. To travel through blood, cholesterol, a fatlike substance, is coated with a protein. The combination of fat and protein is called a *lipoprotein.* If your total cholesterol values are high, your doctor will want to know the amount of LDL (low density lipoprotein) cholesterol and HDL (high density lipoprotein) cholesterol as well.

If too much LDL cholesterol—bad cholesterol—circulates in the blood, it can stick to the walls of the arteries leading to the heart and brain. This eventually forms plaque—thick, hard deposits that clog arteries. Experts believe HDL cholesterol—good cholesterol—carries cholesterol away from the arteries and back to the liver, where it is broken down and removed from the body. This process is called reverse cholesterol transport and it helps prevent the growth of plaque. It may be more important to know if your good HDL cholesterol is too low (less than 40 for men and less than 50 for women) than if your LDL cholesterol is too high.

Easy Steps to Lower Cholesterol

- Use liquid vegetable oils—olive, canola, corn, soybean, sunflower, and safflower—instead of butter, lard, shortening, or stick margarines.
- Limit servings of meat, poultry, fish, and shellfish to 3- to 4-ounce portions.
- Use lean cuts of meat and trim off all visible fat.
- Eat poultry without the skin.
- Don't fry in lard or bacon fat.
- Bake, broil, or roast.
- Use more beans and vegetables to make up for smaller servings of meat, fish, and poultry.
- Substitute two egg whites for one egg with yolk.
- Use lowfat or nonfat milk, cheese, yogurt, and ice cream, and fat free sour cream.
- Use soft margarine instead of stick margarines or butter.
- Use lowfat or fat free salad dressings and gravies.
- Eat fiber-rich foods—beans, whole grains, bran, brown rice, dried fruits, fruits, and vegetables.
- Eat more cholesterol-lowering foods—nuts, soyfoods, and antioxidant-rich fruits and vegetables.
- Eat soy, nuts, and flaxseed with natural cholesterol-lowering plant sterols, or foods fortified with plant sterols—margarines, cereal, chocolate, orange juice, and yogurt.
- If your doctor prescribed a cholesterol-lowering medication, take it daily, even when your cholesterol values return to normal.

PERSPECTIVE ON PROTEIN

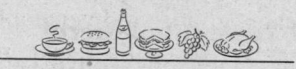

Your body loses millions of cells each day. They are used up, worn out, rubbed off, and even cut off, like your hair or beard. Protein is in almost every cell, tissue, and substance in your body and you need protein to replace these lost or worn out cells.

You lose protein when your body is stressed in any way—physically or mentally. When it's too hot or too cold, you need extra protein. More protein is needed during heavy sweating. Exercise, fever, surgery, injury, infection, and broken bones all increase your need for protein. Even emotional stress, such as losing your job or taking an exam, causes protein loss.

The protein in your body is very similar to the protein found in food. Both are made up of smaller building blocks called *amino acids*. Your body uses a combination of amino acids to build and repair different parts of the body—muscles, glands, skin, bones—just like the letters in the alphabet are used in different combinations to form words. Active tissues—like muscles and glands—contain a lot of protein. Less active tissue—fat—has far less.

Some amino acids can be made in the body, others cannot. The amino acids that can't be made in the body are obtained from the food you eat. When you eat different foods, you get varying amounts of different amino

11

acids. That is one of the reasons it's important to eat a variety of foods.

Almost all foods you eat contain protein—some more, some less. Fruit has very little protein compared to meat, milk, cheese, beans, grains, and vegetables, all of which have more. Whenever you eat a food containing protein you are providing your body with the building blocks—amino acids—to construct and repair your body parts.

CONSIDER THIS

The top 10 sources of protein eaten in the U.S. are beef, poultry, milk, yeast bread, cheese, fish, eggs, fresh pork, ham, and pasta.

A quick way to estimate your daily protein need is to divide your weight by 2.2. For example, if you weigh 150 pounds, you should be eating approximately 68 grams of protein a day (150 ÷ 2.2 = 68). Most people eat more than their recommended level of protein daily.

Meat, fish and poultry are the most obvious protein sources, but many other foods are excellent sources as well.

1 OUNCE PROTEIN EQUALS

1 ounce of meat, fish, or poultry
¼ cup wheat germ
¼ cup canned tuna, salmon, mackerel
8 ounces lowfat yogurt
1 ounce cheese
1 cup lowfat or nonfat milk
¼ cup cottage cheese
3 ounces (¼ block) tofu

¼ cup cooked soybeans
¼ cup tempeh
½ cup cooked dried beans (any variety)
½ cup (2.5 ounces) meat substitute
2 tablespoons of peanut or other nut butter
1 egg
¼ cup egg substitute
¼ cup nuts

WEIGHT LOSS WISDOM

Recent studies have shown that diets with extra protein are more satisfying and result in greater weight loss.

CONSIDERING CARBOHYDRATES

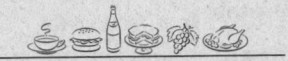

Carbohydrates include all the sugars, starches, and fibers found in foods. Plant foods—fruits, vegetables, beans, and grains—are rich in carbohydrates. Fruits have more sugar. Vegetables, beans, and grains have more starch. Both have some fiber.

Sugars and starches are your body's main source of energy, or calories. When the food you eat is digested, sugar molecules move easily into the bloodstream and travel to cells, where they are burned for energy to keep your body working. Starch molecules are more complex. They are made up of many sugar molecules bound together. During digestion, these larger starch molecules are slowly broken apart to yield smaller sugar fragments, which are sent to the cells to be converted into energy.

YOU SHOULD KNOW

Simple carbohydrates are foods that contain a lot of sugar—syrups, jelly, honey, soda, and molasses—and have few, if any, vitamins and minerals and no fiber.

Complex carbohydrates are foods that contain a lot of starch—whole grains, cereals, vegetables, beans—and are rich in vitamins, minerals, and fiber.

Not too long ago, you were told to eat all the carbohydrates you wanted. In fact, most Americans get 50% or more of their daily calories as carb. Today, however, carbs are being blamed for many of our health concerns, especially obesity. Just as with any other kind of food, if you eat more carbohydrate calories than your body needs for energy, the leftover is stored as fat.

So, how much carb should you be eating?

The National Academy of Sciences' Recommended Dietary Allowance (RDA) for carbohydrate is at least 130 grams a day. The Food and Drug Administration (FDA) has set 300 grams of carb as the Daily Value (DV) for the nutrition facts panel on food labels, the amount recommended for the "typical" American consumer eating 2,000 calories a day.

You can estimate your individual carb intake by first deciding what amount of carb you want to eat each day. Since most Americans get 50% of their calories from carb, let's use 50% as an example. If you eat 1,800 calories a day:

50% of 1,800 calories = 900 carb calories a day

To figure out how many grams of carb to eat each day, you need to know that 1 gram of carb = 4 calories. Continuing to use the example above:

900 carb calories per day ÷ 4 = 225 grams of carb per day

Most food professionals consider a low carb diet one in which 40% or less of your daily calories come from carbohydrates. Now, let's use 40% as an example, if you wish to follow a low carb diet. If you eat 1,800 calories a day:

40% of 1,800 calories = 720 carb calories per day
720 carb calories per day ÷ 4 = 180 grams of carb per day

Both examples more than meet the RDA recommendation of at least 130 grams of carbohydrate a day. To make good carb choices, choose more foods that are higher in starch and fiber, and fewer foods that are high in sugar.

FOCUS ON FIBER

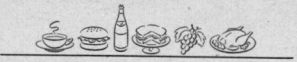

This is one carbohydrate all experts agree on: we need to eat more. Why? Fiber aids in losing weight, managing diabetes, relieving constipation, and protecting against certain cancers. It may even lower the risk for heart disease. All this, without calories!

Fiber is found only in plants, either as the woody part—which helps promote regularity—or as gums and mucilages—which help lower cholesterol. Even though fiber is a carb, your body cannot break it down and use it the way it uses sugar and starch. But, living in your digestive tract are trillions of friendly microbes that use fiber as their main source of nourishment.

These friendly bacteria have been with you since birth to protect you against unfriendly bacteria that could make you sick. When you eat enough fiber, your friendly bacteria are well fed and can put up a good fight. When you eat too little fiber, unfriendly invaders can start to take over. Eating enough fiber stimulates your natural resistance against disease and infection.

Most of us eat too little fiber. We average about 15 grams a day, far less than we should be eating.

DAILY FIBER RECOMMENDATIONS

Men
    19–50 years   38 grams of fiber
    50 and older   30 grams of fiber
Women
    19–50 years   25 grams of fiber
    50 and older   21 grams of fiber
    pregnant   28 grams of fiber

AGE + 5

*Children 2 and older should eat the
amount of fiber daily that equals their age + 5.*

*For a 5-year-old, that would be
at least 10 grams of fiber a day.*

*The rule holds until age 19,
when adult requirements apply.*

Slowly start adding fiber-rich foods to your daily meals—beans, berries, bran, fruits, oatmeal, vegetables, and whole grains. Don't go overboard, because it takes your body a little time to adjust to the extra bulk passing through your digestive tract. And, drink plenty of fluids. Fiber soaks up fluids like a sponge. This not only helps you feel fuller longer, but also helps form soft, easily passed stools.

YOU SHOULD KNOW

*High fiber foods have 5 or more grams of fiber
in a serving.*

*A good source of fiber has 2 or more grams of fiber
in a serving.*

Add a Little Fiber to Your Life
- Eat whole fruits and vegetables instead of drinking juices.
- Eat the fiber-rich skins of cucumbers, apples, pears, potatoes, and zucchini.
- Eat more berries—blueberries, blackberries, raspberries, strawberries.
- Choose whole grains—brown rice, cornmeal, barley, cracked wheat, rye, and whole wheat.
- Eat beans and lentils a few times a week.
- Eat whole grain or high fiber cereals—oatmeal, oat flakes, bran, shredded wheat.
- Eat whole wheat bread, bagels, pasta, pretzels, crackers, and rolls.
- Try soybeans in every form—soynuts, tofu, tempeh, edamame.
- Snack on fig newtons, graham crackers, and popcorn.
- Have vegetarian meals a few times a week.
- Eat dried fruits and raisins.
- Sprinkle ground flaxseed onto cereal or yogurt for a healthy crunch.
- Try some of the new fiber-fortified foods.

BE SENSIBLE WITH SODIUM

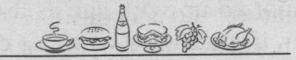

Ever give that salt shaker on your kitchen table a second thought? You should. Once a precious commodity, salt has become ubiquitous in our food supply, to the point where it's estimated we each eat 1¼ to 2½ teaspoons a day—far more than we need.

Salt is made up of 2 minerals, sodium and chloride. One teaspoon of salt has 40% sodium and 60% chloride, or approximately 2,000 milligrams of sodium. It's the sodium we're concerned about.

Sodium regulates the fluid inside cells as well as your total body fluid. This regulates your blood volume, blood pressure, and the acidity of your body. The movement of sodium into and out of cells helps carry other substances that need to get into or be removed from your cells.

WHAT THE EXPERTS ARE SAYING

Americans eat too much salt.

Adults 19–50 should get no more than 1,500 milligrams of sodium a day; those between 50 and 70 should get 1,300 milligrams; and people over 70 should get 1,200 milligrams.

The upper limit of intake for all adults should not exceed 2,300 milligrams.

Ninety-five percent of American adults exceed the recommended upper limit of sodium intake every day, and 90% of adult Americans are at risk for high blood pressure as they get older. In places where little salt is used, blood pressure does not go up with age as it does in the U.S. Logic would say, if you eat less salt, you can prevent high blood pressure. Population studies provide evidence that this is true.

YOU SHOULD KNOW

New research shows lowering high blood pressure reduces the risk for dementia.

You absorb almost all the sodium you eat, and your thirst mechanism is very sensitive to extra sodium, triggering a desire to drink. Your kidneys carefully regulate the amount of sodium needed by the body, excreting the extra in urine. Continually eating a high sodium intake causes your body to hold excess fluid, which puts stress on the kidneys, heart, and blood vessels, and may set the stage for high blood pressure.

YOU SHOULD KNOW

About 10% to 15% of people with high blood pressure are salt-sensitive. If they eat less salt, their blood pressure goes down.

Others with high blood pressure, who are not salt-sensitive, see a less dramatic reduction when they eat less salt.

When people are told to eat less sodium, their first reaction is to empty the salt shaker and stop adding salt in cooking. This may not be the most effective approach, because your daily sodium intake actually comes from:

Salt and **sodium-containing food additives** added in food processing	77%
Sodium naturally occurring in food	12%
Salt added in cooking and at the table	11%

Dumping the salt shaker only reduces your salt intake by slightly more than 10%. Cutting down on processed foods will make a much bigger dent in your sodium intake. What are processed foods? Prepared salad dressing, jarred tomato sauce, canned tuna, marinated fresh meat and poultry, cake mixes, pickles, pretzels, frozen dinners, desserts, canned soup, microwave meals, deli meats, hot dogs—just to name a few.

DID YOU KNOW?

An average dill pickle contains 1,000 milligrams of sodium, two thirds of your day's supply.

Giving up salt isn't easy. Most of us eat between 2,300 to 4,700 milligrams of sodium a day. Many experts believe that healthy adults could do nicely on as little as 500 milligrams of sodium a day. That may be healthy, but would we consider it tasty?

To Lighten Up on Salt
- Don't add salt to restaurant or take-out foods.
- Use naturally low sodium fresh fruits and vegetables, or plain frozen vegetables, to complement take-out or prepared entrees.
- Check the nutrition label—keep snacks and single-serving foods under 400 milligrams a serving; keep main dishes under 600 milligrams a serving.

- Try some low sodium or "no salt added" choices; you might be pleasantly surprised at the taste.
- Fresh salads are naturally low in sodium; just go easy on the dressing.
- Plain frozen vegetables are lower in sodium than sauced and seasoned varieties.
- Almost all frozen vegetables are lower in sodium than canned vegetables.
- Try baldy pretzels and unsalted nuts.
- Reduce salt in recipes by half—swapping ½ teaspoon of salt for 1 teaspoon saves 1,000 milligrams of sodium.
- Rinse canned beans, vegetables, and tuna to reduce the sodium by almost half.
- Don't add salt when cooking rice, pasta, or hot cereal.
- Use fresh pepper or herbs to flavor food instead of salt.
- When you eat a high salt/sodium choice, balance it with lower sodium choices later in the day.

DID YOU KNOW?

1 teaspoon of table salt = 2,400 milligrams of sodium.

Coarser salts, such as kosher salt and sea salt, average between 1,100 and 1,900 milligrams sodium per teaspoon.

USING YOUR COMPLETE FOOD COUNTER

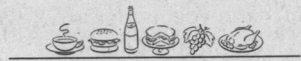

The Complete Food Counter lists the portion size, calories, fat, cholesterol, protein, carbohydrate, fiber, and sodium values for more than 17,000 foods. Now you can compare the values in your favorite foods and, when necessary, choose substitutes before you go out to shop or eat. This will save you time and help you decide what to buy.

The counter section of the book is divided into two parts: Part One: Brand Name, Nonbranded (Generic), and Take-Out Foods (page 33); and Part Two: Restaurant Chains (page 527). Each part lists foods or restaurant chains alphabetically.

In Part One, for each category, you will find nonbranded (generic) foods listed first, in alphabetical order, followed by an alphabetical listing of brand name foods. The nonbranded listing will help you estimate the calories, fat, cholesterol, protein, carbohydrate, fiber, and sodium values when you don't see your favorite brand. They can also help you to evaluate store brands. Large categories are divided into subcategories, such as canned, fresh, frozen, and ready-to-eat, to make it easier to find what you're looking for. Some categories have "see" and "see also" references, to help you find related items.

When a dash (–) appears, it means that no analysis was done for fat, cholesterol, protein, carbohydrate, fiber, or sodium for that food. It is not the same as a "0," which means there is no fat, cholesterol, protein, carbohydrate, fiber, or sodium in the food.

Because we eat out so often, over 700 take-out foods are listed in Part One. These are found in the take-out subcategory in many categories throughout this section. Look there for foods you take-out or order in, since those are not nutrition labeled.

Most foods are listed alphabetically. In some cases, though, foods are grouped by category. For example, a tuna sandwich is found in the SANDWICH category. Other group categories include:

ASIAN FOOD: **Page 42**
Includes all types of Asian foods
except egg rolls and sushi,
which are found in the egg rolls
and sushi categories.

DELI MEATS/COLD CUTS: **Page 197**
Includes all sandwich meats
except chicken, ham, and
turkey, which are found in their
own separate categories.

DINNER: **Page 200**
Includes all by brand name,
except pasta dinners, which
are found in the pasta dinner
category.

LIQUOR/LIQUEUR: Page 298

Includes all alcoholic beverages and mixed drinks except beer, champagne, and wine, which are found in their own separate categories.

NUTRITION SUPPLEMENTS: Page 328

Includes all dieting aids, meal replacements, and drinks, except energy bars and energy drinks, which are found in their own separate categories.

SANDWICHES: Page 421

Includes popular sandwich, calzone, and panini choices.

SNACKS: Page 445

Includes a variety of snack items such as pork rinds and cheese puffs.

SPANISH FOOD: Page 469

Includes all types of Spanish and Mexican foods except salsa and tortillas, which are found in their own separate categories

In Part Two, Restaurant Chains, 100 national and regional restaurant, coffee, doughnut, frozen yogurt, ice cream, pizza, sandwich, soup, and sushi chains are listed. Brand name foods are required by federal law to have nutrition information on labels, but in most areas of the country, restaurants only provide this information voluntarily.

With *The Complete Food Counter* as your guide, you have at your fingertips the most comprehensive guide to calories and important nutrients in all the foods you eat.

DEFINITIONS

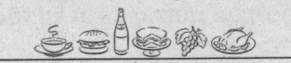

as prep (as prepared)—refers to food that has been prepared according to package directions

lean and fat—describes meat with some fat on its edges that is not cut away before cooking, or poultry prepared with skin and fat as purchased

lean only—refers to lean meat that is trimmed of all visible fat, or poultry without skin

not prep (not prepared)—refers to food that has not been cooked and may require the addition of other ingredients to prepare

shelf-stable—refers to prepared products found on the supermarket shelf that are not canned or frozen, but are packaged and ready-to-eat, or ready to be heated but do not require refrigeration

take-out—describes prepared dishes that you purchase ready-to-eat; those included serve as a guide to the calories, fat, cholesterol, protein, carbohydrate, fiber, and sodium in products you may purchase.

ABBREVIATIONS

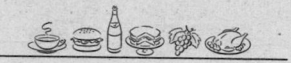

avg	=	average
diam	=	diameter
fl	=	fluid
frzn	=	frozen
g	=	gram
in	=	inch
lb	=	pound
lg	=	large
med	=	medium
mg	=	milligram
oz	=	ounce
pkg	=	package
pt	=	pint
prep	=	prepared
qt	=	quart
reg	=	regular
sec	=	second
serv	=	serving
sm	=	small
sq	=	square
tbsp	=	tablespoon
tr	=	trace
tsp	=	teaspoon
w/	=	with
w/o	=	without
<	=	less than

NOTES

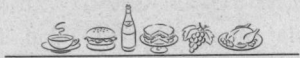

Cals = Calories
   All calorie values have been rounded to the nearest calorie
Fat = Total fat
   All fat values are given in grams (g)
   All values have been rounded to the nearest gram
Chol = Cholesterol
   All cholesterol values are given in milligrams (mg)
   All values have been rounded to the nearest milligram
Prot = protein
   All protein values are given in grams (g)
   All values have been rounded to the nearest gram
Carb = carbohydrate
   All carbohydrate values are given in grams (g)
   All values have been rounded to the nearest gram
Fiber
   All fiber values are given in grams (g).
   All values have been rounded to the nearest gram
Sod = Sodium
   All sodium values are given in milligrams (mg)
   All values have been rounded to the nearest milligram
tr (trace) = less than 0.5 grams of fat, protein, carbohydrate, or fiber, and less than 0.5 milligrams of cholesterol or sodium

- (dash) indicates data was not available

0 (zero) indicates there are no calories, fat, cholesterol, protein, carbohydrate, fiber, or sodium in that food

Discrepancies in figures are due to rounding of values, product reformulation, and reevaluation. The current labeling law allows rounding. Much of the data listed here is analysis data, obtained directly from manufacturers, not from labels; therefore, some values here may differ slightly from labels because they have not been rounded.

PART ONE

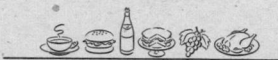

Brand Name, Nonbranded (Generic), and Take-Out Foods

OUR BEST EATING ADVICE IN A NUTSHELL

Calories—go easy, don't overdo, keep portions reasonable

Fat—aim for moderate amounts daily, limit fried foods and fatty add-ons like salad dressing

Cholesterol—aim for 300 milligrams or less a day

Protein—select lean and lowfat choices, eat both animal and vegetable sources

Carbohydrates—limit sugars, and select more complex starches, like grains and vegetables

Fiber—eat more, use whole grains

Sodium—go easy, cut down on processed foods, eat more whole foods naturally lower in salt

FOOD	PORTION	CALS	PROT	FAT	CHOL	CARB	FIBER	SOD
ABALONE								
breaded & fried	1 serv (3 oz)	162	17	6	80	9	tr	980
steamed	1 serv (3 oz)	127	17	3	84	6	0	574
ACAI JUICE								
Zola								
100% Juice	1 box (11 oz)	170	2	2	0	30	1	45
ACEROLA								
fresh	1 (5 g)	2	tr	tr	0	tr	tr	0
ACEROLA JUICE								
juice	1 cup	56	1	1	0	12	1	7
ADZUKI BEANS								
canned sweetened	½ cup	351	6	tr	0	81	–	323
dried cooked w/o salt	½ cup	147	9	tr	0	28	8	9
Arrowhead Mills								
Organic Dried not prep	¼ cup	130	8	0	0	26	5	0
AKEE								
fresh	3.5 oz	223	5	20	0	5	–	–
ALCOHOL (*see* BEER AND ALE, CHAMPAGNE, LIQUOR/LIQUEUR, MALT, WINE)								
ALE (*see* BEER AND ALE)								
ALFALFA								
sprouts	½ cup	40	1	tr	0	1	tr	1
ALLIGATOR								
cooked	3 oz	126	28	2	57	0	0	66
ALLSPICE								
ground	1 tsp	5	tr	tr	0	1	tr	1
ALMONDS								
almond butter w/ salt	2 tbsp	203	5	19	0	7	1	144
almond butter w/o salt	2 tbsp	203	5	19	0	7	1	4
almond extract	1 tsp	38	5	tr	0	–	0	–
almond paste	¼ cup	260	5	16	0	27	3	5
chocolate covered	6 (0.6 oz)	102	3	8	1	6	2	8
dry roasted w/ salt	¼ cup	206	8	18	0	7	4	117
dry roasted w/o salt	¼ cup	206	8	18	0	7	4	0
honey roasted	¼ cup	214	7	18	0	10	5	47

FOOD	PORTION	CALS	PROT	FAT	CHOL	CARB	FIBER	SOD
jordan almonds	6 (0.7 oz)	99	2	4	0	14	1	3
oil roasted w/ salt	¼ cup	238	8	22	0	7	4	133
oil roasted w/o salt	¼ cup	238	8	22	0	7	4	0
praline	17 (1.4 oz)	210	5	12	0	21	3	45
yogurt covered	6 (0.8 oz)	122	3	8	0	10	1	13
American Almond								
Marzipan	2 tbsp	130	2	5	0	19	1	0
Arrowhead Mills								
Organic Almond Butter Creamy	2 tbsp	200	7	17	0	6	4	0
Blue Diamond								
Almond Roca Buttercrunch	3 (1.3 oz)	210	2	14	15	19	0	125
Honey Roasted	¼ cup	170	2	14	0	8	3	35
Jalapeno Smokehouse	28 (1 oz)	170	6	15	0	5	3	180
Jordon Pastels	15 (1.4 oz)	180	3	8	0	28	2	0
Lime 'N Chili	28 (1 oz)	170	6	16	0	5	3	120
Maui Onion & Garlic	28 (1 oz)	170	6	15	0	5	3	170
Milk Chocolate Covered	9 (1.4 oz)	230	5	14	5	19	3	35
Salted	¼ cup	170	5	16	0	6	3	85
Smokehouse	28 (1.3 oz)	170	6	16	0	5	3	150
Wasabi & Soy Sauce	28 (1 oz)	170	6	15	0	6	3	115
Whole Natural	¼ cup	180	6	14	0	6	3	0
Yogurt Covered	12 (1.4 oz)	210	3	14	0	21	0	20
Brach's								
Chocolate Coated	11	220	3	13	10	22	2	10
Eden								
Tamari	3 tbsp (1 oz)	160	8	11	0	8	4	65
Good Sense								
Hickory Smoked	¼ cup	180	6	16	0	4	2	170
Raw Whole	¼ cup	180	6	15	0	6	4	0
Kettle								
Butter Salted	2 tbsp	180	5	17	0	6	2	55
Butter Unsalted	2 tbsp	180	5	17	0	6	2	0
Love'n Bake								
Almond Paste	2 tbsp	140	4	9	0	13	2	0
Almond Schmear	2 tbsp	140	4	8	0	14	2	0
Roasted Butter	2 tbsp	180	6	16	0	6	3	55
Maisie Jane's								
Almond Butter	1 oz	184	5	16	0	6	0	4
Cappuccino	9 (1.4 oz)	220	4	15	5	19	2	20

FOOD	PORTION	CALS	PROT	FAT	CHOL	CARB	FIBER	SOD
Chocolate Toffee	9 (1.4 oz)	210	4	13	5	21	2	45
Coffee Glazed	2 tbsp (1 oz)	150	4	12	0	8	3	15
Cowboy BBQ	2 tbsp (1 oz)	140	4	11	0	8	3	220
Mint Chocolate	9 (1.4 oz)	210	3	15	0	20	2	20
Organic Honey Glazed	2 tbsp (1 oz)	160	6	14	0	12	4	32
Tamari	2 tbsp (1 oz)	160	5	14	0	7	4	60
Mrs. May's								
Almond Crunch	1 oz	156	5	13	0	8	3	37
Odense								
Almond Paste	2 tbsp (1.4 oz)	170	9	7	5	24	0	0
Planters								
Chocolate Lovers Dark Chocolate	11 (1.4 oz)	220	4	17	<5	18	3	15
Dry Roasted	23 (1 oz)	160	6	14	0	6	3	150
Sunkist								
Accents Italian Parmesan	1 tbsp	40	1	4	0	1	0	95
Accents Original Oven Roasted	1 tbsp	40	1	4	0	1	0	70
AMARANTH								
leaves cooked	½ cup	14	1	tr	0	3	–	170
uncooked	½ cup (3.4 oz)	365	14	6	0	65	15	20
Arrowhead Mills								
Organic Whole Grain not prep	¼ cup	180	7	3	0	31	7	10
ANCHOVY								
boneless	1 oz	60	8	3	24	0	0	1042
canned in oil drained	1 can (2 oz)	94	13	4	38	0	0	1651
fresh	1 (4 g)	8	1	tr	3	0	0	147
fresh fillets	3 (0.4 oz)	21	2	1	–	tr	–	–
Brunswick								
Flat Fillets	1 can (2 oz)	25	3	2	10	0	0	980
ANGLERFISH								
raw	3.5 oz	72	15	1	–	0	0	109
ANISE								
seed	1 tsp	7	tr	tr	0	1	tr	0

FOOD	PORTION	CALS	PROT	FAT	CHOL	CARB	FIBER	SOD
ANTELOPE								
roasted	4 oz	215	41	4	127	0	0	304
APPLE								
CANNED								
sliced sweetened	½ cup	68	tr	1	0	17	2	3
Glory								
Fried Apples	½ cup	80	0	0	0	21	1	170
DRIED								
chopped	½ cup	104	tr	tr	0	28	4	37
cooked w/o sugar	½ cup	73	tr	tr	0	20	3	26
rings	5	78	tr	tr	0	21	3	28
Bare Fruit								
Chips Cinnamon	1 pkg (0.6 oz)	43	0	0	0	12	2	15
Crispy Green								
Crispy Apples	1 pkg (0.36 oz)	35	0	0	0	8	1	0
Fruit Ripples								
Cinnamon Apple	1 pkg	50	0	0	0	13	1	75
Strawberry Apple	1 pkg	50	0	0	0	13	1	75
Mrs. May's								
Fruit Chips	1 pkg	35	0	0	0	8	1	0
FRESH								
apple	1 sm	55	tr	tr	0	15	3	1
apple	1 med	72	tr	tr	0	19	3	1
apple	1 lg	110	1	tr	0	29	5	2
candied	1 sm (4.9 oz)	179	2	3	0	40	3	79
candied	1 med (6.5 oz)	234	2	4	0	52	4	103
candied	1 lg (9.8 oz)	357	3	6	6	79	6	157
w/ skin sliced	1 cup	57	tr	tr	0	15	3	1
w/o skin sliced	1 cup	53	tr	tr	0	14	1	0
Earthbound Farm								
Organic Slices	1 pkg (2 oz)	30	0	0	0	7	1	0
Mrs. Prindable's								
Caramel Triple Chocolate	¼ apple (1.7 oz)	120	1	6	5	17	1	10
Caramel Walnut	¼ apple (2 oz)	160	2	10	5	17	1	15

FOOD	PORTION	CALS	PROT	FAT	CHOL	CARB	FIBER	SOD
Rainier								
Apple	1 med (5.5 oz)	80	0	0	0	22	5	0
Sullivan								
McIntosh	1 (5.4 oz)	80	0	1	0	22	4	0
TreeTop								
Slices Red Or Green	1 pkg (2 oz)	35	0	0	0	8	–	0
FROZEN								
sliced w/o sugar	½ cup	42	tr	tr	0	11	2	3
Roast Works								
Flame Roasted Fuji	1 serv (5 oz)	90	0	0	0	23	2	55
TAKE-OUT								
baked	1 (6 oz)	128	tr	tr	0	42	4	2
baked no sugar	1 (5.6 oz)	136	tr	tr	0	24	4	2
fried apple rings	1 serv (2.7 oz)	91	tr	4	0	15	2	33
APPLE JUICE								
cider	1 cup	117	tr	tr	0	29	tr	7
juice + vitamin C & calcium	1 cup	117	tr	tr	0	29	tr	17
mulled cider	1 serv	265	1	1	0	42	6	12
unsweetened w/o vitamin C	1 cup	117	tr	tr	0	29	tr	7
After The Fall								
Organic	8 oz	90	0	0	0	22	–	20
Apple & Eve								
100% Juice	8 oz	110	1	0	0	26	–	5
Celestial Seasonings								
Cider Apple Caramel Kiss as prep	1 cup	80	0	0	0	21	0	0
Eden								
Organic Juice	8 oz	90	0	0	0	24	0	0
Fizz Ed.								
Green Apple	1 can (8.4 oz)	100	0	0	0	25	1	30
Hansen's								
100% Juice	8 oz	120	0	0	0	28	0	15
Hood								
100% Juice	1 cup	120	0	0	0	31	0	5

FOOD	PORTION	CALS	PROT	FAT	CHOL	CARB	FIBER	SOD
Izze								
Sparkling Apple	1 bottle (12 oz)	138	3	0	0	34	–	10
Kedem								
100% Juice	8 oz	110	0	0	0	28	–	15
Langers								
Diet Cocktail 50% Juice	8 oz	60	0	0	0	14	–	10
Harvest Apple 100% Juice	8 oz	120	0	0	0	28	–	0
Minute Maid								
100% Juice	8 oz	100	0	0	0	28	–	20
Mott's								
Hot Spiced Cider All Flavors as prep	1 serv	80	0	0	0	20	–	15
Naked Juice								
Just Apple	8 oz	120	1	0	0	30	0	15
Old Orchard								
Cider 100%	8 oz	120	0	0	0	29	–	25
Healthy Balance Apple	8 oz	30	0	0	0	6	–	9
Organic 100% Juice	8 oz	128	0	0	0	29	–	25
Phat Phruit								
Green Apple	8 oz	40	0	0	0	11	0	30
Red Cheek								
100% Juice	8 oz	120	0	0	0	29	–	20
Seneca								
100% Juice	8 oz	110	0	0	0	28	–	20
Snapple								
Diet	8 oz	15	0	0	0	4	–	10
Tree Ripe								
Organic 100% Juice	6 oz	80	0	0	0	21	0	10
TreeTop								
100% Juice	8 oz	120	0	0	0	29	–	25
Cider 100% Juice No Sugar Added	8 oz	120	0	0	0	29	–	25
Tropicana								
Orchard Style	1 bottle (14 oz)	200	tr	0	0	50	0	20
Walnut Acres								
Organic Juice	8 oz	110	0	0	0	29	0	0

FOOD	PORTION	CALS	PROT	FAT	CHOL	CARB	FIBER	SOD
Zeigler's								
Old Fashioned Cider	8 oz	110	0	0	0	26	1	15
APPLESAUCE								
sweetened	½ cup	97	tr	tr	0	25	2	4
unsweetened	½ cup	52	tr	tr	0	14	2	2
Eden								
Organic	½ cup	60	0	0	0	13	2	10
Organic Apple Cherry	½ cup	70	0	0	0	17	3	10
Organic Apple Strawberry	½ cup	60	0	0	0	13	2	10
Organic Cinnamon	1 pkg (4 oz)	70	0	0	0	17	2	10
Langers								
Unsweetened	½ cup	50	0	0	0	13	2	5
Mott's								
Original	½ cup	110	0	0	0	27	1	0
Single-Serve Cinnamon	1 pkg (4 oz)	100	0	0	0	25	1	0
Single-Serve Natural	1 pkg (4 oz)	50	0	0	0	12	1	0
Musselman's								
Lite	1 pkg (4 oz)	50	0	0	0	12	2	10
White House								
Apple Sauce	1 pkg (4 oz)	90	0	0	0	20	1	15
APRICOT JUICE								
nectar	6 oz	106	1	tr	0	27	1	6
APRICOTS								
canned heavy syrup	½ cup	91	1	tr	0	23	3	4
canned in juice	½ cup	59	1	tr	0	15	2	5
canned in water	½ cup	33	1	tr	0	8	2	4
canned light syrup	½ cup	80	1	tr	0	21	2	5
dried halves	6	51	1	tr	0	13	2	2
dried halves cooked w/o sugar	½ cup	106	2	tr	0	28	3	5
fresh	1	17	tr	tr	0	4	1	0
fresh sliced	½ cup	40	1	tr	0	9	2	1
frozen sweetened	½ cup	119	1	tr	0	30	3	5
Crispy Green								
Crispy Dried	1 pkg (0.36 oz)	40	0	0	0	9	tr	0
Del Monte								
Halves In Heavy Syrup	½ cup	100	0	0	0	26	1	10
Orchard Select Halves	½ cup	80	tr	0	0	21	1	10

FOOD	PORTION	CALS	PROT	FAT	CHOL	CARB	FIBER	SOD
Harvest Bay								
Dried	5 (1.4 oz)	60	2	0	0	15	3	6
Mariani								
Ultimate Dried	¼ cup (1.4 oz)	100	1	0	0	24	6	10
Sunsweet								
Dried	6 pieces (1.4 oz)	100	1	0	0	25	3	25
ARROWHEAD								
corm boiled	1 med	9	1	tr	0	2	–	2
ARROWROOT								
raw	1 root (1.2 oz)	21	1	tr	0	4	tr	9
raw root sliced	1 cup	78	5	tr	0	16	2	31
Bob's Red Mill								
Starch	¼ cup	110	0	0	0	28	1	0
ARTICHOKE								
CANNED								
hearts in oil	1 serv (3 oz)	100	3	7	0	9	4	73
Gertie's Finest								
Tapenade	2 tbsp	29	1	3	0	2	tr	210
Native Forest								
Organic Hearts Quartered	1 serv (4 oz)	35	2	0	0	6	4	390
Progresso								
Hearts	1 piece	15	1	0	0	3	1	120
FRESH								
cooked	1 med	60	4	tr	0	13	7	114
hearts cooked	½ cup	42	3	tr	0	9	5	80
Ocean Mist								
Lemon	1 (4.2 oz)	60	4	0	0	13	6	115
FROZEN								
cooked	1 cup	42	3	tr	0	9	5	80
cooked w/o salt	1 pkg (9 oz)	108	7	1	0	22	11	127
C&W								
Hearts	12 pieces (3 oz)	40	2	1	0	7	5	55
TAKE-OUT								
stuffed	1 (8.8 oz)	397	15	14	8	54	10	1037

FOOD	PORTION	CALS	PROT	FAT	CHOL	CARB	FIBER	SOD
ARUGULA								
fresh	1 cup	3	1	tr	0	1	tr	5

ASIAN FOOD (see also DINNER, EGG ROLLS, SAUCES, SOY SAUCE, SUSHI)

FOOD	PORTION	CALS	PROT	FAT	CHOL	CARB	FIBER	SOD
CANNED								
chow mein chicken no noodles	1 cup	194	20	8	51	10	2	955
FRESH								
wonton wrappers	1	23	1	tr	1	5	–	46
Azumaya								
Round Wraps	10	160	6	1	10	31	1	370
Wrappers Large Square	8	160	6	1	10	31	1	370
Frieda's								
Won Ton Wrappers	4 (1 oz)	80	3	0	0	17	1	160
Nasoya								
Won Ton Wrappers	8	160	6	1	10	31	1	370
FROZEN								
Contessa								
Chow Mein Chicken w/ Sauce not prep	1¾ cups	320	16	3	25	55	3	1060
Curry Chicken w/ Sauce not prep	1¾ cups	240	12	8	25	29	2	330
Fried Rice Chicken w/ Sauce not prep	1¾ cups	260	17	4	100	49	4	680
General Tsao Shrimp w/ Sauce not prep	1¾ cups	270	10	4	35	49	4	930
Kung Pao Shrimp w/ Sauce not prep	1¾ cups	200	10	4	45	30	3	760
Low Mein Shrimp w/ Sauce not prep	1¾ cups	250	11	10	35	29	2	830
Stir-Fry Beef w/ sauce not prep	1¾ cups	190	13	3	20	28	4	820
Stir-Fry Chicken w/ Sauce not prep	1¾ cups	160	16	3	25	18	4	870
Stir-Fry Shrimp w/ Sauce not prep	1¾ cups	120	9	3	40	16	2	980
Sweet & Sour Shrimp w/ Sauce not prep	1½ cups	180	9	0	50	40	3	430
Tandoori Chicken w/ Sauce not prep	1⅓ cups	200	15	4	30	27	3	660

FOOD	PORTION	CALS	PROT	FAT	CHOL	CARB	FIBER	SOD
Glutino								
Gluten Free Chicken Pad Thai Peach	1 pkg (7 oz)	370	17	5	75	65	3	890
Helen's Kitchen								
Thai Yellow Curry w/ Tofu Steaks & Vegetables & Basmati Rice	1 pkg (9 oz)	280	12	5	0	30	2	390
Kahiki								
Beef & Broccoli	1 pkg (10.9 oz)	360	23	10	50	42	2	1060
Chicken Fried Rice	1 pkg (10.9 oz)	460	16	10	85	75	2	1090
General Tso's Chicken	1 pkg (10 oz)	400	12	10	20	66	2	1340
Naturals General Tso's Chicken	1 pkg (10 oz)	330	18	5	35	52	3	1080
Naturals Mandarin Orange Chicken	1 pkg (10 oz)	340	17	5	35	58	3	750
Naturals Szechuan Peppercorn Beef	1 pkg (10 oz)	350	19	14	50	35	3	780
Naturals Teriyaki Mixed Vegetables	1 pkg (10 oz)	260	8	2	0	51	4	750
Sesame Orange Chicken	1 pkg (10.9 oz)	420	15	12	25	60	2	1390
Soothing Lettuce Wraps	4 tbsp (2 oz)	90	5	4	10	9	1	310
Tempura Chicken Nuggets	¾ cup (3.5 oz)	230	13	14	40	10	0	470
Tropical Sweet & Sour Chicken	1 pkg (10.9 oz)	490	14	11	25	82	4	910
Lean Cuisine								
Cafe Classics Asian Style Beef w/ Ginger & Soy	1 pkg (9.25 oz)	210	14	4	25	31	2	570
Cafe Classics Bowl Chicken Fried Rice	1 pkg (10 oz)	310	17	7	50	45	3	690
Cafe Classics Bowl Chicken Teriyaki	1 pkg (11 oz)	320	16	3	30	58	3	690
Cafe Classics Bowl Teriyaki Steak	1 pkg (10.5 oz)	340	21	7	30	47	4	690
Cafe Classics Chicken Teriyaki Stir Fry	1 pkg (10 oz)	300	17	5	30	49	3	690

FOOD	PORTION	CALS	PROT	FAT	CHOL	CARB	FIBER	SOD
Cafe Classics Hunan Beef & Broccoli	1 pkg (8.5 oz)	230	12	4	15	36	1	680
Cafe Classics Thai-Style Chicken	1 pkg (9 oz)	230	18	4	30	30	2	620
One Dish Favorites Asian Style Pot Stickers	1 pkg (9 oz)	320	11	6	20	55	3	610
One Dish Favorites Chicken Chow Mein	1 pkg (9 oz)	200	13	3	25	31	2	650
Skillet Asian Style Chicken & Vegetables	1 serv	160	12	3	20	22	2	610
Organic Classics								
Thai Chicken Curry	1 pkg (10 oz)	420	19	17	40	50	3	510
Seeds Of Change								
Asian Stir-Fry Noodles	1 pkg (11 oz)	290	11	4	5	55	4	720
Spicy Peanut Noodles	1 pkg (11 oz)	370	15	12	5	53	4	650
Teriyaki Stir Fried Rice	1 pkg (11 oz)	340	10	8	5	56	6	650
Tyson								
Meal Kit Chicken Fried Rice	2½ cups	440	27	6	30	69	5	1810
MIX								
Annie Chun's								
Meal Kit Chow Mein Noodles w/ Garlic Black Bean Sauce	⅓ pkg	230	8	3	0	42	2	690
Meal Kit Chow Mein Noodles w/ Peanut Sesame Sauce	⅓ pkg	270	9	7	0	42	2	600
Meal Kit Chow Mein Noodles w/ Scallion Sauce	⅓ pkg	240	8	5	0	39	2	940
Meal Kit Chow Mein Noodles w/ Teriyaki Sauce	⅓ box	210	8	1	0	43	2	870
Meal Kit Pad Thai Noodles w/ Pad Thai Sauce	⅓ pkg	210	3	1	0	48	–	570
Meal Kit Soba Noodles w/ Soy Ginger Sauce	⅓ pkg	210	8	2	0	41	3	920

FOOD	PORTION	CALS	PROT	FAT	CHOL	CARB	FIBER	SOD
Nissin								
Chow Mein Chicken as prep	½ pkg (2 oz)	240	6	9	0	34	2	660
Chow Mein Thai Peanut as prep	½ pkg (2 oz)	270	6	12	0	35	tr	780
SHELF-STABLE								
Fantastic								
Pad Thai w/ Rice Noodles	1 pkg (7 oz)	400	18	11	0	59	5	680
Thai Lemon Grass w/ Rice Noodles	1 pkg (7.4 oz)	340	8	10	0	48	5	690
TAKE-OUT								
beef & broccoli	1 cup	221	18	12	54	10	3	399
buddha's delight w/ cellophane noodles fat choi jai	1 serv (7.6 oz)	211	7	4	tr	44	2	772
cha siu bao steamed buns w/ chicken filling	1 (2.3 oz)	160	5	3	15	26	tr	300
chinese style fried egg noodles w/ seafood & lettuce	1 serv (14 oz)	694	27	37	257	63	8	1563
chow mein beef no noodles	1 cup	271	22	15	51	12	3	922
chow mein noodles	1 cup	237	4	14	0	26	2	198
chow mein pork no noodles	1 cup	284	22	16	55	12	3	889
chow mein shrimp no noodles	1 cup	154	16	5	92	11	2	737
chow mein vegetable no noodles	1 cup	224	5	15	0	16	4	1014
dim sum meat filled	3 pieces (4 oz)	124	13	3	54	11	1	484
egg foo yung beef	1 patty (6 oz)	243	17	16	336	7	1	243
egg foo yung chicken	1 patty (3 oz)	121	8	8	166	4	1	121
egg foo yung pork	1 patty (3 oz)	125	8	8	166	4	1	120
egg foo yung shrimp	1 patty (3 oz)	153	8	12	184	3	1	483

FOOD	PORTION	CALS	PROT	FAT	CHOL	CARB	FIBER	SOD
filipino chicken adobo (15 oz)	1 serv	555	33	26	116	45	1	468
foochow fish ball	1 (1 oz)	36	2	2	6	3	1	163
fried rice	1 cup	333	12	12	103	42	1	834
fried rice beef	1 cup	346	12	14	107	42	1	649
fried rice chicken	1 cup	329	12	12	105	42	1	602
fried rice pork	1 cup	335	12	13	103	42	1	602
fried rice shrimp	1 cup	323	11	12	115	42	1	851
general tsao's chicken	1 cup	296	19	17	66	16	1	844
green beans szechuan style	1 cup	176	4	12	0	16	6	446
indian style fried egg noodles w/ eggs tomato sauce & lime	1 serv (15 oz)	721	29	31	377	80	8	2418
kung pao beef	1 cup	410	28	30	62	9	2	645
kung pao chicken	1 cup	434	29	31	65	12	2	907
kung pao pork	1 cup	460	26	34	60	12	2	862
kung pao shrimp	1 cup	345	30	20	191	11	2	791
lo mein beef	1 cup	286	14	11	26	31	3	594
lo mein chicken	1 cup	262	15	9	26	31	3	538
lo mein meatless	1 cup	234	8	6	0	38	3	366
lo mein pork	1 cup	314	13	14	22	34	3	508
lo mein shrimp	1 cup	236	11	7	48	33	4	180
moo goo gai pan chicken	1 cup	272	15	19	35	12	3	305
moo shu pork w/o pancake	1 cup	512	19	46	172	5	1	1048
phad thai	1 serv (9.2 oz)	232	11	9	0	30	1	426
sesame seed paste bun	1 (2.5 oz)	220	5	6	0	39	2	53
shrimp chips banh phong tom	6 med	214	3	14	21	20	tr	456
shrimp w/ lobster sauce	1 cup	298	35	12	259	8	1	1030
shu mai chicken & vegetable dumplings	6 (3.6 oz)	160	10	5	35	18	1	910
spring roll	1 (3.5 oz)	112	12	2	–	37	5	670
sukiyaki beef	1 cup	165	19	7	130	6	1	654
sweet & sour chicken w/o rice	1 cup	670	45	37	169	36	2	1819
sweet & sour pork w/ rice	1 cup	268	13	6	29	40	2	898
sweet & sour pork w/o rice	1 cup	231	15	8	38	25	2	1209
sweet & sour shrimp	1 cup	480	12	30	70	46	1	2020
sweet red bean bun	1 (2.5 oz)	130	4	1	0	38	2	95

FOOD	PORTION	CALS	PROT	FAT	CHOL	CARB	FIBER	SOD
szechuan chicken	1 cup	190	16	9	42	9	2	620
szechuan shrimp & vegetables	1 cup	159	14	7	94	10	2	629
tempura vegetable	8 pieces	90	2	6	36	8	1	20
tempura hawaiian fish tofu vegetable	2 cups	285	11	22	200	13	2	430
teriyaki beef	1 cup	454	51	19	149	13	tr	1386
teriyaki chicken plain	¾ cup	399	30	27	92	7	–	2190
teriyaki chicken w/ rice	1 serv (11 oz)	430	19	6	25	77	1	1210
teriyaki shrimp	1 cup	271	39	3	269	14	1	3103
thai style pineapple rice w/ ham & pork floss	1 serv (7.7 oz)	408	13	14	63	60	6	1277
wonton fried meat filled	1 (0.7 oz)	54	3	3	20	5	tr	111
wonton meat & shrimp boiled	1 (0.5 oz)	19	1	1	3	2	tr	48

ASPARAGUS
CANNED

FOOD	PORTION	CALS	PROT	FAT	CHOL	CARB	FIBER	SOD
spears	1 cup	46	5	2	0	6	4	695
spears	1	3	tr	tr	0	tr	tr	52
Del Monte								
Cuts & Tips	½ cup	20	2	0	0	3	1	365
Spears	½ cup	20	2	0	0	3	1	365
Tips	½ cup	20	2	0	0	3	1	365
Gertie's Finest								
White	1 oz	15	1	0	0	3	1	340
Green Giant								
Spears Extra Long	5	20	2	0	0	3	1	430
Native Forest								
White	1 serv (4 oz)	20	2	0	0	3	1	550
Tillen Farms								
Crispy Asparagus Pickled	3 spears	10	1	0	0	1	0	75
FRESH								
cooked	½ cup	20	2	tr	0	4	2	13
cooked	4 spears	13	1	tr	0	2	1	8
spears raw	4	10	1	tr	0	2	1	1
Apline Fresh								
Fresh Green	5 spears (3.3 oz)	20	2	0	0	5	2	0

FOOD	PORTION	CALS	PROT	FAT	CHOL	CARB	FIBER	SOD
Frieda's								
White	⅔ cup	20	2	0	0	4	2	0
Ocean Mist								
Spears	5 (3.3 oz)	25	2	0	0	4	2	0
FROZEN								
cooked	1 pkg (10 oz)	53	9	1	0	6	5	9
cooked	4 spears	11	2	tr	0	1	1	2
C&W								
Spears	7 (3 oz)	20	2	0	0	3	tr	0
Europe's Best								
Spears	7 spears	15	2	1	0	3	2	0
ATEMOYA								
fresh	½ cup	94	1	1	–	24	–	2
AVOCADO								
california mashed	¼ cup	96	1	9	0	5	4	5
california peeled & pitted	1	289	3	27	0	15	12	14
florida mashed	¼ cup	69	1	6	0	5	1	1
florida peeled & pitted	1	365	7	31	0	24	17	6
Calavo								
Fresh	⅕ med (1 oz)	55	tr	5	0	3	3	0
Earthbound Farm								
Organic Fresh	⅕ med (1 oz)	55	1	5	0	3	3	0
Frieda's								
Fresh Cocktail	1 (1.4 oz)	60	0	6	0	3	2	0
TAKE-OUT								
guacamole	1 serv (2.2 oz)	105	1	10	0	5	2	187
BACON								
bacon grease	1 tbsp	116	0	13	12	0	0	19
beef breakfast strips cooked	3 strips	153	11	12	40	tr	0	766
gammon lean & fat grilled	4.2 oz	274	35	15	–	0	0	–
pan fried	3 strips	109	6	9	16	tr	0	303
turkey	2 (0.8 oz)	84	7	6	22	1	0	503
Boar's Head								
Fully Cooked Slices	3 (0.5 oz)	70	4	6	15	0	0	260

FOOD	PORTION	CALS	PROT	FAT	CHOL	CARB	FIBER	SOD
Jennie-O								
Turkey Bacon	1 slice (0.5 oz)	35	2	3	10	0	0	170
Oscar Mayer								
Bacon Bits	1 tbsp (7 g)	25	3	2	5	0	0	220
Center Cut cooked	2 slices (0.4 oz)	50	4	4	15	0	0	270
Hardwood Smoked	2 slices (0.5 oz)	70	4	6	15	0	0	290
Lower Sodium	3 slices (0.5 oz)	70	4	6	10	0	0	170
Ready To Serve	3 slices	70	5	5	15	0	0	220
Uncured	3 slices (0.5 oz)	60	7	5	15	1	0	400
Tyson								
Hickory Thick Cut	2 pieces (0.8 oz)	140	8	11	25	0	0	380
Wellshire								
Beef Uncured	2 oz	114	9	3	50	0	0	225
Panchetta Sliced	1 slice (0.4 oz)	60	4	3	10	0	0	200
Pork Range Sliced Dry Rubbed	2 slices	30	4	3	10	0	0	220
Uncured Turkey	1 slice (1 oz)	20	3	1	10	0	0	180
BACON SUBSTITUTES								
bacon bits meatless	1 tbsp	33	2	2	0	2	1	124
meatless	1 strip	16	1	1	0	tr	tr	73
Bob's Red Mill								
Bac'Ums	4 tsp	25	3	1	0	2	0	140
Lightlife								
Organic Tempeh Smokey Strips	3 slices (2 oz)	80	8	3	0	6	1	230
Smart Bacon	2 strips (0.8 oz)	45	6	2	0	1	1	350
Worthington								
Stripples	2 strips (0.5 oz)	60	2	5	0	2	tr	220
BAGEL								
cinnamon raisin	1 mini	71	3	tr	0	14	1	84

FOOD	PORTION	CALS	PROT	FAT	CHOL	CARB	FIBER	SOD
cinnamon raisin	1 lg (4 in)	244	9	2	0	49	2	287
egg	1 lg (4.5 in)	364	14	3	31	69	3	662
low carb	1 (4 oz)	216	12	0	10	42	14	360
mini onion	1 (1.4 oz)	100	4	0	0	20	1	90
oat bran	1 lg (4 in)	227	10	1	0	47	3	451
plain	1 sm (3 in)	190	7	1	0	37	2	368
plain	1 med (3.5 in)	289	11	2	0	56	2	561
plain	1 lg (4.5 in)	360	14	2	0	70	3	700
Alvarado Street Bakery								
Sprouted Wheat Cinnamon Raisin	1 (3.3 oz)	280	9	1	0	59	3	270
David's								
Deli Bagels	1 (2.8 oz)	230	8	1	0	46	2	360
Enjoy Life								
Nut Gluten Free Classic Original	1 (3 oz)	270	5	7	0	46	3	380
New York Style								
Crisps Natural Whole Wheat	6	120	4	6	0	16	2	180
Crisps Plain	7	140	3	6	0	17	1	70
Pepperidge Farm								
100% Whole Wheat	1	250	11	2	0	49	6	450
Everything	1	260	9	2	0	53	2	400
Mini 100% Whole Wheat	1	100	4	1	0	20	3	180
Mini Plain	1	110	4	1	0	22	1	200
Sara Lee								
Apple Cinnamon	1 (4 oz)	310	11	2	0	64	3	430
Banana Walnut	1 (4 oz)	350	12	7	0	61	4	440
Blueberry Deluxe	1 (3.3 oz)	260	9	1	0	53	2	490
Blueberry Junior	1 (1 oz)	70	3	0	0	15	tr	140
Blueberry Toaster Size	1 (2.1 oz)	160	6	1	0	34	1	310
Cinnamon Raisin Deluxe	1 (3.3 oz)	260	9	1	0	55	4	460
Heart Healthy 100% Whole Wheat	1 (3.3 oz)	220	11	2	0	47	6	490
Heart Healthy Cinnamon Raisin	1 (3.3 oz)	250	11	2	0	50	7	340
Plain	1 (2.1 oz)	160	6	1	0	33	1	320
Sundried Tomato & Basil	1 (4 oz)	300	11	2	0	61	2	480
Whole Grain Plain	1 (3.3 oz)	240	10	1	0	50	3	510

FOOD	PORTION	CALS	PROT	FAT	CHOL	CARB	FIBER	SOD
Thomas'								
Bagelbread Mini Squares 100% Whole Wheat	1 (2 oz)	150	7	1	0	30	4	240
Carb Consider Plain	1	150	11	3	0	24	6	340
Carb Consider Whole Wheat	1	140	11	3	0	23	7	320
Weight Watchers								
Original	1 (2.8 oz)	190	10	2	0	44	10	520
BAKING POWDER								
baking powder	1 tsp	2	0	0	0	1	0	488
low sodium	1 tsp	5	tr	tr	0	2	tr	4
Bob's Red Mills								
Baking Powder	1 tsp	5	0	0	0	1	0	590
Calumet								
Double Acting	1/8 tsp	0	0	0	0	0	0	60
BAKING SODA								
baking soda	1 tsp	0	0	0	0	0	0	1259
Bob's Red Mill								
Baking Soda	1/4 tsp	0	0	0	0	0	0	270
BALSAM PEAR (BITTER GOURD)								
leafy tips cooked w/o salt	1 cup	20	2	tr	0	4	1	8
leafy tips raw	1 cup	14	3	tr	0	2	–	5
pods raw sliced	1 cup	16	1	tr	0	3	3	5
pods sliced cooked w/ salt	1 cup	24	1	tr	0	5	3	300
BAMBOO SHOOTS								
canned sliced	1/2 cup	12	1	tr	0	2	1	5
fresh sliced cooked w/ salt	1/2 cup	7	1	tr	0	1	1	144
raw sliced	1/2 cup	20	2	tr	0	4	2	3
BANANA								
banana chips	1 oz	147	1	10	0	17	2	2
fresh baby	1 extra sm (<6 in)	72	1	tr	0	19	2	1
fresh	1 sm (6 in)	90	1	tr	0	23	3	1
fresh	1 med (7 in)	105	1	tr	0	27	3	1
fresh	1 lg (8 in)	121	1	tr	0	31	4	1
fresh mashed	1/2 cup	100	1	tr	0	26	3	1
fresh sliced	1 cup	134	2	1	0	34	4	2

FOOD	PORTION	CALS	PROT	FAT	CHOL	CARB	FIBER	SOD
powder	1 tbsp	21	tr	tr	0	5	1	0
whole dried	1 piece (1.2 oz)	130	1	1	0	33	2	0
Bob's Red Mill								
Chips	25 (1.4 oz)	210	0	11	0	26	0	1
Frieda's								
Burro	1 (3 oz)	80	1	0	0	20	1	0
Dried	1 piece (1.2 oz)	130	1	1	0	33	2	0
Goodniks								
Nutty Bananas Crunchy Snack	⅔ cup	230	1	16	5	21	3	10
TAKE-OUT								
fritter	1 (2.3 oz)	197	1	5	0	36	2	103

BARBECUE SAUCE

FOOD	PORTION	CALS	PROT	FAT	CHOL	CARB	FIBER	SOD
barbecue	2 tbsp	52	0	tr	0	13	tr	392
low sodium	2 tbsp	52	0	tr	0	13	tr	47
Annie's Naturals								
Organic Orignal	2 tbsp	45	0	1	–	9	–	240
Bone Suckin'								
Sauce	2 tbsp	40	0	0	0	10	0	110
Cattlemen's								
Classic	2 tbsp	60	tr	0	0	15	tr	400
Honey	2 tbsp	70	0	0	0	17	tr	370
Smokehouse	2 tbsp	60	tr	0	0	14	tr	490
Consorzio								
Organic Original	1 tbsp	50	0	0	0	11	0	280
Organic Spicy	1 tbsp	50	1	0	0	11	0	280
David Burke								
Flavor Spray Memphis BBQ	2 sprays	0	0	0	0	0	0	10
Emeril's								
Original BBQ	2 tbsp	45	0	0	0	12	–	390
Hunt's								
Hickory	2 tbsp	45	0	0	0	11	tr	290
Hickory & Brown Sugar	2 tbsp	70	0	0	0	16	1	360
Honey Hickory	2 tbsp	50	0	0	0	12	tr	380
Honey Mustard	2 tbsp	50	0	0	0	12	1	310
Hot & Spicy	2 tbsp	45	0	0	0	11	tr	440
Mesquite	2 tbsp	40	0	0	0	9	tr	360

FOOD	PORTION	CALS	PROT	FAT	CHOL	CARB	FIBER	SOD
Original	2 tbsp	50	0	0	0	13	tr	280
Original Bold	2 tbsp	45	0	0	0	11	tr	290
Nando's								
Barbecue	1 tbsp	7	0	0	0	2	0	34
San-J								
Asian BBQ	2 tbsp	40	2	0	0	7	–	840
Wellshire								
Original	2 tbsp	39	1	0	0	10	0	278
BARLEY								
flour	1 cup	511	16	2	0	110	15	6
pearled cooked	1 cup (5.5 oz)	193	4	1	0	44	6	5
pearled uncooked	¼ cup	176	5	1	0	39	8	5
Arrowhead Mills								
Organic Pearled not prep	¼ cup	160	5	1	0	32	8	5
Robinsons								
Barley Water Lemon as prep	9 oz	48	tr	5	–	tr	–	–
BARRACUDA								
broiled	4 oz	239	27	14	62	tr	0	480
cooked flaked	1 cup	287	32	16	75	1	0	575
poached	4 oz	227	29	11	67	0	0	111
TAKE-OUT								
breaded & fried	4 oz	282	26	17	59	5	tr	432
BASIL								
fresh chopped	2 tbsp	1	tr	tr	0	tr	tr	0
ground	1 tsp	4	tr	tr	0	1	1	tr
leaves fresh	5	1	tr	tr	0	tr	tr	0
Dorot								
Chopped Cube frzn	1 cube (4 g)	5	tr	tr	0	tr	tr	12
Eden								
Shiso Leaf Powder	1 tsp	0	0	0	0	0	0	200
BASS								
breaded baked	4 oz	205	25	7	129	10	1	506
pickled mero en escabeche	2 oz	156	7	14	16	tr	tr	114
striped baked	3 oz	105	19	3	88	0	0	75
striped bass farm raised	4 oz	110	20	3	90	0	0	80

FOOD	PORTION	CALS	PROT	FAT	CHOL	CARB	FIBER	SOD
BAY LEAF								
crumbled	1 tsp	2	tr	tr	0	tr	tr	0
BEANS (see also individual names)								
CANNED								
baked beans plain	½ cup	119	6	tr	0	27	5	428
baked beans vegetarian	½ cup	119	6	tr	0	27	5	428
baked beans w/ franks	½ cup	184	9	9	8	20	9	557
baked beans w/ pork	½ cup	134	7	2	9	25	7	524
baked beans w/ pork & tomato sauce	½ cup	119	7	1	9	24	5	553
refried beans	½ cup	134	8	1	–	23	–	534
B&M								
Bacon & Onion	½ cup	190	8	2	<5	36	8	450
Bush's								
Barbecue	½ cup	150	6	1	0	32	5	510
Boston Recipe	½ cup	150	6	1	0	31	5	440
Homestyle	½ cup	140	6	1	0	29	5	550
Onion 98% Fat Free	½ cup	140	6	1	0	29	5	550
Vegetarian Fat Free	½ cup	130	6	0	0	29	5	550
Campbell's								
Pork & Beans	½ cup	140	6	2	5	25	7	440
Eden								
Organic Baked w/ Sorghum	½ cup	150	8	0	0	27	7	130
Green Giant								
Three Bean Salad	½ cup	80	3	0	0	18	3	470
Heinz								
Vegetarian	1 cup	250	11	1	0	48	9	840
Las Palmas								
Refried	½ cup	150	8	3	0	23	2	540
Old El Paso								
Refried Fat Free	½ cup	100	6	0	0	18	6	580
Refried Fat Free Spicy	½ cup	100	6	0	0	18	6	570
Pace								
Refried Salsa	½ cup	70	4	0	0	14	4	590
Ranch Style								
Original Texas	½ cup	138	6	3	0	20	6	590
Read								
3 Bean Salad	½ cup	60	1	0	0	13	2	300

FOOD	PORTION	CALS	PROT	FAT	CHOL	CARB	FIBER	SOD
Rosarita								
Refried Traditional 98% Fat Free	½ cup	100	6	2	0	18	5	510
Van Camp's								
Baked Beans w/ Chicken	1 cup	360	23	2	20	62	0	1060
Pork And Beans	½ cup	110	6	1	0	23	6	420
FROZEN								
Lean Cuisine								
Cafe Classics Sante Fe Style Rice & Beans	1 pkg (10.4 oz)	290	11	5	15	50	5	580
MIX								
Fantastic								
Instant Black Beans not prep	⅓ cup	160	10	2	0	29	7	310
Instant Refried Beans not prep	¼ cup	130	7	2	0	23	8	330
TAKE-OUT								
baked beans	½ cup	191	7	7	6	27	7	534
barbecue beans	3.5 oz	120	4	tr	0	26	–	460
frijolas a la charra w/ pork tomatoes & chili peppers	1 cup	341	14	22	27	23	5	719
refried beans	½ cup	43	2	2	2	5	–	104
three bean salad	1 cup	114	4	5	0	15	5	651

BEAN SPROUTS (see ALFALFA, SPROUTS)

BEAR

simmered	3 oz	220	28	11	83	0	0	60

BEAVER

roasted	4 oz	240	39	8	132	0	0	67

BEECHNUTS

dried	1 oz	163	2	14	0	10	–	11

BEEF (see also BEEF DISHES, MEAT STICKS, MEATBALLS, VEAL)

CANNED

corned beef	1 oz	71	8	4	24	0	0	285
FRESH								
arm pot roast trim 0 in fat braised	3.5 oz	297	29	19	95	0	0	47

FOOD	PORTION	CALS	PROT	FAT	CHOL	CARB	FIBER	SOD
arm pot roast trim ⅛ in fat braised	3.5 oz	302	30	19	79	0	0	50
beef crumbles 70% lean pan browned	3 oz	230	22	15	75	0	0	82
bottom round roast trim 0 in fat braised	4 oz	253	38	10	112	0	0	50
bottom round roast trim 0 in fat roasted	3.5 oz	187	8	8	86	0	0	36
bottom round roast trim ½ in fat braised	4 oz	337	22	22	109	0	0	57
bottom round roast trim ⅛ in fat braised	4 oz	280	37	13	86	0	0	49
bottom round roast trim ⅛ in fat roasted	4 oz	247	30	13	85	0	0	40
bottom sirloin butt roast trim 0 in fat roasted	3.5 oz	182	27	8	71	0	0	55
brisket flat half trim ⅛ in fat braised	3.5 oz	298	29	19	80	0	0	46
brisket flat trim 0 in fat braised	3.5 oz	221	32	9	46	0	0	52
brisket point half trim 0 in fat braised	3.5 oz	358	24	29	92	0	0	68
brisket point half trim ¼ in fat braised	3.5 oz	404	22	22	92	0	0	65
brisket point half trim ⅛ in fat braised	3.5 oz	349	24	27	92	0	0	69
chuck boston cut roast trim 0 in fat roasted	3.5 oz	207	26	11	69	0	0	71
chuck boston cut roast trim ¼ in fat roasted	3.5 oz	242	24	15	75	0	0	67
chuck bottom roast trim 0 in fat braised	3.5 oz	334	27	24	104	0	0	65
chuck bottom roast trim ¼ in fat braised	3.5 oz	345	27	26	104	0	0	64
chuck fillet steak trim 0 in fat broiled	4 oz	181	29	6	71	0	0	80
chuck top roast trim 0 in fat broiled	4 oz	245	29	13	69	0	0	76
club steak trim ½ in fat broiled	4 oz	384	28	29	91	0	0	70

FOOD	PORTION	CALS	PROT	FAT	CHOL	CARB	FIBER	SOD
corned beef brisket cooked	3 oz	213	15	16	83	tr	0	964
crosscut shank trim ¼ in fat stewed	1 serv (6.8 oz)	510	60	28	155	0	0	118
delmonico steak trim ¼ in fat broiled	4 oz	409	27	33	95	0	0	70
entrecote steak trim ½ in fat broiled	4 oz	413	27	33	95	0	0	70
eye round roast trim 0 in fat roasted	4 oz	190	33	5	61	0	0	43
eye round roast trim ¼ in fat roasted	4 oz	283	31	17	82	0	0	67
eye round roast trim ⅛ in fat roasted	4 oz	236	32	11	70	0	0	42
filet mignon roast trim ¼ in fat roasted	4 oz	376	27	29	97	0	0	63
filet mignon roast trim ⅛ in fat roasted	4 oz	367	27	28	96	0	0	65
filet mignon trim 0 in fat broiled	4 oz	247	31	13	95	0	0	63
filet mignon trim ⅛ in fat broiled	4 oz	303	30	19	102	0	0	61
ground 70% lean broiled	3.5 oz	273	25	18	82	0	0	81
ground 75% lean broiled	2.5 oz	195	18	13	62	0	0	55
ground 80% lean broiled	3 oz	234	22	15	77	0	0	64
ground 85% lean pan fried	3 oz	197	21	12	73	0	0	67
ground 90% lean pan fried	3 oz	173	21	9	70	0	0	64
ground 95% lean pan fried	3 oz	139	22	5	65	0	0	60
ground low-fat w/ carrageenan raw	4 oz	160	20	7	53	tr	–	70
london broil trim 0 in fat broiled	3.5 oz	188	28	8	45	0	0	56
london broil trim ¼ in fat broiled	4 oz	260	35	12	95	0	0	68
new york strip steak trim 0 in fat broiled	4 oz	219	33	9	66	0	0	67
oxtails cooked	6 pieces (6.3 oz)	472	56	26	191	0	0	419
porterhouse steak trim 0 in fat broiled	1 lb	1252	109	87	304	0	0	295

FOOD	PORTION	CALS	PROT	FAT	CHOL	CARB	FIBER	SOD
porterhouse steak trim ¼ in fat broiled	1 lb	1492	102	117	327	0	0	281
porterhouse steak trim ⅛ in fat broiled	1 lb	1324	107	99	322	0	0	290
porterhouse steak trim ⅛ in fat broiled	4 oz	337	27	25	80	0	0	73
rib eye roast trim ¼ in fat roasted	3.5 oz	365	23	30	85	0	0	64
rib eye steak trim ⅛ in fat broiled	4 oz	221	34	9	81	0	0	70
rib roast trim ¼ in fat roasted	4 oz	406	26	33	95	0	0	71
rib steak trim ¼ in fat broiled	4 oz	388	25	31	93	0	0	71
round tip roast trim 0 in fat roasted	4 oz	213	30	9	105	0	0	40
sandwich steaks thinly sliced	1 serv (2 oz)	173	9	15	40	0	0	38
shell steak trim ¼ in fat broiled	4 oz	366	29	27	90	0	0	71
short ribs lean & fat braised	1 serv (7.8 oz)	1060	49	94	212	0	0	113
skirt steak trim 0 in fat broiled	4 oz	289	27	19	67	0	0	104
t-bone steak trim 0 in fat broiled	4 oz	280	27	18	68	0	0	76
t-bone steak trim ¼ in fat broiled	1 lb	1388	106	103	295	0	0	304
t-bone steak trim ⅛ in fat broiled	1 lb	804	70	56	178	0	0	489
tip round roast trim ⅛ in fat roasted	4 oz	248	31	13	93	0	0	71
top loin steak boneless trim ⅛ in fat broiled	4 oz	299	30	19	100	0	0	61
top round roast trim 0 in fat braised	4 oz	237	40	7	102	0	0	51
top round roast trim ¼ in fat braised	4 oz	281	38	13	102	0	0	51
top round roast trim ¼ in fat roasted	4 oz	265	31	15	93	0	0	71

FOOD	PORTION	CALS	PROT	FAT	CHOL	CARB	FIBER	SOD
top round steak trim ¼ in fat pan fried	4 oz	314	37	17	110	0	0	77
top sirloin steak trim ⅛ in fat broiled	4 oz	275	31	16	85	0	0	63
top sirloin steak trim ⅛ in fat pan fried	4 oz	355	33	24	111	0	0	80
tri-tip roast trim 0 in fat roasted	3.5 oz	218	26	12	94	0	0	50
tri-tip steak trim 0 in fat broiled	4 oz	300	34	17	77	0	0	82
Laura's Lean								
Eye Of Round	4 oz	135	25	4	50	0	0	75
Flank Steak	4 oz	140	–	5	55	–	–	85
Ground Beef 92% Lean	4 oz	160	21	9	60	0	0	70
Ground Beef Patties	1 (4 oz)	160	21	9	60	0	0	70
Ground Round 96% Lean	4 oz	140	24	5	60	0	0	85
Ribeye Steak	4 oz	175	–	9	60	–	–	–
Sirloin Steak	4 oz	145	–	5	65	–	–	70
Sirloin Tip	4 oz	130	24	4	60	0	0	65
Strip Steak	4 oz	150	–	5	55	–	–	70
Tenderloin Filet	4 oz	145	–	5	55	–	–	80
Top Round	4 oz	135	25	4	55	0	0	55
Organic Prairie								
90% Lean Ground	4 oz	250	30	13	95	0	0	75
Shady Brook								
Tri-Tip Roast Rosemary Garlic & Chardonnay	4 oz	180	18	9	50	4	0	550
Tri-Tip Roast Sizzling Ginger	4 oz	210	20	10	50	9	0	390
FROZEN								
patty broiled medium	3 oz	240	21	17	80	0	0	65
Organic Prairie								
Rib Eye Steak	1 (6 oz)	470	47	31	160	0	0	100
Soy Lean								
Beef Patty	1 (2.5 oz)	90	14	4	20	1	–	–
READY-TO-EAT								
dried beef smoked chopped	1 oz	37	6	1	13	1	0	352
roast beef spread	¼ cup	127	9	9	40	2	tr	413
smoked beef cooked	1 sausage (1.4 oz)	134	–	12	29	–	–	–

FOOD	PORTION	CALS	PROT	FAT	CHOL	CARB	FIBER	SOD
Boar's Head								
Corned Beef Brisket	2 oz	80	12	4	40	0	0	460
Top Round Deluxe	2 oz	80	15	2	30	tr	0	80
Top Round Oven Roasted No Salt Added	2 oz	90	14	3	30	0	0	40
Healthy Ones								
Deli Roast Beef	2 oz	70	9	2	0	1	0	480
Laura's Lean								
Beef Pot Roast Au Jus	3 oz	110	17	4	45	3	–	380
Oscar Mayer								
Slow Roasted Shaved	¼ pkg (1.8 oz)	60	10	3	30	0	0	520
Sara Lee								
Roast Beef Medium or Rare	2 oz	60	11	2	30	1	0	420
Tyson								
Beef Strips Seasoned	1 serv (3 oz)	130	18	6	55	1	0	420
TAKE-OUT								
roast beef rare	2 oz	70	12	2	30	0	0	210

BEEF DISHES
CANNED

FOOD	PORTION	CALS	PROT	FAT	CHOL	CARB	FIBER	SOD
corned beef hash	3 oz	155	10	10	–	9	–	–
Hormel								
Corned Beef Hash 50% Reduced Fat	1 cup	290	21	12	60	24	2	1070
FROZEN								
Quaker Maid								
Sandwich Steaks Pure Beef	1 serv (1.8 oz)	120	8	10	30	0	0	35
Tyson								
Steak Country Fried	1 (3.2 oz)	310	10	23	25	15	1	710
REFRIGERATED								
Chi Chi's								
For Tacos! Ground Beef	¼ cup	90	5	4	15	5	0	360
Hormel								
Beef Tips & Gravy	½ cup	170	21	8	60	4	1	700
Huxtable's								
Shepherds Pie Beef	1 pkg (10 oz)	270	17	11	35	27	3	1030

FOOD	PORTION	CALS	PROT	FAT	CHOL	CARB	FIBER	SOD
Laura's Lean								
Meatloaf w/ Tomato Sauce	1 serv (5 oz)	230	19	8	60	27	–	580
Shredded Beef w/ Barbecue Sauce	1 serv (5 oz)	245	22	5	65	27	–	390
Tyson								
Chuck Roast w/ Vegetables	1 serv (4 oz)	320	18	21	70	14	2	340
Seasoned Meatloaf	1 serv (5 oz)	320	14	23	60	16	0	600
Steak Tips In Bourbon Sauce	1 serv (5 oz)	180	20	5	45	12	0	480
TAKE-OUT								
beef bourguignonne	1 cup	339	36	12	85	10	1	124
beef satay + peanut sauce	2 skewers	253	25	16	62	6	1	433
bool kogi korean marinated beef ribs	4 oz	190	18	10	55	6	0	580
bracciola	1 roll (4.7 oz)	276	27	14	76	8	1	485
bubble & squeak	5 oz	186	2	13	–	16	3	–
bulgoghi korean grilled beef	1 serv (5.2 oz)	256	23	15	67	5	tr	834
chipped beef on toast	1 slice (5 oz)	226	11	10	22	22	1	715
cornish pasty	1 (8 oz)	847	20	52	–	79	3	–
goulash w/ potatoes	1 cup	298	27	12	66	19	2	437
greek moussaka	1 serv (8.5 oz)	450	24	33	179	12	1	763
irish stew	1 cup (7 oz)	280	23	16	–	10	–	–
kebab indian	1 (5.4 oz)	553	47	40	–	2	–	–
kheena	6.7 oz	781	34	71	–	1	tr	–
koftas	5	280	18	22	–	3	tr	–
meatloaf	1 lg slice (5 oz)	294	23	17	114	9	1	596
pepper steak	1 cup	317	28	20	69	5	1	562
pot roast w/ gravy	1 serv (6 oz)	320	54	10	110	4	0	620
samosa	2 (4 oz)	652	6	62	–	20	2	–
shepherds pie	1 serv (7 oz)	282	16	16	70	20	2	840
sloppy joes	1 serv (9 oz)	398	39	6	67	48	12	88
steak & kidney pie w/ top crust	1 slice (5 oz)	400	21	26	–	23	1	–
stew w/ potatoes & vegetables	1 cup	199	16	5	30	22	3	504
stroganoff	1 cup	394	26	25	69	15	1	1155

FOOD	PORTION	CALS	PROT	FAT	CHOL	CARB	FIBER	SOD
swiss steak w/ sauce	1 serv (8 oz)	234	26	10	66	8	1	563
toad in the hole	1 (4.7 oz)	383	10	29	–	23	1	–

BEEFALO
roasted	4 oz	213	35	7	66	0	0	93

BEER AND ALE
alcohol free beer	7 oz	50	1	tr	–	11	–	3
ale brown	10 oz	77	1	0	0	8	0	–
ale pale	10 oz	88	1	0	0	12	0	–
beer cooler	1 (16 oz)	194	1	0	0	34	1	43
beer light	12 oz can	103	1	0	0	6	0	14
beer regular	12 oz can	153	2	0	0	13	0	14
black & tan	1 serv (12 oz)	146	1	0	0	13	1	18
black velvet	1 (10 oz)	160	1	0	0	8	1	10
boilermaker	1 serv	216	1	0	0	13	1	18
lager	10 oz	80	1	0	0	4	0	–
lager & black	1 (14 oz)	241	1	0	0	39	–	31
mead	1 serv	250	1	0	0	13	1	18
pilsener lager	7 oz	85	1	tr	–	13	–	4
shandy	1 serv	125	1	0	0	12	1	16
stout	10 oz	102	1	0	0	6	0	–
trojan horse	1 (16 oz)	189	1	0	0	35	–	57
Beck's								
Premium Light	1 bottle	64	–	0	0	–	–	–

BEET JUICE
juice	7 oz	72	2	0	0	16	–	400

BEETS
CANNED
harvard	½ cup	90	1	tr	0	22	3	199
pickled	½ cup	74	1	tr	0	18	3	300
sliced	½ cup	37	1	tr	0	9	2	176
Del Monte								
Pickled Sliced	½ cup	35	1	0	0	8	2	290
Sliced	½ cup	35	1	0	0	8	2	290
Greenwood								
Harvard	1 serv (4.4 oz)	100	1	0	0	27	1	370
Pickled	1 oz	25	0	0	0	6	0	100

FOOD	PORTION	CALS	PROT	FAT	CHOL	CARB	FIBER	SOD
FRESH								
greens cooked w/o salt	½ cup	19	2	tr	0	4	2	174
sliced cooked	½ cup	37	1	tr	0	8	2	65
whole cooked	2 med (3.5 oz)	44	2	tr	0	10	2	77
Frieda's								
Beets	½ cup	35	1	0	0	8	2	65

BEVERAGES (*see* BEER AND ALE, CHAMPAGNE, COFFEE, DRINK MIXERS, ENERGY DRINKS, FRUIT DRINKS, ICED TEA, LIQUOR/LIQUEUR, MALT, MILKSHAKE, SMOOTHIES, SODA, TEA/HERBAL TEA, WATER, WINE, YOGURT DRINKS)

BISCUIT

FOOD	PORTION	CALS	PROT	FAT	CHOL	CARB	FIBER	SOD
MIX								
plain as prep	1 (2 oz)	190	4	7	2	27	1	541
Bisquick								
Heart Smart	⅓ cup	140	3	3	0	27	1	430
Jiffy								
Buttermilk as prep	1	170	3	4	<5	29	tr	380
King Arthur								
Whole Grain Buttermilk not prep	¼ cup	100	4	1	0	19	2	125
REFRIGERATED								
plain baked	1 (1 oz)	93	2	4	0	13	tr	325
TAKE-OUT								
buttermilk	1 lg (2.7 oz)	280	5	13	1	37	1	810
oatcakes	2 (4 oz)	115	3	5	–	16	1	–
plain	1 sm (1.2 oz)	127	2	6	0	17	1	368
tea biscuit	1 (3 oz)	210	5	3	0	30	1	370
w/ egg	1 (4.8 oz)	373	12	22	245	32	1	891
w/ egg & bacon	1 (5.3 oz)	458	17	31	353	29	1	999
w/ egg & ham	1 (6.7 oz)	442	20	27	300	30	1	1382
w/ egg & sausage	1 (6.3 oz)	581	19	39	302	11	1	1141
w/ egg & steak	1 (5.2 oz)	410	18	28	272	21	–	888
w/ egg cheese & bacon	1 (5.1 oz)	477	16	31	261	33	–	1260
w/ ham	1 (4 oz)	386	13	18	25	44	1	1433
w/ sausage	1 (4.4 oz)	485	12	32	35	40	1	1071

BITTERMELON

FOOD	PORTION	CALS	PROT	FAT	CHOL	CARB	FIBER	SOD
Frieda's								
Foo Qua	1 cup	15	1	0	0	3	2	0

FOOD	PORTION	CALS	PROT	FAT	CHOL	CARB	FIBER	SOD
BLACK BEANS								
dried cooked	1 cup	227	15	1	0	41	15	1
Eden								
Organic Caribbean	½ cup	90	7	1	–	20	7	135
Organic Refried	½ cup	110	6	2	–	18	7	180
BLACKBERRIES								
canned in heavy syrup	½ cup	118	2	tr	0	30	4	4
fresh	½ cup	31	1	tr	0	7	4	1
unsweetened frzn	½ cup	48	1	tr	0	12	4	1
Cascadian Farm								
Organic frzn	1 cup	80	1	1	0	22	7	0
Oregon								
In Light Syrup	½ cup	120	1	0	0	29	6	10
BLACKBERRY JUICE								
canned	6 oz	65	1	1	0	13	tr	2
Izze								
Sparkling Blackberry	8 oz	140	1	0	0	34	–	–
BLACKEYE PEAS								
catjang dried cooked	1 cup (2.9 oz)	200	14	1	0	35	–	32
cowpeas canned	1 cup	184	11	1	0	33	–	718
cowpeas frozen cooked	½ cup	112	7	tr	0	20	–	5
cowpeas leafy tips chopped cooked	1 cup	12	2	tr	0	1	–	3
cowpeas leafy tips raw chopped	1 cup	10	1	tr	0	2	–	2
CANNED								
w/pork	½ cup	199	7	4	17	40	–	840
Eden								
Organic	½ cup	90	6	1	0	16	4	25
DRIED								
cooked	1 cup	198	13	1	0	36	16	6
FROZEN								
McKenzie								
Blackeye Peas	1 serv (2.8 oz)	110	7	1	0	18	–	10
TAKE-OUT								
blackeye peas & pork	1 cup	236	24	5	27	25	8	1303

FOOD	PORTION	CALS	PROT	FAT	CHOL	CARB	FIBER	SOD
BLINTZE								
Golden								
Cheese	1 (2.1 oz)	80	6	2	15	13	2	135
Ratner's								
Cheese	1 (2.2 oz)	100	5	2	30	16	0	140
TAKE-OUT								
cheese	1 (2.7 oz)	160	5	9	65	15	tr	240
BLUEBERRIES								
canned in heavy syrup	½ cup	113	1	tr	0	28	2	4
fresh	½ cup	41	1	tr	0	11	2	1
fresh	1 pt	229	3	1	0	58	10	4
frzn unsweetened	½ cup	40	tr	1	0	9	2	1
C&W								
Ultimate	¾ cup	70	0	0	0	16	3	0
De-Lite								
Dried Sweetened	1 oz	86	1	1	0	23	4	4
Eden								
Organic Dried Wild	¼ cup	150	tr	0	0	35	5	15
Europe's Best								
Woodland frzn	¾ cup	70	1	1	0	17	4	0
Frieda's								
Dried	¼ cup (1.4 oz)	140	0	0	0	33	4	0
Hodgson Mill								
Dried Wild	¼ cup	120	1	1	0	32	6	0
LiteHouse								
Glaze	3 tbsp	70	0	0	0	17	0	45
Marie's								
Glaze	2 tbsp	40	0	0	0	10	0	35
Oregon								
In Light Syrup	½ cup	110	tr	0	0	26	2	5
Sunsweet								
Dried	¼ cup (1.4 oz)	140	1	0	0	33	3	0
BLUEBERRY JUICE								
Izze								
Sparkling Blueberry	8 oz	100	1	0	0	23	–	10
Van Dyk's								
100% Juice	6 oz	74	tr	0	0	18	0	7

FOOD	PORTION	CALS	PROT	FAT	CHOL	CARB	FIBER	SOD
Walnut Acres								
Organic	8 oz	130	0	0	0	31	tr	15
BLUEFIN								
fillet baked	4.1 oz	186	30	6	88	0	0	90
BLUEFISH								
fresh baked	3 oz	135	22	5	64	0	0	65
BOAR								
wild roasted	3 oz	136	24	4	–	0	0	–
BOK CHOY (see CABBAGE)								
BONITO								
dried	1 oz	50	8	2	13	0	0	14
fresh	3 oz	117	20	4	–	0	0	–
BORAGE								
fresh chopped	1 cup	19	2	tr	0	3	–	71
BOTTLED WATER (see WATER)								
BOYSENBERRIES								
frzn unsweetened	½ cup	33	1	tr	0	8	4	1
in heavy syrup	½ cup	113	1	tr	0	29	3	4
BRAINS								
beef pan-fried	3 oz	167	11	13	1696	0	0	134
beef simmered	3 oz	123	10	9	2635	0	0	92
lamb braised	3 oz	123	11	9	1737	0	0	114
lamb fried	3 oz	232	14	19	2128	0	0	133
pork braised	3 oz	117	10	8	2169	0	0	77
veal braised	3 oz	116	10	8	2635	0	0	133
veal fried	3 oz	181	12	14	1802	0	0	150
BRAN								
corn	1 cup (2.7 oz)	170	6	1	0	65	65	5
oat	½ cup (1.6 oz)	116	8	3	0	31	7	2
oat cooked	½ cup (3.8 oz)	44	4	1	0	13	3	1
rice	½ cup (2.1 oz)	187	8	12	0	29	12	3

FOOD	PORTION	CALS	PROT	FAT	CHOL	CARB	FIBER	SOD
wheat	½ cup (2 oz)	63	5	1	0	19	12	1
Bob's Red Mill								
Rice Bran	2 tbsp	60	2	3	0	8	3	0
BRAZIL NUTS								
dried unblanched	1 oz	186	4	19	0	4	–	0
BREAD								
CANNED								
boston brown	1 slice (1.6 oz)	88	2	1	0	19	2	284
FROZEN								
Alexia								
Baguette Garlic	2 pieces (1.6 oz)	130	4	5	10	19	tr	250
Cedarlane								
Organic Mediterranean Stuffed Focaccia	1 piece (4 oz)	295	13	10	22	37	1	485
Corbi's								
Chee-Zee Bread Original	½ piece (1.8 oz)	180	6	8	10	21	1	330
Pepperidge Farm								
Garlic	1 slice (2.5 in)	170	4	7	0	24	2	250
Texas Toast Five Cheese	1 slice	150	4	7	<5	18	1	200
Whole Grain Texas Toast	1 slice	150	4	8	0	14	2	250
MIX								
cornbread	1 piece (2 oz)	188	4	6	37	29	1	467
Buitoni								
Focaccia Italian Herb & Cheese	1 slice	110	3	2	0	21	0	390
Focaccia Rosemary & Garlic	1 piece (1 oz)	110	4	1	0	22	1	250
READY-TO-EAT								
anadama	1 piece (1.1 oz)	87	2	1	1	16	1	272
baguette whole wheat	2 oz	140	6	0	0	29	1	360
challah	1 slice (1.4 oz)	115	4	2	20	19	1	197

FOOD	PORTION	CALS	PROT	FAT	CHOL	CARB	FIBER	SOD
cinnamon	1 slice (0.9 oz)	69	2	1	0	13	1	177
cracked wheat	1 slice (1.1 oz)	78	3	1	0	15	2	161
cuban bread	1 slice (1.1 oz)	83	3	1	0	16	1	163
french	1 slice (1.1 oz)	88	3	1	0	17	1	195
italian	1 loaf (1 lb)	1255	41	4	0	256	–	2656
jewish rye	1 slice	90	2	2	0	17	1	240
navajo fry	1 piece	281	6	10	6	41	–	280
oat bran	1 slice (1.1 oz)	71	3	1	0	12	1	122
oatmeal	1 slice (0.9 oz)	73	2	1	0	13	1	162
pan criollo	1 piece (0.9 oz)	69	2	1	0	13	tr	136
pannetone	1 slice (0.9 oz)	86	2	2	18	15	1	92
pita	1 sm (1 oz)	77	3	tr	0	16	1	150
pita	1 lg (2 oz)	165	5	1	0	33	1	322
pita whole wheat	1 sm (1 oz)	74	3	1	0	15	2	149
pita whole wheat	1 lg (2.2 oz)	170	6	2	0	35	5	340
potato scallion	1 slice (2 oz)	120	4	1	0	24	0	340
pumpernickel	1 slice (0.9 oz)	65	2	1	0	12	2	174
raisin	1 slice (1.1 oz)	88	3	1	0	17	1	125
rye	1 slice (1.1 oz)	83	3	1	0	15	2	211
seven grain	1 slice (1.1 oz)	80	3	1	0	15	2	456
wheat berry	1 slice (0.9 oz)	65	2	1	0	12	1	133
wheat bran	1 slice (1.3 oz)	89	3	1	0	17	1	175
wheat germ	1 slice (1 oz)	73	3	1	0	14	1	155
white cubed	1 cup	93	3	1	0	18	1	238
whole wheat	1 slice (1 oz)	69	3	1	0	13	2	148

FOOD	PORTION	CALS	PROT	FAT	CHOL	CARB	FIBER	SOD
Alvarado Street Bakery								
Sprouted Whole Wheat	1 slice	90	4	1	0	19	3	170
Arnold								
Bakery Light 100% Whole Wheat	1 slice	80	5	1	0	18	5	160
Country Classics Wheat	1 slice	100	4	2	0	19	2	190
Smart & Healthy Omega-3 100% Whole Wheat	1 slice	80	4	1	0	16	2	180
Smart & Healthy Sugar Free 100% Whole Wheat	1 slice	80	4	1	0	15	2	180
Whole Grains 12 Grain	1 slice	110	4	2	0	21	3	200
Whole Grains 7 Grain	1 slice	110	4	2	0	22	3	190
Baker's Inn								
9 Grain	1 slice	100	5	2	0	18	2	210
Cracked Wheat	1 slice	100	4	2	0	18	2	190
Honey White Made w/ Whole Grain	1 slice	110	4	2	0	19	1	250
Honey Whole Wheat	1 slice	100	4	2	0	19	2	250
Potato Made w/ Whole Grain	1 slice	100	4	2	0	18	1	220
Damascus								
Roll-Up Flax	1 (2 oz)	110	12	3	0	15	9	360
Roll-Up Whole Wheat	1 (2 oz)	110	10	3	0	17	7	370
Earth Grains								
100% Multi Grain Extra Fiber	1 slice	110	5	2	0	19	5	180
Oat & Nut	1 slice	120	4	3	0	20	1	210
Potato	1 slice	110	4	1	0	20	tr	190
Whole Grain Honey	1 slice	110	5	2	0	19	2	160
Whole Wheat Honey	1 slice	110	5	2	0	20	5	180
Ecce Panis								
Country Wheat	1 slice (2 oz)	150	4	0	0	32	2	320
Food For Life								
Brown Rice Bread Yeast Free	1 slice	100	2	1	0	20	1	260
Rice Bread Fruit & Seed Yeast Free	1 slice	140	2	1	0	35	0	45
Rice Bread Multi Seed Yeast Free	1 slice	120	2	1	0	26	1	170
White Rice Bread Yeast Free	1 slice	100	2	0	0	23	tr	150

FOOD	PORTION	CALS	PROT	FAT	CHOL	CARB	FIBER	SOD
French Meadow Bakery								
Healthy Hemp	1 slice	110	7	3	0	14	5	150
Organic Men's Bread	1 slice	120	9	5	0	10	4	135
Kangaroo								
Bread Wraps	1 (2.6 oz)	140	3	3	0	30	5	285
Greek Pita Flat	1 (2.6 oz)	200	6	2	0	38	3	380
Greek Pita Flat Wheat	1 (2.4 oz)	145	6	2	0	30	3	320
Pita Pockets Onion	½ (1.2 oz)	90	3	0	0	18	1	140
Pita Pockets Wheat N'Honey	½ (1.2 oz)	90	3	0	0	16	4	140
Pita Pockets White	½ (1.2 oz)	90	3	0	0	18	1	140
Salad Pockets	1 (1.2 oz)	90	3	0	0	16	1	140
Sandwich Pockets Whole Grain	1 (1.2 oz)	80	4	1	0	16	5	100
La Tortilla Factory								
Wraps Smart & Delicious Gluten Free Dark Teff	1 (2.3 oz)	180	2	5	5	31	3	320
Wraps Smart & Delicious Gluten Free Ivory Teff	1 (2.3 oz)	180	2	5	0	30	3	320
Matthew's								
All Natural Cinnamon Raisin	1 slice	80	3	1	0	17	1	115
Milton's								
100% Whole Wheat	1 slice	110	5	1	0	22	5	220
Buttermilk	1 slice	90	3	1	0	19	1	160
Gourmet White	1 slice	110	4	1	0	23	1	110
Original Multi-Grain	1 slice	120	4	1	0	26	3	140
Potato	1 slice	90	3	1	0	19	1	160
Whole Grain	1 slice	90	4	1	0	16	5	125
Nature's Own								
100% Whole Wheat	1 slice	50	4	1	0	10	2	115
9 Grain	1 slice	120	4	2	0	24	2	190
Hearty Oatmeal	1 slice	100	5	2	0	18	3	170
Wheat Double Fiber	1 slice	10	4	1	0	10	5	150
Wheat Light	2 slices	80	5	1	0	19	5	200
Wheat N' Fiber	1 slice	60	6	1	0	7	2	105
Whole Wheat w/ Organic Flour	1 slice	100	5	2	0	21	3	240
Nature's Path								
Manna Carrot Raisin	1 slice	130	5	0	0	27	5	6

FOOD	PORTION	CALS	PROT	FAT	CHOL	CARB	FIBER	SOD
Manna Millet Rice	1 slice	130	5	0	0	28	5	3
Manna SunSeed	1 slice	160	6	2	0	29	7	3
Pepperidge Farm								
100% Natural Whole Grain German Dark Wheat	1 slice	100	4	2	0	20	3	210
Canadian White	1 slice	100	3	2	0	18	1	180
Carb Style 7 Grain	1 slice	60	5	2	0	8	3	150
Farmhouse Hearty White	1 slice	120	4	2	0	22	1	250
Farmhouse Honey Wheatberry	1 slice	120	4	2	0	22	2	190
Farmhouse Soft 100% Whole Wheat	1 slice	110	5	2	0	19	3	150
Farmhouse Soft Oatmeal	1 slice	120	4	2	0	21	1	200
Farmhouse Whole Grain White	1 slice	110	4	2	0	21	3	180
Hot & Crusty Italian	1 slice (2 in thick)	150	5	2	0	29	1	250
Jewish Rye Seeded	1 slice	80	3	1	0	15	2	170
Light Style 7 Grain	1 slice	45	2	0	0	9	1	90
Light Style Oatmeal	3 slices	140	7	1	0	27	2	260
Party Pumpernickel	5 slices	130	5	2	0	23	3	320
Very Thin White	3 slices	120	4	1	0	24	1	250
Whole Grain Honey Oat	1 slice	110	4	2	0	20	3	170
Whole Grain Honey Whole Wheat	1 slice	110	4	2	0	20	3	170
Whole Grain Swirl Cinnamon	1 slice	100	4	2	0	17	3	150
Whole Grain Swirl Cinnamon Raisin	1 slice	100	4	2	0	17	3	140
Rudi's Organic Bakery								
100% Whole Wheat	1 slice	100	4	1	0	19	3	150
14 Grain	1 slice	90	4	1	0	19	4	150
Artisan Country French	1 slice	100	4	1	0	20	tr	210
Artisan Rosemary Olive Oil	1 slice	100	3	1	0	19	tr	230
Low Carb Right Choice	1 slice	45	4	1	0	7	2	105
Spelt Ancient Grain	1 slice	120	4	3	0	20	2	170
Whole Grain Apple N Spice	1 slice	110	4	1	0	24	5	190
Sara Lee								
100% Whole Wheat	1 slice	70	3	1	0	13	2	135
Blueberry Crumble	1 slice	180	5	3	0	33	4	210

FOOD	PORTION	CALS	PROT	FAT	CHOL	CARB	FIBER	SOD
Cinnamon Raisin	1 slice	190	6	4	0	32	3	160
Classic Wheat	1 slice	70	3	1	0	13	2	150
Delightful Wheat	1 slice	45	3	0	0	9	2	120
Delightful White	1 slice	90	5	1	0	15	4	250
Heart Healthy 100% Whole Wheat Essentials	1 slice	80	4	1	0	14	4	135
Heart Healthy Multigrain	1 slice	100	4	1	0	19	2	180
Honey Wheat	1 slice	70	2	1	0	14	1	140
Honey White	1 slice	100	3	1	0	22	tr	210
Multigrain	1 slice	100	5	2	0	19	2	190
Soft & Smooth 100% Whole Wheat	1 slice	70	3	1	0	12	2	135
Soft & Smooth Whole Grain White	2 slices	150	6	2	0	28	3	250
Sonoma								
Wraps Organic Multi Grain	1 (2.4 oz)	180	6	7	0	27	6	330
Wraps Organic Wheat	1 (2.4 oz)	190	5	7	0	30	4	380
Wraps Original White Whole Wheat	1 (2.4 oz)	200	6	5	0	33	4	360
Stroehmann								
100% Whole Wheat	1 slice	90	4	2	0	17	3	180
Family Grains Twisted Bread	1 slice	70	3	1	0	14	2	140
Potato	1 slice	100	3	2	0	18	1	170
Soft Rye Seeded	1 slice	90	3	2	0	16	1	230
Super Bakery								
Athlete's Formula	1 slice (1.5 oz)	100	7	4	0	12	7	160
Fitness Formula	1 slice (1.5 oz)	90	7	3	0	12	7	160
Wrap Organic	1 (4 oz)	340	16	8	0	56	20	520
The Baker								
Yoga Bread	1 slice	70	3	1	0	13	2	80
Thomas'								
Breakfast Original	1 slice	90	4	1	0	17	1	190
Corn	1 slice	110	4	2	0	19	1	210
Swirl Cinnamon Raisin	1 slice	120	3	2	0	21	1	160
Toasting Cinnamon	1 slice	130	3	5	0	20	1	170

FOOD	PORTION	CALS	PROT	FAT	CHOL	CARB	FIBER	SOD
Tumaro's								
Wraps Chipotle Chili & Peppers	1 (2.3 oz)	170	4	2	0	34	2	200
Wraps Sun Dried Tomato & Basil	1 (2.3 oz)	170	5	2	0	34	2	210
TAKE-OUT								
banana	1 slice (2 oz)	196	3	6	26	33	1	181
chapatis as prep w/ fat	1 (1.6 oz)	95	3	2	3	18	3	180
chapatis as prep w/o fat	1 (2.5 oz)	141	5	1	–	31	5	–
cornbread	1 piece (2.3 oz)	183	4	6	26	27	2	317
cornstick	1 (1.4 oz)	118	3	4	17	18	1	204
focaccia onion	1 piece (4.6 oz)	282	6	10	0	43	2	536
focaccia rosemary	1 piece (3.5 oz)	251	6	7	0	40	2	535
focaccia tomato olive	1 piece (4.7 oz)	270	6	8	0	42	2	683
garlic bread	1 slice (1 oz)	96	2	4	0	13	1	177
irish soda bread	1 slice (3 oz)	247	6	4	15	48	2	338
italian garlic	1 loaf (11 oz)	990	23	38	0	137	8	1830
naan	1 bread (3.5 oz)	286	7	9	46	43	2	546
papadums fried	2 (1.5 oz)	81	4	4	–	9	2	–
paratha	1 bread (2.1 oz)	201	4	10	27	23	2	268
poori indian puffed bread	1 piece (1.3 oz)	112	3	4	0	16	2	226
zucchini	1 slice (1.4 oz)	150	2	7	26	19	1	115

BREAD COATING
Don's Chuck Wagon

FOOD	PORTION	CALS	PROT	FAT	CHOL	CARB	FIBER	SOD
Chicken Baking Mix	¼ cup	95	3	0	0	21	1	665
Fish Mix	¼ cup	95	4	0	0	21	1	710
Onion Ring Mix	¼ cup	100	3	0	0	21	1	690

FOOD	PORTION	CALS	PROT	FAT	CHOL	CARB	FIBER	SOD
Fryin' Magic								
Cornmeal	1 tbsp	30	1	0	0	6	0	390
Hodgson Mill								
Vidalia Sweet Onion Mix not prep	¼ cup	100	3	0	0	21	1	690

BREADCRUMBS

FOOD	PORTION	CALS	PROT	FAT	CHOL	CARB	FIBER	SOD
dry seasoned	¼ cup	115	4	2	0	21	2	528
fresh	¼ cup	30	1	tr	0	6	tr	77
plain	¼ cup	107	4	1	0	19	1	198
4C								
Carb Careful Seasoned	⅓ cup	110	15	1	0	9	5	340
Salt Free Seasoned	⅓ cup	110	4	1	0	23	2	5
Edward & Sons								
Organic Lightly Salted	⅓ cup	110	7	1	0	21	1	110
Organic Panko	⅓ cup	110	2	1	0	21	1	110
Ian's								
Panko Italian	¼ cup	70	2	1	0	15	2	137
Panko Original	¼ cup	71	2	0	0	15	1	32
Panko Whole Wheat	¼ cup	70	3	1	0	14	2	23
Progresso								
Italian Style	¼ cup	110	4	2	0	20	1	470
Rienzi								
Italian Style	¼ cup	120	5	2	0	20	2	480

BREADFRUIT

FOOD	PORTION	CALS	PROT	FAT	CHOL	CARB	FIBER	SOD
fresh	1 sm (13.5 oz)	396	4	1	0	104	19	8
fried	1 cup	379	2	21	0	52	9	3
raw	1 cup	227	2	1	0	60	11	4

BREADNUTTREE SEEDS

FOOD	PORTION	CALS	PROT	FAT	CHOL	CARB	FIBER	SOD
dried	1 oz	104	2	tr	0	23	–	–

BREADSTICKS

FOOD	PORTION	CALS	PROT	FAT	CHOL	CARB	FIBER	SOD
plain	1 sm	21	1	tr	0	3	tr	33
plain	1 lg	41	1	1	0	7	tr	66
Fattorie & Pandea								
Grissini Sesame	3	70	2	2	0	12	tr	125
Pepperidge Farm								
Garlic frzn	1	160	5	5	0	25	1	320

FOOD	PORTION	CALS	PROT	FAT	CHOL	CARB	FIBER	SOD
Stella D'Oro								
Mini Cracked Pepper	4 (0.5 oz)	70	2	2	0	11	0	80
Original	1 (0.3 oz)	40	1	1	0	6	0	40
Roasted Garlic	1	45	1	1	0	7	0	80
Sesame	1 (0.4 oz)	50	2	3	0	6	0	50
Sodium Free	1 (0.3 oz)	40	1	1	0	6	0	0

BREAKFAST BARS (see CEREAL BARS, ENERGY BARS)

BREAKFAST DRINKS

FOOD	PORTION	CALS	PROT	FAT	CHOL	CARB	FIBER	SOD
Carnation								
Instant Breakfast Chocolate Malt as prep w/ fat free milk	1 serv	220	13	1	6	39	tr	120
Instant Breakfast Classic French Vanilla as prep w/ fat free milk	1 serv	220	13	1	9	39	tr	80
Instant Breakfast Ready-To-Drink Carb Conscious French Vanilla	1 pkg	150	12	5	10	13	0	200
Instant Breakfast Ready-To-Drink Carb Conscious Milk Chocolate	1 pkg	150	12	5	10	15	2	230
Instant Breakfast Ready-To-Drink Strawberry Creme	1 pkg	250	13	5	10	37	0	200
Instant Breakfast Strawberry as prep w/ fat free milk	1 serv	220	13	6	9	39	0	160
Instant Breakfast Junior Vanilla	1 box (8.8 oz)	250	8	12	–	27	0	210

BROAD BEANS

FOOD	PORTION	CALS	PROT	FAT	CHOL	CARB	FIBER	SOD
canned	½ cup	91	7	tr	0	16	–	580
fava fresh cooked	½ cup	94	6	tr	0	17	5	4

BROCCOFLOWER

FOOD	PORTION	CALS	PROT	FAT	CHOL	CARB	FIBER	SOD
fresh raw	½ cup (1.8 oz)	16	1	tr	0	3	–	12

FOOD	PORTION	CALS	PROT	FAT	CHOL	CARB	FIBER	SOD
BROCCOLI								
FRESH								
chinese broccoli (gai lan) cooked	½ cup	10	1	tr	0	2	1	3
raab cooked	½ cup	28	3	tr	0	3	2	48
raw	1 bunch (1.3 lbs)	207	17	2	0	40	16	201
raw flower	1 piece	3	tr	tr	0	1	–	3
raw flowers	1 cup	20	2	tr	0	4	–	19
BroccoSprouts								
Broccoli Sprouts	½ cup	16	1	0	0	2	1	3
Mann's								
Broccoli Wokly	1 serv (3 oz)	25	3	0	0	4	2	25
Broccolini	8 stalks (3 oz)	35	3	0	0	6	1	25
Ocean Mist								
Rapini Broccoli Rabe Chopped Raw	1 cup	9	1	0	0	1	1	13
River Ranch								
Broccoli Slaw	1 cup	25	2	0	0	5	2	25
Florets	1¼ cups	25	3	0	0	4	3	25
FROZEN								
chopped cooked	½ cup	26	3	tr	0	5	3	10
spears cooked	½ cup	26	3	tr	0	5	3	22
spears cooked	1 pkg (10 oz)	70	8	tr	0	13	8	60
Birds Eye								
Broccoli & Cheese Sauce	½ cup	90	3	5	5	8	1	490
Steamfresh Cuts	1 cup	30	2	0	0	4	2	20
C&W								
Broccoli & Cheddar Cheese Sauce	1⅓ cups	70	4	3	5	7	2	370
Florets	1 cup	30	1	0	0	4	2	20
Cascadian Farm								
Organic Florets	⅔ cup	20	2	0	0	4	2	20
Green Giant								
Broccoli & Cheese Sauce	⅔ cup	60	2	3	0	7	2	460
Butter Sauce Low Fat	3 spears (4 oz)	40	2	2	<5	6	2	330
Cuts as prep	⅔ cup	25	1	0	0	4	2	20
Pasta Broccoli & Alfredo Sauce as prep	1 cup	210	9	4	<5	34	3	780

FOOD	PORTION	CALS	PROT	FAT	CHOL	CARB	FIBER	SOD
TAKE-OUT								
batter dipped & fried	4 pieces	77	2	5	9	6	1	83
w/ cheese sauce	1 cup	242	12	15	32	16	5	426
BROWNIE								
brownie	1 (2 oz)	227	3	9	10	36	1	175
butterscotch	1 (1.2 oz)	151	2	8	20	19	tr	95
Arrowhead Mills								
Gluten Free as prep	1	160	1	8	21	21	tr	40
Bob's Red Mill								
Gluten Free as prep	1	140	2	5	0	27	2	180
Foxy's Bake Shop								
Milk Chocolate	½ (1.7 oz)	200	3	11	55	23	0	65
White Chocolate	½ (1.7 oz)	200	3	12	0	23	0	70
French Meadow Bakery								
Gluten Free Fudge	1 (1.3 oz)	150	2	5	15	23	1	25
Glenny's								
100 Calorie 75% Organic	1 (1.45 oz)	100	4	4	–	12	7	85
Jiffy								
Fudge as prep	1	160	1	5	30	28	1	150
Joseph's								
Sugar Free	1 (1.5 oz)	150	2	7	0	26	1	59
Laura's Wholesome Junk Food								
Gluten Free Better Brownie	2	120	2	6	0	16	2	80
Nature's Path								
Organic Double Fudge	1/10 pkg	150	4	3	0	31	3	65
Organic HempPlus	1/10 pkg	140	4	2	0	31	3	55
No Pudge!								
All Flavors as prep	1	100	2	0	0	21	tr	90
Sara Lee								
Brownie Bites Chocolate Dipped	1 (0.7 oz)	90	1	4	5	12	1	30
VitaBrownie								
Dark Chocolate Pomegranate	1 (2 oz)	100	3	2	0	21	6	140
Deep Velvety Chocolate	1 (2 oz)	100	4	3	0	23	6	240
BRUSSELS SPROUTS								
FRESH								
cooked	6 pieces	45	3	1	0	9	3	26
Ocean Mist								
Brussels Sprouts	4 (2 oz)	40	2	1	0	6	3	25

FOOD	PORTION	CALS	PROT	FAT	CHOL	CARB	FIBER	SOD
Select Gourmet								
Fresh	½ cup	35	3	0	0	8	3	21
FROZEN								
cooked	1 cup	65	6	1	0	13	6	23
C&W								
Petite	10 (3 oz)	45	3	0	0	8	3	15
Green Giant								
Baby & Butter Sauce as prep	½ cup	60	3	1	<5	9	3	320

BUCKWHEAT

FOOD	PORTION	CALS	PROT	FAT	CHOL	CARB	FIBER	SOD
groats roasted cooked	½ cup	323	3	1	0	17	2	3
groats roasted uncooked	½ cup	292	11	3	0	61	9	1
Bob's Red Mill								
Organic Kernels	¼ cup	142	5	1	0	31	3	4

BUFFALO (see also MEAT STICKS)

FOOD	PORTION	CALS	PROT	FAT	CHOL	CARB	FIBER	SOD
burger	3 oz	202	20	13	71	0	0	62
chuck braised	4 oz	205	36	6	118	0	0	61
top round steak broiled	3 oz	313	54	9	153	0	0	74
water buffalo roasted	3 oz	111	23	2	52	0	0	48

BULGUR

FOOD	PORTION	CALS	PROT	FAT	CHOL	CARB	FIBER	SOD
cooked	½ cup	76	3	tr	0	17	4	5
uncooked	½ cup	239	9	1	0	53	13	12
Bob's Red Mill								
From Soft White Wheat	¼ cup	150	4	1	0	32	4	0
Fantastic								
Tabouli Mix not prep	2 tbsp	70	2	0	0	15	4	280
Sabra								
Black Bean & Wheat Pilaf	2 oz	45	2	2	0	7	2	130
Cracked Wheat Salad	2 oz	80	2	3	0	12	1	220
Tabouli	2 oz	70	2	4	0	6	1	100
TAKE-OUT								
tabbouleh	1 cup	198	3	15	0	16	4	797

BURBOT (FISH)

FOOD	PORTION	CALS	PROT	FAT	CHOL	CARB	FIBER	SOD
fresh baked	3 oz	98	65	1	65	0	0	106

BURDOCK ROOT

FOOD	PORTION	CALS	PROT	FAT	CHOL	CARB	FIBER	SOD
cooked w/o salt	1 cup	110	3	tr	0	26	2	5
cooked w/o salt	1 root (5.8 oz)	146	3	tr	0	35	3	7

FOOD	PORTION	CALS	PROT	FAT	CHOL	CARB	FIBER	SOD
Frieda's								
Gobo Root	¾ cup	60	1	0	0	15	3	0
BUTTER								
clarified butter	3.5 oz	876	tr	99	256	0	0	–
ghee cow's milk	1 tbsp	126	–	14	39	–	0	0
ghee vegetable oil	1 tbsp	126	–	14	0	–	0	0
stick	1 pat (5 g)	36	tr	4	11	tr	–	41
stick	1 stick (4 oz)	813	1	92	248	tr	–	937
whipped	1 pat (4 g)	27	tr	3	8	tr	–	31
whipped	1 tbsp	70	0	7	20	0	0	0
whipped	4 oz	542	1	61	165	tr	–	625
Cabot								
Salted	1 tbsp	100	0	11	30	0	0	90
Crystal Farms								
Butter	1 tbsp	100	0	11	30	0	0	90
Whipped	1 tbsp	70	0	7	20	0	0	55
Deerfield								
Creamy	1 tbsp	100	0	11	30	0	0	0
Horizon Organic								
European	1 tbsp	100	0	12	30	0	0	0
Land O Lakes								
Unsalted	1 tbsp	100	0	11	30	0	0	0
Organic Valley								
European Style	1 tbsp	110	0	12	25	0	0	0
BUTTER SUBSTITUTES								
stick	1 stick	811	1	91	99	1	–	1013
Butter Buds								
Granules	1 pkg (2 g)	5	0	0	0	2	–	75
Sunsweet								
Lighter Bake	1 tbsp	35	0	0	0	9	–	0
BUTTERBUR								
canned fuki chopped	1 cup	3	tr	tr	0	tr	–	5
fresh fuki	1 cup	13	tr	tr	0	3	–	7
BUTTERFISH								
baked	3 oz	159	19	9	71	0	0	97
fillet baked	1 oz	47	6	3	21	0	0	29
BUTTERNUTS								
dried	1 oz	174	7	16	0	3	–	0

FOOD	PORTION	CALS	PROT	FAT	CHOL	CARB	FIBER	SOD
BUTTERSCOTCH (see also CANDY)								
E. Guittard								
Baking Chips	33 (0.5 oz)	80	tr	5	0	10	0	15
CABBAGE (see also COLESLAW)								
chinese bok choy shredded cooked w/o salt	1 cup	20	3	tr	0	3	2	58
chinese pe-tsai shredded cooked w/o salt	1 cup	17	2	tr	0	3	2	11
green raw shredded	1 cup	19	1	tr	0	4	2	13
green shredded cooked w/o salt	1 cup	34	2	tr	0	8	3	12
japanese pickled	½ cup	22	1	tr	0	4	2	208
red raw shredded	1 cup	22	1	tr	0	5	2	19
red shredded cooked w/o salt	1 cup	44	2	tr	0	10	4	42
savoy shredded cooked w/o salt	1 cup	35	3	tr	0	8	4	35
Aunt Nellie's								
Sweet & Sour Red	¼ cup	40	0	0	0	10	0	220
Frieda's								
Baby Bok Choy	⅔ cup	10	1	0	0	2	1	35
Bok Choy	1 cup	10	1	0	0	2	1	55
Gai Choy	1 cup (3 oz)	20	2	0	0	4	2	20
Napa	1 cup (3 oz)	15	0	0	0	3	1	10
Salad Savoy	⅔ cup (3 oz)	25	2	0	0	5	3	25
Tuscan	⅔ cup (3 oz)	20	1	0	0	5	2	15
Glory								
Country Cabbage	½ cup	25	1	0	0	6	1	350
Greenwood								
Red	½ cup	100	1	0	0	24	0	380
River Ranch								
Angel Hair	1½ cups	20	1	0	0	5	2	15
TAKE-OUT								
creamed	1 cup	158	5	10	6	13	2	610
kimchee	1 cup	32	2	tr	0	6	2	996
stuffed cabbage w/ rice & beef	1 (3.6 oz)	117	9	5	42	9	1	369
sweet & sour red cabbage	4 oz	61	1	3	–	8	3	–

FOOD	PORTION	CALS	PROT	FAT	CHOL	CARB	FIBER	SOD
CACAO								
Navitas Naturals								
Butter	1 tbsp	120	0	14	0	0	0	0
Nibs	1 oz	130	4	12	0	10	9	0
Powder	1 oz	120	5	3	0	18	7	20
CACTUS								
fresh cooked w/ fat	1 pad (1 oz)	11	tr	1	0	1	1	84
fresh cooked w/o fat	1 cup (5.2 oz)	22	2	tr	0	5	3	399
pricklypear fresh	1 cup (5.3 oz)	56	2	1	0	13	4	–
Frieda's								
Cactus Pads	¾ cup (3 oz)	20	1	0	0	4	1	5
CAKE (see also CAKE MIX)								
battenburg cake	1 slice (2 oz)	204	3	10	–	28	1	–
cream puff shell	1 (2.3 oz)	239	6	17	129	15	–	368
crumpet	1 (2.3 oz)	131	4	1	0	31	2	535
eccles cake	1 slice (2 oz)	285	2	16	–	36	1	–
madeira cake	1 slice (1 oz)	98	1	4	–	15	1	–
sponge	1 piece (1.3 oz)	110	2	1	39	23	tr	93
sponge cake dessert shell	1 (0.8 oz)	70	1	2	20	12	0	150
treacle tart	1 slice (2.5 oz)	258	3	10	–	42	1	–
Arnold								
Date Nut Loaf	1 slice (2 oz)	190	3	5	0	32	2	350
Aunt Trudy's								
Organic Baklava Soy Nut	1 (1.8 oz)	190	4	6	0	29	2	60
Balocco								
Il Panettone	1 serv (3.5 oz)	380	7	15	120	54	2	75
Boboli								
Mini Eclairs Custard Filled	4 (2.3 oz)	224	4	12	35	22	0	29
Chudleigh's								
Apple Blossoms	1 (4 oz)	350	3	19	10	43	2	290
Drake's								
Coffee Cake Low Fat	2 (2.3 oz)	210	3	2	20	44	1	220
Entenmann's								
All Butter French Crumb	⅛ cake (1.8 oz)	210	2	10	50	29	tr	230

FOOD	PORTION	CALS	PROT	FAT	CHOL	CARB	FIBER	SOD
Cheese Cake Deluxe French	⅙ cake (3.8 oz)	390	6	24	40	39	tr	400
Coffee Cake Crumb	1 serv (2 oz)	260	3	12	10	34	1	230
Danish Twist Raspberry	⅛ cake	220	3	11	20	28	tr	180
Fudge Iced Golden Cake	⅛ cake	290	3	13	35	41	1	220
Loaf All Butter	⅙ cake (2.4 oz)	220	3	9	70	31	0	280
Louisiana Crunch	⅑ cake (2.9 oz)	330	3	14	45	49	tr	35
Marble Loaf	⅛ cake	190	2	8	40	28	tr	260
Marshmallow Iced Devil's Food	⅛ cake	280	2	14	15	40	tr	270
Mini's Carrot Cake	1 (1.4 oz)	160	1	7	20	22	tr	140
Strawberry Cheese Buns	1 (3 oz)	320	4	14	35	45	1	270
Fillo Factory								
Organic Apple Strudel	1 (4.4 oz)	290	3	10	0	47	2	110
Organic Apple Turnovers	1 (3 oz)	180	2	6	0	30	1	90
Glenny's								
Blondie 100 Calorie 75% Organic	1 (1.45 oz)	100	4	3	–	12	7	100
Goody Man								
Happy Birthday Cupcake White	1 (1.75 oz)	190	2	5	20	37	0	230
Gourmet Pastries								
Baklava Walnut	1 piece (1.8 oz)	240	3	11	5	30	0	100
Guiltless Gourmet								
Dessert Bowl Bananas Foster Cake	1 pkg (2 oz)	200	3	2	15	42	tr	250
Dessert Bowl Black Velvet Cake	1 pkg (2 oz)	200	4	3	20	42	3	190
Hostess								
100 Calorie Pack Mini Carrot Cake	1 pkg (1.2 oz)	100	2	3	5	20	4	120
100 Calorie Pack Mini Chocolate Cupcakes	1 pkg (1.3 oz)	100	2	3	10	22	5	140
100 Calorie Pack Mini Coffee Cake Cinnamon Streusel	1 pkg (1.2 oz)	100	2	3	10	21	5	135

FOOD	PORTION	CALS	PROT	FAT	CHOL	CARB	FIBER	SOD
100 Calorie Pack Mini Golden Cupcakes	1 pkg (1.2 oz)	100	2	3	5	20	3	150
Cup Cakes Chocolate	1 (1.8 oz)	170	1	6	5	30	1	250
Ho Ho's	1	120	1	6	0	18	0	75
Twinkies	1 (1.5 oz)	150	1	5	20	27	0	220
Kellogg's								
Pop-Tarts Apple Cinnamon	1 (1.8 oz)	210	2	6	0	37	tr	180
Pop-Tarts French Toast	1	220	3	8	0	35	tr	180
Pop-Tarts Frosted Cookies & Cream	1	200	2	5	0	35	tr	260
Pop-Tarts Low Fat Frosted Brown Sugar Cinnamon	1 (1.8 oz)	190	2	3	0	38	tr	210
Pop-Tarts Yogurt Blast Strawberry	1 (1.8 oz)	210	2	6	0	37	tr	190
Mrs. Smith's								
Carrot	⅙ cake (2.9 oz)	300	3	16	30	37	2	320
Cobbler Blackberry	1 serv (4 oz)	260	2	10	0	43	2	250
Nature's Path								
Organic Toaster Pastry Apple Cinnamon	1 (2 oz)	210	3	5	0	40	1	150
Organic Toaster Pastry Blueberry	1 (2 oz)	210	3	5	0	40	1	150
Organic Toaster Pastry Frosted Apple Cinnamon	1 (2 oz)	210	2	5	0	39	1	130
Organic Toaster Pastry Frosted Blueberry	1 (2 oz)	200	2	4	0	38	1	125
Organic Toaster Pastry Frosted Strawberry	1 (2 oz)	210	3	4	0	40	1	140
Neuman's								
Date Nut Bread	1 oz	90	2	2	<5	17	1	154
Pepperidge Farm								
Chocolate Coconut 3 Layer	⅛ cake	240	2	10	20	33	tr	130
Devil's Food 3 Layer	⅛ cake	220	2	9	20	34	tr	170
Golden 3 Layers	⅛ cake	230	2	9	15	34	1	130
Lemon 3 Layer	⅛ cake	240	2	11	25	34	tr	130
Turnover Apple	1	290	4	15	0	36	2	230
Philadelphia								
Snack Bars Classic Cheesecake	1 (1.5 oz)	190	2	11	15	22	0	85

FOOD	PORTION	CALS	PROT	FAT	CHOL	CARB	FIBER	SOD
Snack Bars Strawberry Cheesecake	1 bar (1.5 oz)	190	2	9	10	22	0	80
Sara Lee								
Cheesecake Classic French	1 piece (4.7 oz)	410	6	25	25	41	1	330
Cheesecake French Strawberry	1 piece (4.3 oz)	320	4	14	20	43	1	230
Cheesecake French Chocolate	1 piece (4.2 oz)	430	5	22	15	52	2	340
Cheesecake Strawberry Swirl	1 piece (2.9 oz)	290	4	11	60	44	1	140
Cobbler Anytime Apple	1 (4 oz)	350	3	17	10	47	1	240
Coffee Cake Butter Streusel	1 piece (2 oz)	190	3	9	35	25	1	190
Coffee Cake Crumb	1 serv (2 oz)	190	2	8	20	30	1	150
Layer Cake Coconut	1 slice (2.8 oz)	260	2	14	15	33	1	210
Layer Cake Double Chocolate	1 slice (2.8 oz)	260	3	13	10	33	2	230
Layer Cake Fudge Golden	1 slice (2.8 oz)	260	2	13	15	34	1	200
Layer Cake Vanilla	1 slice (2.8 oz)	260	2	14	15	32	0	210
Pound Cake All Butter	1 slice (0.6 oz)	240	4	16	115	37	1	160
Pound Cake Free & Light	1 slice (2.5 oz)	200	3	4	0	39	1	290
Weight Watchers								
Lemon w/ Lemon Icing	1 (1 oz)	80	1	3	5	14	2	90
TAKE-OUT								
angelfood	1 slice (2 oz)	143	3	tr	0	33	tr	283
apple crisp	1 serv (8.6 oz)	384	4	8	0	76	4	502
apple turnover	1 (6.6 oz)	661	7	34	0	83	3	614
baklava	1 piece (2.7 oz)	334	5	23	35	29	2	253
basbousa namoura	1 piece (1 oz)	60	2	3	0	10	2	144
bean cake	1 cake (1.1 oz)	130	2	7	0	16	1	60

FOOD	PORTION	CALS	PROT	FAT	CHOL	CARB	FIBER	SOD
black forest chocolate cherry	1 piece (2.5 oz)	187	2	9	30	27	1	160
boston cream pie	1 slice (3.2 oz)	232	2	8	34	39	1	132
cannoli w/ cannoli cream	1	369	6	21	–	42	–	–
carrot w/ icing	1 slice (4.7 oz)	543	5	28	80	70	2	245
cheesecake	1 slice (4.5 oz)	410	11	25	86	37	tr	484
cheesecake chocolate	1 slice (4.5 oz)	489	8	32	118	49	2	384
chinese moon cake	1 (4.8 oz)	458	9	6	69	92	4	119
coconut mochiko filipino cake	1 piece (2.7 oz)	252	3	12	0	35	2	76
coffeecake iced	1 piece (1.6 oz)	175	3	8	31	24	1	180
cream puff custard filled chocolate frosted	1 (3.9 oz)	293	7	18	142	27	1	377
dutch honey cake	1 slice (0.8 oz)	70	1	0	0	17	0	25
eclair	1 (3.5 oz)	262	6	16	127	24	1	337
french apple tart	1 (3.5 oz)	302	4	15	60	37	2	326
fruitcake	1 slice (1.5 oz)	139	1	4	2	26	2	116
funnel cake	1 (3.2 oz)	276	7	14	62	29	1	269
gingerbread	1 piece (2.4 oz)	213	3	7	24	35	1	316
jelly roll	1 slice (1.8 oz)	146	3	2	93	28	tr	92
jelly roll lemon filled	1 slice (3 oz)	210	3	2	35	48	tr	300
napoleon	1 mini (1 oz)	123	2	9	14	9	tr	51
napoleon	1 (3 oz)	348	5	25	39	25	1	144
panettone	1/12 cake (2.9 oz)	300	6	12	90	43	2	120
petit fours	2 (0.9 oz)	120	1	7	0	15	0	15
pineapple upside down	1 piece (4.2 oz)	387	4	15	27	61	1	385
pound	1 slice (1 oz)	120	2	5	32	15	–	96
pound fat free	1 slice (2 oz)	160	3	1	0	35	1	193

FOOD	PORTION	CALS	PROT	FAT	CHOL	CARB	FIBER	SOD
sacher torte	1 slice (2.2 oz)	240	4	11	50	30	4	120
sacher torte chocolate + apricot jam	1 serv	430	–	12	–	23	–	–
strawberry shortcake	1 serv (4.1 oz)	211	4	5	109	40	1	112
strudel apple	1 piece (2.2 oz)	175	2	7	4	26	1	172
strudel cheese	1 piece (2.2 oz)	195	6	8	42	24	tr	111
strudel cherry	1 piece (2.2 oz)	179	3	6	9	29	1	82
tiramisu	1 piece (5.1 oz)	409	7	30	171	31	tr	79
tiramisu	1 cake (4.4 lbs)	5732	101	421	2395	439	3	1107
torte chocolate ganache	1 slice (3.5 oz)	400	7	26	90	40	6	120
trifle w/ cream	6 oz	291	4	16	–	34	1	–
white w/ coconut icing	1 slice (3.9 oz)	399	5	12	1	71	1	318
zucchini bread	1 slice (1.4 oz)	150	2	7	26	19	1	115

CAKE ICING

FOOD	PORTION	CALS	PROT	FAT	CHOL	CARB	FIBER	SOD
chocolate	¼ cup	269	1	7	1	53	1	125
vanilla	¼ cup	322	tr	8	0	64	0	152
Jiffy								
Fudge Frosting	¼ cup	150	tr	4	0	28	1	150
White Frosting	¼ cup	150	0	5	0	27	0	150

CAKE MIX

FOOD	PORTION	CALS	PROT	FAT	CHOL	CARB	FIBER	SOD
Bisquick								
Heart Smart	⅓ cup	140	3	3	0	27	1	430
Don's Chuck Wagon								
All Purpose Batter Mix	¼ cup	100	4	0	0	20	1	580
Jiffy								
Devil's Food as prep	⅕ cake	220	3	6	42	40	1	528
Golden Yellow as prep	⅕ cake	220	2	5	36	39	tr	340
White Cake as prep	⅕ cake	210	2	5	3	39	tr	320

FOOD	PORTION	CALS	PROT	FAT	CHOL	CARB	FIBER	SOD
King Arthur								
Cinnamon Buns Kit not prep	½ cup	240	6	1	0	52	3	15
CALABAZA								
fresh	½ cup	32	1	tr	–	8	–	3
CALZONE (*see* SANDWICHES)								
CANADIAN BACON								
grilled	2 slices (1.6 oz)	87	11	4	27	1	0	727
Boar's Head								
Canadian Bacon	2 oz	70	12	2	35	1	0	570
Celebrity								
98% Fat Free	3 slices (1.8 oz)	60	10	1	30	1	0	350
Organic Prairie								
Hardwood Smoked	1 oz	40	7	1	15	1	0	250
Wellshire								
Sliced	2 oz	20	13	3	30	10	0	250
CANADIAN BACON SUBSTITUTES								
Yves								
Meatless Canadian Bacon	2 slices (2 oz)	80	17	1	0	2	0	400
CANDY								
butterscotch	1 piece (6 g)	24	0	tr	1	6	–	3
candied cherries	1 (4 g)	12	0	tr	0	3	–	–
candied citron	1 oz	89	tr	tr	0	23	–	82
candied lemon peel	1 oz	90	tr	tr	0	23	–	14
candied orange peel	1 oz	90	tr	tr	0	23	–	14
candied pineapple slice	1 slice (2 oz)	179	tr	tr	0	45	–	–
candy corn	1 oz	105	tr	0	0	27	–	57
caramels	1 piece (8 g)	31	tr	1	1	6	–	20
caramels chocolate	1 piece (6 g)	22	tr	tr	0	6	–	–
carob bar	1 (3.1 oz)	453	11	28	–	42	–	–
crisped rice bar almond	1 bar (1 oz)	130	2	6	0	18	1	66
crisped rice bar chocolate chip	1 bar (1 oz)	115	4	4	0	21	1	79
dark chocolate	1 oz	150	1	10	0	16	–	5

FOOD	PORTION	CALS	PROT	FAT	CHOL	CARB	FIBER	SOD
fondant	1 piece (0.6 oz)	57	0	0	0	15	–	6
fondant chocolate coated	1 piece (0.4 oz)	40	tr	1	0	9	–	3
fondant mint	1 oz	105	tr	0	0	27	–	57
fruit pastilles	1 tube (1.4 oz)	101	2	0	–	25	–	–
fudge brown sugar w/ nuts	1 piece (0.5 oz)	56	tr	1	1	11	–	14
fudge chocolate marshmallow	1 piece (0.7 oz)	84	1	3	5	14	–	21
fudge chocolate marshmallow w/ nuts	1 piece (0.8 oz)	96	1	4	5	15	–	21
fudge chocolate w/ nuts	1 piece (0.7 oz)	81	1	3	3	14	–	11
fudge peanut butter	1 piece (0.6 oz)	59	1	1	1	13	–	12
fudge vanilla w/ nuts	1 piece (0.5 oz)	62	tr	2	2	11	–	9
gumdrops	10 sm (0.4 oz)	135	0	0	0	35	–	15
gumdrops	10 lg (3.8 oz)	420	0	0	0	108	–	48
hard candy	1 oz	106	0	0	0	28	–	11
jelly beans	10 sm (0.4 oz)	40	0	tr	0	10	–	3
jelly beans	10 lg (1 oz)	104	0	tr	0	26	–	7
lollipop	1 (6 g)	22	0	0	0	6	–	2
marzipan	1 oz	128	3	7	0	15	2	5
milk chocolate	1 bar (1.55 oz)	226	3	14	10	26	–	36
milk chocolate crisp	1 bar (1.45 oz)	203	3	11	8	28	–	59
milk chocolate w/ almonds	1 bar (1.45 oz)	215	4	14	8	22	–	30
nougat nut cream	0.5 oz	49	1	4	–	8	–	–
organic dark chocolate w/ raisins & pecans	1.4 oz	220	2	14	0	22	3	0
peanut bar	1 (1.4 oz)	209	6	14	–	19	–	91
peanut brittle	1 oz	128	2	5	4	20	–	128

FOOD	PORTION	CALS	PROT	FAT	CHOL	CARB	FIBER	SOD
peanuts chocolate covered	10 (1.4 oz)	208	5	13	4	20	–	16
peanuts chocolate covered	1 cup (5.2 oz)	773	19	50	13	74	–	61
praline	1 piece (1.4 oz)	177	1	10	0	24	–	24
pretzels chocolate covered	1 (0.4 oz)	50	1	2	–	8	–	10
pretzels chocolate covered	1 oz	130	2	5	–	20	–	–
sesame crunch	20 pieces (1.2 oz)	181	4	12	0	18	–	–
sweet chocolate	1 oz	143	1	10	0	17	–	5
sweet chocolate	1 bar (1.45 oz)	201	2	14	0	25	–	7
taffy	1 piece (0.5 oz)	56	0	1	1	14	–	13
toffee	1 piece (0.4 oz)	65	tr	4	13	8	–	22
truffles	1 piece (0.4 oz)	59	1	4	6	5	–	8
3 Musketeers								
Bar	1 (2.1 oz)	260	2	8	5	46	1	110
Fun Size	3 bars (1.6 oz)	190	1	6	5	34	1	85
Miniatures	7 (1.4 oz)	170	1	5	5	32	1	80
Anastasia								
Coco Rhum Bites	2 pieces (1 oz)	110	2	5	0	16	1	45
Andes								
Dark Chocolate Covered Cherries	2 (1 oz)	110	1	5	0	19	tr	10
Thins Cherry Jubilee	8 pieces (1.3 oz)	200	2	13	0	22	1	20
Thins Creme De Menthe	8 pieces (1.3 oz)	200	2	13	0	22	tr	20
Baby Ruth								
Fun Size	2 bars (1.3 oz)	170	2	8	0	24	tr	85
Snack Bars	2 (1.3 oz)	170	2	8	0	24	tr	85
Bartons								
Cashew Toppers	1 (1 oz)	140	3	9	5	14	1	20

FOOD	PORTION	CALS	PROT	FAT	CHOL	CARB	FIBER	SOD
Benecol								
Smart Chews Caramel	1 piece	20	0	0	0	4	–	15
Blow Pop								
Regular	1 (0.6 oz)	60	0	0	0	16	0	0
Brach's								
Bridge Mix	16 pieces	190	2	8	5	26	tr	40
Candy Corn	26 pieces	140	0	0	0	35	0	115
Caramel Clusters	3 pieces	210	4	13	5	23	1	80
Circus Peanuts	6 pieces	160	tr	0	0	39	0	0
Fruit Rippers Berry Punch	1 pkg (0.5 oz)	60	2	0	0	11	0	15
Fruit Slices	3 pieces	150	0	0	0	38	0	10
Malts	15 pieces	190	2	7	10	30	1	25
Mellowcreme Pumpkins	6 pieces	130	0	0	0	33	0	130
Milk Maid Caramels	4 pieces	160	1	5	0	30	0	80
Mint Patties	3 pieces	140	0	3	0	29	0	0
Orange Slices	2 pieces	130	0	0	0	32	0	10
Peanut Butter Meltaways	3 pieces	200	3	13	0	19	1	90
Root Beer Barrels	3 pieces	70	0	0	0	17	0	5
Spearmint Leaves	5 pieces	130	0	0	0	34	0	15
Spice Drops	12 pieces	130	0	0	0	33	0	15
Sprinkles	17 pieces	200	2	9	15	29	1	35
Star Brites Butterscotch	3 pieces	60	0	0	0	16	0	80
Stars	10 pieces	200	2	11	0	24	0	25
Wild'N Fruity Gummi Bears	14 pieces	140	2	0	0	32	0	15
Breath Savers								
Sugar Free Peppermint	1 piece	5	0	0	0	2	–	0
Butterfinger								
Bar	1 (2.1 oz)	270	4	11	0	43	1	135
Crisps	1 bar (1.8 oz)	250	3	13	0	33	1	140
Minis	4 (1.4 oz)	180	2	7	0	29	tr	90
Cadbury								
Milk Chocolate Fruit & Nut	10 blocks (1.4 oz)	200	4	10	5	24	1	30
Royal Dark	10 blocks (1.4 oz)	220	2	13	<5	24	3	0
Cella's								
Milk Chocolate Covered Cherries	2 (1 oz)	120	1	5	5	20	1	20

FOOD	PORTION	CALS	PROT	FAT	CHOL	CARB	FIBER	SOD
Chargers								
Chocolate Covered Expresso Beans	1 pkg (0.5 oz)	60	1	3	0	9	tr	0
Charleston Chews								
Chocolate	1 bar (1.9 oz)	230	2	6	0	43	1	30
Vanilla	1 bar (1.9 oz)	230	2	8	0	44	0	30
Charms								
Fluffy Stuff Cotton Candy	1 pkg (0.6 oz)	70	0	0	0	17	0	0
Sour Balls	1 (5 g)	20	0	0	0	5	0	0
Squares	2 pieces	20	0	0	0	6	0	0
Chew-ets								
Peanut Chews Original Dark	3 pieces	170	3	9	0	22	2	55
CocoaVia								
Dark Chocolate Blueberry & Almond Bar	1 (0.8 oz)	100	1	6	0	12	2	0
Dark Chocolate Covered Almonds	1 pkg (1 oz)	140	3	11	0	12	3	0
Dark Chocolate Crispy Bar	1 (0.7 oz)	90	2	5	0	11	2	10
Dark Chocolate Original Bar	1 (0.8 oz)	80	1	6	0	12	2	0
Milk Chocolate Almond Bar	1 (0.8 oz)	110	2	7	5	12	1	15
Milk Chocolate Bar	1 (0.8 oz)	110	1	6	5	13	0	15
Milk Chocolate Covered Raisins	1 pkg (1 oz)	150	2	6	0	22	1	15
Coffee Rio								
Coffee Candy All Flavors	4 pieces	60	0	2	5	10	0	20
Crispy Cat								
Roasted Peanut	1 bar (1 oz)	220	4	10	0	29	2	125
Dare								
RealFruit Gummies All Flavors	8 pieces (1.4 oz)	120	2	0	0	28	0	5
Dots								
All Flavors	12 (1.5 oz)	140	0	0	0	35	0	10
Dove								
Dark Chocolate	⅓ bar	170	2	11	5	20	3	0

FOOD	PORTION	CALS	PROT	FAT	CHOL	CARB	FIBER	SOD
Dark Chocolate Covered Almonds	13 pieces	210	3	15	5	19	3	10
Dark Chocolate Miniatures	5 pieces	210	2	13	5	24	3	0
Milk Chocolate	⅓ bar	180	2	11	5	20	1	20
Milk Chocolate Covered Almonds	13 pieces	220	4	15	5	19	2	20
Milk Chocolate Minatures w/ Caramel	5 pieces	200	2	11	5	24	1	45
Milk Chocolate Miniatures	5	220	2	13	5	24	1	25
Milk Chocolate w/ Almonds	⅓ bar	190	3	12	5	19	2	20
E. Guittard								
Bar Quevedo Bittersweet 65% Cocoa	1 (2 oz)	290	3	23	0	29	5	0
Bar Sur Del Lago Bittersweet 65% Cocoa	1 (2 oz)	290	3	23	0	29	5	0
Eclipse								
Mints Sugarless All Flavors	3 pieces	5	0	0	0	2	–	0
Endangered Species								
Dark Chocolate w/ Espresso Beans	½ bar (1.5 oz)	200	4	15	0	13	5	10
Dark Chocolate w/ Hazelnut Toffee	½ bar (1.5 oz)	220	3	15	5	15	4	5
Milk Chocolate w/ Cherries	½ bar (1.5 oz)	230	3	14	15	22	1	0
Organic Dark Chocolate	½ bar (0.7 oz)	100	1	6	0	12	1	1
Organic Dark Chocolate w/ Tangerine	½ bar (0.7 oz)	100	1	6	0	12	1	1
Organic Milk Chocolate w/ Key Lime	½ bar (0.7 oz)	110	1	7	5	11	0	1
Equal Exchange								
Organic Chocolate Expresso Bean	1 bar (1.4 oz)	216	2	15	0	22	3	2
Organic Milk Chocolate	1 bar (1.4 oz)	230	4	16	12	19	1	40
Organic Very Dark Chocolate	1 bar (1.4 oz)	220	3	17	0	18	5	5
Estee								
Fructose Sweetened Peanut Butter Cups	5	200	5	12	<5	19	1	70

FOOD	PORTION	CALS	PROT	FAT	CHOL	CARB	FIBER	SOD
Fructose Sweetened Milk Chocolate w/ Crisp Rice	½ bar (1.2 oz)	370	7	26	30	29	0	110
Sugar Free Assorted Fruit	3	15	0	0	0	16	14	0
Sugar Free Butterscotch	4	15	0	0	0	16	14	50
Sugar Free Gourmet Jelly Beans	26	70	0	0	0	24	0	30
Sugar Free Gum Drops Assorted Fruit	11	110	0	0	0	34	0	70
Sugar Free Gummy Bears Assorted Fruit	17	70	3	0	0	30	0	5
Sugar Free Peppermint	3	15	0	0	0	14	13	0
Sugar Free Sour Citrus Slices	9	60	0	0	0	30	0	50
Sugar Free Toffee	4	15	0	0	0	16	14	95
Sugar Free Tropical Fruit	3	15	0	0	0	16	14	0
Ethel's								
Truffles Assorted	4	200	2	14	15	17	1	30
Fauchon								
Assortment Truffles	3 pieces (1.3 oz)	160	2	11	<5	19	2	15
Chocolate Assortment	3 pieces (1.1 oz)	170	3	11	<5	19	2	15
Ferrero Rocher								
Candy	3 pieces (1.3 oz)	220	4	15	0	17	1	35
Figamajigs								
Fig Candy Drops Dark Chocolate Covered	1 pkg (1.4 oz)	150	2	4	0	29	3	15
Fig Candy Drops Orange & Yellow Chocolate Covered	1 pkg (1.4 oz)	150	1	3	0	32	2	10
Frooties								
Chewy Candy Fruit Flavored	12 pieces (1.3 oz)	104	0	3	0	29	0	20
Fruitzels								
Assorted	7 pieces	120	2	0	0	29	0	10
Ghirardelli								
Squares Milk Chocolate w/ Caramel Filling	3 (1.6 oz)	220	2	12	10	27	tr	60
Squares Mint Indulgence	3 (1.6 oz)	210	1	11	0	30	2	0

FOOD	PORTION	CALS	PROT	FAT	CHOL	CARB	FIBER	SOD
Squares 60% Cacao Dark Chocolate	4 (1.5 oz)	220	2	17	0	23	3	0
Squares 60% Cacao Dark Chocolate w/ Caramel	3 (1.6 oz)	220	2	15	5	25	3	35
Godiva								
Sugar Free Chocolate	1 bar (1.5 oz)	190	1	15	5	24	tr	0
Sugar Free Chocolate w/ Almonds	1 bar (1.5 oz)	200	2	15	5	23	1	0
Sugar Free Dark Chocolate	1 bar (1.5 oz)	190	3	14	<5	25	4	10
Truffles Assorted	2 pieces (1.4 oz)	210	3	13	10	20	2	20
Green & Black's								
Organic Chocolate Fairtrade Maya Gold	1 bar (3.5 oz)	526	7	34	–	48	8	14
Organic Dark Chocolate	1 bar (3.5 oz)	551	9	41	–	36	12	16
Organic Dark Chocolate Mint	1 bar (3.5 oz)	478	7	27	–	51	9	42
Organic Dark Chocolate w/ Hazelnuts & Currants	1 bar (3.5 oz)	513	8	34	–	45	9	16
Organic Milk Chocolate	1 bar (3.5 oz)	523	10	30	–	54	4	65
Organic Milk Chocolate Caramel	1 bar (3.5 oz)	495	8	26	–	56	3	15
Organic Milk Chocolate Raisins & Hazelnuts	1 bar (3.5 oz)	556	9	37	–	47	3	58
Organic Milk Chocolate Whole Almonds	1 bar (3.5 oz)	578	12	42	–	38	5	71
Organic White Chocolate	1 bar (3.5 oz)	573	7	37	–	54	tr	81
Guylian								
Twists Milk Chocolate Truffle	5 pieces (1.2 oz)	230	2	19	10	15	1	20
Twists Original Praline	4 pieces (1.2 oz)	200	3	13	10	19	1	20
Hershey's								
Chocolate Miniatures Sugar Free	5 pieces (1.4 oz)	170	1	13	10	25	2	10

FOOD	PORTION	CALS	PROT	FAT	CHOL	CARB	FIBER	SOD
Chocolate w/ Almonds Miniatures Sugar Free	5 pieces (1.4 oz)	180	2	14	10	23	3	10
Cacao Reserve 65% Cacao Dark	3 blocks (1.3 oz)	180	4	15	<5	18	4	0
Cacao Reserve 35% Cacao Milk Chocolate w/ Hazelnuts	3 sq (1.3 oz)	220	3	15	10	18	1	25
Dark Chocolate Miniatures Sugar Free	5 pieces (1.4 oz)	190	2	15	5	23	3	0
Milk Chocolate	1 bar (1.4 oz)	210	3	12	10	23	1	35
Milk Chocolate w/ Almonds	1 bar (1.4 oz)	230	4	14	5	21	1	30
Nuggets Cookies 'N' Creme	4	190	3	10	5	22	0	75
Nuggets Dark Chocolate w/ Almonds	4	220	3	14	<5	20	3	0
Nuggets Milk Chocolate	4	230	3	13	10	24	1	35
Pot Of Gold	3 pieces	130	1	5	<5	21	tr	45
Sticks Special Dark	1 (0.4 oz)	60	tr	4	0	7	tr	15
Jay's								
Cotton Candy	1 pkg (2 oz)	220	3	0	0	56	–	0
Jelly Belly								
Jelly Beans Sugar Free	35	80	0	0	0	37	8	0
Jolly Rancher								
All Flavors	4 pieces	60	0	0	0	15	0	0
Sugar Free	4 pieces (0.6 oz)	35	0	0	0	13	0	0
Joyva								
Halvah Chocolate Covered	1 serv (2 oz)	380	5	25	0	20	3	95
Junior								
Caramels	1 box (1.4 oz)	170	1	3	0	35	tr	30
Mints	1 box (1.4 oz)	170	1	3	0	35	tr	30
Kellogg's								
Fruit Flavored Snacks Hello Kitty	10 pieces	100	0	0	0	26	0	25
Fruit Flavored Snacks Winnie The Pooh	1 pkg	80	0	0	0	21	0	20

FOOD	PORTION	CALS	PROT	FAT	CHOL	CARB	FIBER	SOD
Fruit Streamers Watermelon Madness	1 pkg (0.8 oz)	80	1	1	0	17	0	80
Fruit Twistables Triple Cherry Explosion	1 pkg (0.8 oz)	70	tr	1	0	17	0	55
Gamester Rolls All Varieties	1 pkg (0.7 oz)	80	0	2	0	16	0	20
Yogos Crazy Berries	1 pkg (0.8 oz)	90	0	2	0	18	0	15
KitKat								
Bar	1 (0.5 oz)	73	1	4	tr	9	tr	10
Legacy Chocolates								
Truffles Assorted	1 piece (0.5 oz)	90	1	6	tr	6	1	0
Let's Do Organic								
Black Licorice Bars	1 (0.9 oz)	80	1	0	0	20	tr	20
Black Licorice Chews	8 (1.4 oz)	130	2	0	0	30	tr	30
Gummi Bears	1 pkg (0.9 oz)	80	0	0	0	22	0	15
Lifesavers								
Variety	4 pieces	60	0	0	0	16	–	0
Lindt								
Lindor Truffles 60% Extra Dark	3 pieces	210	2	19	<5	15	tr	0
Love Candy								
Dark Chocolate	1 bar (1.5 oz)	190	2	11	20	21	1	55
Milk Chocolate	1 bar (1.5 oz)	200	1	11	25	22	tr	65
Yogurt Supreme	1 bar (1.5 oz)	190	1	11	20	23	tr	60
M&M's								
Almond	1 pkg (1.3 oz)	200	3	11	5	21	2	15
Dark Chocolate	1 pkg (1.7 oz)	240	2	11	5	33	2	10
Milk Chocolate	1 pkg (1.7 oz)	240	2	10	5	34	1	30
Minis	1 pkg (1.1 oz)	150	1	7	5	21	1	20

FOOD	PORTION	CALS	PROT	FAT	CHOL	CARB	FIBER	SOD
Peanut	1 pkg (1.7 oz)	250	5	13	5	30	2	25
Peanut Butter	1 pkg (1.6 oz)	240	5	14	5	26	2	100
Mentos								
Sugar Free Mixed Berries	1 piece	5	0	0	0	3	–	0
Mike & Ike								
All Flavors	1 pkg (2 oz)	200	0	0	0	50	–	–
Milky Way								
Bar	1 (2 oz)	260	2	10	5	41	1	95
Fun Size	2 bars (1.2 oz)	150	1	6	5	24	0	55
Midnight	1 bar (1.8 oz)	220	2	8	5	36	1	90
Midnight Minis	5 (1.4 oz)	180	1	7	5	29	1	70
Milk Chocolate Covered Caramels	5 (1.5 oz)	200	2	8	10	30	0	120
Minis	5 (1.5 oz)	190	2	7	5	30	0	70
Mr. Goodbar								
Bar	1 (1.75 oz)	270	5	16	5	27	2	20
Mrs. Fields								
Decadent Chocolates	3 pieces (1.8 oz)	240	3	12	10	29	2	70
Munch								
Nut Bar	1 (1.42 oz)	220	6	15	10	18	2	140
Necco								
Mint	1 piece	12	–	tr	0	–	–	–
Nestle								
Crunch Stix	1 (0.6 oz)	90	tr	5	0	12	0	30
Turtles Original	3 pieces	240	3	14	5	30	1	65
Newman's Own								
Organic Chocolate Cups Dark Chocolate Peanut Butter	1 pkg (1.2 oz)	180	3	12	0	18	1	50
Organic Chocolate Cups Milk Chocolate Peanut Butter	1 pkg (1.2 oz)	180	4	12	0	17	1	70
Organic Chocolate Cups Peppermint	1 pkg (1.2 oz)	170	2	11	0	20	1	0

FOOD	PORTION	CALS	PROT	FAT	CHOL	CARB	FIBER	SOD
Organic Chocolate Sweet Dark	½ bar (¼ oz)	200	2	13	0	24	2	0
Organic Chocolate Sweet Dark Expresso	½ bar (1.4 oz)	200	2	14	0	20	2	0
Organic Chocolate Sweet Dark Orange	½ bar (1.4 oz)	200	2	13	0	24	2	0
Organic Milk Chocolate	½ bar (1.4 oz)	210	3	13	9	22	1	34
Nutty Ducky's								
Cashew Brittle	4 pieces (1.6 oz)	240	4	14	5	22	2	55
Cashew Brittle Dark Chocolate	2 pieces (1.5 oz)	220	3	14	5	23	2	30
Peanut Brittle	4 pieces (1.6 oz)	230	6	12	5	23	4	50
Peanut Brittle Milk Chocolate	2 pieces (1.5 oz)	220	5	12	5	23	2	40
Odense								
Marzipan	2 tbsp (1.4 oz)	170	3	4	0	29	0	0
Raisinets								
Candy	3 pkg (1.7 oz)	200	2	8	5	34	1	15
Reese's								
Bites	16 pieces	220	4	12	<5	23	1	70
FastBreak	1 bar (0.7 oz)	90	2	5	0	11	–	65
Miniatures Peanut Butter Cups Sugar Free	5 pieces (1.4 oz)	170	2	12	5	24	5	110
Peanut Butter Cups Miniatures	5 (1.4 oz)	210	4	12	<5	22	1	115
Peanut Butter Cups Snack Size	1 piece (0.5 oz)	80	1	5	–	8	–	45
Peanut Butter Cups Sugar Free	1 piece (1.5 oz)	180	2	13	5	26	5	120
White Miniatures Peanut Butter Cups	4 pieces (1.4 oz)	210	7	12	<5	21	tr	125
White Miniatures Peanut Butter Cups Sugar Free	5 pieces (1.4 oz)	180	4	13	0	21	3	125
Russell Stover								
Assorted	3 pieces (1.4 oz)	170	1	7	5	27	1	50

FOOD	PORTION	CALS	PROT	FAT	CHOL	CARB	FIBER	SOD
Low Carb Pecan Delights	1 piece (1 oz)	130	2	9	0	15	2	25
Private Reserve Triple Chocolate Mousse	3 pieces (1.3 oz)	220	2	17	<5	19	2	15
Private Reserve Vanilla Bean Brulee	3 pieces (1.3 oz)	180	3	13	<5	19	3	25
Scharffen Berger								
Semisweet 60% Cacao	1 bar (2 oz)	320	4	20	0	32	tr	0
Skittles								
Original Fruit	1 pkg (2.2 oz)	250	0	3	0	56	0	10
Slim-Fast								
Protein Snack Chews Peanut Butter	1 pkg (0.9 oz)	100	6	4	0	12	0	90
Smucker's								
Jelly Beans	25	150	0	0	0	37	0	10
Snickers								
Almond	1 (1.8 oz)	230	3	11	5	32	2	115
Bar	1 bar (2.07 oz)	280	4	14	5	35	1	140
Cruncher	1 bar (1.6 oz)	220	3	11	5	28	1	85
Cruncher	3 fun size (1.4 oz)	230	4	13	5	25	1	140
Miniatures	4 (1.3 oz)	170	3	9	5	22	1	90
Sour Patch								
Connectors	1.5 oz	150	0	0	0	37	–	25
Kids	1.5 oz	140	0	0	0	36	–	30
Starburst								
Baja California	1 pkg	240	0	5	0	48	0	0
Jellybeans	¼ cup	160	0	0	0	39	0	15
Original Fruit	1 pkg	240	0	0	0	48	0	0
Sour Fruit	1 pkg	240	0	5	0	47	0	0
Sugar Babies								
Candy	30 pieces (1.5 oz)	180	0	2	0	41	0	40
Chocolate	19 pieces (1.4 oz)	180	1	5	5	33	0	35
Sugar Daddy								
Pop	1 lg (1.7 oz)	200	1	3	0	43	0	65

FOOD	PORTION	CALS	PROT	FAT	CHOL	CARB	FIBER	SOD
Swedish Fish								
Aqua Life	1.5 oz	140	0	0	0	36	–	30
Original	20 pieces (1.5 oz)	140	0	0	0	36	–	30
Take 5								
Snack Size	2 pieces	220	4	11	<5	25	1	180
The Chocolate Traveler								
Wedges Bittersweet	4 pieces	130	3	10	0	10	4	20
Wedges Dark Chocolate Coffee	4 pieces	130	1	8	0	15	2	0
Wedges Dark Chocolate Mint	4 pieces	130	1	8	0	15	2	0
Wedges Dark Chocolate Orange	4 pieces	120	1	8	0	15	2	0
Wedges Dark Chocolate Raspberry	4 pieces	120	1	8	0	15	2	0
Wedges Dark Chocolate Tiramisu	4 pieces	120	1	8	0	15	2	0
Wedges Milk Chocolate	4 pieces	130	1	8	5	15	0	10
Wedges Milk Chocolate Dulce De Leche	4 pieces	120	1	7	5	17	tr	10
Wedges White Chocolate	4 pieces	140	2	9	5	14	14	25
Wedges White Chocolate Creme Brulee	4 pieces	140	2	9	0	14	0	25
Toblerone								
Bittersweet Chocolate w/ Honey & Almond Nugget	⅓ bar (1.2 oz)	170	1	9	<5	20	2	5
Tootsie Roll								
Midgees	6	140	0	3	0	28	0	10
Mini Chews	30 pieces (1.4 oz)	170	2	7	5	27	1	20
Pops	1 (0.6 oz)	60	0	0	0	15	0	0
Pops Caramel Apple	1 (0.6 oz)	60	0	1	0	15	0	15
Twix								
Fun Size	1 (0.6 oz)	80	1	4	0	10	0	70
Peanut Butter	1 bar	280	5	17	5	28	2	120
Twizzlers								
Sugar Free	4 pieces (1.5 oz)	130	1	1	0	33	0	105

FOOD	PORTION	CALS	PROT	FAT	CHOL	CARB	FIBER	SOD
Vere								
75% Chocolate Gluten Free	1 sm bar	80	1	6	0	6	2	0
Brownie Box Coconut Gluten Free Vegan	3 pieces (1.4 oz)	210	3	18	0	13	5	10
Brownie Box Peanut Butter Gluten Free	3 pieces (1.3 oz)	180	4	14	20	12	3	35
Brownie Box Walnut Gluten Free	3 pieces (1.3 oz)	190	4	15	30	12	3	10
Clusters Chocolate Coconut Gluten Free Vegan	3 pieces (1.7 oz)	280	4	23	0	18	6	10
Clusters Chocolate Almond Gluten Free Vegan	2 pieces (1.3 oz)	210	7	16	0	11	4	5
Clusters Chocolate Rice Gluten Free Vegan	3 pieces (1.3 oz)	170	3	8	0	22	3	80
Clusters Chocolate Seed Gluten Free Vegan	2 pieces (1.3 oz)	210	7	16	0	11	4	5
Wafers Cacao Nibs Gluten Free Vegan	2 (1.1 oz)	170	3	12	0	15	4	0
Wafers Espresso Gluten Free Vegan	3 (1.6 oz)	250	5	19	0	21	8	0
Wafers Pink Peppercorn Gluten Free Vegan	3 (1.6 oz)	250	5	19	0	21	6	5
Wafers Spicy Pepita Gluten Free	2 (1.1 oz)	170	4	13	0	14	4	15
Wafers Tamari Almond Gluten Free Vegan	2 (1.2 oz)	170	4	11	0	18	5	20
Weight Watchers								
English Toffee Squares	3 pieces	160	2	10	10	23	6	80
Mint Patties	2	100	1	6	5	15	5	35
Peanut Butter Crunch	4 pieces	180	2	8	5	31	6	85
Pecan Crowns	3 pieces	150	2	9	5	21	8	20
Whitman's								
Sampler	3 pieces (1.4 oz)	220	2	10	5	31	tr	65
Whoppers								
Malted Milk Balls	18 pieces	190	1	7	0	31	tr	135
York								
Peppermint Patty	3 (1.4 oz)	150	tr	3	0	29	tr	10
Peppermint Patty Sugar Free	3 (1.3 oz)	110	1	4	0	28	1	0

FOOD	PORTION	CALS	PROT	FAT	CHOL	CARB	FIBER	SOD
Yummy Earth								
Organic Lollipops All Flavors	3	70	0	0	0	17	0	0
CANTALOUPE								
dried	3.5 pieces (1.4 oz)	140	0	0	0	34	1	110
fresh cubed	1 cup	57	1	tr	0	13	1	14
fresh half	½	94	2	1	0	22	2	23
Del Monte								
Fresh	¼ melon (4.7 oz)	50	1	0	0	12	1	25
CAPERS								
capers	1 tbsp	2	tr	tr	0	tr	tr	255
CARAWAY								
seed	1 tbsp	22	1	1	0	3	3	1
CARDAMOM								
ground	1 tsp	6	tr	tr	0	1	1	0
CARDOON								
fresh cooked w/o salt	1 serv (3.5 oz)	22	1	tr	0	5	2	176
fresh shredded	1 cup (6.2 oz)	30	1	tr	0	7	3	303
Frieda's								
Cardoon	1 cup	15	1	0	0	4	1	140
Ocean Mist								
Cardone Fresh Shredded	1 cup (6.2 oz)	36	1	tr	0	9	3	303
CARIBOU								
roasted	3 oz	142	25	4	93	0	0	51
CARISSA								
fresh	1	12	tr	tr	0	3	–	1
CAROB								
carob mix	3 tsp	45	tr	0	0	11	–	12
carob mix as prep w/ whole milk	9 oz	195	8	8	33	23	–	132
flour	1 tbsp	14	tr	tr	0	7	–	3
flour	1 cup	185	5	1	0	92	–	36

FOOD	PORTION	CALS	PROT	FAT	CHOL	CARB	FIBER	SOD
Bob's Red Mill								
Powder Toasted	2 tsp	25	1	0	0	11	2	5
CARP								
fresh cooked	3 oz	138	19	6	72	0	0	54
fresh cooked	1 fillet (6 oz)	276	39	12	143	0	0	107
fresh raw	3 oz	108	15	5	56	0	0	42
roe raw	1 oz	37	7	tr	103	tr	–	–
roe salted in olive oil	2 tbsp (1 oz)	40	–	–	100	6	0	1400
CARROT JUICE								
canned	6 oz	73	2	tr	0	17	–	54
Bolthouse Farms								
Carrot Juice	8 oz	70	2	0	0	14	tr	150
Hollywood								
100% Juice	1 can (12 oz)	120	2	1	0	27	1	250
Lakewood								
Organic	6 oz	73	2	0	0	17	2	45
Luvli Juices								
Zingy Carrot	1 bottle (10 oz)	145	2	0	0	35	2	45
Naked Juice								
Just Carrot	8 oz	80	2	0	0	13	0	90
Odwalla								
100% Juice	8 oz	70	2	0	0	15	1	160
CARROTS								
CANNED								
slices	½ cup	17	tr	tr	0	4	1	176
slices low sodium	½ cup	17	tr	tr	0	4	1	31
Del Monte								
Savory Sides Honey Glazed	½ cup	70	1	0	0	18	tr	440
Sliced	½ cup	35	0	0	0	8	3	300
Glory								
Seasoned Honey	½ cup	50	0	0	0	12	2	220
Tillen Farms								
Crispy Carrots Pickled	5 pieces (1 oz)	30	0	0	0	7	1	5
FRESH								
baby raw	1 (0.5 oz)	6	tr	tr	0	1	–	5
raw	1 (2.5 oz)	31	1	tr	0	7	2	25

FOOD	PORTION	CALS	PROT	FAT	CHOL	CARB	FIBER	SOD
raw shredded	½ cup	24	1	tr	0	6	2	19
slices cooked	½ cup	35	1	tr	0	8	–	52
Bolthouse Farms								
Matchstix	3 oz	35	1	0	0	9	2	45
Earthbound Farm								
Organic Tops On	1 (2.7 oz)	35	1	0	0	8	2	40
Organic w/ Organic Ranch Dip	1 pkg (2.2 oz)	90	1	8	5	5	1	180
Frieda's								
Gold	⅔ cup (3 oz)	35	1	0	0	9	3	30
Grimmway								
Baby	3 oz	38	1	0	0	9	2	30
Nature's Gold								
Fresh	1 med (2.7 oz)	40	1	0	0	9	3	50
River Ranch								
Shredded	¾ cup	35	tr	0	0	9	3	30
FROZEN								
slices cooked	½ cup	26	1	tr	0	6	–	43
Birds Eye								
Steam & Serve Carrots & Cranberries	1 cup	130	1	5	10	20	3	230
C&W								
Whole Baby	⅔ cup	35	tr	0	0	7	2	60
Green Giant								
Honey Glazed	1 cup	90	1	3	0	15	3	190
CASABA								
cubed	1 cup	45	2	tr	0	11	–	20
fresh	1/10	43	1	tr	0	10	–	20
CASHEWS								
cashew butter w/o salt	1 tbsp	94	3	8	0	4	–	2
dry roasted w/ salt	18 (1 oz)	160	4	13	0	9	1	180
dry roasted w/ salt	1 oz	163	4	13	0	9	–	213
oil roasted w/ salt	1 oz	163	5	14	0	8	–	209
oil roasted w/o salt	1 oz	163	5	14	0	8	–	5
Arrowhead Mills								
Organic Cashew Butter	2 tbsp	160	4	13	0	9	tr	0

FOOD	PORTION	CALS	PROT	FAT	CHOL	CARB	FIBER	SOD
Frito Lay								
Salted	3 tbsp	160	4	13	0	7	1	115
Good Sense								
Jumbo Honey Roasted	¼ cup	170	6	11	0	13	1	65
Jumbo Roasted & Salted	¼ cup	190	5	16	0	9	1	115
Kettle								
Butter Creamy Unsalted	2 tbsp	160	5	14	0	8	1	0
Navitas Naturals								
Cashews	1 oz	160	5	12	0	9	1	0
Peeled Snacks								
Nut Picks Cashew Later	1 pkg (1 oz)	180	4	14	0	9	tr	120
Planters								
Chocolate Lovers Milk Chocolate	10 pieces (1.5 oz)	230	5	16	5	20	tr	25
Dry Roasted	19 pieces (1 oz)	160	5	12	0	9	tr	140
Organic	23 pieces (1 oz)	170	5	13	0	8	1	115
Sunfood								
Organic	1 oz	164	5	12	0	9	1	3
CASSAVA								
fresh	3.5 oz	120	3	tr	0	27	–	8
CATFISH								
channel breaded & fried	3 oz	194	15	11	69	7	–	238
wolffish atlantic baked	3 oz	105	19	3	50	0	0	93
Simmons								
Farm Raised	4 oz	140	17	6	50	0	0	40
CAULIFLOWER								
FRESH								
cooked	½ cup (2.2 oz)	14	1	tr	0	3	1	9
flowerets cooked	3 (2 oz)	12	1	tr	0	2	1	8
flowerets raw	3 (2 oz)	14	1	tr	0	3	1	17
green cooked	1½ cups (3.2 oz)	29	3	tr	0	6	3	21
green raw	1 cup (2.2 oz)	20	2	tr	0	4	2	15
green raw	1 head 7 in diam (18 oz)	158	15	2	0	31	16	118

FOOD	PORTION	CALS	PROT	FAT	CHOL	CARB	FIBER	SOD
green raw floweret	1 (0.9 oz)	8	1	tr	0	2	1	6
raw	½ cup (1.8 oz)	13	1	tr	0	3	1	15
Mann's								
Cauliettes	1 serv (3 oz)	20	2	0	0	4	2	25
River Ranch								
Florets	1 cup	20	1	0	0	4	2	25
FROZEN								
cooked	½ cup	17	1	tr	0	3	–	16
Green Giant								
Cheese Sauce	½ cup	50	2	3	<5	6	1	420
CAVIAR								
black or red	2 tbsp	81	8	6	188	1	0	480
CELERY								
fresh	1 lg stalk (2.2 oz)	9	tr	tr	0	2	1	51
pickled	½ cup	10	tr	tr	0	2	1	192
raw diced	½ cup	8	tr	tr	0	2	1	48
seed	1 tsp	1	tr	tr	0	tr	tr	0
strips	1 cup	17	1	tr	0	4	2	99
Dole								
Stalks	2 med (3 oz)	20	1	0	0	5	2	100
Earthbound Farm								
Organic Hearts	2 stalks (3.9 oz)	20	1	0	0	5	2	100
Frieda's								
Celery Root	¾ cup	35	1	0	0	8	3	85
River Ranch								
Sticks Fresh	4 (3 oz)	15	tr	0	0	3	1	75
TAKE-OUT								
creamed	½ cup	87	3	6	3	7	1	383
stir fried	½ cup	30	1	2	0	3	1	238
stuffed w/ cheese	1 (5 inch)	38	1	3	10	1	tr	84
CELERY JUICE								
juice	1 cup	42	2	tr	0	9	4	215
CELTUCE								
raw	3.5 oz	22	1	tr	0	4	–	11

FOOD	PORTION	CALS	PROT	FAT	CHOL	CARB	FIBER	SOD
CEREAL								
bran flakes	¾ cup	90	4	1	0	22	–	264
corn flakes	1¼ cups	110	2	tr	0	24	–	351
farina as prep w/ water	¾ cup	88	2	tr	0	19	2	0
granola	½ cup	285	9	15	0	32	6	15
oatmeal instant as prep w/ water	1 cup (8.2 oz)	138	6	2	0	24	4	377
oatmeal regular & quick as prep w/ water	¾ cup (6.1 oz)	149	5	2	0	19	3	2
oatmeal regular & quick not prep	⅓ cup (0.9 oz)	104	4	2	0	18	3	1
puffed rice	1 cup	56	1	tr	0	13	tr	0
puffed wheat	1 cup	44	2	tr	0	10	1	0
shredded mini wheats	1 cup	107	3	1	0	24	3	3
shredded wheat rectangular	1 biscuit (0.8 oz)	85	3	tr	0	19	2	0
Alti Plano								
Hot Cereal Chai Almond	1 pkg	210	5	7	0	33	5	200
Hot Cereal Oaxacan Chocolate	1 pkg	170	6	3	0	30	5	120
Hot Cereal Orange Date	1 pkg	180	4	3	0	36	6	200
Hot Cereal Regular	1 pkg	190	6	3	0	32	7	5
Hot Cereal Spiced Apple Raisin	1 pkg	160	3	2	0	35	5	110
Alti Plano Gold								
Instant Quinoa Hot Cereal Spiced Apple Raisin	1 pkg	160	3	2	0	35	5	110
Instant Quinoa Organic Hot Cereal Oaxacan Chocolate	1 pkg	170	6	3	0	30	5	120
Alvarado Street Bakery								
Plain Granola	½ cup	220	4	5	0	38	4	0
Arrowhead Mills								
Organic Amaranth Flakes	1 cup	140	4	2	0	26	3	0
Organic Kamut Flakes	1 cup	120	4	1	0	25	2	70
Organic Multigrain Flakes	1 cup	170	5	2	0	33	3	180
Organic Nature O's	1 cup	130	4	2	0	25	2	0
Organic Puffed Corn	1 cup	60	2	1	0	12	2	5
Organic Puffed Millet	1 cup	60	2	1	0	11	1	0
Organic Puffed Wheat	1 cup	60	3	0	0	12	2	0

FOOD	PORTION	CALS	PROT	FAT	CHOL	CARB	FIBER	SOD
Organic Rice Flakes Sweetened	1 cup	180	3	1	0	40	1	190
Organic Shredded Wheat	1 cup	190	7	1	0	38	6	5
Organic Spelt Flakes	1 cup	120	4	1	0	24	3	100
Back To Nature								
Energy Start Hi Protein Crunch	½ cup	170	15	2	0	28	3	110
Flax & Fiber Crunch	1 cup	200	9	3	0	41	9	150
Granola Apple Blueberry	½ cup	200	6	3	0	39	4	20
Granola Classic	½ cup	180	6	3	0	36	4	5
Granola French Vanilla	½ cup	220	6	6	0	35	4	50
Heart Basics Organic Apple Cinnamon Harvest	¾ cup	180	4	2	0	45	10	100
Multigrain Harvest	1 cup	210	7	3	0	46	9	140
Oat & Soy Crisp	¾ cup	180	8	3	0	33	3	20
Strawberry & Seven Grains	1 cup	210	5	1	0	50	5	5
Barbara's Bakery								
Alpen No Sugar Added	⅔ cup	200	7	3	0	40	4	30
Organic Breakfast O's Fruit Juice Sweetened	1 cup	120	4	2	0	22	3	125
Organic Brown Rice Crisps Fruit Juice Sweetened	1 cup	120	2	1	0	25	1	125
Organic Corn Flakes Fruit Juice Sweetened	1 cup	110	2	1	0	25	1	140
Organic Wild Puffs	1 cup	100	2	1	0	23	tr	40
Organic Wild Puffs Fruity Punch	1 cup	110	2	1	0	26	1	55
Organic Ultima High Fiber	½ cup	90	3	1	0	24	8	130
Organic Ultima Pomegranate	½ cup	100	3	1	0	24	5	85
Puffins Cinnamon	⅔ cup	100	2	1	0	26	6	150
Puffins Originals	¾ cup (0.9 oz)	90	2	1	0	23	5	190
Shredded Wheat	2 biscuits (1.4 oz)	140	4	1	0	31	5	0
Bear Naked								
Apple Cinnamon	¼ cup	140	3	7	0	17	3	0
Banana Nut	¼ cup	140	3	7	0	17	3	5
Fruit And Nut	¼ cup	140	3	7	0	16	3	0
Peak Protein	½ cup	200	10	8	0	24	2	25

FOOD	PORTION	CALS	PROT	FAT	CHOL	CARB	FIBER	SOD
Bob's Red Mill								
Farina Creamy Brown Rice not prep	¼ cup	150	3	1	0	32	2	5
Muesli Old Country	¼ cup	110	4	3	0	21	4	0
Natural Granola No Fat	½ cup	180	5	3	0	35	4	10
Organic Right Stuff Hot Cereal 6 Grain not prep	¼ cup	140	6	2	0	27	4	0
Rolled Oats Gluten Free not prep	½ cup	160	7	3	0	27	4	0
Cascadian Farm								
Organic Clifford Crunch	1 cup	100	2	1	0	25	5	160
Organic Granola Oats & Honey	⅔ cup	230	5	6	0	42	3	110
CoCo Wheats								
Hot Cereal	⅓ cup	200	7	1	0	41	2	15
Country Choice Naturals								
Instant Oatmeal Organic Plus Golden Brown Sugar	1 pkg	180	7	3	0	32	3	140
Instant Oatmeal Regular	1 pkg	110	4	2	0	19	3	0
Oatmeal Steel Cut not prep	½ cup	150	5	3	0	27	4	0
Oats Old Fashioned not prep	½ cup	150	5	3	0	27	4	0
Earthbound Farm								
Organic Granola Maple Almond	½ cup	260	6	14	0	31	4	0
Enjoy Life								
Allergen Gluten Free Granola Cinnamon	½ cup	160	3	3	0	31	5	10
EnviroKidz								
Organic Orangutan O's	¾ cup	120	20	1	0	26	2	65
Fantastic								
Oatmeal Big Cup Apple Cinnamon	1 pkg	270	8	4	0	54	6	320
Oatmeal Big Cup Maple Raisin 3 Grain	1 pkg	270	7	2	0	60	8	310
General Mills								
Cheerios	1 cup	110	3	2	0	22	3	210
Cheerios Crunch Oat Cluster	¾ cup	100	2	1	0	22	2	140

FOOD	PORTION	CALS	PROT	FAT	CHOL	CARB	FIBER	SOD
Cheerios Yogurt Burst Strawberry	¾ cup	120	2	2	0	24	2	170
Cheerios Yogurt Burst Vanilla	¾ cup	120	2	2	0	24	2	170
Chex Whole Grain Chocolate	¾ cup	130	2	3	0	26	tr	230
Curves	¾ cup	100	2	1	0	22	2	180
Total Honey Clusters	¾ cup	170	3	2	0	39	3	260
Total Raisin Bran	1 cup	170	3	1	0	42	5	240
Glucerna								
Crunchy Flakes 'N Raisins	1 bowl (1.6 oz)	140	4	1	0	36	6	270
Crunchy Flakes 'N Strawberries	1 bowl (1.5 oz)	150	4	1	0	37	7	320
Glutino								
Gluten Free Apple Cinnamon	½ cup	120	1	2	0	24	1	180
Gluten Free Honey Nut	½ cup	130	2	3	0	24	1	150
Grandy Oats								
Organic Granola Classic	½ cup	252	8	14	0	27	5	75
Organic Granola Low Fat Cranberry Chew	½ cup	191	5	1	0	41	3	53
Organic Granola Mainely Maple	½ cup	204	6	7	0	31	4	109
Hodgson Mill								
Hot Cereal Bulgur Wheat w/ Soy not prep	¼ cup	115	10	1	0	22	3	0
Hot Cereal Oat Bran not prep	¼ cup	120	6	3	0	23	6	3
Honest Foods								
Granola Planks Maple Almond Crunch	½ bar (2 oz)	250	6	10	0	37	5	150
Kashi								
7 Whole Grain Flakes	1 cup	180	6	1	0	41	6	150
7 Whole Grain Honey Puffs	1 cup	120	3	1	0	25	2	6
7 Whole Grain Nuggets	½ cup	210	7	2	0	47	7	260
7 Whole Grain Pilaf as prep	½ cup	170	6	3	0	30	6	15
7 Whole Grain Puffs	1 cup	70	2	1	0	15	1	0
GoLean	1 cup	140	13	1	0	30	10	85
GoLean Crunch!	1 cup	190	9	3	0	36	8	95

FOOD	PORTION	CALS	PROT	FAT	CHOL	CARB	FIBER	SOD
GoLean Crunch Honey Almond Flax	1 cup	200	9	5	0	34	8	140
GoLean Instant Hot Cereal Creamy Truly Vanilla	1 pkg	150	9	2	0	25	7	100
GoLean Instant Hot Cereal Hearty Honey & Cinnamon	1 pkg	150	8	2	0	26	5	100
Good Friends	1 cup	170	5	2	0	43	12	130
Granola Mountain Medley	½ cup	220	6	7	0	37	6	10
Heart To Heart Instant Oatmeal Golden Brown Maple	1 pkg	160	4	2	0	33	5	100
Heart To Heart Instant Oatmeal Raisin Spice	1 pkg	150	3	2	0	33	4	100
Heart To Heart Oat Flakes & Blueberry Clusters	1¼ cups	200	6	3	0	42	4	130
Heart To Heart Toasted Oat	¾ cup	110	4	2	0	25	5	90
Mighty Bites All Flavors	1 cup	110	5	2	0	23	3	160
Organic Promise Autumn Wheat	1 cup	190	5	1	0	45	6	0
Organic Promise Cinnamon Harvest	1 cup	190	4	1	0	44	5	0
Organic Promise Strawberry Fields	1 cup	120	2	0	0	28	1	200
Vive Probiotic Digestive Wellness	1¼ cups	170	4	3	0	43	12	60
Kellogg's								
All-Bran	½ cup	80	4	1	0	23	10	80
All-Bran Extra Fiber	½ cup	50	3	1	0	20	13	120
Apple Jacks	1 cup	130	1	1	0	30	1	150
Caramel Nut Crunch	1 cup	210	3	4	0	41	1	310
Cocoa Krispies	¾ cup	120	1	1	0	27	1	190
Complete Oat Bran Flakes	¾ cup	110	3	1	0	23	1	210
Corn Flakes	1 cup	100	2	0	0	24	1	200
Corn Pops	1 cup	120	1	0	0	28	tr	120
Cracklin' Oat Bran	¾ cup	200	4	7	0	35	6	150
Crispix	1 cup	110	2	0	0	25	tr	210
Frosted Flakes	¾ cup	120	1	0	0	28	1	150
Frosted Flakes ⅓ Less Sugar	1 cup	120	1	0	0	28	tr	180
Fruit Harvest	¾ cup	120	2	2	0	25	1	140

FOOD	PORTION	CALS	PROT	FAT	CHOL	CARB	FIBER	SOD
Fruit Loops	1 cup	120	1	1	0	28	1	150
Fruit Loops ⅓ Less Sugar	1¼ cups	120	2	1	0	28	1	180
Granola Low Fat w/ Raisins	⅔ cup	230	4	3	0	49	3	150
Honey Smacks	¾ cup	100	2	1	0	24	1	50
Mini-Wheat Frosted	5 (1.8 oz)	180	5	1	0	41	5	5
Mueslix Raisins Dates & Almonds	⅔ cup	200	5	3	0	40	4	170
Organic Mini Wheats Frosted	24 pieces	190	4	1	0	44	5	0
Organic Raisin Bran	1 cup	190	5	1	0	46	8	380
Organic Rice Krispies	1¼ cups	120	2	0	0	29	0	320
Product 19	1 cup	100	2	0	0	25	1	210
Raisin Bran	1 cup	190	5	2	0	45	7	350
Rice Krispies	1¼ cups	120	2	0	0	29	0	320
Smart Start Antioxidants	1 cup	190	3	1	0	43	3	280
Smart Start Healthy Heart	1¼ cups	230	6	2	0	49	5	140
Smorz	1 cup	120	1	2	0	25	tr	140
Special K	1 cup	110	7	0	0	22	tr	220
Special K Fruit & Yogurt	¾ cup	120	2	1	0	27	1	135
Special K Low Carb Lifestyle Protein Plus	¾ cup	100	10	3	0	14	5	110
Special K Red Berries	1 cup	110	2	0	0	25	1	220
Special K Vanilla Almond	¾ cup	110	2	2	0	25	1	160
Liquid Cereal								
Apple & Cinnamon	1 can (11 oz)	160	7	1	5	32	1	170
Chocolate	1 can (11 oz)	170	7	1	5	33	1	125
Fruit	1 can (11 oz)	150	7	0	5	31	tr	135
Peanut Butter	1 can (11 oz)	170	7	2	5	32	1	110
Lundberg								
Purely Organic Hot 'n Creamy Rice	⅓ cup	190	4	2	0	43	3	0
Malt-O-Meal								
Balance	¾ cup	120	3	1	0	26	3	220
Cinnamon Toasters	¾ cup	130	1	4	0	24	1	104
Colossal Crunch	¾ cup	120	1	2	0	26	0	230
Creamy Hot Wheat not prep	3 tbsp	130	4	0	0	27	1	0
Crispy Rice	1¼ cups	130	2	0	0	29	0	300
Frosted Flakes	¾ cup	120	2	0	0	28	1	180
Frosted Mini Spooners	1 cup	190	5	1	0	45	6	10

FOOD	PORTION	CALS	PROT	FAT	CHOL	CARB	FIBER	SOD
Honey & Oat Blenders	¾ cup	120	2	2	0	25	1	150
Honey Buzzers	1⅓ cup	110	1	1	0	26	1	220
Instant Oatmeal Apple & Cinnamon	1 pkg	130	3	2	0	27	3	170
Instant Oatmeal Cinnamon & Spice	1 pkg	170	4	2	0	36	3	240
Instant Oatmeal Maple & Brown Sugar	1 pkg	160	4	2	0	33	3	240
Original Hot Wheat not prep	3 tbsp	130	5	1	0	27	1	0
Puffed Rice	1 cup	60	1	0	0	13	0	0
Raisin Bran	1 cup	220	5	1	0	47	7	350
Mom's Best Naturals								
Oatmeal Instant	1 pkg	160	4	2	0	33	3	240
Raisin Bran	1 cup	230	5	2	0	49	6	340
Toasted Wheat-fuls	1 cup	200	8	1	0	44	7	10
Toasty O's	1 cup	120	4	2	0	23	3	200
Nature's Path								
Optimum Organic ReBound	¾ cup	190	10	6	0	35	6	140
Organic Flax Plus Pumpkin Raisin Crunch	¾ cup	200	6	4	0	41	9	150
Organic Smart Bran	⅔ cup	90	3	1	0	24	13	130
Organic Granola Pomegran Plus	½ cup	140	2	5	0	21	2	35
Organic Zen Instant Oatmeal Cranberry Ginger	1 pkg	150	5	3	0	30	3	170
Nature's Plus								
Organic Oatmeal Hemp Plus	1 pkg	160	5	3	0	30	4	105
Perky's								
Nutty Flax	¾ cup	230	6	5	0	41	7	110
PerkyO's Original	¾ cup	120	2	1	0	28	3	70
Post								
100% Bran	1 (0.8 oz)	80	4	1	0	22	9	0
Bran Flakes	1 cup	100	3	1	0	24	5	220
Cocoa Pebbles	¾ cup (1 oz)	110	1	2	0	26	3	180
Golden Crisp	¾ cup (1 oz)	110	1	0	0	25	1	25
Grape-Nuts O's	1 cup (1 oz)	120	2	0	0	28	2	140
Grape-Nuts	2 oz	200	7	1	0	47	6	310

FOOD	PORTION	CALS	PROT	FAT	CHOL	CARB	FIBER	SOD
Grape-Nuts Trail Mix Crunch	1 cup (1.7 oz)	170	4	2	0	37	5	210
Great Grains Crunchy Pecan	1.8 oz	220	5	6	0	38	4	150
Honey Bunches Of Oats	¾ cup	130	2	2	0	25	2	150
Honey Bunches Of Oats Peaches	1 cup	120	2	2	0	26	2	135
Honey Bunches Of Oats Strawberry	¾ cup	120	2	2	0	26	2	140
Honeycomb	1⅓ cups (1 oz)	120	2	1	0	28	3	170
LiveActive Mixed Berry Crunch	1 cup	190	4	2	0	43	7	250
LiveActive Nut Harvest Crunch	1 cup	220	5	6	0	39	8	270
Oreo O's	1 cup	110	1	2	0	22	1	90
Raisin Bran	1 cup (2 oz)	190	4	1	0	46	8	300
Selects Blueberry Morning	2 oz	220	3	3	0	45	2	280
Shredded Wheat Frosted	2 oz	180	4	1	0	43	5	0
Shredded Wheat 'N Bran	2 oz	200	6	1	0	49	8	0
Shredded Wheat Original	2 biscuits (1.6 oz)	160	5	1	0	37	6	0
Shredded Wheat Spoon Size	1 cup	170	6	1	0	40	6	0
Toasties Corn Flakes	1 cup (1 oz)	100	2	0	0	24	1	260
Quaker								
Instant Oatmeal Cinnamon & Spice	1 pkg	170	4	2	0	35	3	250
Instant Oatmeal Cinnamon Roll	1 pkg	160	4	2	0	33	3	240
Instant Oatmeal Crunch Mixed Berry	1 pkg	190	4	3	0	39	3	250
Instant Oatmeal Express Baked Apple	1 pkg	200	4	3	0	42	4	320
Instant Oatmeal For Kids Dinosaur Eggs	1 pkg	190	4	4	0	37	3	260
Instant Oatmeal Lower Sugar Maple & Brown Sugar	1 pkg	120	4	2	0	24	3	290
Instant Oatmeal Maple Brown Sugar w/ Pecans	1 pkg	160	4	4	0	30	4	75

FOOD	PORTION	CALS	PROT	FAT	CHOL	CARB	FIBER	SOD
Instant Oatmeal Nutrition For Women Golden Brown Sugar	1 pkg	170	5	2	0	32	3	330
Instant Oatmeal Organic Regular	1 pkg	100	4	2	0	19	3	0
Instant Oatmeal Regular	1 pkg	100	4	2	0	19	3	80
Instant Oatmeal Simple Harvest Apples w/ Cinnamon	1 pkg	150	4	2	0	32	4	90
Instant Oatmeal Strawberries & Cream	1 pkg	130	3	3	0	27	2	190
Instant Oatmeal Supreme Apple Raisin	1 pkg	150	4	2	0	32	3	290
Instant Oatmeal Supreme Cinnamon Pecan	1 pkg	180	4	4	0	33	3	290
Instant Oatmeal Take Heart Golden Maple	1 pkg	160	4	3	0	33	5	110
Instant Oatmeal Weight Control Banana Bread	1 pkg	160	7	3	0	29	6	260
Instant Oatmeat Crunch Maple & Brown Sugar	1 pkg	190	4	3	0	39	3	220
Life	¾ cup	120	3	2	0	25	2	160
Life Cinnamon	¾ cup	120	3	2	0	25	2	150
Life Honey Graham	¾ cup	120	3	2	0	25	2	160
Life Vanilla Yogurt Crunch	1¼ cups	210	5	3	0	43	4	250
Oat Bran Hot Cereal not prep	½ cup	150	7	3	0	25	6	0
Old Fashioned Oats not prep	½ cup	150	5	3	0	27	4	0
Quick Oats Sun Country Iron Fortified	1 pkg	150	5	3	0	27	4	0
Ralston								
100% Hot Wheat	⅓ cup	150	5	1	0	31	5	0
Apple Dapples	1 cup	120	2	1	0	30	tr	105
Cocoa Crumbles	1 cup	120	1	1	0	26	0	170
Confruity Crisp	¾ cup	110	1	1	0	25	0	150
Corn Biscuits	1 cup	110	2	0	0	26	tr	280
Corn Flakes	1 cup	100	2	0	0	24	tr	200
Crisp Crunch	¾ cup	120	0	1	0	27	tr	210
Crisp Crunch Berry Treats	1 cup	120	1	1	0	27	tr	190

FOOD	PORTION	CALS	PROT	FAT	CHOL	CARB	FIBER	SOD
Crisp Rice	1¼ cups	120	2	0	0	29	0	310
Enriched Bran Flakes	¾ cup	90	3	1	0	23	5	210
Farina	3 tbsp	120	0	0	0	25	1	90
Freaky Fruits	1 cup	120	1	1	0	27	0	140
Frosted Flakes	¾ cup	120	1	0	0	28	tr	150
Fruit Rings	1 cup	120	1	1	0	28	0	120
Grits	¼ cup	140	3	1	0	32	1	0
Instant Oats Bananas & Cream	1 pkg	130	3	4	0	27	2	170
Magic Stars	¾ cup	120	2	1	0	27	1	160
Oats & More W/ Almonds	¾ cup	130	3	2	0	27	1	140
Oats Instant	1 pkg	100	4	2	0	19	3	80
Oats Instant Apples & Cinnamon	1 pkg	130	3	2	0	26	3	170
Oats Instant Blueberries & Cream	1 pkg	130	3	3	0	26	2	160
Oats Instant Cinnamon & Spice	1 pkg	170	4	2	0	34	3	240
Oats Instant For Kids Cinnawow	1 pkg	140	3	2	0	30	3	125
Oats Instant For Kids Maplicious & Brown Sugar	1 pkg	150	4	2	0	31	3	150
Oats Instant For Kids Roarin' Raspberry	1 pkg	150	4	3	0	29	3	150
Oats Instant For Kids Strawberries & Stars	1 pkg	140	3	2	0	30	3	170
Oats Instant Maple Brown Sugar	1 pkg	160	4	2	0	32	3	230
Oats Instant Peaches & Cream	1 pkg	130	3	3	0	36	2	170
Oats Instant Raisins & Spice	1 pkg	150	3	2	0	32	3	230
Oats Instant Strawberries & Cream	1 pkg	140	4	3	0	26	2	160
Oats Old Fashioned	½ cup	150	5	3	0	27	4	0
Oats Quick	½ cup	140	5	3	0	26	4	0
Raisin Bran	1 cup	200	6	2	0	47	8	370
Rice Biscuits	1¼ cups	120	2	0	0	27	0	290
Shredded Wheat Frosted Bite Size	1¼ cups	200	5	1	0	47	5	0

FOOD	PORTION	CALS	PROT	FAT	CHOL	CARB	FIBER	SOD
Silly Spheres	1½ cups	110	2	1	0	25	0	260
Tasteeos	1 cup	110	4	2	0	22	3	240
Tasteeos Apple Cinnamon	¾ cup	120	2	2	0	26	1	120
Tasteeos Honey Nut	1 cup	120	3	2	0	24	2	210
South Beach								
Crunch Strawberry Harvest	1 cup	170	7	2	0	37	8	290
Crunch Vanilla Almond	1 cup	180	8	4	0	35	8	280
Granola Clusters Cherry Almond	1 pkg (1 oz)	130	6	4	0	18	6	55
Granola Clusters Mixed Berry	1 pkg (1 oz)	130	6	4	0	18	6	55
Stark Sisters								
Granola Lo-Fat Raspberry Blueberry	½ cup	230	4	7	0	38	4	0
Granola Nutty Maple	½ cup	250	6	11	0	32	4	5
Granola Original Maple Almond	½ cup	240	6	10	0	33	5	0
Sunbelt								
Granola Low Fat Cinnamon & Raisins	½ cup	250	4	3	0	52	3	90
Weetabix								
Organic	2 biscuits (1.2 oz)	120	4	1	0	28	4	130
Organic Crispy Flakes	¾ cup	110	3	1	0	24	4	180
Wheatena								
Toasted Wheat	⅓ cup	160	5	1	0	33	5	0
Zoe's								
Granola Cinnamon Raisin	½ cup	190	7	5	0	32	7	65
Granola Cranberries Currants	½ cup	190	7	5	0	32	7	65
Granola Honey Almond	½ cup	190	8	5	0	32	7	70
O's Cinnamon	¾ cup	120	4	2	0	25	5	150
O's Honey	¾ cup	120	4	2	0	25	5	150
O's Natural	¾ cup	120	5	2	0	23	tr	180

CEREAL BARS (see also ENERGY BARS)
Attune

FOOD	PORTION	CALS	PROT	FAT	CHOL	CARB	FIBER	SOD
Wellness Yogurt & Granola Lemon Creme	1 (1.4 oz)	180	5	7	0	24	2	60

FOOD	PORTION	CALS	PROT	FAT	CHOL	CARB	FIBER	SOD
Wellness Yogurt & Granola Strawberry Bliss	1 (1.4 oz)	180	5	7	0	24	5	60
Back To Nature								
Bakery Squares Banana Walnut	1 (1.1 oz)	130	3	5	0	19	2	60
Chewy Trail Mix Cherry Pecan	1 (1 oz)	120	2	5	0	19	2	70
Fruit & Grain Apple	1 (1.1 oz)	110	2	2	0	20	tr	85
Barbara's Bakery								
Fruit & Yogurt Cherry Apple	1	150	3	3	0	29	1	125
Nature's Choice Blueberry	1 (1.3 oz)	150	2	2	0	29	2	85
Organic Crunchy Granola Cinnamon Crisp	2 (1.5 oz)	190	4	8	0	27	3	10
Cascadian Farm								
Organic Chewy Granola Fruit & Nut	1 (1.2 oz)	140	2	4	0	24	1	110
CocoaVia								
Dark Chocolate Almond	1 (0.8 oz)	90	1	2	0	13	1	60
Enjoy Life								
Allergen Gluten Free Caramel Apple	1 (1 oz)	110	2	3	0	21	2	95
Entenmann's								
Multi-Grain Real Strawberry	1 (1.3 oz)	140	1	3	0	26	tr	110
EnviroKidz								
Crispy Rice Panda Peanut Butter	1 (1 oz)	110	2	3	0	20	tr	80
Estee								
Rice Crunchy Chocolate	1	60	1	1	0	14	tr	65
Rice Crunchy Chocolate Chip	1	70	1	1	0	15	0	70
Rice Crunchy Vanilla	1	70	1	0	0	15	tr	70
General Mills								
Team Cheerios Strawberry	1	160	2	4	0	30	2	130
Trix	1	160	2	4	0	30	2	160
Glenny's								
Organic Muesli Raisins & Dates	1 (1.6 oz)	170	3	3	0	34	3	50
Organic Museli Chocolate Chip	1 (1.6 oz)	170	3	3	0	34	3	50

FOOD	PORTION	CALS	PROT	FAT	CHOL	CARB	FIBER	SOD
Slim Carb Bars Brownie Cheesecake	1 (1.3 oz)	130	12	3	–	19	1	180
Slim-1 w/ Acai Very Berry Blast	1 (1.1 oz)	100	2	3	–	21	2	40
Slim-1 w/ Green Tea Double Fudge	1 (1.1 oz)	100	3	3	–	20	2	90
Slim-1 w/ Hoodia Peanut Butter Caramel	1 (1.1 oz)	100	2	4	–	20	2	35
Glutino								
Gluten Free Breakfast Bar Apple	1 (1.4 oz)	120	2	1	0	25	3	10
Gluten Free Breakfast Bar Chocolate	1 (1.4 oz)	110	2	1	0	25	4	10
Gluten Free Organic Chocolate & Peanut	1 (1 oz)	110	2	3	0	19	1	50
Gluten Free Organic Wildberry	1 (1 oz)	100	1	1	0	21	1	65
Honest Foods								
Cran Lemon Zest	1 (2.2 oz)	240	6	9	0	35	4	150
Farmer's Trail Mix	1 (2.2 oz)	240	6	9	0	35	4	150
Kashi								
TLC Chewy Granola Honey Almond Flax	1 (1.2 oz)	140	5	5	0	19	4	115
TLC Chewy Granola Peanut Peanut Butter	1 (1.2 oz)	140	7	5	0	19	4	90
TLC Chewy Trail Mix	1 (1.2 oz)	140	6	5	0	20	4	105
Kellogg's								
All-Bran Brown Sugar Cinnamon	1	130	2	3	0	27	5	180
All-Bran Honey Oat	1	130	2	3	0	27	5	170
All-Bran Oatmeal Raisin	1	120	2	3	0	26	5	170
Crunchy Nut Sweet & Salty Chocolatey Almond	1 (1.1 oz)	160	5	8	0	16	2	150
Nutri-Grain Apple Cinnamon	1	140	1	3	0	26	1	105
Nutri-Grain Banana Muffin	1	170	3	4	0	30	1	110
Nutri-Grain Chewy Granola Chocolatey Chunk	1	110	1	4	0	18	tr	55
Nutri-Grain Cinnamon Raisin Muffin	1	170	2	4	0	32	1	100

FOOD	PORTION	CALS	PROT	FAT	CHOL	CARB	FIBER	SOD
Nutri-Grain Yogurt Vanilla	1	140	1	3	0	26	tr	105
Smart Start Healthy Heart Cinnamon	1 (1.4 oz)	150	3	3	0	30	2	85
Snack Bites	1 pkg (0.8 oz)	90	1	2	0	18	tr	125
Special K Chocolatey Drizzle	1 (0.8 oz)	90	1	2	0	17	tr	105
Special K Meal Bar Chocolate Peanut Butter	1 (1.6 oz)	190	10	6	5	23	2	220
Special K Snack Bar Chocolate Peanut	1 (0.9 oz)	110	4	4	0	15	1	60
Special K Strawberry	1 (0.8 oz)	90	1	2	0	18	tr	95
Special K Vanilla Crisp	1 (0.8 oz)	90	2	2	0	17	tr	100
Kind								
Almond & Coconut	1	193	4	14	0	14	4	25
Almonds & Apricot In Yogurt	1	208	4	13	2	19	3	32
Banana & Oatbran	1	160	2	7	0	23	4	30
Nut Delight	1	203	7	15	0	12	3	13
Walnut & Date	1	150	2	7	0	22	3	39
Kudos								
Granola Chocolate Chip	1	120	1	4	0	20	1	70
Granola Peanut Butter	1	130	2	6	0	18	1	75
Granola w/ M&M's	1	100	1	3	0	17	1	80
Granola w/ Snickers	1	100	1	3	0	16	1	70
Nature Valley								
Chewy Granola Blueberry Yogurt	1	140	2	4	0	26	1	130
Chewy Granola Lemon Yogurt	1	140	2	4	0	26	1	130
Chewy Granola Vanilla Yogurt	1	140	2	4	0	26	1	130
Chewy Trail Mix Granola Apple Cinnamon	1	140	2	4	0	259	1	120
Chewy Trail Mix Granola Fruit & Nut	1	140	3	4	0	25	2	95
Chewy Trail Mix Granola Mixed Berry	1	140	2	4	0	26	1	90
Crunchy Granola Apple Crisp	1	104	2	4	0	26	1	130

FOOD	PORTION	CALS	PROT	FAT	CHOL	CARB	FIBER	SOD
Crunchy Granola Banana Nut	2	190	4	7	0	28	2	160
Crunchy Granola Maple Brown Sugar	2	180	4	6	0	29	2	160
Crunchy Granola Peanut Butter	2	160	5	7	0	30	2	190
Crunchy Granola Roasted Almond	2	190	4	7	0	28	2	180
Heart Healthy Chewy Granola Honey Nut	1	160	3	4	0	28	3	115
Sweet & Salty Granola Almond	1	160	3	7	0	22	2	170
Sweet & Salty Granola Peanut	1	170	4	9	0	19	2	150
Nutri-Grain								
Nutri-Grain Blueberry	1	140	1	3	0	26	tr	105
Nutri-Grain Mixed Berry	1	140	1	3	0	26	tr	105
Post								
Honey Bunches Of Oats Banana Nut	1 (1.2 oz)	140	2	4	0	24	1	115
Honey Bunches Of Oats Oatmeal Raisin	1 (1.2 oz)	130	2	3	0	25	2	105
Quaker								
Breakfast Bar Apple Crisp	1 (1.3 oz)	130	1	3	0	27	1	90
Breakfast Bar Iced Raspberry	1 (1.3 oz)	130	1	3	0	26	1	100
Breakfast Bites Iced Raspberry	1 pkg (1.3 oz)	130	1	3	0	28	3	75
Breakfast Bites Strawberry	1 pkg (1.3 oz)	130	1	3	0	27	2	90
Chewy Chocolate Chip	1 (0.8 oz)	100	1	3	0	18	1	75
Chewy Cookies & Cream	1 (0.8 oz)	90	1	3	0	18	2	85
Chewy 90 Calorie Cinnamon Sugar	1 (1 oz)	90	1	2	0	19	1	80
Chewy 90 Calorie Honey Nut	1 (0.8 oz)	90	1	2	0	19	1	80
Chewy Dipps Peanut Butter	1 (1 oz)	150	3	7	0	18	1	105
Chewy Low Fat S'mores	1 (1 oz)	110	1	2	0	22	1	70
Crunchy Granola Oats & Berries	1 (1 oz)	130	2	4	0	23	1	125

FOOD	PORTION	CALS	PROT	FAT	CHOL	CARB	FIBER	SOD
Oatmeal To Go Oatmeal Raisin	1 (2.1 oz)	220	4	4	15	43	5	240
Oatmeal To Go Raspberry Streusel	1 (2.1 oz)	220	4	4	15	43	5	220
Q-Smart Cranberry Vanilla Almond	1 (1 oz)	120	10	6	0	9	2	106
Trail Mix Cranberry Raisin & Almond	1 (1.2 oz)	150	2	5	0	24	1	50
Rice Krispies								
Split Stix Chocolatey	1 (1 oz)	130	1	5	–	19	1	95
Split Stix Original	1 (1 oz)	120	1	5	–	20	1	95
Treats Original	1 (0.8 oz)	90	tr	3	0	17	0	105
South Beach								
100 Calorie Chocolate Delight	1 (1 oz)	100	3	3	0	18	3	150
100 Calorie Peanut Butter Chocolate Chip	1 (1 oz)	100	3	3	0	18	3	160
100 Calorie Snack Bar Mixed Berry	1 (1 oz)	100	3	3	0	18	3	140
High Protein Chocolate	1 (1.2 oz)	140	10	5	0	15	3	150
High Protein Cranberry Almond	1 (1.2 oz)	140	10	5	0	15	3	135
High Protein Maple Nut	1 (1.2 oz)	140	10	5	5	15	3	160
High Protein Peanut Butter	1 (1.2 oz)	140	10	5	0	15	3	160
Wings Of Nature								
Organic Apple Cinnamon	1 (1.2 oz)	119	3	4	0	21	3	13
Organic Cafe Mocha Coffee	1 (1.2 oz)	153	3	9	0	18	3	26
Organic Cappuccino Coffee	1 (1.2 oz)	153	3	9	0	17	2	21

CHAMPAGNE

FOOD	PORTION	CALS	PROT	FAT	CHOL	CARB	FIBER	SOD
mimosa	1 serv	117	1	tr	0	12	tr	1
punch	1 serv	113	0	0	0	5	0	tr
sekt german champagne	3.5 oz	84	tr	0	0	5	–	–

CHAYOTE

FOOD	PORTION	CALS	PROT	FAT	CHOL	CARB	FIBER	SOD
fresh cooked	1 cup	38	1	1	0	8	–	1
raw	1 (7 oz)	49	2	1	0	11	–	8
raw cut up	1 cup	32	1	tr	0	7	–	198

FOOD	PORTION	CALS	PROT	FAT	CHOL	CARB	FIBER	SOD

CHEESE (see also CHEESE DISHES, CHEESE SUBSTITUTES, COTTAGE CHEESE, CREAM CHEESE, NEUFCHATEL)

FOOD	PORTION	CALS	PROT	FAT	CHOL	CARB	FIBER	SOD
american	1 oz	93	6	7	18	2	–	337
american cheese spread	1 oz	82	5	6	16	2	–	381
beaufort	1 oz	115	8	9	34	tr	0	128
bel paese	1 oz	112	7	9	–	0	0	–
blue	1 oz	100	6	8	21	1	–	396
blue crumbled	1 cup (4.7 oz)	477	29	39	102	3	–	1884
bocconcini smoked	1 oz	90	6	6	25	1	0	90
brick	1 oz	105	7	8	27	1	–	159
brie	1 oz	95	8	8	28	tr	–	178
cacio di roma sheep's milk cheese	1 oz	130	8	10	30	0	0	170
caerphilly	1.4 oz	150	9	13	–	0	0	–
camembert	1 oz	85	6	7	20	tr	–	239
cantal	1 oz	105	7	9	26	tr	0	269
caraway	1 oz	107	7	8	–	1	–	196
chabichou	1 oz	95	6	8	23	tr	0	189
chaource	1 oz	83	5	7	20	tr	0	230
cheddar	1 oz	114	7	9	30	tr	–	176
cheddar low fat	1 oz	49	9	2	6	1	–	174
cheddar low sodium	1 oz	113	7	9	28	1	–	6
cheddar reduced fat	1.4 oz	104	13	6	–	0	0	–
cheddar shredded	1 cup	455	28	37	119	1	–	701
cheshire	1 oz	110	7	9	29	1	–	198
cheshire reduced fat	1.4 oz	108	13	6	–	tr	0	–
colby	1 oz	112	7	9	27	1	–	171
colby low fat	1 oz	49	9	2	6	1	–	174
colby low sodium	1 oz	113	7	9	28	1	–	6
comte	1 oz	114	8	9	34	tr	0	105
coulommiers	1 oz	88	6	7	23	tr	0	195
crottin	1 oz	105	6	9	23	tr	0	133
derby	1.4 oz	161	10	14	–	0	0	–
edam	1 oz	101	7	8	25	tr	–	274
edam reduced fat	1.4 oz	92	13	4	–	tr	0	–
emmentaler	1 oz	115	8	9	26	tr	–	129
feta	1 oz	75	4	6	25	1	–	316
fontina	1 oz	110	7	9	33	tr	–	–
frais	1.6 oz	51	3	3	–	3	0	–
gjetost	1 oz	132	3	8	–	12	–	170

FOOD	PORTION	CALS	PROT	FAT	CHOL	CARB	FIBER	SOD
gloucester double	1.4 oz	162	10	14	–	0	0	–
goat fresh	1 oz	23	1	2	5	tr	0	18
goat hard	1 oz	128	9	10	30	1	–	98
gorgonzola	1 oz	107	5	9	–	tr	–	–
gouda	1 oz	101	7	8	32	1	–	232
grana padano parmesan shaved	1 tbsp	20	2	2	5	0	0	45
gruyere	1 oz	117	8	9	31	tr	–	95
lancashire	1.4 oz	149	9	12	–	0	0	–
leicester	1.4 oz	160	10	14	–	0	0	–
limburger	1 oz	93	8	8	26	tr	–	227
lymeswold	1.4 oz	170	6	16	–	tr	0	–
maroilles	1 oz	97	6	8	26	tr	0	300
monterey	1 oz	106	7	9	–	tr	–	152
morbier	1 oz	99	7	8	23	tr	0	283
mozzarella	1 oz	80	6	6	22	1	–	106
mozzarella fresh	1 oz	80	6	6	20	tr	0	160
mozzarella part skim	1 oz	72	7	5	16	1	–	132
muenster	1 oz	104	7	9	27	tr	–	178
parmesan grated	1 tbsp	23	2	2	4	tr	–	93
parmesan hard	1 oz	111	10	7	19	1	–	454
picodon	1 oz	99	6	8	23	tr	0	–
pimento	1 oz	106	6	9	27	tr	–	405
pont l'eveque	1 oz	86	6	7	20	tr	0	191
port du salut	1 oz	100	7	8	35	tr	–	151
provolone	1 oz	100	7	8	20	1	–	248
pyrenees	1 oz	101	6	8	26	tr	0	235
quark 20% fat	1 oz	33	4	1	5	1	–	10
quark 40% fat	1 oz	48	3	3	11	1	–	10
quark made w/ skim milk	1 oz	22	4	tr	tr	1	–	11
queso anego	1 oz	106	6	9	30	1	–	321
queso asadero	1 oz	101	6	8	30	1	–	186
queso chichuahua	1 oz	106	6	8	30	2	–	175
queso fresco	1 oz	41	4	2	–	1	0	–
queso manchego	1 oz	107	8	8	27	tr	0	341
queso panela	1 oz	74	6	5	–	1	0	–
raclette	1 oz	102	7	8	26	tr	0	217
reblochon	1 oz	88	6	7	23	tr	0	240
ricotta part skim	½ cup (4.4 oz)	171	14	10	38	6	–	155

FOOD	PORTION	CALS	PROT	FAT	CHOL	CARB	FIBER	SOD
ricotta whole milk	½ cup (4.4 oz)	216	14	16	63	4	–	104
romadur 40% fat	1 oz	83	7	6	–	tr	–	–
romano	1 oz	110	9	8	29	1	–	340
roquefort	1 oz	105	6	9	26	1	–	513
rouy	1 oz	95	7	8	23	tr	0	138
saint marcellin	1 oz	94	5	8	23	tr	0	171
saint nectaire	1 oz	97	6	8	23	tr	0	169
saint paulin	1 oz	85	7	6	20	tr	0	174
sainte maure	1 oz	99	6	8	23	tr	0	411
selles sur cher	1 oz	93	5	8	20	tr	0	181
stilton blue	1.4 oz	164	9	14	–	0	0	–
stilton white	1.4 oz	145	8	13	–	0	0	–
swiss	1 oz	107	8	8	26	1	–	74
swiss processed	1 oz	95	7	7	24	1	–	388
tilsit	1 oz	96	7	7	29	1	–	213
tome	1 oz	92	6	7	23	tr	0	231
triple creme	1 oz	113	3	11	34	tr	0	86
vacherin	1 oz	92	5	8	23	tr	0	129
wensleydale	1.4 oz	151	9	13	–	0	0	–
whey cheese	1 oz	126	4	8	–	9	0	146
yogurt cheese	1 oz	80	6	7	15	0	0	60
Athenos								
Traditional	¼ cup	90	7	7	25	2	tr	390
Traditional Reduced Fat	¼ cup	70	7	5	10	1	tr	470
Back To Nature								
Organic American Slices	1 slice (0.7 oz)	80	4	7	20	tr	0	340
Organic Cheddar Cubes	8 pieces (1.1 oz)	130	7	11	30	0	0	210
Organic Cheddar Shredded	¼ cup	110	6	10	30	tr	0	180
Organic Mozzarella Shredded	¼ cup	80	7	5	15	tr	0	200
Organic White Cheddar Slices Reduced Fat	1 slice (0.7 oz)	60	5	4	10	0	0	340
Bel Gioioso								
Mozzarella Fresh	1 in cube (1 oz)	80	5	6	20	0	0	85
Boar's Head								
American	1 oz	100	6	9	25	1	0	380

FOOD	PORTION	CALS	PROT	FAT	CHOL	CARB	FIBER	SOD
American 25% Lower Sodium 25% Lower Fat	1 oz	90	6	6	20	1	0	300
ButterKase	1 oz	100	6	9	30	0	0	180
Cheddar Sharp	1 oz	110	7	9	30	tr	0	190
Colby Jack	1 oz	110	6	9	25	0	0	180
Cream Havarti	1 oz	110	6	10	35	0	0	210
Creamy Blue	1 oz	90	6	8	30	0	0	310
Double Glouster Yellow	1 oz	110	7	10	35	0	0	200
Edam	1 oz	90	7	7	20	0	0	280
Feta	1 oz	60	5	4	10	1	0	360
Gouda	1 oz	110	6	9	30	0	0	280
Lacey Swiss	1 oz	90	9	6	15	0	0	35
Longhorn Colby	1 oz	110	7	9	30	tr	0	170
Monterey Jack	1 oz	100	6	9	25	0	0	180
Mozzarella	1 oz	90	6	7	20	1	0	150
Muenster	1 oz	100	6	8	25	0	0	180
Muenster Low Sodium	1 oz	100	6	8	20	0	0	75
Provolone 42% Lower Sodium	1 oz	100	7	8	20	1	0	140
Provolone Picante Sharp	1 oz	100	7	8	25	1	0	250
Swiss No Salt Added	1 oz	110	8	8	25	tr	0	10
Cabot								
Cheddar Shake	2 tsp	25	1	2	5	1	0	210
Cantare								
Baked Brie En Croute	1 oz	100	5	7	30	4	0	180
Connoisseur								
Asiago Spread	1 tbsp	90	5	7	20	2	0	240
Brie Spread	2 tbsp	90	4	7	25	2	0	250
Gorgonzola Spread	1 tbsp	90	5	7	20	2	0	340
Wheel Asiago Pesto	2 tbsp	90	5	6	20	4	0	240
Wheel Swiss Bacon	2 tbsp	90	5	7	25	2	0	260
Cracker Barrel								
Fontina	1 slice (0.7 oz)	80	6	7	15	tr	0	230
Sharp Cheddar 2% Milk	1 oz	90	7	6	20	tr	0	240
Crystal Farms								
American Singles	1 slice (0.7 oz)	70	4	5	15	2	0	340
American Singles 2%	1 slice (0.7 oz)	50	4	3	10	2	0	340

FOOD	PORTION	CALS	PROT	FAT	CHOL	CARB	FIBER	SOD
American Singles Fat Free	1 slice (0.7 oz)	30	5	0	<5	2	0	360
Blue Crumbled	2 tbsp	100	7	8	25	0	0	260
Cheese Curds	8 pieces (1 oz)	110	7	9	15	1	0	250
Cheezoids Sticks	1 piece (0.8 oz)	70	6	5	15	tr	0	170
Danish Havarti	1 oz	110	6	10	25	0	0	160
Deli Slices Muenster	1 slice (0.8 oz)	80	6	7	16	0	0	200
Deli Slices Swiss	1 slice (0.7 oz)	80	6	6	20	0	0	50
Feta Crumbled	¼ cup	90	5	7	20	2	tr	360
Gorgonzola Crumbled	2 tbsp	100	7	8	25	0	0	260
It's So Cheesy Cheddar Aerosol	2 tbsp	90	4	7	15	3	0	440
Little Chunks To Go	1 pkg (0.7 oz)	80	5	7	20	tr	0	135
Marble Jack	1 oz	110	6	9	30	tr	0	180
Parmesan Grated	2 tsp	25	2	2	<5	0	0	70
Pepper Jack	1 oz	110	6	9	30	tr	0	200
Ricotta	¼ cup	90	6	6	30	4	0	150
Shredded Mexican 4 Cheese	¼ cup	100	67	8	25	tr	0	170
Shredded Mozzarella	¼ cup	80	7	6	20	tr	0	180
Shredded Pizza Blend	¼ cup	100	7	8	25	tr	0	180
Shredded Sharp Cheddar	¼ cup	110	6	9	30	tr	0	180
Smoked Gouda	1 oz	100	6	8	25	tr	0	360
String	1 piece (1 oz)	80	8	5	15	1	0	150
Dragone								
Mozzarella Whole Milk	1 oz	90	6	7	20	tr	0	170
Parmesan Wedge	1 oz	100	9	7	20	tr	0	390
Ricotta Part Skim	¼ cup (2.2 oz)	90	6	6	30	4	0	85
Easy Cheese								
American	2 tbsp (1.1 oz)	90	5	6	20	2	0	410
Cheddar	2 tbsp (1.1 oz)	90	5	6	20	2	0	410

FOOD	PORTION	CALS	PROT	FAT	CHOL	CARB	FIBER	SOD
Fage								
Feta	1 oz	80	5	7	4	0	0	180
Finlandia								
Muenster	1 slice (1.1 oz)	120	8	10	30	tr	0	200
Formaggio								
Fresh Mozzarella	1 oz	90	6	6	20	1	0	150
Friendship								
Farmer	2 tbsp (1 oz)	50	5	3	10	0	0	120
Frigo								
Mozzarella Part Skim	1 oz	80	7	6	15	tr	0	210
Parmesan Shredded	¼ cup (1 oz)	100	9	7	20	1	tr	430
Ricotta Whole Milk	¼ cup (2.2 oz)	110	7	8	35	2	0	150
Romano Shredded	¼ cup (1 oz)	100	8	7	20	1	tr	460
Heluva Good Cheese								
Cheddar Extra Sharp	1 oz	110	7	9	30	1	0	180
Horizon Organic								
American	1 slice (0.7 oz)	60	4	5	15	1	0	250
Cheddar	1 oz	110	7	9	30	tr	0	180
Montery Jack	1 oz	100	7	8	30	0	0	170
Shred Mexican	¼ cup	110	7	9	30	tr	0	180
Shred Parmesan	1 tbsp	20	2	2	5	0	0	70
Slice Provolone	1 slice (0.7 oz)	70	5	6	15	0	0	140
Sticks Colby	1 (1 oz)	110	7	9	30	tr	0	180
String Mozzarella	1 stick (1 oz)	80	8	5	15	tr	0	170
J.L. Kraft								
Spreadable Feta & Spinach	2 tbsp	80	3	7	25	1	0	160
Jordan's								
Provolone	1 slice (1 oz)	100	7	8	20	0	0	240
Kraft								
Cheddar Extra Sharp	1 oz	120	6	10	30	0	0	180
Cheddar Sharp Shredded 2% Milk	¼ cup	80	7	6	20	tr	0	230
LiveActive 2% Milk Marbled Colby & Monterey Jack	1 stick (1 oz)	90	8	6	20	tr	0	240

FOOD	PORTION	CALS	PROT	FAT	CHOL	CARB	FIBER	SOD
LiveActive Cheddar Cheese Sticks	1 (1 oz)	120	6	10	30	0	0	180
LiveActive Colby & Monterey Jack Cubes	7 (1 oz)	110	7	9	30	tr	0	200
LiveActive Mozzarella Sticks	1 (1 oz)	80	8	5	15	tr	0	200
Shredded Mexican Style Cheddar & Monterey Jack	¼ cup	110	6	9	25	1	0	190
Singles American 2%	1 (0.7 oz)	50	4	3	10	2	0	290
Land O Lakes								
Cheddar Mild	1 slice (1 oz)	110	7	9	30	0	0	190
Co-Jack	1 slice (1 oz)	110	7	9	25	0	0	190
Swiss	1 slice (1 oz)	110	8	8	30	1	0	115
Laughing Cow								
Creamy French Onion Light	1 wedge	35	3	2	10	1	0	260
Creamy Garlic & Herb Light	1 wedge (0.7 oz)	35	3	2	10	1	0	260
Creamy Swiss Light Original	1 wedge (0.7 oz)	35	3	2	10	1	0	260
Creamy Swiss Original	1 wedge (0.7 oz)	50	2	4	15	1	0	250
Mini Babybel Bonbel	1 piece (0.7 oz)	70	5	6	20	0	0	170
Mini Babybel Gouda	1 piece (0.7 oz)	80	5	6	20	0	0	170
Mini Babybel Light Original	1 piece (0.7 oz)	50	6	3	15	0	0	160
Mini Babybel Mild Cheddar	1 piece (0.7 oz)	70	5	5	20	1	0	140
Mini Babybel Original	1 piece (0.7 oz)	70	5	6	20	0	0	170
Lifeway								
Farmer's Kefir	2 tbsp	25	3	2	6	4	0	10
Farmer's Kefir Lite	2 tbsp	25	3	1	<5	2	0	10
Sweet Kiss Peach	1 oz	45	3	1	<5	6	0	5
Meza								
Baked Brie In Pastry w/ Cranberries & Spiced Almonds	1 oz	110	4	7	30	8	tr	120
Miller's								
Mozzarella	1 slice (1 oz)	81	8	5	20	0	0	160

FOOD	PORTION	CALS	PROT	FAT	CHOL	CARB	FIBER	SOD
Mont Chevre								
Assorted Crottins	1 oz	70	4	6	10	1	0	130
Mt Vikos								
Feta Sheep & Goat Milk	1 oz	80	5	7	19	1	0	270
Organic Valley								
Blue Crumbles	1 oz	100	6	8	25	1	0	380
Cheddar Mild	1 oz	110	7	9	30	0	0	170
Feta	1 oz	60	5	4	10	tr	0	430
Monterey Jack Shredded	¼ cup	80	8	5	15	1	0	180
Muenster	1 slice (0.7 oz)	80	5	6	20	0	0	160
Provolone	1 slice (0.7 oz)	70	5	6	15	0	0	190
Swiss	1 oz	110	7	9	25	0	0	125
Polly-O								
Mozzarella Part Skim	1 oz	70	6	5	15	tr	0	200
Mozzarella Shredded	¼ cup	90	6	7	20	tr	0	190
Ricotta Part Skim	¼ cup	90	8	6	20	2	0	65
Sargento								
4 Cheese Italian Shredded	¼ cup	80	8	5	15	1	0	220
4 Cheese Mexican Reduced Fat Shredded	¼ cup (1 oz)	80	8	6	20	tr	0	200
American Burger	1 slice (0.7 oz)	70	4	6	20	tr	0	240
Bistro Blends Shredded Mozzarella w/ Sun Dried Tomato & Basil	¼ cup	90	7	6	20	1	0	220
Blue Crumbled	¼ cup (1 oz)	100	6	8	25	1	0	380
Cheddar Chipotle Shredded	¼ cup	100	6	8	15	1	0	190
Cheddar Chipotle Sticks	1 (0.7 oz)	80	5	6	0	1	0	150
Cheddar Mild Cubes	7 (1 oz)	120	7	10	30	tr	0	190
Cheddar Mild Shredded Reduced Fat	¼ cup (1 oz)	80	7	6	20	tr	0	180
Cheddar White Vermont Sharp	1 slice (0.7 oz)	80	5	7	20	0	0	125
Cheddar White Vermont Sharp Shredded	¼ cup (1 oz)	110	7	9	25	1	0	190
Cheese Dips Cheddar & Buttery Pretzels	1 pkg (3.8 oz)	360	9	16	15	47	2	1430

FOOD	PORTION	CALS	PROT	FAT	CHOL	CARB	FIBER	SOD
Cheese Dips Cheddar & Tortilla Chips	1 pkg (3 oz)	320	7	21	15	26	1	880
Colby-Jack Shredded	¼ cup (1 oz)	110	6	9	25	1	0	190
Fancy 6 Cheese Italian Shredded	¼ cup	90	7	7	20	1	0	200
Jarlsberg	1 slice (0.8 oz)	80	6	6	15	tr	0	110
Monterey Jack Shredded	¼ cup (1 oz)	110	7	9	30	1	0	190
Mozzarella Reduced Fat Shredded	¼ cup (1 oz)	80	8	5	10	tr	0	200
Mozzarella Shredded	¼ cup (1 oz)	80	7	6	15	1	0	190
Muenster	1 slice (0.7 oz)	80	5	6	20	0	0	135
Nacho & Taco Shredded	¼ cup (1 oz)	110	7	9	30	1	0	200
Parmesan Grated	2 tsp (5 g)	25	2	2	5	0	0	80
Parmesan Shredded	2 tsp	20	2	2	<5	0	0	55
Pepper Jack	1 slice (0.7 oz)	80	6	6	20	0	0	140
Provolone	1 slice (0.7 oz)	70	5	5	15	0	0	125
Provolone Reduced Fat	1 slice (0.7 oz)	50	5	4	10	0	0	140
Ricotta Fat Free	¼ cup	50	5	0	10	5	0	65
Ricotta Light	¼ cup	60	5	3	15	3	0	55
Ricotta Whole Milk	¼ cup	90	7	8	25	3	0	75
String	1 piece (1 oz)	80	8	6	15	tr	0	240
String Light	1 piece (0.7 oz)	50	6	3	10	tr	0	180
Swiss Reduced Fat	1 slice (0.7 oz)	80	7	4	10	1	0	30
Swiss Shredded	¼ cup (1 oz)	110	8	8	25	tr	0	60
Swiss Thick Slice	1 slice (1 oz)	110	8	8	25	1	0	60

FOOD	PORTION	CALS	PROT	FAT	CHOL	CARB	FIBER	SOD
Swiss Thin Sliced	1 slice (0.6 oz)	70	5	5	20	0	0	40
Smart Balance								
Cheddar Shredded	1 oz	80	7	5	5	tr	0	200
Mozzarella Shredded	1 oz	80	7	5	5	tr	0	260
Sorrento								
Mozzarella Fresh	1 oz	90	5	6	30	0	0	130
Stella								
3 Cheese Italian Shredded	¼ cup	100	8	7	25	1	tr	410
Asiago Wedge	1 oz	110	6	9	30	tr	0	280
Gorgonzola Wedge	1 oz	100	6	9	25	tr	0	390
Kasseri Wedge	1 oz	110	6	9	30	tr	0	280
Treasure Cave								
Blue Cheese Crumbled	¼ cup (1 oz)	100	6	8	20	tr	–	400
Feta Crumbled	¼ cup (1 oz)	60	4	5	15	tr	–	420
Gorgonzola Crumbled	¼ cup (1 oz)	100	6	8	20	tr	–	310
Wholesome Valley								
Organic American	1 slice (0.7 oz)	50	3	4	10	tr	0	210

CHEESE DISHES
Alexia

FOOD	PORTION	CALS	PROT	FAT	CHOL	CARB	FIBER	SOD
Mozzarella Stix	2 pieces	120	5	7	15	13	tr	220
Farm Rich								
Cheese Sticks Breaded	2 (2.1 oz)	210	9	12	15	17	tr	290
Mozzarella Bites Breaded	4 (2.2 oz)	150	8	7	10	13	1	270
Original Cheese Bites Breaded	7 (2.1 oz)	180	9	11	15	13	tr	440
Fillo Factory								
Tyropita Cheese Fillo Appetizers	3 (3 oz)	230	7	14	40	19	0	310
Stouffer's								
Welsh Rarebit	¼ pkg (2.5 oz)	140	6	10	20	6	0	270
TAKE-OUT								
fondue	½ cup (3.8 oz)	247	15	15	49	4	–	142

FOOD	PORTION	CALS	PROT	FAT	CHOL	CARB	FIBER	SOD
fried mozzarella sticks	3 (4.6 oz)	503	33	32	107	20	1	759
souffle	1 serv (7 oz)	504	23	38	370	18	1	848
welsh rarebit	1 slice	228	8	16	–	14	1	–

CHEESE SUBSTITUTES

FOOD	PORTION	CALS	PROT	FAT	CHOL	CARB	FIBER	SOD
mozzarella	1 oz	70	3	3	0	7	–	194
Playfood								
Cheesey Cheese	1 oz	60	2	5	0	4	1	190
Rice								
Shreds Mozzarella Flavor	⅓ cup (1 oz)	70	6	4	0	3	0	370
Vegan American Flavor	1 slice (0.7 oz)	45	1	3	0	0	0	130
Sheese								
Blue Style	1 oz	100	4	8	0	3	0	340
Cheddar Style Medium	1 oz	100	4	8	0	3	0	340
Creamy Mexican	2 tbsp	80	2	7	0	2	0	140
Creamy Original	2 tbsp	80	2	7	0	2	0	140
Super Stix								
Mozzarella Flavor	1 (1 oz)	70	6	5	0	0	0	370
Veggie								
American Flavor	1 slice (0.6 oz)	40	3	3	0	tr	0	220
Greated Parmesan Flavor	2 tsp	15	2	1	0	0	0	90
Pepper Jack Flavor	1 oz	60	6	4	0	2	0	390
Shreds Cheddar Flavor	1 oz	70	6	4	0	0	0	260
Veggy								
Mozzarella Flavor	1 slice (0.7 oz)	40	4	3	0	tr	0	230

CHERIMOYA

FOOD	PORTION	CALS	PROT	FAT	CHOL	CARB	FIBER	SOD
fresh	1	515	7	2	0	131	–	–

CHERRIES
CANNED

FOOD	PORTION	CALS	PROT	FAT	CHOL	CARB	FIBER	SOD
maraschino	1 (4 g)	7	tr	tr	0	2	tr	0
maraschino	¼ cup (1.4 oz)	66	tr	tr	0	17	1	2
sour in light syrup	½ cup	94	1	tr	0	24	1	9
sour water packed	½ cup	44	1	tr	0	11	1	9
sweet juice pack	½ cup	68	1	tr	0	17	2	4

FOOD	PORTION	CALS	PROT	FAT	CHOL	CARB	FIBER	SOD
sweet pitted in heavy syrup	½ cup	105	1	tr	0	27	2	4
sweet water pack	½ cup	57	1	tr	0	15	2	1
Del Monte								
Sweet Dark Pitted In Heavy Syrup	½ cup	100	tr	0	0	24	tr	10
DRIED								
bing unsulfured	¼ cup	130	0	0	0	31	2	10
montmorency tart pitted	⅓ cup	160	2	1	0	36	2	0
tart	½ cup	200	2	1	0	49	2	0
yogurt covered	¼ cup	170	1	6	0	29	5	20
Bob's Red Mill								
Tart	⅓ cup	140	1	0	0	33	11	0
De-Lite								
Tart	1 oz	95	1	tr	0	23	1	14
Eden								
Montmorency	¼ cup	140	0	0	0	36	3	15
Frieda's								
Bing	¼ cup (1.4 oz)	120	2	0	0	26	3	5
Tart	⅓ cup (1.4 oz)	150	2	0	0	33	2	0
Good Sense								
Cherries	⅓ cup	145	2	0	0	33	2	0
Peeled Snacks								
Fruit Picks Cherry-Go-Round	1 pkg (1.5 oz)	130	2	0	0	30	4	0
Sunsweet								
Tart & Sweet	¼ cup (1.4 oz)	100	1	0	0	30	2	5
FRESH								
sour	1 cup	52	1	tr	0	13	2	3
sour pitted	1 cup	78	2	tr	0	19	3	5
sweet	20	86	1	1	0	22	3	0
Rainier								
Sweet Premium Northwest	1 cup	90	2	1	0	22	3	0
FROZEN								
sour unsweetened	½ cup	36	1	tr	0	9	1	1
sweet sweetened	½ cup	115	2	tr	0	29	3	1

FOOD	PORTION	CALS	PROT	FAT	CHOL	CARB	FIBER	SOD
CHERRY JUICE								
tart cherry concentrate	1 cup	140	1	0	0	34	0	25
Eden								
Organic Montmorency	8 oz	140	1	1	0	33	0	30
Froose								
Cheerful Cherry	1 box (4.2 oz)	80	0	0	0	19	3	15
HP								
Tart Montmorency Concentrate	1 oz	80	tr	0	0	19	0	15
L&A								
Black Cherry 100% Juice	8 oz	180	0	0	0	45	–	10
Old Orchard								
100% Pure Tart Cherry	8 oz	140	0	0	0	34	–	25
CHERVIL								
seed	1 tsp	1	tr	tr	0	tr	–	tr
CHESTNUTS								
chinese steamed	3 (1 oz)	43	1	tr	0	10	–	1
creme de marrons	1 oz	73	1	tr	0	18	1	1
japanese roasted	1 oz	57	1	tr	0	13	–	5
ready-to-eat vacuum packed	5 (1 oz)	40	tr	0	0	8	0	10
roasted	3 (1 oz)	70	1	1	0	15	1	1
CHEWING GUM								
bubble gum	1 block	20	0	tr	0	5	tr	0
stick	1 piece	7	0	tr	0	2	tr	0
sugarless	1 piece	5	0	tr	0	2	0	0
Bazooka								
Bubble Gum	1 piece (4 g)	15	0	0	0	4	–	0
Big Red								
Gum	1 piece	10	0	0	0	2	–	0
Brach's								
Abra Cabubble	1 piece	45	0	0	0	10	0	0
Doublemint								
Gum	1 piece	10	0	0	0	2	–	0
Dubble Bubble								
Gumball	1 piece	10	0	0	0	2	0	0

FOOD	PORTION	CALS	PROT	FAT	CHOL	CARB	FIBER	SOD
Eclipse								
Flash All Flavors	1 piece	0	0	0	0	2	–	0
Sugarless All Flavors	2 pieces	5	0	0	0	2	–	0
Extra								
Sugar Free All Flavors	1 piece	5	0	0	0	2	–	0
Sugar Free Bubble Gum	1 piece	5	0	0	0	1	–	0
Flare								
Warming Cinnamon	1 piece	5	0	0	0	2	–	0
Juicy Fruit								
Gum	2 pieces	10	0	0	0	2	–	0
Orbit								
Sugarless All Flavors	2 pieces	5	0	0	0	2	–	0
White Melon Breeze	2 pieces	5	0	0	0	2	0	0
Skittles								
Bubble Gum	2 pieces	10	0	0	0	2	–	0
SteviaDent								
Gum	2 pieces	3	0	0	0	1	0	0
Stride								
All Flavors	1 piece	<5	0	0	0	1	–	0
Winterfresh								
Gum	1 stick	10	0	0	0	2	–	0
Thin Ice Mountain Rush	1 piece	0	0	0	0	2	–	0
Wrigley's								
Spearmint	1 stick	10	0	0	0	2	–	0
CHIA SEEDS								
dried	1 oz	134	5	7	0	14	–	–

CHICKEN (see also CHICKEN DISHES, CHICKEN SUBSTITUTES, DINNER, HOT DOGS)
CANNED

FOOD	PORTION	CALS	PROT	FAT	CHOL	CARB	FIBER	SOD
breast meat in water	2 oz	70	13	1	25	0	0	230
w/ broth	½ can (2.5 oz)	117	15	6	–	0	0	357
Swanson								
Chunk Breast In Water	2 oz	50	9	1	25	1	0	300
Tyson								
Premium Chunk Breast	½ can (2 oz)	60	13	1	30	0	0	200
Premium Chunk	½ can (2 oz)	60	10	3	30	0	0	200

FOOD	PORTION	CALS	PROT	FAT	CHOL	CARB	FIBER	SOD
Valley Fresh								
Chunk White	2 oz	70	15	1	25	0	0	180
White & Dark Chunk	2 oz	80	15	2	50	0	0	130
FRESH								
broiler/fryer breast w/ skin batter dipped & fried	½ breast (4.9 oz)	364	35	18	119	13	–	385
broiler/fryer breast w/ skin roasted	½ breast (3.4 oz)	193	29	8	83	0	0	69
broiler/fryer breast w/ skin stewed	½ breast (3.9 oz)	202	30	8	83	0	0	68
broiler/fryer breast w/o skin fried	½ breast (3 oz)	161	29	4	78	tr	–	68
broiler/fryer breast w/o skin roasted	½ breast (3 oz)	142	27	3	73	0	0	63
broiler/fryer drumstick w/ skin batter dipped & fried	1 (2.6 oz)	193	16	11	62	6	–	194
broiler/fryer drumstick w/ skin floured & fried	1 (1.7 oz)	120	13	7	44	1	–	44
broiler/fryer drumstick w/ skin roasted	1 (1.8 oz)	112	14	6	48	0	0	47
broiler/fryer drumstick w/ skin stewed	1 (2 oz)	116	14	6	48	0	0	43
broiler/fryer drumstick w/o skin fried	1 (1.5 oz)	82	12	3	40	0	0	40
broiler/fryer drumstick w/o skin roasted	1 (1.5 oz)	76	12	2	41	0	0	42
broiler/fryer drumstick w/o skin stewed	1 (1.6 oz)	78	13	3	40	0	0	37
broiler/fryer leg w/ skin batter dipped & fried	1 (5.5 oz)	431	34	26	142	14	–	442
broiler/fryer leg w/ skin floured & fried	1 (3.9 oz)	285	30	16	105	3	–	99
broiler/fryer leg w/ skin roasted	1 (4 oz)	265	30	15	105	0	0	99
broiler/fryer leg w/ skin stewed	1 (4.4 oz)	275	30	16	105	0	0	92
broiler/fryer leg w/o skin fried	1 (3.3 oz)	195	27	9	93	1	–	90

FOOD	PORTION	CALS	PROT	FAT	CHOL	CARB	FIBER	SOD
broiler/fryer leg w/o skin roasted	1 (3.3 oz)	182	26	8	89	0	0	87
broiler/fryer leg w/o skin stewed	1 (3.5 oz)	187	26	8	90	0	0	78
broiler/fryer neck w/ skin stewed	1 (1.3 oz)	94	7	7	27	0	0	20
broiler/fryer neck w/o skin stewed	1 (.6 oz)	32	4	1	14	0	0	12
broiler/fryer skin floured & fried	from ½ chicken (2 oz)	281	24	24	41	5	–	30
broiler/fryer skin roasted	from ½ chicken (2 oz)	254	11	23	46	0	0	36
broiler/fryer skin stewed	from ½ chicken (2.5 oz)	261	11	24	45	0	0	40
broiler/fryer thigh w/ skin batter dipped & fried	1 (3 oz)	238	19	14	80	8	–	248
broiler/fryer thigh w/ skin floured & fried	1 (2.2 oz)	162	17	9	60	2	–	55
broiler/fryer thigh w/ skin roasted	1 (2.2 oz)	153	16	10	58	0	0	52
broiler/fryer thigh w/ skin stewed	1 (2.4 oz)	158	16	10	57	0	0	49
broiler/fryer thigh w/o skin fried	1 (1.8 oz)	113	15	5	53	1	–	49
broiler/fryer thigh w/o skin roasted	1 (1.8 oz)	109	13	6	49	0	0	46
broiler/fryer thigh w/o skin stewed	1 (1.9 oz)	107	14	5	49	0	0	41
broiler/fryer w/ skin floured & fried	½ chicken (11 oz)	844	90	47	283	10	–	264
broiler/fryer w/ skin fried	½ chicken (16.4 oz)	1347	81	81	404	44	–	1360
broiler/fryer w/ skin roasted	½ chicken (10.5 oz)	715	82	41	263	0	0	244
broiler/fryer w/ skin stewed	½ chicken (11.7 oz)	730	82	42	262	0	0	224

FOOD	PORTION	CALS	PROT	FAT	CHOL	CARB	FIBER	SOD
broiler/fryer w/ skin neck & giblets batter dipped & fried	1 chicken (2.3 lbs)	2987	235	180	1054	93	–	2921
broiler/fryer w/ skin neck & giblets roasted	1 chicken (1.5 lbs)	1598	183	90	730	tr	–	536
broiler/fryer w/ skin neck & giblets stewed	1 chicken (1.6 lbs)	1625	184	93	726	tr	–	494
broiler/fryer w/o skin fried	1 cup	307	43	13	131	2	–	127
broiler/fryer w/o skin roasted	1 cup (5 oz)	266	41	10	125	0	0	120
broiler/fryer w/o skin stewed	1 cup (5 oz)	248	38	9	116	0	0	98
broiler/fryer wing w/ skin batter dipped & fried	1 (1.7 oz)	159	10	11	39	5	–	157
broiler/fryer wing w/ skin floured & fried	1 (1.1 oz)	103	8	7	26	1	–	25
broiler/fryer wing w/ skin roasted	1 (1.2 oz)	99	9	7	29	0	0	28
broiler/fryer wing w/ skin stewed	1 (1.4 oz)	100	9	7	28	0	0	27
capon w/ skin neck & giblets roasted	1 chicken (3.1 lbs)	3211	402	165	1458	1	–	704
cornish hen w/ skin roasted	1 hen (8 oz)	595	51	42	299	0	0	146
cornish hen w/o skin & bone roasted	½ hen (2 oz)	72	13	2	57	0	0	34
cornish hen w/o skin & bone roasted	1 hen (3.8 oz)	144	25	4	113	0	0	67
cornish hen w/skin roasted	½ hen (4 oz)	296	25	21	149	0	0	73
roaster dark meat w/o skin roasted	1 cup (5 oz)	250	33	12	104	0	0	133
roaster light meat w/o skin roasted	1 cup (5 oz)	214	38	6	105	0	0	71
roaster w/ skin neck & giblets roasted	1 chicken (2.4 lbs)	2363	257	140	1003	1	–	760
roaster w/ skin roasted	½ chicken (1.1 lbs)	1071	115	64	365	0	0	349
roaster w/o skin roasted	1 cup (5 oz)	469	9	28	160	0	0	105
stewing dark meat w/o skin stewed	1 cup (5 oz)	361	39	21	132	0	0	133

FOOD	PORTION	CALS	PROT	FAT	CHOL	CARB	FIBER	SOD
stewing w/ skin neck & giblets stewed	1 chicken (1.3 lbs)	1636	157	107	603	tr	–	419
stewing w/ skin stewed	½ chicken (9.2 oz)	744	70	49	205	0	0	190
Tyson								
Breasts Boneless Skinless	4 oz	110	23	3	65	0	0	180
Cornish Hen	1 serv (4 oz)	200	19	14	130	0	0	65
Drumsticks	4 oz	150	18	9	95	0	0	180
Thigh Cutlets Boneless Skinless	4 oz	130	18	7	90	0	0	160
Whole Cut Up	4 oz	220	19	16	80	0	0	170
Wings	4 oz	220	17	17	105	0	0	190
FROZEN								
Barber								
Buffalo Fingers	1 (3.3 oz)	160	15	4	35	18	tr	380
Nuggets 4 Cheese Stuffed	3 (3 oz)	230	14	16	45	9	tr	570
Nuggets Cheddar & Bacon Stuffed	3 (3 oz)	240	14	17	45	8	tr	520
Potato Chip Sticks	2 (4.5 oz)	350	18	24	60	16	tr	950
Ian's								
Fingers	3	190	15	8	40	14	0	460
Nuggets	5	190	15	8	40	14	0	250
Nuggets Allergy Free	5	190	15	8	40	14	0	250
Patties	1 (3.4 oz)	220	18	9	40	16	0	300
Organic Prairie								
Ground	4 oz	200	21	12	95	1	–	90
Tyson								
Any'tizers Barbeque Style Wings	3 (3.2 oz)	200	19	13	110	7	0	380
Any'tizers Homestyle Chicken Fries	7 (3.2 oz)	230	13	11	25	19	1	590
Any'tizers Popcorn Chicken	6 (2.8 oz)	220	12	10	25	19	1	670
Breast Pattie	1 (2.6 oz)	180	10	11	25	12	1	300
Cordon Bleu	1 (5.9 oz)	380	22	24	80	20	1	790
Diced Strips	1 serv (3 oz)	90	20	1	45	0	0	250
Kiev	1 (5.9 oz)	480	17	37	150	19	1	420
Weaver								
Breast Strips	3	230	12	14	35	14	1	620
Breast Tenders	5	240	14	15	35	15	0	330
Buffalo Popcorn Chicken	7	230	14	14	35	13	1	900

FOOD	PORTION	CALS	PROT	FAT	CHOL	CARB	FIBER	SOD
Crispy Breast Strips	2	220	8	14	20	13	2	410
Crispy Mini Drums	5	250	14	16	40	14	1	410
Croquettes	2 + gravy	230	11	14	30	15	0	950
Honey Batter Breast Tenders	5	220	13	13	30	13	2	250
Hot Wings Buffalo Style	3	190	18	13	95	0	0	370
Nuggets	4	210	11	15	35	9	1	360
Patties Italian	1	210	10	14	20	12	1	470
Patties Breast	1	170	10	10	20	10	1	410
Patties Original	1	180	10	11	30	10	1	430
Wings Honey BBQ	3	200	17	11	95	7	–	430
Wellshire								
Chicken Bites Dinosaur Shaped Gluten Free	5	160	9	10	30	15	2	300
READY-TO-EAT								
chicken salad sandwich spread	¼ cup	104	6	7	16	4	0	196
Boar's Head								
Breast Hickory Smoked	2 oz	60	13	1	35	0	0	360
Breast Oven Roasted	2 oz	60	13	1	35	0	0	350
Carl Buddig								
Chicken Sliced	2 oz	85	10	5	–	1	–	–
Healthy Ones								
Oven Roasted 97% Fat Free	4 slices (2 oz)	60	9	2	25	2	0	410
Hillshire Farm								
Smoked Breast	6 slices (2 oz)	60	11	1	25	2	0	600
Oscar Mayer								
Breast Oven Roasted Thin Sliced	⅓ pkg (2 oz)	60	10	2	30	1	0	710
Breast Strips Breaded	½ pkg (3 oz)	170	15	6	30	14	–	800
Breast Strips Grilled	½ pkg (3 oz)	110	19	3	55	1	–	770
Perdue								
Short Cuts Chicken Breast Honey Roasted	½ cup (2.5 oz)	90	13	3	35	5	–	480
Short Cuts Chicken Strips Fajita Style	½ cup	90	13	3	35	3	–	480

FOOD	PORTION	CALS	PROT	FAT	CHOL	CARB	FIBER	SOD
Short Cuts Grilled Chicken Breast	½ cup (2.5 oz)	90	16	2	40	1	–	510
Short Cuts Grilled Italian	½ cup	90	13	3	35	4	–	480
Short Cuts Grilled Lemon Pepper	½ cup (2.5 oz)	80	15	1	40	3	–	480
Sara Lee								
Breast Oven Roasted	4 slices (2 oz)	45	10	1	25	0	0	430
Tyson								
Chicken Strips Fajita	1 serv (3 oz)	110	19	2	60	3	0	450
Honey Roasted Breast	2 slices (1.6 oz)	50	8	1	15	3	0	530
Hot Wings Buffalo Style	4	220	20	15	110	1	0	560
Roasted Whole Chicken Lemon Pepper	1 serv (3 oz)	120	17	6	75	1	0	510
Salad Kit Chunk Chicken	1 pkg (3.4 oz)	210	18	9	50	15	1	640
TAKE-OUT								
oven roasted breast of chicken	2 oz	60	11	1	25	0	0	470

CHICKEN DISHES
FROZEN
Barber

FOOD	PORTION	CALS	PROT	FAT	CHOL	CARB	FIBER	SOD
Broccoli & Cheese Reduced Fat	1 (5.5 oz)	250	25	13	55	11	tr	610
Cordon Bleu	1 (6 oz)	370	28	23	95	14	0	840
Cordon Bleu Reduced Fat	1 (5.5 oz)	260	27	13	75	11	0	700
Creme Brie & Apple	1 (6 oz)	350	25	21	90	18	tr	830
Kiev	1 (6 oz)	430	27	29	110	15	tr	720
Mashed Potato Stuffed	1 (6 oz)	340	21	18	85	21	tr	630
Skinless Breast Stuffed	1 (6 oz)	280	21	11	45	24	tr	860
Maple Leaf Farms								
Chicken Breast Stuffed Broccoli & Cheese	1 (6 oz)	340	22	19	40	20	0	870
REFRIGERATED								
Lunchables								
Chicken Shake-Up	1 pkg	220	12	6	30	29	tr	480

FOOD	PORTION	CALS	PROT	FAT	CHOL	CARB	FIBER	SOD
Tyson								
Chicken Breast Medallions In White Wine & Garlic Sauce	1 serv (5 oz)	140	19	6	45	3	1	500
Ventera								
Rollatini w/ Rice Stuffing & Marsala Wine Sauce	1 serv + sauce (6 oz)	230	24	10	70	9	0	590
Wellshire								
Shredded Chicken In BBQ Sauce	¼ cup	70	6	3	20	8	0	270
TAKE-OUT								
arroz con pollo	1 serv (16 oz)	579	48	14	126	62	2	1433
barbecued pulled chicken	1 serv (9 oz)	312	36	2	147	37	2	794
boneless breast w/ apple stuffing	1 serv (5 oz)	260	32	9	80	10	1	250
breast & wing breaded & fried	2 pieces (5.7 oz)	494	36	30	149	20	–	975
chicken & dumplings	¾ cup	256	23	12	109	12	tr	1283
chicken & noodles	1 cup	365	22	18	103	26	–	600
chicken a la king	1 cup	470	27	34	221	12	–	760
chicken cacciatore	¾ cup	394	33	24	99	9	2	671
chicken paprikash	1½ cups	296	–	10	90	–	–	–
chicken pie w/ top crust	1 slice (5.6 oz)	472	19	31	–	32	1	–
chicken cordon bleu	1 serv (5 oz)	280	29	13	70	10	0	800
chicken meatloaf	1 lg slice (5 oz)	243	29	9	122	11	1	658
chicken satay + peanut sauce	2 skewers	239	27	12	64	6	1	439
drumstick breaded & fried	2 pieces (5.2 oz)	430	30	27	165	16	–	756
grilled breast strips	4 strips (3 oz)	100	20	2	50	0	0	310
groundnut stew hkatenkwan	1 serv (15.7 oz)	576	38	40	116	18	4	1009
jamaican jerk wings	4 wings (9.9 oz)	709	57	51	172	3	tr	1045
kobete turkish chicken w/ pastry	1 serv	513	–	13	71	–	–	551

FOOD	PORTION	CALS	PROT	FAT	CHOL	CARB	FIBER	SOD
sancocho de pollo dominican chicken stew	1 serv	702	71	30	195	34	1	653
sukiyaki	1 serv (18 oz)	436	71	8	175	19	4	1048
tandoori chicken breast	1 serv	260	–	13	–	5	–	–
tandoori chicken leg & thigh	1 serv	300	–	17	–	6	–	–
thigh breaded & fried	2 pieces (5.2 oz)	430	30	27	165	16	–	756

CHICKEN SUBSTITUTES

Boca

Chik'n Nuggets	1 serv (3 oz)	180	14	7	0	17	3	500
Chik'n Patties	1 (2.5 oz)	160	11	6	0	15	2	430

Gardenburger

Chik'n Grill	1 patty (2.5 oz)	100	13	3	0	5	5	360

Lightlife

Smart Cutlet Seasoned Chicken	1 (4 oz)	180	27	4	0	11	4	670
Smart Menu Chick'n Nuggets	4 pieces	220	14	11	0	16	2	520
Smart Menu Chick'n Patties	1 patty	160	11	7	0	14	2	540
Smart Menu Chick'n Strips	1 serv (3 oz)	80	15	0	0	5	3	530

Loma Linda

Fried Chik'n w/ Gravy	2 pieces (2.8 oz)	150	12	10	0	5	2	430

Morningstar Farms

Chik'n Roasted Herb	1 pattie (2.2 oz)	110	13	3	0	9	2	380
Meal Starters Chik'n Strips	12 pieces (3 oz)	140	23	4	0	6	1	510

Quorn

Cutlets	1 (3.5 oz)	200	10	8	0	20	4	610
Gruyere Cutlet	1 (4 oz)	260	11	15	20	23	3	510
Naked Cutlet	1 (2.4 oz)	80	11	3	5	5	2	420
Nuggets	3–4 pieces (3 oz)	180	8	8	0	18	3	650
Patties	1 patty (2.6 oz)	160	8	7	0	12	3	525

FOOD	PORTION	CALS	PROT	FAT	CHOL	CARB	FIBER	SOD
Tenders	1 cup (3 oz)	90	12	2	0	8	3	350
Viana								
Veggie Chickin Fillets	1 (3.7 oz)	260	29	14	0	8	4	890
Veggie Chickin Nuggets	3 pieces (2.6 oz)	200	16	12	0	8	2	590
Worthington								
FriChik Original	2 pieces (3.2 oz)	140	12	8	0	3	1	430
Meatless Chicken Style	1 slice (2 oz)	90	9	5	0	2	1	240
Yves								
Meatless Chicken Burger	1 (2.6 oz)	100	15	3	0	5	2	420
Meatless Smoked Chicken Slices	4 (2.2 oz)	100	14	2	0	5	0	460

CHICKPEAS
CANNED

FOOD	PORTION	CALS	PROT	FAT	CHOL	CARB	FIBER	SOD
chickpeas	1 cup	285	12	3	0	54	–	718
Eden								
Organic Garbanzo	½ cup	130	7	1	0	23	5	30
Green Giant								
Garbanzo Beans	½ cup	100	5	2	0	17	4	430
Progresso								
ChickPeas	½ cup	100	5	2	0	17	4	280
DRIED								
cooked	1 cup	269	15	4	0	45	–	11
Arrowhead Mills								
Organic Dried Chickpeas not prep	¼ cup	160	9	3	0	27	8	10
REFRIGERATED								
Sabra								
Balela Vinaigrette	2 oz	100	4	5	0	11	3	220
Spicy Armenian Salad	2 oz	50	2	3	0	5	1	230

CHICORY

FOOD	PORTION	CALS	PROT	FAT	CHOL	CARB	FIBER	SOD
endive fresh chopped	½ cup	4	tr	tr	0	1	–	6
greens raw chopped	½ cup	21	2	tr	0	4	–	41
root raw	1 (2.1 oz)	44	1	tr	0	11	–	30
roots raw cut up	½ cup (1.6 oz)	33	1	tr	0	8	–	23
witloof head raw	1 (1.9 oz)	9	tr	tr	0	2	–	1

FOOD	PORTION	CALS	PROT	FAT	CHOL	CARB	FIBER	SOD
witloof raw	½ cup (1.6 oz)	8	tr	tr	0	2	–	1
Frieda's								
Belgian Endive	2 cups	115	1	0	0	3	3	20

CHILI

FOOD	PORTION	CALS	PROT	FAT	CHOL	CARB	FIBER	SOD
powder	1 tbsp	24	1	1	0	4	3	76
Boca								
Chili w/ Ground Burger	1 pkg (9.4 oz)	150	20	1	0	25	12	650
Bush's								
ChiliMagic Chili Starter as prep	1 cup	250	19	11	55	17	4	910
Original No Beans	1 cup	240	13	14	25	16	3	1380
Del Monte								
Sauce	1 tbsp	20	0	0	0	5	0	480
Fantastic								
3 Bean	1 pkg (8 oz)	180	10	4	0	28	5	680
Vegetarian Mix not prep	¼ cup	100	8	1	0	17	4	480
Hunt's								
Family Favorites Chili	¼ cup (2.2 oz)	25	1	0	0	9	1	400
Lean Cuisine								
Cafe Classics Three Bean Chili	1 pkg (10 oz)	260	9	7	10	40	8	600
Lightlife								
Smart Chili	1 pkg	200	14	0	0	34	12	1120
McIhenny								
Original Recipe	½ cup	50	2	1	0	10	3	610
Mimi's Gourmet								
Organic Vegan Gluten Free 3 Bean w/ Rice	1 pkg (11.5 oz)	270	10	6	0	46	10	670
Organic Vegan Gluten Free Black Bean & Corn	1 pkg (10.5 oz)	250	10	6	0	40	11	680
Organic Vegan Gluten Free White Bean	1 pkg (10.5 oz)	230	10	6	0	35	9	660
Pacific Foods								
Beef Steak w/ Beans	1 cup	250	20	7	35	29	8	800
Ro-Tel								
Chili Fixin's	½ cup	35	2	1	0	8	3	540

FOOD	PORTION	CALS	PROT	FAT	CHOL	CARB	FIBER	SOD
Spice Hunter								
Powder Blend Salt Free	¼ tsp	0	0	0	0	0	0	0
Stagg								
Chunkero w/ Beans	1 cup	300	16	15	45	26	5	830
Classic w/ Beans	1 cup	330	17	17	45	28	5	820
Country Blend	1 cup	330	16	17	40	30	6	1100
Country Blend w/ Beans	1 cup	330	16	17	40	30	6	1100
Ranch House Chicken w/ Beans	1 cup	290	19	9	50	32	6	810
Silverado Beef w/ Beans	1 cup	230	18	3	45	33	6	880
Turkey Ranchero w/ Beans	1 cup	240	22	3	35	31	6	880
Vegetable Garden Four Bean	1 cup	200	10	1	0	37	7	870
Worthington								
Vegetarian	1 cup	280	24	10	0	25	8	1130
TAKE-OUT								
chiles rellenos cheese filled	1 (5 oz)	365	17	30	167	8	1	496
chili con carne w/ beans	1 cup	264	21	11	53	22	7	1275
con carne w/ beans & rice	1 cup	298	11	9	28	45	7	1172
vegetarian con carne	1 cup	272	19	7	0	35	11	1090

CHILI PEPPER (see PEPPERS)

CHINESE FOOD (see ASIAN FOOD)

CHINESE PRESERVING MELON

cooked	½ cup	11	tr	tr	0	3	–	93

CHIPS (see also SNACKS)

apple chips	10	101	tr	5	0	16	2	22
corn	1 oz	153	2	10	0	16	1	179
corn barbecue	1 oz	148	2	9	0	16	1	216
corn cones	1 oz	145	2	8	0	18	–	290
corn cones nacho	1 oz	152	2	9	–	17	–	270
corn onion	1 oz	142	2	6	0	19	–	278
potato	1 oz	152	2	10	0	15	–	168
potato cheese	1 oz	140	2	8	–	16	–	225
potato cheese	1 bag (6 oz)	842	14	46	–	98	–	1348
potato light	1 oz	134	2	6	0	19	–	139
potato sour cream & onion	1 oz	150	2	10	2	15	–	177
potato sticks	1 pkg (1 oz)	148	2	10	0	15	–	71

FOOD	PORTION	CALS	PROT	FAT	CHOL	CARB	FIBER	SOD
potato sticks	½ cup (0.6 oz)	94	1	6	0	10	1	45
taco	1 bag (8 oz)	1089	18	55	–	143	–	1788
taco	1 oz	136	2	7	–	18	–	223
taro	1 oz	141	1	7	0	19	–	97
taro	10 (0.8 oz)	115	1	6	0	16	–	79
tortilla	1 oz	142	2	7	0	18	2	150
tortilla nacho	1 oz	141	2	7	0	18	2	201
tortilla nacho light	1 oz	126	3	4	0	20	–	284
tortilla ranch	1 oz	139	2	7	0	18	–	174
Bachman								
Potato Golden Crips	1 pkg (1 oz)	150	2	9	0	16	0	115
Bravos!								
Tortilla Nacho Cheese	1 oz	150	2	8	0	17	1	180
Cape Cod								
Potato 40% Reduced Fat	19	130	2	6	0	18	1	110
Potato Beachside BBQ	19	150	2	8	0	17	1	160
Potato Classic	19	150	2	8	0	17	1	110
Potato Fresh Garden Herb Reduced Fat	19	130	2	6	0	19	1	160
Potato Jalapeno & Cheddar	19	140	2	8	0	16	3	260
Potato No Salt	19	150	2	10	0	14	tr	0
Potato Robust Russet	19	150	2	8	0	16	1	150
Potato Salt & Vinegar	19	150	2	8	0	17	1	130
Potato Sea Salt & Cracked Pepper	19	140	2	7	0	16	1	160
Tortilla Reduced Carb	10	140	9	6	0	11	2	110
Tortilla Veggie	12	140	2	6	0	18	1	110
Corazonas								
Tortilla Jalapeno Jack	1 oz	140	3	7	0	16	3	115
Tortilla Original	1 oz	140	2	7	0	16	3	70
Tortilla Salsa Picante	1 oz	140	2	7	0	16	3	110
Doritos								
Baked Cooler Ranch	15 (1 oz)	120	2	4	0	21	2	200
Baked Nacho Cheesier	15	120	2	4	0	21	2	220
Cooler Ranch	12	140	2	7	0	18	1	170
Four Cheese	12	140	2	8	0	17	1	240
Guacamole	12	150	4	8	0	16	1	230

FOOD	PORTION	CALS	PROT	FAT	CHOL	CARB	FIBER	SOD
Light Nacho Cheesier	11	90	2	1	0	18	1	240
Natural White Nacho Cheese	11	150	2	8	0	17	1	190
Ranchero	12	150	2	1	0	17	1	290
Rollitos Cooler Ranch	17	140	2	8	0	17	1	250
Rollitos Zesty Taco	17	150	2	8	0	17	1	140
Toasted Corn	13	140	2	7	0	18	1	120
Eatsmart								
Cafe Fries Malt Vinegar & Sea Salt	1 oz	150	1	7	0	20	–	290
Cafe Fries Tangy Tomato & Spices	1 oz	150	1	7	0	20	–	290
CheddAirs	1 oz	135	3	5	0	20	–	90
Soy Crisps Parmesan Garlic & Olive Oil	1 oz	160	8	9	0	11	–	340
Soy Crisps Tomato Romano & Olive Oil	1 oz	160	8	9	0	11	–	360
Veggie Crisps	1 oz	140	1	7	0	18	–	290
Veggie Crisps Cheddar & Jalapeno	1 oz	130	1	7	0	18	–	430
Veggie Crisps Sundried Tomato & Pesto	1 oz	140	1	7	0	19	–	390
Eden								
Brown Rice Chips	25	150	2	7	0	19	0	100
Sea Vegetable Chips	25	140	tr	5	0	23	0	220
Vegetable	25	130	tr	4	0	24	0	260
Wasabi	25	130	tr	4	0	24	0	260
Flat Earth								
Baked Fruit Crisps Apple Cinnamon Grove	14 (1 oz)	130	1	5	0	21	2	35
Baked Fruit Crisps Peach Mango Paradise	14 (1 oz)	130	1	5	0	21	1	35
Baked Fruit Crisps Wild Berry Patch	14 (1 oz)	130	1	5	0	21	1	40
Baked Veggie Crisps Farmland Cheddar	14 (1 oz)	130	2	5	0	19	2	190
Baked Veggie Crisps Garlic & Herb Field	14 (1 oz)	130	2	5	0	19	2	190
Baked Veggie Crisps Tangy Tomato Ranch	14 (1 oz)	130	2	5	0	19	2	210

FOOD	PORTION	CALS	PROT	FAT	CHOL	CARB	FIBER	SOD
French's								
Potato Sticks Barbecue	¾ cup	160	2	10	0	16	1	190
Potato Sticks Cheddar	¾ cup	170	2	12	0	14	tr	200
Potato Sticks Original	¾ cup	190	2	12	0	16	1	190
Fritos								
Corn Chips King Size	12	160	2	10	0	16	1	150
Original	32	160	2	10	0	16	2	160
Scoops	10	160	2	10	0	16	1	110
Twists	23	150	2	9	0	17	1	230
Garden Of Eatin'								
Organic Pita Baked Brown Sugar & Cinnamon	8	120	3	3	0	22	1	70
Organic Tortilla Blue Corn	7	140	2	7	0	18	2	60
Organic Tortilla Blue No Salt Added	16	140	2	7	0	18	2	10
Organic Tortilla White Corn	7	140	2	6	0	19	2	70
Glenny's								
Organic Soy Barbeque	1 oz	110	8	3	–	13	3	350
Organic Soy Creamy Ranch	1 oz	110	9	3	–	12	3	300
Soy Crisps Apple Cinnamon	½ pkg (0.6 oz)	70	5	2	–	10	2	90
Soy Crisps Caramel	½ pkg (1.3 oz)	70	5	2	0	9	1	125
Soy Crisps Low Fat Lightly Salted	½ pkg (0.6 oz)	70	5	1	–	9	2	170
Soy Crisps No Salt	½ pkg (0.6 oz)	70	5	1	–	9	2	100
Soy Crisps Salt & Pepper	½ pkg (0.6 oz)	70	5	1	–	9	2	190
Soy Crisps White Cheddar	½ pkg (0.6 oz)	70	5	2	–	9	2	180
Spud Delites Sea Salt	1 pkg (1.1 oz)	100	2	1	–	21	1	270
Veggie Fries	½ pkg (0.6 oz)	70	1	1	0	13	0	120
Zen Health Tortilla Crisps Original	1 oz	110	9	3	0	12	tr	250
Guiltless Gourmet								
Potato Au Gratin	1 oz	100	7	3	0	14	3	340
Potato Pico De Gallo	1 oz	100	7	3	0	14	3	390

FOOD	PORTION	CALS	PROT	FAT	CHOL	CARB	FIBER	SOD
Potato Sea Salt	1 oz	90	8	2	0	15	3	280
Tortilla Chili Lime	18 (1 oz)	110	2	2	0	22	2	200
Tortilla Chili Verde	18 (1 oz)	120	2	2	0	22	2	200
Tortilla Chipotle	18 (1 oz)	120	2	2	0	22	2	200
Tortilla Red Corn	18 (1 oz)	110	3	2	0	22	2	160
Tortilla Spicy Black Bean	18 (1 oz)	110	3	2	0	22	2	200
Tortilla Sweet White Corn	18 (1 oz)	110	3	2	0	22	2	160
Tortilla Yellow Corn Unsalted	18 (1 oz)	110	2	1	0	22	2	26
Jay's								
Potato	1 oz	150	2	10	0	14	1	190
Kettle								
Bakes Potato Aged White Cheddar	1 oz	120	3	3	0	20	2	170
Bakes Potato Hickory Honey Barbeque	1 oz	120	3	3	0	21	2	160
Bakes Potato Lightly Salted	1 oz	120	3	3	0	21	2	115
Krinkle Cut Potato Barbeque	1 oz	150	2	9	0	16	2	170
Krinkle Cut Potato Dill & Sour Cream	1 oz	150	2	9	0	16	2	170
Krinkle Cut Potato Lightly Salted	1 oz	150	2	9	0	15	2	115
Krinkle Cut Potato Salt & Fresh Ground Pepper	1 oz	150	2	9	0	16	2	200
Organic Tortilla Blue Corn	1 oz	140	3	6	0	18	2	80
Organic Tortilla Brown Rice & Black Bean w/ Garlic & Onions	1 oz	120	3	6	0	16	2	85
Organic Tortilla Fire Roasted Chili	1 oz	140	3	7	0	18	2	150
Organic Tortilla Five Grain Yellow Corn	1 oz	140	2	6	0	18	2	80
Organic Tortilla Lightly Salted Yellow Corn	1 oz	140	2	6	0	19	2	80
Organic Tortilla Little Dippers	1 oz	140	2	6	0	19	2	80
Organic Tortilla Sesame Blue Moons	1 oz	150	3	8	0	18	2	80
Potato Cheddar Beer	1 oz	150	2	9	0	15	1	180

FOOD	PORTION	CALS	PROT	FAT	CHOL	CARB	FIBER	SOD
Potato Honey Dijon	1 oz	150	2	9	0	16	1	150
Potato Sea Salt & Vinegar	1 oz	150	2	9	0	16	1	160
Potato Spicy Thai	1 oz	150	2	9	0	15	1	180
Potato Unsalted	1 oz	150	2	9	0	15	2	0
Potato Yogurt & Green Onion	1 oz	150	2	9	0	15	1	190
Lay's								
Deli Style Original	17 (1 oz)	150	1	10	0	16	1	180
Dill Pickle	20 (1 oz)	160	2	10	0	13	1	360
Kettle Cooked Jalapeno	15 (1 oz)	140	2	8	0	16	1	170
Kettle Cooked Mesquite BBQ	18 (1 oz)	140	2	8	0	16	tr	210
Kettle Cooked Original	22 (1 oz)	150	2	8	0	16	1	190
Light Fat Free KC Masterpiece	20 (1 oz)	75	2	0	0	17	1	250
Light Fat Free Original	20 (1 oz)	75	2	0	0	18	1	200
Limon	17 (1 oz)	150	2	10	0	15	1	370
Natural Country BBQ	14 (1 oz)	150	2	9	0	16	1	150
Natural Sea Salted	16 (1 oz)	150	2	9	0	15	tr	320
Original Baked	11 (1 oz)	110	2	2	0	23	2	150
Stax	13 (1 oz)	160	1	10	0	15	1	160
Wavy Au Gratin	13 (1 oz)	150	2	10	<5	14	1	200
Wavy Hickory Barbecue	13 (1 oz)	150	2	9	0	16	1	210
Wavy Ranch	12 (1 oz)	150	2	10	0	16	1	200
Lundberg								
Rice Chips Original Sea Salt	1 oz	140	2	7	0	18	tr	110
Rice Chips Sesame Seaweed	1 oz	140	2	7	0	18	tr	90
Rice Chips Wasabi	1 oz	140	2	6	0	18	1	210
Madhouse Munchies								
Potato Sea Salt	16	150	2	9	0	16	1	80
Potato Sea Salt & Vinegar	16	150	2	9	0	16	2	130
Tortilla White	9	140	2	6	0	19	1	110
Manny's								
Organic Tortilla Blues	1 oz	150	2	7	0	20	3	140
Tortilla No Salt Added	1 oz	150	2	7	0	20	3	0
Maui								
Shrimp Chips	17	140	tr	8	0	19	tr	220

FOOD	PORTION	CALS	PROT	FAT	CHOL	CARB	FIBER	SOD
Moore's								
Corn Chips	1 oz	160	1	10	0	16	1	180
New York Deli								
Potato Kettle Cooked	1 oz	150	2	9	0	15	1	170
Popchips								
Corn Hint Of Butter	23 (1 oz)	120	2	5	0	17	2	190
Potato Barbeque	19 (1 oz)	120	1	5	0	20	1	230
Potato Original	22 (1 oz)	120	1	5	0	20	1	290
Rice Sea Salt	19 (1 oz)	120	2	5	0	17	1	160
Rice Wasabi	20 (1 oz)	120	2	5	0	17	1	160
Pringles								
Jalapeno	15 (1 oz)	150	1	10	0	14	tr	190
Loaded Baked Potato	15 (1 oz)	150	1	10	0	14	tr	170
Minis Cheddar Cheese	1 pkg	120	1	7	0	12	tr	220
Minis Original	1 pkg	120	1	7	0	13	tr	140
Original	14 (1 oz)	160	1	11	0	14	tr	170
Pizza	15 (1 oz)	150	1	10	0	14	tr	190
Select Cinnamon Sweet Potato	28 (1 oz)	150	1	9	0	16	1	15
Select Parmesan Garlic	28 (1 oz)	140	1	9	0	15	tr	180
Snack Stacks Original	1 pkg	140	1	10	0	12	tr	150
Ruffles								
Baked Original	10	120	2	3	0	21	2	200
Cheddar & Sour Cream	11	160	2	10	0	14	1	230
KC Masterpiece Mesquite BBQ	11	150	2	10	0	15	1	190
Light Cheddar & Sour Cream	15	75	3	0	0	16	1	230
Original	12	160	2	10	0	14	1	160
Potato Crisps	16	160	1	10	0	16	1	230
Sour Cream & Onion	11	160	2	10	0	14	1	190
Santitas								
White Corn	9	130	2	6	0	19	1	110
Yellow Corn	9	130	2	6	0	19	1	110
Snyder's Of Hanover								
Kosher Dill	1 oz	140	2	6	0	20	4	360
MultiGrain Sunflower	1 oz	140	2	6	0	20	2	190
MultiGrain Sunflower Southwestern Cheddar	1 oz	140	2	6	0	20	2	190

FOOD	PORTION	CALS	PROT	FAT	CHOL	CARB	FIBER	SOD
MultiGrain Tortilla Lightly Salted	1 oz	130	2	5	0	20	3	110
MultiGrain Tortilla Strips Flaxseed Gold	1 oz	140	2	6	0	18	2	230
Organic Veggie Crisps	1 oz	140	1	7	0	18	2	290
Potato Original	1 oz	150	2	7	0	19	3	90
Sweet Potato Baked	1 oz	110	1	2	0	23	1	310
Tortilla White Corn	1 oz	140	2	5	0	23	2	110
Tortilla Pounder Multi-Grain	1 oz	130	2	5	0	20	2	110
Solea								
Polenta Corn	1 oz	120	2	4	0	20	0	250
Potato Olive Oil Sea Salt	1 oz	120	2	6	0	14	1	110
Stacy's								
Pita Chips Multigrain	1 pkg	140	3	6	0	17	2	240
Pita Chips Parmesan Garlic & Herb	1 oz	140	4	5	0	19	2	200
Pita Chips Texarkana Hot	1 oz	130	3	5	0	19	2	260
Soy Thin Chips Sticky Bun	18 (1 oz)	130	6	5	0	15	3	180
Soy Thin Crisps Simply Cheese	18 (1 oz)	130	7	6	0	13	3	230
SunChips								
French Onion	10	140	2	6	0	18	2	160
Original	1 pkg (1 oz)	140	2	6	0	18	2	120
Tastee								
Potato Yukon Gold	1 oz	130	3	5	0	19	1	160
Terra								
Exotic Vegetable Original	14 (1 oz)	150	7	9	0	16	3	150
Exotic Vegetable Zesty Tomato	14 (1 oz)	150	1	9	0	16	3	190
Kettles Potato Sea Salt & Pepper	15 (1 oz)	140	2	6	0	18	tr	65
Parsnip Chips	12 (1 oz)	150	2	10	0	13	5	50
Potato Au Natural	18 (1 oz)	150	2	9	0	15	2	0
Potato Blues	1 oz	130	2	6	0	19	3	115
Potato Golds Original	1 oz	130	2	5	0	19	0	80
Potato Potpourri	1 oz	140	2	7	0	17	4	110
Potato Red Bliss	1 oz	140	1	7	0	18	2	110
Potato Frites Sea Salt & Vinegar	1 oz	150	2	8	0	18	3	200

FOOD	PORTION	CALS	PROT	FAT	CHOL	CARB	FIBER	SOD
Stix Original Exotic Vegetable	1 oz	150	1	9	0	16	3	110
Sweet Potato	17 (1 oz)	160	1	11	0	15	3	10
Sweets & Beets	16 (1 oz)	150	2	9	0	15	1	5
Taro	1 oz	140	1	6	0	19	4	110
Tostitos								
Blue Corn	6	140	2	6	0	19	1	80
Crispy Rounds	13	140	2	7	0	18	1	120
Gold	6	140	2	7	0	19	1	110
Light Restaurant Style	6	90	2	1	0	20	1	105
Original Bite Size	20	110	3	1	0	24	2	200
Restaurant Style	6	130	2	6	0	19	1	80
Santa Fe	7	140	1	6	0	19	1	80
Scoops	13	140	2	7	0	18	1	120
Yellow Corn	6	140	2	6	0	19	1	80
Utz								
Pita Natural w/ Sea Salt	1 oz	120	3	5	0	18	tr	140
Potato	20 (1 oz)	150	2	9	0	14	1	95
Potato Baked	1 oz	110	2	2	0	23	2	170
Potato BBQ	20 (1 oz)	150	2	10	0	14	1	200
Potato Grandma Kettle	1 oz	140	2	8	5	14	1	120
Potato Homestyle Kettle	1 oz	140	2	8	0	14	1	120
Potato Kettle Classics	20 (1 oz)	150	2	9	0	15	1	120
Potato Mystic Kettle	1 oz	150	2	9	0	15	1	120
Potato Mystic Kettle Reduced Fat	1 oz	130	2	6	0	18	1	120
Potato Natural Lightly Salted Kettle	1 oz	140	2	8	0	15	1	95
Potato No Salt Added	20 (1 oz)	150	2	9	0	14	1	5
Potato Onion & Garlic	1 oz	150	2	9	0	14	1	180
Potato Ripple	20 (1 oz)	150	2	10	0	14	1	95
Sweet Potato Kettle Classics	20 (1 oz)	150	1	9	0	16	2	65
Tortilla Baked	10	120	2	2	0	23	1	125
Tortilla Organic Yellow Corn	1 oz	140	2	6	0	19	2	100
Vegetable Natural Exotic Medley	1 oz	160	2	10	0	15	2	110
Wise								
Dipsy Doodles Corn Chips	1 oz	160	1	10	0	16	1	180
Potato	1 pkg (1 oz)	150	2	10	0	14	1	190
Potato Lightly Salted	1 oz	150	2	10	0	14	1	80

FOOD	PORTION	CALS	PROT	FAT	CHOL	CARB	FIBER	SOD
Potato Ridgies	1 oz	150	2	10	0	14	1	190
Potato Unsalted	1 oz	150	2	10	0	14	1	0

CHITTERLINGS
pork cooked	3 oz	258	9	24	122	0	0	33

CHIVES
freeze-dried	1 tbsp	1	tr	tr	0	tr	–	–
fresh chopped	1 tbsp	1	tr	tr	0	tr	–	0
fresh chopped	1 tsp	0	tr	tr	0	tr	–	0

CHOCOLATE (see also CANDY, CHOCOLATE SPREAD, CHOCOLATE SYRUP, COCOA, HOT COCOA, ICE CREAM TOPPINGS, MILK DRINKS)

FOOD	PORTION	CALS	PROT	FAT	CHOL	CARB	FIBER	SOD
baking	1 oz	145	3	15	0	8	–	1
baking grated unsweetened	¼ cup	165	4	17	0	10	6	8
baking liquid unsweetened	1 oz	134	3	14	0	10	5	3
baking squares unsweetened	1 square (1 oz)	145	4	15	0	9	5	7
chips milk chocolate	1 cup (6 oz)	862	12	52	38	100	–	138
chips semisweet	60 pieces (1 oz)	136	1	9	0	18	–	3
chips semisweet	1 cup (6 oz)	804	7	50	0	106	–	19
drink mix powder	2–3 heaping tsp	75	1	1	0	20	–	45
mexican baking	1 sq (0.7 oz)	85	1	3	0	15	1	1
Baker's								
Chips Chocolate Chunks	13 pieces (0.5 oz)	70	tr	5	0	9	tr	5
E. Guittard								
Chips Cappuccino	30 (0.5 oz)	80	tr	5	0	9	0	15
Chips Milk Chocolate	12 (0.5 oz)	80	1	5	5	9	0	10
Chips Semisweet	30 (0.5 oz)	70	tr	4	0	10	tr	0
Love'n Bake								
Chocolate Schmear	2 tbsp	140	4	8	0	14	2	0
M&M's								
Baking Bits Milk Chocolate	1 tbsp	70	1	4	5	10	0	10
Baking Bits Semi-Sweet Chocolate	1 tbsp	70	1	4	0	9	1	0
Sunfood								
Organic Cacao Beans	1 oz	171	4	13	0	8	6	15
Organic Cacao Nibs	1 oz	171	4	13	0	8	6	15
Organic Powder	2 tbsp (1 oz)	120	6	4	0	15	9	6

FOOD	PORTION	CALS	PROT	FAT	CHOL	CARB	FIBER	SOD
CHOCOLATE MILK (see MILK DRINKS)								
CHOCOLATE SYRUP								
chocolate fudge	1 tbsp (0.7 oz)	73	1	3	–	12	–	27
chocolate fudge	1 cup (11.9 oz)	1176	15	46	–	200	–	442
syrup	2 tbsp	82	1	tr	0	22	–	36
syrup	1 cup	653	6	3	0	177	–	287
syrup as prep w/ whole milk	9 oz	232	9	9	33	34	–	156
Hershey's								
Syrup	2 tbsp	100	tr	0	0	25	–	25
Nesquik								
Calcium Fortified	2 tbsp	100	0	0	0	27	1	55
Smucker's								
Sundae Syrup Chocolate	2 tbsp	110	1	0	0	26	1	20
CHUTNEY								
apple	1.2 oz	68	tr	0	–	18	1	–
coconut	2 oz	87	1	9	0	1	3	217
fresh mint	2 oz	18	1	0	0	3	1	432
mango	1 tbsp	54	tr	2	0	10	tr	207
tomato	1 oz	90	1	7	6	6	2	269
Patak's								
Major Grey	1 tbsp	60	0	0	0	14	0	290
Mango Hot	1 tbsp	60	0	0	0	14	0	300
Mango Sweet	1 tbsp	60	0	1	0	14	0	310
Robert Rothchild Farm								
Hot Peach & Apple	2 tbsp	45	0	0	0	12	tr	35
School House Kitchen								
Bardshar	1 oz	80	0	0	0	20	1	240
CILANTRO								
fresh	¼ cup	1	tr	tr	0	tr	tr	2
fresh sprigs	5 (5 g)	1	tr	tr	0	tr	tr	3
Dorot								
Chopped Cube frzn	1 cube (4 g)	5	tr	tr	0	tr	tr	17
CINNAMON								
cinnamon sugar	1 tsp	16	tr	tr	0	4	tr	0
ground	1 tsp	6	tr	tr	0	2	1	0
sticks	0.5 oz	39	1	tr	–	8	3	4

FOOD	PORTION	CALS	PROT	FAT	CHOL	CARB	FIBER	SOD
CISCO								
raw	3 oz	84	16	2	–	0	0	47
smoked	1 oz	50	5	3	9	0	0	135
CLAMS								
CANNED								
liquid only	1 cup	6	1	tr	–	tr	–	516
liquid only	3 oz	2	tr	tr	–	tr	–	183
meat only	3 oz	126	22	2	57	4	–	95
meat only	1 cup	236	41	3	107	8	–	179
Brunswick								
Baby	2 oz	50	8	1	25	0	0	360
Bumble Bee								
Baby	¼ cup	50	9	1	40	2	0	270
Chopped Or Minced	¼ cup	25	4	0	10	2	0	320
Smoked	¼ cup	130	11	9	40	1	0	460
Chicken Of The Sea								
Chopped	¼ cup	30	5	0	12	2	0	370
Minced	¼ cup	30	5	0	12	2	–	370
Whole Baby	¼ cup	30	6	0	10	1	0	290
Orleans								
Clam Juice	1 tbsp	0	1	0	0	0	0	100
FRESH								
cooked	3 oz	126	22	2	57	4	–	95
cooked	20 sm	133	23	2	60	5	–	100
raw	9 lg (6.3 oz)	133	23	2	60	5	–	100
raw	3 oz	63	11	1	29	2	–	47
raw	20 sm (6.3 oz)	133	23	2	60	5	–	100
FROZEN								
Mrs. Paul's								
Fried	18 (3 oz)	270	9	13	20	29	1	690
TAKE-OUT								
breaded & fried	20 sm	379	27	21	115	19	–	684
CLEMENTINE JUICE								
Izze								
Sparkling Clementine	8 oz	100	0	0	0	23	–	10

FOOD	PORTION	CALS	PROT	FAT	CHOL	CARB	FIBER	SOD
CLEMENTINES								
Sunkist								
Fresh	2	80	1	0	0	17	4	0
Tina								
Fresh	1	50	1	1	0	15	3	0
CLOVES								
ground	1 tsp	7	tr	tr	0	1	1	5
COCOA (see also HOT COCOA)								
powder unsweetened	1 tbsp (5 g)	11	1	1	0	3	2	1
powder unsweetened	1 cup (3 oz)	197	17	12	0	47	29	18
COCONUT								
dried sweetened shredded	¼ cup	116	1	8	0	11	1	61
dried toasted	1 oz	168	2	13	0	13	–	10
dried unsweetened	1 oz	187	2	18	0	7	5	10
fresh from 1 coconut	14 oz	1405	13	133	0	60	36	79
fresh shredded	¼ cup	71	1	7	0	3	2	4
Bob's Red Mill								
Shredded	3 tbsp	120	1	11	0	4	2	5
Frieda's								
White	¼ cup (1.4 oz)	140	1	13	0	6	4	10
Let's Do Organic								
Organic Reduced Fat Shredded	1 can (0.5 oz)	70	1	6	0	4	2	0
Shredded	3 tbsp (0.5 oz)	110	1	10	0	4	2	5
Prosperity								
Organic Coconut Flax Butter Garlic & Onion	1 tbsp	140	0	15	0	0	0	0
COCONUT JUICE								
coconut water fresh	½ cup	23	1	tr	0	4	1	126
milk canned	½ cup	276	3	29	0	7	3	18
A Taste Of Thai								
Coconut Milk	⅓ cup	140	1	15	0	3	0	20
Lite Coconut Milk	⅓ cup	45	1	4	0	3	0	20
Goya								
Coconut Water	1 can (11.8 oz)	120	0	1	0	29	tr	130

FOOD	PORTION	CALS	PROT	FAT	CHOL	CARB	FIBER	SOD
Let's Do Organic								
Creamed	1 oz	220	4	19	0	8	6	10
Milk	¼ cup	100	1	11	0	2	0	5
O.N.E.								
Natural Coconut Water	1 box (11 oz)	60	1	0	0	15	0	35
Vita Coco								
Coconut Water	1 box (11 oz)	65	0	0	0	17	–	65
Coconut Water w/ Fruit Juice All Flavors	1 box (11 oz)	110	0	0	0	27	5	35
COD								
atlantic canned	3 oz	89	19	1	47	0	0	185
atlantic canned	1 can (11 oz)	327	71	3	171	0	0	680
atlantic dried	3 oz	246	53	2	129	0	0	5973
atlantic fresh cooked	1 fillet (6.3 oz)	189	41	2	99	0	0	141
atlantic fresh cooked	3 oz	89	19	1	47	0	0	66
atlantic fresh raw	3 oz	70	15	1	37	0	0	46
pacific fresh baked	3 oz	95	21	1	43	0	0	82
roe canned	1 oz	34	6	1	–	tr	–	–
roe tarama	3.5 oz	547	8	55	–	6	–	600
Mrs. Paul's								
Filets Lightly Breaded	1 (4 oz)	220	12	11	40	17	1	430
TAKE-OUT								
roe baked w/ butter & lemon juice	1 oz	36	6	1	–	tr	–	21
COFFEE (see also COFFEE BEVERAGES, COFFEE SUBSTITUTES)								
INSTANT								
decaffeinated as prep	8 oz	2	tr	0	0	0	0	5
decaffeinated powder	1 rounded tsp	4	tr	0	0	1	0	0
powder	1 rounded tsp	4	tr	tr	0	1	0	64
REGULAR								
brewed	8 oz	2	tr	tr	0	0	0	5
roasted beans	1 oz	64	4	4	–	18	2	–
Flavia								
English Breakfast	1 bag	0	0	0	0	0	0	0
Espresso Roast	1 bag	0	0	0	0	0	0	0
French Roast	1 bag	0	0	0	0	0	0	0
French Vanilla	1 bag	0	0	0	0	0	0	0

FOOD	PORTION	CALS	PROT	FAT	CHOL	CARB	FIBER	SOD
Soy Java								
All Flavors	1 tbsp	20	5	0	0	0	0	0
Spava								
Calm Decaffeinated	1 cup	0	0	0	0	0	0	0

COFFEE BEVERAGES

FOOD	PORTION	CALS	PROT	FAT	CHOL	CARB	FIBER	SOD
America's Best Brew								
Iced Coffee All Flavors	8 oz	110	3	2	0	25	–	15
Cafe Sepia								
House Blend	1 bottle (6.2 oz)	80	2	0	5	15	0	70
Mocha	1 bottle (6.2 oz)	70	1	0	0	14	0	40
Cinnabon								
Lattes All Flavors	1 can (9.5 oz)	190	4	5	15	32	1	260
Cool Java								
Cappuccino Dark Roast	1 bottle (11 oz)	190	4	3	15	39	0	240
Cappuccino French Vanilla	1 bottle (11 oz)	190	4	3	15	38	0	210
Cappuccino Mocha	1 bottle (11 oz)	190	4	3	15	38	0	190
Double Bean Elixir								
Coffee Soda All Flavors	8 oz	90	0	0	0	23	–	0
Double Hit								
Maximum Energy Coffee Drink	1 can (12 oz)	80	0	0	0	20	–	65
Frappio								
Iced Coffee Energy Drink	1 can (15 oz)	260	6	4	30	42	0	270
Froid								
Original or French Vanilla	1 bottle (11 oz)	180	6	3	10	34	1	260
General Foods								
International Coffees Cafe Francais	1 serv	60	0	3	0	8	–	90
International Coffees Cafe Vienna	1 serv	70	0	2	0	12	–	110

FOOD	PORTION	CALS	PROT	FAT	CHOL	CARB	FIBER	SOD
International Coffees Cafe Vienna Sugar Free	1 serv	30	0	2	0	2	–	60
International Coffees Creme Caramel	1 serv	60	0	2	–	12	–	50
International Coffees French Vanilla Cafe	1 serv	60	0	3	0	10	–	55
International Coffees French Vanilla Sugar & Fat Free Decaffeinated	1 serv	30	0	3	0	2	–	50
International Coffees French Vanilla Sugar Free	1 serv	30	0	3	0	2	–	50
International Coffees Italian Cappuccino	1 serv	50	0	2	0	10	–	45
International Coffees Orange Cappuccino	1 serv	70	0	2	0	12	–	100
International Coffees Suisse Mocha	1 serv	60	0	2	0	10	–	40
International Coffees Suisse Mocha Decaffeinated Sugar Free	1 serv	30	0	5	0	2	–	30
International Coffees Suisse Mocha Sugar Free	1 serv	30	0	2	0	2	–	30
International Coffees Swiss White Chocolate	1 serv	70	0	3	0	12	–	30
International Coffees Vanilla Creme Decaffeinate Sugar Free	1 serv	35	0	3	0	3	–	50
International Coffees Vanilla Creme Decaffeinated	1 serv	60	1	3	0	11	–	25
International Coffees Viennese Chocolate Cafe	1 serv	50	0	2	0	11	–	25
Godiva								
Latte French Vanilla	1 bottle (12 oz)	200	6	4	15	36	0	140
Mocha Dark Chocolate	1 bottle (16 oz)	200	6	4	15	37	1	160
Iced 'Spresso								
Ultra Light American Vanilla	1 bottle (9.5 oz)	90	6	3	10	11	0	180

FOOD	PORTION	CALS	PROT	FAT	CHOL	CARB	FIBER	SOD
Ultra Light Expresso Latte	1 bottle (9.5 oz)	70	6	0	0	11	0	190
Loco-Joe								
Iced Coffee	1 box (8.25 oz)	160	6	4	15	26	0	120
Shock								
Latte	8 oz	150	4	3	7	28	tr	110
Triple Latte	1 can (8 oz)	125	4	2	–	27	0	125
Triple Mocha	1 can (8 oz)	125	4	2	–	27	0	125
Starbucks								
DoubleShot	1 (6.5 oz)	140	4	6	20	18	–	70
Stomping Grounds								
Latte Caramel not prep	⅓ cup	70	0	0	0	18	0	0
Latte Espresso not prep	⅓ cup	35	0	0	0	9	0	0
Latte Mocha not prep	⅓ cup	60	0	0	0	15	0	0
Latte Vanilla not prep	⅓ cup	60	0	0	0	14	0	0
Tully's Coffee								
Bellaccino All Flavors	1 bottle (9.5 oz)	210	6	4	20	36	0	100
Wolfgang Puck								
Gourmet Heated Lattes All Flavors	1 can (10 oz)	100	5	5	25	9	0	105
TAKE-OUT								
cafe amaretto w/ alcohol	1 serv	192	1	9	33	15	0	14
cafe au lait	1 cup (8 oz)	77	4	4	17	6	–	62
cafe brulot	1 cup	48	tr	0	0	3	–	2
cafe brulot w/ alcohol	1 serv	130	1	tr	0	16	3	4
cappuccino	1 cup (8 oz)	77	4	4	17	6	–	62
coffee con leche	1 cup (6 oz)	104	3	4	10	16	0	36
cuban coffee w/ rum & creme de cacao	1 (9 oz)	112	3	2	–	6	0	–
dutch coffee w/ gin	1 (7 oz)	181	1	10	29	6	0	19
espresso	1 cup (4 oz)	2	tr	tr	0	0	0	17
french coffee w/ orange liqueur & kahlua	1 (8 oz)	232	1	10	29	24	0	–
irish coffee	1 serv (8 oz)	209	1	11	38	5	0	13
italian coffee w/ strega	1 (7 oz)	163	1	10	–	12	0	19
latte w/ skim milk	1 serv (13 oz)	88	8	tr	4	12	0	128

FOOD	PORTION	CALS	PROT	FAT	CHOL	CARB	FIBER	SOD
latte w/ whole milk	1 serv (14 oz)	143	9	6	20	15	0	126
mocha	1 serv (17 oz)	403	11	9	29	69	2	199
puerto rican coffee w/ rum & kahlua	1 (8 oz)	166	1	10	29	9	0	–
turkish	1 cup (4 oz)	50	tr	1	0	12	0	1

COFFEE SUBSTITUTES
Pixie
Mate Latte Chai	½ cup (4 oz)	80	0	0	0	18	tr	5
Mate Latte Dark Roast	½ cup (4 oz)	70	0	0	0	16	tr	0
Mate Latte Mocha	½ cup (4 oz)	70	0	0	0	18	0	0
Mate Latte Original	½ cup (4 oz)	70	0	0	0	17	0	0

Teeccino
Herbal Coffee All Flavors	1 cup	15	0	0	0	3	1	2

COFFEE WHITENERS
Coffee-Mate
Half & Half Original	2 tbsp	40	tr	4	15	1	–	70
Half & Half Vanilla	2 tbsp	60	tr	4	15	7	–	60
Latte Classic	2 tbsp	100	1	6	0	12	–	125
Latte Mocha	2 tbsp	90	tr	4	0	14	–	125
Latte Vanilla	2 tbsp	90	0	4	0	14	–	125
Liquid All Flavors	1 tbsp	40	0	2	0	5	–	5
Liquid French Vanilla Fat Free	1 tbsp	10	0	0	5	2	–	0
Liquid Original	1 tbsp	20	0	1	0	2	–	0
Liquid Original Fat Free	1 tbsp	10	0	0	0	2	–	0
Liquid Original Low Fat	1 tbsp	10	1	1	0	–	–	5
Original Powder	1 tsp	10	0	0	0	1	–	0
Original Lite Powder	1 tsp	10	0	0	0	2	–	0
Sugar Free All Flavors	1 tbsp	15	0	1	0	1	–	5

Farmland
Nondairy Creamer	2 tbsp	40	1	3	15	2	0	15

FOOD	PORTION	CALS	PROT	FAT	CHOL	CARB	FIBER	SOD
Hood								
Country Creamer Non Dairy	1 tbsp	20	0	2	0	2	0	0
International Delight								
Amaretto	1 tbsp	40	0	2	0	7	0	0
Fat Free Amaretto	1 tbsp	30	0	0	0	7	0	5
Fat Free French Vanilla	1 tbsp	30	0	0	0	7	0	5
Fat Free Irish Creme	1 tbsp	30	0	0	0	7	0	5
French Vanilla	1 tbsp	45	0	2	0	7	0	5
Sugar Free French Vanilla	1 tbsp	20	0	2	0	1	0	5
WildWood								
Soymilk Creamer Plain	1 tbsp	15	0	2	0	1	0	0
COLESLAW								
Dole								
Classic Cole Slaw	1½ cups (3 oz)	25	1	0	0	5	2	25
Fresh Express								
3 Color Deli	1½ cups	20	1	0	0	5	2	20
Mann's								
Broccoli Cole Slaw w/o Dressing	1 serv (3 oz)	25	2	0	0	5	3	25
River Ranch								
Country Homestyle Kit	1 cup	140	1	9	6	14	2	160
Honey Dijon Peppercorn Kit	1 cup	120	1	8	9	11	2	220
Mix	1¼ cups	25	1	0	0	5	2	15
TAKE-OUT								
coleslaw w/ dressing	¾ cup	147	1	11	5	13	–	267
vinegar & oil coleslaw	3.5 oz	150	1	9	0	16	–	480
COLLARDS								
fresh cooked	½ cup	17	1	tr	0	4	–	10
frzn chopped cooked	½ cup	31	3	tr	0	6	–	42
raw chopped	½ cup	6	tr	tr	0	1	–	4
Allens								
Seasoned Southern Style	½ cup	35	3	1	0	5	1	830
Glory								
Green Fresh	2 cups	25	2	0	0	5	3	15
Seasoned canned	½ cup	35	2	0	0	5	2	490
Sensibly Seasoned canned	½ cup	20	2	0	0	4	2	240

FOOD	PORTION	CALS	PROT	FAT	CHOL	CARB	FIBER	SOD
COOKIES								
MIX								
chocolate chip	1 (0.56 oz)	79	1	4	7	10	–	47
oatmeal	1 (0.6 oz)	74	1	3	7	10	tr	75
oatmeal raisin	1 (0.6 oz)	74	1	3	7	10	tr	75
Bob's Red Mill								
Gluten Free Chocolate Chip as prep	2	260	2	10	39	41	2	180
King Arthur								
Chocolate Chip Whole Grain not prep	2 tbsp	90	2	3	0	16	1	35
Nature's Path								
Organic Chocolate Chip	1/10 pkg	150	4	2	0	31	3	260
Pillsbury								
Ready To Bake Chocolate Chip Sugar Free	1	90	1	4	–	16	3	85
READY-TO-EAT								
animal	11 (1 oz)	126	2	4	–	21	–	112
animal crackers	1 box (2.4 oz)	299	4	9	11	51	–	274
animal crackers	1 (2.5 g)	11	tr	tr	–	2	–	10
australian anzac biscuit	1	98	1	3	0	17	1	59
butter	1 (5 g)	23	tr	1	–	3	tr	18
chocolate chip	1 (0.4 oz)	48	1	2	–	7	tr	32
chocolate chip	1 box (1.9 oz)	233	3	12	12	36	–	188
chocolate chip low fat	1 (0.25 oz)	45	1	2	0	7	–	38
chocolate chip low sugar low sodium	1 (0.24 oz)	31	tr	1	0	5	–	1
chocolate chip soft-type	1 (0.5 oz)	69	1	4	0	9	tr	49
chocolate w/ creme filling	1 (0.35 oz)	47	1	2	–	7	tr	36
chocolate w/ creme filling chocolate coated	1 (0.60 oz)	82	1	5	–	11	–	55
chocolate w/ creme filling sugar free low sodium	1 (0.35 oz)	46	1	2	–	7	–	24
chocolate w/ extra creme filling	1 (0.46 oz)	65	1	3	–	9	–	64
chocolate wafer	1 (0.2 oz)	26	tr	1	0	4	–	35
cream cheese	1 (1.1 oz)	141	2	9	25	14	tr	53
digestive biscuits plain	2	141	2	7	–	21	1	–

FOOD	PORTION	CALS	PROT	FAT	CHOL	CARB	FIBER	SOD
fig bars	1 (0.56 oz)	56	1	1	–	11	1	56
fortune	1 (0.28 oz)	30	tr	tr	–	7	tr	22
fudge	1 (0.73 oz)	73	1	1	–	17	tr	40
gingersnaps	1 (0.24 oz)	29	tr	1	0	5	–	48
graham	1 square (0.24 oz)	30	1	1	0	5	–	42
graham chocolate covered	1 (0.49 oz)	68	1	3	0	9	–	41
graham honey	1 (0.24 oz)	30	1	1	0	5	tr	42
hermits	1 (1 oz)	117	2	5	23	18	1	54
jumbles coconut	1 (1 oz)	121	1	7	26	13	1	19
ladyfingers	1 (0.38 oz)	40	1	1	40	7	–	16
macaroons	1 (0.8 oz)	97	1	3	0	17	–	59
madeleines	1 (0.8 oz)	86	2	5	46	10	tr	34
marshmallow chocolate coated	1 (0.46 oz)	55	1	2	–	9	–	22
marshmallow pie chocolate coated	1 (1.4 oz)	165	2	7	–	26	–	66
molasses	1 (0.5 oz)	65	1	2	0	11	–	69
oatmeal	1 (0.6 oz)	81	1	3	0	12	1	69
oatmeal soft-type	1 (0.5 oz)	61	1	2	–	10	tr	52
oatmeal raisin	1 (0.6 oz)	81	1	3	0	12	1	69
oatmeal raisin low sugar no sodium	1 (0.24 oz)	31	tr	1	0	5	–	1
oatmeal raisin soft-type	1 (0.5 oz)	61	1	2	–	10	tr	52
peanut butter sandwich	1 (0.5 oz)	67	1	3	0	9	–	52
peanut butter sandwich sugar free low sodium	1 (0.35 oz)	54	1	3	–	5	–	41
peanut butter soft-type	1 (0.5 oz)	69	1	4	0	9	tr	50
pinenut cookies	1 (1.1 oz)	134	4	9	0	11	1	11
raisin soft-type	1 (0.5 oz)	60	1	2	0	10	–	51
reginette queen's biscuit	1 (0.8 oz)	86	2	3	tr	13	tr	83
shortbread	1 (0.28 oz)	40	1	2	2	5	–	36
shortbread pecan	1 (0.49 oz)	79	1	5	5	8	tr	39
spritz	1 (0.4 oz)	42	1	2	6	6	tr	9
sugar	1 (0.52 oz)	72	1	3	8	10	–	53
sugar low sugar	1 (0.24 oz)	30	1	1	0	5	–	0
sugar wafers w/ creme filling	1 (0.12 oz)	18	tr	1	0	3	–	5
sugar wafers w/ creme filling sugar free sodium free	1 (0.14 oz)	20	tr	1	0	3	–	0

FOOD	PORTION	CALS	PROT	FAT	CHOL	CARB	FIBER	SOD
toll house original	1 (0.8 oz)	105	2	6	15	13	tr	57
vanilla sandwich	1 (0.35 oz)	48	tr	2	0	7	tr	35
vanilla wafers	1 (0.21 oz)	28	tr	1	–	4	–	18
zeppole	1 (0.8 oz)	78	1	6	24	6	tr	14
ABC								
Vegan Colossal Chocolate Chip	1 (2.1 oz)	240	3	7	0	41	1	190
Vegan Double Chocolate Decadence	1 (2.1 oz)	240	3	8	0	39	2	120
Vegan Luscious Lemon Poppyseed	1 (2.1 oz)	240	3	7	0	40	0	125
Vegan Mac The Chip	1 (2.1 oz)	250	4	10	0	35	3	200
Vegan Peanut Butter Chocolate Chip	1 (2.1 oz)	240	4	8	0	39	1	160
Vegan Phenomenal Pumpkin Spice	1 (2.1 oz)	220	4	7	0	39	3	115
Alex & Dani's								
Original Hazelnut	3 (1 oz)	130	3	6	25	17	1	55
Annie's Homegrown								
Bunny Grahams All Flavors	26	130	2	4	0	20	tr	150
Archway								
Frosty Lemon	1 (0.9 oz)	110	1	5	0	18	0	105
Fruit Filled Raspberry	1 (0.8 oz)	90	1	3	<5	15	0	80
Arico								
Gluten Free Casein Free Almond Cranberry	1 bar (1.4 oz)	140	3	6	25	22	4	120
Gluten Free Casein Free Double Chocolate	1 (0.9 oz)	100	2	5	15	15	3	70
Gluten Free Casein Free Lemon Ginger	1 (0.9 oz)	90	2	4	15	15	3	85
Gluten Free Casein Free Peanut Butter	1 bar (1.4 oz)	160	5	7	25	19	4	140
Arrowroot								
Biscuit	1 (5 g)	20	0	1	0	4	0	15
Back To Nature								
Chocolate Chunk	2	130	1	6	0	17	tr	110
Crispy Oatmeal	2	120	1	5	0	18	tr	100
Sandwich Chocolate & Mint Creme	2	130	tr	6	0	18	tr	125
Sandwich Classic Creme	2	130	tr	6	0	18	tr	125

FOOD	PORTION	CALS	PROT	FAT	CHOL	CARB	FIBER	SOD
Bahlsen								
Hanover Waffelin	5 (1 oz)	160	1	10	0	16	0	35
Nuss Dessert	3 (1.1 oz)	170	2	11	10	17	0	75
Barbara's Bakery								
Fig Bars Traditional	1	60	0	1	0	14	–	20
Fig Bars Wheat Free	1	60	0	0	0	13	1	25
Organic 100 Calorie Mini Ginger	1 pkg (0.9 oz)	100	1	2	5	19	–	150
Snackimals Chocolate Chip	10	120	1	4	0	19	–	80
Snackimals Wheat Free Oatmeal	10	120	1	5	0	17	1	130
Barnum's								
Animal Crackers	10 (1 oz)	120	2	4	0	22	1	140
Bolands								
Custard Creams	1	62	1	3	–	8	tr	25
Cameo								
Sandwich Creme	2 (1 oz)	130	1	5	0	21	0	105
Chips Ahoy!								
Chocolate Chip	1 pkg (1.4 oz)	190	2	9	0	27	1	140
Reduced Fat	1 pkg (1.1 oz)	140	2	5	0	23	1	150
Country Choice Naturals								
Double Fudge Brownie	1 (0.8 oz)	90	1	3	5	16	tr	85
Ginger Snaps	5	120	1	5	0	19	2	85
Oatmeal Raisin	1 (0.8 oz)	100	1	3	5	16	1	70
Old Fashioned Oatmeal	1 (0.8 oz)	100	2	3	5	16	1	90
Sandwich Cremes Ginger Lemon	2	130	1	5	0	19	0	130
Sandwich Cremes Mint Creme	2	130	1	5	0	19	0	100
Sandwich Cremes Vanilla	2	130	1	5	0	19	0	125
Vanilla Wafers	7	120	1	5	5	19	2	100
Crummy								
Organic Chocolate Chip	1 (2 oz)	240	4	10	30	34	0	230
Organic Lavender Chocolate Chip	1 (2 oz)	240	4	10	30	34	0	220
Dare								
Breaktime Coconut	4	140	2	5	0	22	1	105
Breaktime Ginger	4	130	2	4	0	23	0	100

FOOD	PORTION	CALS	PROT	FAT	CHOL	CARB	FIBER	SOD
Creme Chocolate Fudge	1	100	1	5	0	13	0	60
Maple Leaf Creme	1	80	1	4	0	12	0	60
Whipper	2	130	1	5	0	21	0	45
David's								
Hamantash Raspberry	1 (0.7 oz)	85	7	6	7	12	7	60
De Beukelaer								
Pirouline	8 (1 oz)	130	3	4	15	23	tr	50
DiCamillo								
Biscotti DiPrato	5 (1 oz)	130	3	4	15	21	tr	130
Doritos								
Barras De Coco	5	120	2	4	0	21	tr	130
Dove								
Beyond Chocolate Chunk	1 (0.7 oz)	110	1	5	10	13	1	100
Chocolate Walnut Rendezous	1 (0.7 oz)	110	1	6	10	13	1	100
Milk Chocolate Moment	3 (1.1 oz)	160	2	9	5	20	1	45
Mint Chocolate Serenade	3 (1.1 oz)	160	2	8	0	19	1	70
Earthbound Farm								
Organic Ginger Snaps	2	120	2	6	20	18	0	70
Enjoy Life								
Allergen Gluten Free Gingerbread Spice	2 (1 oz)	100	1	4	0	19	2	120
Allergen Gluten Free No Oats Oatmeal	2 (1 oz)	120	1	4	0	21	1	50
Allergen Gluten Free Snickerdoodle	2 (1 oz)	130	1	5	0	21	2	110
Snack Bar Sunbutter Crunch	1 (1 oz)	140	3	5	0	20	3	110
Entenmann's								
Original Chocolate Chip	3	140	1	7	<5	20	tr	80
Soft Baked Chocolate Chunk	1 (1.3 oz)	190	2	9	15	25	0	140
Estee								
Fructose Sweetened Chocolate Chip	4	160	2	8	0	21	1	40
Fructose Sweetened Lemon	4	160	2	6	0	20	2	40
Fructose Sweetened Sandwich Chocolate	3	170	2	6	0	26	tr	40

FOOD	PORTION	CALS	PROT	FAT	CHOL	CARB	FIBER	SOD
Fructose Sweetened Sandwich Original	3	170	2	6	0	26	0	25
Fructose Sweetened Sandwich Peanut Butter	3	190	4	8	0	25	tr	50
Fructose Sweetened Vanilla	4	160	2	7	0	21	1	45
Fructose Sweetened Vanilla Sandwich	3	170	2	6	0	27	0	20
Sugar Free Chocolate Chip	3	110	2	4	0	22	1	70
Sugar Free Wafer Chocolate Creme	4	150	2	8	0	20	0	35
Sugar Free Wafer Lemon Creme	4	150	1	9	0	21	0	30
Sugar Free Wafer Peanut Butter Creme	4	150	tr	9	0	20	0	40
Sugar Free Wafer Strawberry Creme	4	150	1	9	0	21	0	25
Fauchon								
Assorted Chocolate	4 (2 oz)	330	4	15	55	34	5	165
Fox's								
Golden Crunch Creams	1	75	1	4	–	9	tr	200
French Meadow Bakery								
Gluten Free Chocolate Chip	1 (1.3 oz)	190	1	10	15	26	1	150
Frieda's								
Asian Almond	2 (1 oz)	170	2	10	0	19	0	75
Gak's Snacks								
Organic Brownie Chip	1 (1 oz)	130	2	5	0	20	1	115
Organic Chocolate Chip	1 (1 oz)	140	1	6	0	21	1	95
Organic Oatmeal	1 (1 oz)	120	2	4	0	19	2	75
Gamesa								
Animalitos	14	110	2	1	0	25	tr	160
Arcoiris Marshmallow	2	120	1	5	0	18	tr	50
Arcoiris Merengue	6	200	3	3	0	43	1	170
Emperador Chocolate	2	120	1	4	0	19	tr	105
Emperador Fresa	2	120	2	4	<5	19	tr	65
Emperador Limon	6	270	3	8	0	45	1	260
Emperador Vanilla	2	120	2	4	<5	19	0	75
Sugar Wafers Chocolate	3	160	1	7	0	23	0	30
Sugar Wafers Strawberry	3	160	1	6	0	24	0	25
Sugar Wafers Vanilla	3	160	1	7	0	25	0	25

FOOD	PORTION	CALS	PROT	FAT	CHOL	CARB	FIBER	SOD
Ginger Snaps								
Cookies	4 (1 oz)	120	1	3	0	23	0	190
Girl Scout								
Cafe Cookies	5	150	3	7	0	20	1	65
Lemon Cooler Reduced Fat	5	130	1	4	0	22	0	115
Samoas	2	150	1	8	0	19	tr	55
Tagalongs	2	130	2	9	0	13	1	90
Thin Mints	4	140	1	7	0	18	tr	100
Trefoils	4	130	2	6	0	17	0	85
Gluten-Free Pantry								
Gluten Free Buckwheat Raisin	1 (1 oz)	140	1	6	5	21	1	135
Gluten Free Chocolate Chunk	1 (1 oz)	140	1	8	5	19	1	120
Glutino								
Gluten Free Wafers Chocolate	4	160	1	8	5	19	3	25
Gluten Free Wafers Lemon	3	150	0	6	0	24	0	25
Gottena								
Exquisit	5	170	2	10	0	19	1	25
Gourmet Pastries								
Kourabiethes Butter Almond	1 (1.1 oz)	150	2	9	25	15	1	110
Phoenicia Honey & Spice	1 (1.3 oz)	140	2	5	0	20	0	60
Grandma's								
Homestyle Big Oatmeal Raisin	1 (1.4 oz)	180	2	6	10	30	1	240
Vanilla Creme Sandwich	5	210	2	10	5	30	tr	125
Healthy Handfuls								
Organic Crocodile Cookies	1 pkg (1 oz)	130	2	5	0	20	7	75
Organic Koala Krackers	1 pkg (1 oz)	120	2	4	5	21	2	35
Honey Maid								
Grahams Honey	1 (1.1 oz)	130	2	4	0	24	1	180
Grahams Honey Low Fat	1 (1.1 oz)	120	2	2	0	25	1	190
Jacob's								
Oat Crumbles Chocolate & Pecan	1	107	1	6	–	13	1	40
Joseph's								
Almond Sugar Free	4	100	1	5	0	13	1	20
Chocolate Chip Sugar Free	4	95	1	5	0	13	1	40

FOOD	PORTION	CALS	PROT	FAT	CHOL	CARB	FIBER	SOD
Lemon Sugar Free	4	95	1	4	0	15	0	30
Oatmeal Chocolate Chip w/ Pecans Sugar Free	4	100	1	6	0	14	1	40
Peanut Butter Sugar Free	4	95	1	5	0	14	0	40
Kashi								
TLC Happy Trail Mix	1 (1 oz)	130	2	5	0	21	4	80
TLC Oatmeal Raisin Flax	1 (1 oz)	130	2	5	0	20	4	75
TLC Oatmeal Dark Chocolate	1 (1 oz)	130	2	5	0	21	3	70
Keebler								
100 Calorie Pack Sandies Shortbread	1 pkg	100	0	3	0	17	tr	90
Chocolate Dip & Cookie Sticks	1 pkg (1 oz)	130	1	6	0	18	tr	65
Sandies Fruit Delights Lemon	1 (0.6 oz)	80	0	4	<5	11	0	55
Sandies Fudge Drops	4 (1 oz)	140	1	7	0	18	tr	60
S'mores Snack	1 pkg (0.8 oz)	110	1	6	0	14	0	40
Soft Batch Chocolate Chip	1 (0.6 oz)	80	tr	4	0	10	tr	70
Laura's Wholesome Junk Food								
Anna Banana Split	1	105	2	5	0	13	1	90
Gluten Free Charlotte's Chocolate Chip	2	120	2	6	0	16	1	90
Gluten Free Sally's Raisin	2	110	2	5	0	16	tr	90
Lemon Vanilla	2	120	2	6	0	15	1	90
Oatmeal Chocolate Chip	2	110	2	5	0	14	1	88
Oatmeal Raisin	2	100	2	4	0	11	1	88
Wheat Free X-Treme Chocolate Fudge	2	110	2	5	0	13	2	95
Lee's								
Dreamy Mallows	2	150	1	5	0	25	0	10
Leibniz								
Butter Biscuits	6	130	2	3	10	23	1	190
Liz Lovely								
Vegan Cowboy	½ cookie (1.3 oz)	190	3	9	0	24	2	90
Vegan Cowgirl	½ cookie (1.5 oz)	210	2	9	0	30	0	130

FOOD	PORTION	CALS	PROT	FAT	CHOL	CARB	FIBER	SOD
Vegan Ginger Snapdragons	½ cookie (1.5 oz)	190	2	7	0	29	0	230
Lorna Doone								
Shortbread	4 (1 oz)	140	1	7	0	20	0	150
LU								
Le Chocolatier	3 (1 oz)	150	1	9	0	17	1	5
Le Fondant	4 (1.1 oz)	170	2	10	0	19	1	5
Le Petit Beurre	4 (1.2 oz)	140	3	4	10	28	tr	170
Le Petit Ecolier Milk Chocolate	2 (0.9 oz)	130	2	6	5	17	tr	55
Shortbread	2	140	1	8	25	16	tr	95
Mallomars								
Cookies	2	120	1	5	0	18	1	40
Miss Meringue								
Chocolatette Strawberry Vanilla	4	130	2	4	0	24	1	25
Chocolettes Crunchy Chocolate	4	110	–	110	4	2	21	25
Classiques Cappuccino	4	110	1	0	0	26	0	20
Classiques Chocolate Chip	4	120	1	2	0	25	1	15
Classiques Dulce De Leche Artisan	4	110	1	0	0	26	0	20
Macaroons Traditional	1 (1.3 oz)	180	2	10	0	20	1	20
Madeleines Traditional	2 (1.2 oz)	160	2	9	55	19	0	20
Minis Vanilla	13 (1.1 oz)	110	1	0	0	27	0	20
Minis Vanilla Sugar Free	13	35	4	0	0	9	3	60
Murray's								
Sugar Free Chocolate Sandwich	3 (1 oz)	130	1	7	0	19	1	55
Sugar Free Chocolate Chip	3 (1.1 oz)	160	2	9	<5	20	1	130
Sugar Free Fudge Dipped Grahams	4 (1 oz)	150	2	8	0	19	1	80
Sugar Free Ginger Snap	7 (1.1 oz)	130	2	5	0	23	2	115
Sugar Free Oatmeal	3 (1.1 oz)	140	2	7	0	21	3	130
Sugar Free Shortbread	8 (1 oz)	130	2	5	0	21	2	140
Nabisco								
100 Calorie Barnum's Animal Choco	1 pkg	100	1	3	0	17	tr	115
100 Calorie Pack Alpha-Bits Mini	1 pkg	100	1	3	0	16	0	120

FOOD	PORTION	CALS	PROT	FAT	CHOL	CARB	FIBER	SOD
100 Calorie Pack Lorna Doone	1 pkg	100	1	3	0	16	0	120
100 Calorie Pack Teddy Grahams Mini Cinnamon	1 pkg	100	1	3	0	16	1	115
Biscos Sugar Wafers	8 (1 oz)	140	tr	6	0	21	0	25
Social Tea	6	140	2	4	0	24	1	125
Nana's								
No Gluten Berry Vanilla	1 bar (1.2 oz)	130	1	4	0	22	tr	135
No Gluten Chocolate	1 (3.5 oz)	360	4	12	0	62	2	380
No Gluten Ginger	1 (3.5 oz)	360	4	10	0	64	2	170
No Gluten Nana Banana	1 bar (1.2 oz)	130	1	5	0	23	0	130
No Wheat Oatmeal Raisin	1 (3.5 oz)	280	6	10	0	46	6	150
Vegan Chocolate Chip	1 (4 oz)	320	6	14	0	48	6	210
Vegan Peanut Butter	1 (4 oz)	360	8	16	0	46	4	220
Vegan Sunflower	1 (3.5 oz)	380	8	14	0	60	6	360
Nature's Path								
Organic Signature Lemon Poppyseed	4	130	2	4	0	23	tr	60
Organic Animal Vanilla	9	120	2	4	0	20	tr	80
New York Style								
Biscotti Almond	3 (1 oz)	130	3	5	25	20	1	35
Newman's Own								
Organic Champion Chip Chocolate Chocolate Chip	4	160	2	8	0	20	1	70
Organic Champion Chip Chocolate Chip	4	160	2	7	0	21	1	100
Organic Champion Chip Double Chocolate Mint Chip	4	160	2	8	0	21	1	70
Organic Champion Chip Expresso Chocolate Chip	4	150	2	7	0	21	1	100
Organic Champion Chip Orange Chocolate Chip	4	160	2	7	0	20	1	105
Organic Champion Chip Wheat Free Dairy Free	4	160	tr	8	0	21	0	110
Organic Fig Newmans Fat Free	2	120	2	0	0	28	1	140

FOOD	PORTION	CALS	PROT	FAT	CHOL	CARB	FIBER	SOD
Organic Fig Newmans Low Fat	2	140	2	2	0	28	1	170
Organic Fig Newmans Wheat Free Dairy Free	2	120	2	2	0	26	1	170
Organic Newman-O's Chocolate Creme	2	130	2	5	0	20	1	85
Organic Newman-O's Ginger-O's	2	120	2	5	0	19	0	160
Organic Newman-O's Mint Creme	2	130	2	5	0	20	1	85
Organic Newman-O's Original	2	130	2	5	0	20	1	85
Organic Newman-O's Tops & Bottoms	6	120	2	3	0	21	1	110
Organic Newman-O's Wheat Free Dairy Free	2	130	1	5	0	21	0	80
Newtons								
Fig	2 (1.1 oz)	110	1	2	0	22	1	125
Fig 100% Whole Grain	2 (1.3 oz)	130	1	3	0	26	3	135
Fig Fat Free	2 (1 oz)	90	1	0	0	22	1	130
Raspberry	2 (1 oz)	100	1	2	0	21	0	110
Nilla Wafers								
Cookies	1 oz	140	1	6	0	21	0	115
Reduced Fat	1 oz	110	1	2	0	24	0	110
Nonni's								
Biscotti Cioccolati	1 (0.8 oz)	110	2	5	20	17	1	70
Biscotti Limone	1 (0.8 oz)	110	2	5	20	17	0	75
Biscotti Original	1 (0.7 oz)	90	2	3	20	14	0	65
NutraBalance								
High Fibre	1 (0.7 oz)	90	1	4	0	13	3	85
Nutter Butter								
Sandwich Cookie	1 (1 oz)	130	2	6	0	19	1	110
Oreo								
Cakesters	2 (2 oz)	250	2	12	5	36	1	260
Oreo Double Stuff	1 (1 oz)	140	1	7	0	21	1	120
Sandwich Cookie	2 (1.2 oz)	160	2	7	0	25	1	190
Pepperidge Farm								
Chantilly Raspberry	2	120	1	3	0	23	tr	115
Chessmen	3 (0.9 oz)	120	2	5	20	18	tr	80

FOOD	PORTION	CALS	PROT	FAT	CHOL	CARB	FIBER	SOD
Dark Chocolate Mint Chocolate Chunk	1	140	2	7	10	16	0	80
Gingerman	4	130	2	4	10	21	tr	100
Medallion Milk Chocolate	5	160	2	8	10	20	0	40
Milano	3	180	2	10	10	21	tr	80
Milano French Vanilla	2	130	1	5	<5	18	tr	65
Milano Mint Chocolate Covered	4	130	2	6	<5	18	1	40
Milano Sugar Free	3	170	2	9	5	21	tr	65
Nantucket Chocolate Dipped	1	150	2	8	10	20	tr	100
Nantucket Dark Chocolate Chunk	1	140	2	7	10	16	0	80
Pirouettes Cappuccino	2	120	1	5	<5	18	0	40
Pirouettes Chocolate Mint	2	120	1	5	<5	18	tr	40
Sausalito Milk Chocolate Macadamia Nut	1	140	2	8	10	16	0	80
Shortbread	2	140	2	7	10	16	tr	105
Soft Baked Milk Chocolate	1	150	1	7	5	21	tr	70
Soft Baked Oatmeal Cranberry	1	130	2	4	5	22	tr	110
Soft Baked Sugar	1	140	2	5	10	22	0	90
Tahiti	2	170	2	10	5	17	2	40
Verona Apricot Raspberry	3	140	2	5	10	22	tr	100
Quaker								
Breakfast Cookie Oatmeal Raisin	1	180	3	5	0	33	5	200
Right Direction								
Chocolate Chip	1	60	2	6	10	24	5	150
SnackWell's								
Cookie Cakes Chocolate Mint	1 (0.6 oz)	50	1	1	0	12	0	40
Creme Sandwich	1 pkg (1.7 oz)	210	2	5	0	38	tr	200
Devil's Food Fat Free	1 (0.5 oz)	50	1	0	0	12	0	25
Sugar Free Lemon Creme	2 (1.1 oz)	130	1	6	0	23	2	135
Sugar Free Shortbread	2 (1 oz)	130	2	6	5	21	2	140
South Beach								
Wafer Sticke Dark Chocolate Hazelnut Creme	1 pkg	100	5	6	0	10	3	70

FOOD	PORTION	CALS	PROT	FAT	CHOL	CARB	FIBER	SOD
Wafer Sticke Dark Chocolate Peanut Butter	1 pkg	100	5	6	0	10	3	75
Stella D'Oro								
Almond Delight	1 (1 oz)	150	2	8	10	18	tr	85
Angelica Goodies	1 (0.7 oz)	90	1	3	10	15	0	45
Anginetti	4 (1.1 oz)	130	1	3	25	25	0	5
Biscotti Almond	1 (0.7 oz)	90	2	4	5	15	1	40
Biscotti French Vanilla	1 (0.7 oz)	90	1	3	5	15	0	50
Breakfast Treats Chocolate	1 (0.9 oz)	110	1	4	20	19	tr	70
Breakfast Treats Original	1 (0.7 oz)	90	1	3	20	14	0	65
Coffee Treats Almond Toast	2 (0.9)	100	2	2	25	20	tr	90
Coffee Treats Angel Wings	3 (1 oz)	160	2	10	0	16	0	90
Coffee Treats Anisette Sponge	2 (0.9 oz)	90	2	1	40	18	0	80
Coffee Treats Anisette Toast	3 (1.2 oz)	130	2	1	35	27	tr	110
Coffee Treats Roman Egg Biscuits	1 (1.1 oz)	130	3	5	15	19	0	125
Egg Jumbo	3 (1.2 oz)	120	2	2	50	25	0	85
Lady Stella	3 (1 oz)	130	1	5	<5	19	tr	60
Margherite	2 (1 oz)	130	2	5	20	20	0	85
Swiss Fudge	3 (1.2 oz)	170	2	9	<5	22	tr	80
Teddy Grahams								
Chocolate	24 (1.1 oz)	130	2	5	0	22	2	160
Honey	24 (1 oz)	130	2	4	0	23	1	150
Temptations								
Chocolate Alps	1 bar (1.6 oz)	170	2	7	0	28	1	130
Chocolate Mocha	1 bar (1.6 oz)	170	2	6	0	27	1	130
No Gluten Chocolate Rush	1 bar (1.6 oz)	170	1	9	0	25	1	90
Zwieback								
Toast	1 (8 g)	35	1	1	0	6	0	10
REFRIGERATED								
chocolate chip	1 (0.42 oz)	59	1	3	3	8	–	28
chocolate chip unbaked	1 oz	126	1	6	7	17	–	59
oatmeal	1 (0.4 oz)	56	1	3	3	8	–	39
oatmeal raisin	1 (0.4 oz)	56	1	3	3	8	–	39
peanut butter	1 (0.4 oz)	60	1	3	4	7	–	52

FOOD	PORTION	CALS	PROT	FAT	CHOL	CARB	FIBER	SOD
peanut butter dough	1 oz	130	2	7	8	15	–	112
sugar	1 (0.42 oz)	58	1	3	4	8	–	56
sugar dough	1 oz	124	1	6	8	17	–	120
TAKE-OUT								
biscotti w/ nuts chocolate dipped	1 (1.3 oz)	117	2	6	18	16	1	33
black & white	1 lg (3 oz)	302	4	9	58	52	1	72
finikia	1 (1.2 oz)	171	2	5	27	16	1	26
koulourakia butter cookie twist	1 (0.9 oz)	113	2	6	32	14	tr	59
linzer tart	1 (2.4 oz)	280	2	14	40	34	0	130

CORIANDER

FOOD	PORTION	CALS	PROT	FAT	CHOL	CARB	FIBER	SOD
cilantro fresh	1 tsp (2 g)	tr	tr	tr	0	tr	tr	1
leaf dried	1 tsp	2	tr	tr	0	tr	tr	1
leaf fresh	¼ cup	1	tr	tr	0	tr	–	1
seed	1 tsp	5	tr	tr	0	1	1	1

CORN
CANNED

FOOD	PORTION	CALS	PROT	FAT	CHOL	CARB	FIBER	SOD
cream style	½ cup	93	2	1	0	23	–	365
w/ red & green peppers	½ cup	86	3	1	0	21	–	396
white	½ cup	66	2	1	0	15	–	–
yellow	½ cup	66	2	1	0	15	1	–
Del Monte								
Cream Style	½ cup	60	1	1	0	14	2	360
Cream Style No Salt Added	½ cup	60	1	1	0	14	2	10
Fiesta	½ cup	50	2	1	0	12	2	310
Gold & White	½ cup	80	2	1	0	18	2	360
Savory Sides In Butter Sauce	½ cup	90	2	3	5	14	tr	530
Savory Sides Santa Fe	½ cup	70	3	1	0	16	1	510
Summer Crisp	½ cup	70	2	1	0	13	3	270
White	½ cup	60	2	1	0	11	3	360
Green Giant								
Mexicorn	⅓ cup	70	2	1	0	14	1	250
Super Sweet Yellow & White	⅓ cup	60	2	1	0	12	1	200
FRESH								
white cooked	½ cup	89	3	1	0	21	–	14

FOOD	PORTION	CALS	PROT	FAT	CHOL	CARB	FIBER	SOD
white raw	½ cup	66	2	1	0	15	–	12
yellow cooked	½ cup	89	3	1	0	21	–	14
yellow cooked	1 ear (2.7 oz)	83	3	1	0	19	–	13
yellow raw	1 ear (3 oz)	77	3	1	0	17	–	14
yellow raw	½ cup	66	2	1	0	15	–	12
FROZEN								
cooked	½ cup	67	2	tr	0	17	–	4
on the cob cooked	1 ear (2.2 oz)	59	2	tr	0	14	–	3
Birds Eye								
Steamfresh Southwestern	⅔ cup	90	2	2	0	16	1	260
Steamfresh Super Sweet	⅔ cup	70	3	1	0	14	2	0
Steamfresh Sweet Mini Corn On The Cob	1	90	3	1	0	19	1	0
C&W								
Cheddar Bacon	½ cup	130	4	5	10	18	3	210
Early Harvest Supersweet Petite	⅔ cup	70	3	1	0	14	2	0
Salsa Corn	1 cup	90	3	1	0	17	3	250
Europe's Best								
Baby Sweet	⅔ cup	50	2	1	0	9	2	0
Glory								
Savory Accents Fried Corn	½ cup	110	3	2	0	24	2	470
Green Giant								
Cream Style	½ cup	110	2	1	0	24	2	320
Nibblers On-The-Cob	1 (2.1 oz)	70	2	1	0	14	1	5
Niblets & Butter Sauce Low Fat	⅔ cup	110	3	2	<5	21	2	370
Pictsweet								
Cut Corn	⅔ cup	100	3	1	0	21	1	0
Roast Works								
Flame Roasted Cob Corn	1 cob (3 oz)	130	4	1	0	25	4	15
Stouffer's								
Souffle	½ pkg (6 oz)	150	5	5	65	22	2	490
TAKE-OUT								
fritters	1 (1 oz)	62	2	2	12	9	1	126
on the cob w/ butter cooked	1 ear	155	4	3	6	32	–	30
scalloped	1 cup	257	10	11	152	34	3	666

CORN CHIPS (see CHIPS)

FOOD	PORTION	CALS	PROT	FAT	CHOL	CARB	FIBER	SOD
CORNISH HEN (see CHICKEN)								
CORNMEAL								
cornmeal mush as prep w/ water	1 cup	223	5	1	0	47	5	523
cornmeal yellow	1 cup	505	12	2	0	107	10	4
Indian Head								
Stone Ground	¼ cup	100	3	1	0	20	2	0
McKenzie's								
Hush Puppies	1 serv (1.9 oz)	190	2	10	0	23	2	470
Quaker								
Quick Grits not prep	¼ cup	130	3	1	0	29	2	0
TAKE-OUT								
corn pone	1 piece (2.1 oz)	128	2	3	0	23	2	275
fritter puerto rican style	1 (1.4 oz)	109	3	7	8	8	1	223
harina de maíz con coco	½ cup	383	4	27	0	36	4	287
harina de maize con leche	1 cup	295	8	7	25	51	7	300
hush puppies	1 (0.8 oz)	74	2	3	10	10	1	147
johnnycake	1 piece (1.7 oz)	134	4	4	35	21	2	432
CORNSTARCH								
cornstarch	1 cup (4.5 oz)	488	tr	tr	0	117	1	12
Argo								
Cornstarch	1 tbsp	30	0	0	0	7	–	0
Bob's Red Mill								
Cornstarch	1 tbsp	30	0	0	0	7	0	0
Kingsford's								
Cornstarch	1 tbsp	30	0	0	0	7	–	0
COTTAGE CHEESE								
creamed	1 cup (7.4 oz)	217	26	9	31	6	–	850
creamed	4 oz	117	14	5	17	3	–	457
creamed w/ fruit	4 oz	140	11	4	13	15	–	457
dry curd	1 cup (5.1 oz)	123	25	1	10	3	–	19
dry curd	4 oz	96	20	tr	8	2	–	14

FOOD	PORTION	CALS	PROT	FAT	CHOL	CARB	FIBER	SOD
lowfat 1%	1 cup (7.9 oz)	164	28	2	10	6	–	918
lowfat 1%	4 oz	82	14	1	5	3	–	459
lowfat 2%	1 cup (7.9 oz)	203	31	4	19	8	–	918
lowfat 2%	4 oz	101	16	2	9	4	–	459
Breakstone's								
Fat Free	½ cup	80	12	0	10	8	0	450
LiveActive	1 pkg (4 oz)	90	10	2	15	8	3	380
LiveActive Mixed Berries	1 pkg (4 oz)	120	8	2	10	18	3	310
Hood								
4% Fat w/ Pineapple	½ cup	130	10	4	20	15	0	320
Fat Free	½ cup	80	14	0	10	6	0	410
Low Fat	½ cup	90	14	1	15	5	0	440
Low Fat No Salt Added	½ cup	90	14	1	15	6	0	55
Low Fat w/ Peaches	½ cup	110	10	1	10	18	0	310
Horizon Organic								
Lowfat	½ cup	100	13	3	15	4	0	390
Regular	½ cup	120	13	5	20	4	0	390
Knudsen								
LiveActive Pineapple	1 pkg (4 oz)	110	8	2	10	17	3	310
Light N'Lively								
Lowfat	½ cup	80	12	2	10	6	0	420
Organic Valley								
Low Fat	½ cup	100	15	2	10	4	0	450

COTTONSEED

FOOD	PORTION	CALS	PROT	FAT	CHOL	CARB	FIBER	SOD
kernels roasted	1 tbsp	51	3	4	0	2	–	3

COUSCOUS

FOOD	PORTION	CALS	PROT	FAT	CHOL	CARB	FIBER	SOD
cooked	1 cup (5.5 oz)	176	6	tr	0	36	2	8
dry	1 cup (6.1 oz)	650	22	1	0	134	9	17
Hodgson Mill								
Whole Wheat not prep	⅓ cup	210	8	1	0	47	5	0
Marrakesh Express								
Mango Salsa as prep	1 cup	190	7	0	0	38	1	380
Mushroom as prep	1 cup	190	8	1	0	39	1	600
Plain as prep	1 cup	270	10	0	0	57	2	10

FOOD	PORTION	CALS	PROT	FAT	CHOL	CARB	FIBER	SOD
Rice Select								
All Varieties not prep	¼ cup	150	4	0	0	31	–	0
CRAB								
CANNED								
blue	½ cup	67	14	1	60	0	0	225
blue drained	1 can (6.5 oz)	124	26	2	111	0	0	416
Ace Of Diamonds								
Fancy w/ Leg Meat	¼ cup (2 oz)	40	7	0	50	2	0	400
Brunswick								
Crabmeat 15% Leg	2 oz	40	9	1	50	1	0	240
Fancy Lump	2 oz	45	9	1	50	1	0	350
Bumble Bee								
Lump	¼ cup	40	8	1	50	0	0	300
Pink	¼ cup	35	7	1	50	0	0	300
White	¼ cup	40	8	1	50	0	0	300
Chicken Of The Sea								
Fancy	½ can (2 oz)	40	7	0	50	2	0	400
Lump	½ can (2 oz)	35	7	1	50	1	0	400
Madam								
Crab Meat	½ cup	40	8	1	55	12	0	370
Terry's								
Crabmeat	¼ cup	40	7	0	50	2	0	400
FRESH								
alaska king meat only steamed	3 oz	82	16	1	45	0	0	911
blue cooked flaked	1 cup (4 oz)	120	24	2	118	0	0	329
dungeness steamed	3 oz	94	19	1	65	1	0	321
queen steamed	3 oz	98	20	1	60	0	0	587
FROZEN								
Margaritaville								
Coral Reef Cakes + Sauce	1	200	17	10	71	4	0	490
Mrs. Paul's								
Deviled Crab Cakes	1 (3 oz)	220	20	12	60	12	3	320
Phillips Seafood								
Crab Cakes	1 (3 oz)	160	12	10	85	7	–	560

FOOD	PORTION	CALS	PROT	FAT	CHOL	CARB	FIBER	SOD
Crab Meat Stuffing	1 serv (3.5 oz)	170	13	4	85	15	–	850
Mini Cakes	4	160	12	10	85	7	–	560
Slammers	2	150	6	9	40	12	–	280
TAKE-OUT								
alaska king leg steamed	1 leg (4.7 oz)	130	26	2	71	0	0	1436
baked	1 (3.8 oz)	160	29	2	184	4	–	550
cakes	2 (4.2 oz)	186	24	9	180	1	0	396
crab imperial	1 crab (6.8 oz)	289	30	15	242	6	0	782
crab salad	1 serv (5.5 oz)	285	21	21	109	3	1	736
crab thermidor	1 serv (6.4 oz)	456	22	37	313	8	tr	664
deviled	1 serv (4.5 oz)	254	17	13	126	17	1	825
dungeness steamed	1 crab (4.5 oz)	140	28	2	97	1	0	480
empanada de jueyes	1 (4.4 oz)	341	12	16	45	38	2	680
fried crab puffs	4 (3.2 oz)	323	10	18	85	30	1	792
kenagi korean crab cooked	1 serv (3 oz)	71	16	tr	–	0	0	204
salmorejo de jueyes (in tomato sauce)	1 serv (4.5 oz)	215	20	14	99	3	tr	785
soft-shell breaded & fried	1 med (2.3 oz)	216	13	13	79	11	1	353
taco de jueyes	1 (4.2 oz)	266	16	14	79	18	2	800

CRACKER CRUMBS

FOOD	PORTION	CALS	PROT	FAT	CHOL	CARB	FIBER	SOD
cracker meal	1 cup	440	11	2	0	93	3	32
graham cracker crumbs	1 cup	355	6	8	0	65	2	508
Kellogg's								
Corn Flake Crumbs	6 tbsp (1.2 oz)	120	2	0	0	29	tr	240

CRACKERS

FOOD	PORTION	CALS	PROT	FAT	CHOL	CARB	FIBER	SOD
melba toast round	1	12	tr	tr	0	2	tr	25
oyster cracker	¼ cup	48	1	1	0	8	tr	121
saltines	1	13	tr	tr	0	2	tr	32
water biscuits	3	92	2	3	–	16	1	–
zwieback	1 oz	107	3	1	–	21	1	75

FOOD	PORTION	CALS	PROT	FAT	CHOL	CARB	FIBER	SOD
Annie's Homegrown								
Cheddar Bunnies BBQ	50	130	3	6	0	18	2	250
Cheddar Bunnies Original	50	150	3	7	<5	19	1	250
Cheddar Bunnies Ranch	50	130	3	6	0	17	2	250
Cheddar Bunnies Whole Wheat	50	130	3	6	0	17	2	250
Athenos								
Pita Chips Whole Wheat	11 (1 oz)	120	4	4	0	18	2	270
Back To Nature								
Classic Rounds	5	70	1	2	0	11	0	150
Crispy Wheats	17	130	3	4	0	22	1	290
Rice Thin Sesame Ginger	16	120	2	3	0	23	0	180
Rice Thin White Cheddar	16	120	2	3	0	23	0	250
Barbara's Bakery								
Rite Rounds Lite Original	5 (0.5 oz)	60	1	2	0	11	–	200
Wheatines Original	4	60	1	1	0	11	tr	80
Better Cheddars								
Original	1.1 oz	160	3	8	5	18	1	360
Blue Diamond								
Nut-Thins Almond	16	130	3	3	0	23	1	115
Nut-Thins Hazelnut	16	130	2	3	0	23	tr	115
Nut-Thins Pecan	16	130	2	4	0	23	tr	130
Bremner Wafers								
Cracked Wheat	7	70	2	2	0	11	0	100
Low Sodium	7	70	2	2	0	12	0	10
Original	7	70	2	2	0	11	0	105
Brown Rice Snaps								
Cheddar	6	60	1	1	0	12	tr	40
Original Tamari Seaweed	9	60	1	0	0	12	tr	120
Unsalted Plain	8	60	1	0	0	13	tr	0
Cheese Nips								
Cheddar	1 pkg (1.2 oz)	170	3	7	0	22	1	400
Cheetos								
Cheddar	1 pkg	240	4	14	5	25	1	440
Chicken Biskit								
Original	1.1 oz	160	2	8	0	19	1	300
Dare								
Breton Minis	13	80	2	4	0	9	0	130
Breton Multigrain	3 (0.5 oz)	80	2	4	0	10	1	160

FOOD	PORTION	CALS	PROT	FAT	CHOL	CARB	FIBER	SOD
Breton Original	3	60	1	3	0	8	0	110
Breton Reduced Fat & Sodium	7	120	2	2	0	22	2	150
Cabaret	3	70	1	4	0	9	0	70
Crispy Baguettes Original	9	110	3	2	0	22	1	160
Crispy Baguettes Three Cheese	8	130	3	5	0	19	tr	350
Grainsfirst	4	90	2	3	0	12	2	125
Vinta	2 (0.5 oz)	70	1	3	0	8	0	110
Vivant	3	60	1	3	0	9	0	120
Water Crackers Original	5	60	2	2	0	11	0	120
Doritos								
Jalapeno Cheese	1 pkg	230	3	13	<5	26	1	450
Nacho Cheesier	1 pkg	240	4	14	<5	25	1	390
Dr. Kracker								
Flatbread Klassic Seed	1 (1 oz)	120	6	5	0	13	4	220
Flatbread Pumpkin Seed Cheddar	1 (1 oz)	120	5	5	<5	12	4	220
Flatbread Seeded Spelt	1 (1 oz)	120	5	6	0	12	4	200
Flatbread Seedlander	1 (1 oz)	120	5	5	0	15	3	220
Flatbread Spelt Sunflower Cheddar	1 (1 oz)	120	5	6	<5	12	4	220
Krispy Grahams	5 (1 oz)	110	2	3	4	17	2	120
Eden								
Brown Rice	8 (1.1 oz)	120	3	2	0	22	2	230
Nori Nori Rice	15 (1 oz)	110	3	0	0	24	2	160
Foods Alive								
Golden Flax Maple & Cinnamon	5	150	6	8	0	12	8	15
Golden Flax Mexican Harvest	5	150	8	8	0	10	9	270
Golden Flax Onion Garlic	5	140	8	7	0	11	9	380
Golden Flax Organic Hemp	5	130	7	6	0	12	11	310
Golden Flax Regular	5	150	6	9	0	11	11	270
Gamesa								
Sabrisas	11	150	2	2	0	20	0	190
Glutino								
Gluten Free	4 (0.5 oz)	70	tr	2	5	12	0	120
Gluten Free Rusks	2 (0.7 oz)	80	0	2	0	15	2	140

FOOD	PORTION	CALS	PROT	FAT	CHOL	CARB	FIBER	SOD
Healthy Handfuls								
Lucky Duckies Cheddar Cheese	1 pkg (1 oz)	100	2	4	0	14	1	180
Jacob's								
Table Cracker Bran	1	33	1	1	–	5	tr	37
Kashi								
TLC Country Cheddar	18 (1 oz)	130	3	5	0	20	tr	220
TLC Honey Sesame	15 (1 oz)	130	3	3	0	22	2	160
TLC Natural Ranch	15 (1 oz)	130	4	3	0	22	2	200
TLC Original 7 Grain	15 (1 oz)	130	3	3	0	22	2	160
TLC Party Mediterranean Bruschetta	4	120	3	4	0	18	3	140
TLC Snack Fire Roasted Vegetable	5	130	3	4	0	21	2	210
Kitchen Table Bakers								
Aged Parmesan	3	80	7	6	15	tr	0	150
Everything	3	80	7	6	15	tr	0	150
Garlic	3	80	6	6	15	tr	0	150
Jalapeno	3	80	6	6	15	2	1	150
Lance								
Cheese On Wheat	1 pkg (1.4 oz)	190	4	9	<5	24	2	290
Mary's Gone Crackers								
Wheat Free Gluten Free Black Pepper	13 (1 oz)	140	3	5	0	21	3	180
Wheat Free Gluten Free Onion	13 (1 oz)	140	3	5	0	21	3	190
Wheat Free Gluten Free Original Seed	13 (1 oz)	140	3	5	0	21	3	190
Milton's								
Multi-Grain	2	70	1	4	0	10	0	180
Nabisco								
Garden Harvest Apple Cinnamon	16 (1 oz)	120	2	3	0	22	3	65
Garden Harvest Banana	16 (1 oz)	120	2	3	0	22	3	60
Garden Harvest Tomato Basil	16 (1 oz)	120	2	4	0	20	3	220
Garden Harvest Vegetable Medley	16 (1 oz)	120	2	4	0	20	3	240
Vegetable Thins	21 (1 oz)	150	2	7	0	20	tr	330

FOOD	PORTION	CALS	PROT	FAT	CHOL	CARB	FIBER	SOD
Water Original	4	60	1	1	0	11	0	75
Wheat	4	90	2	4	0	12	tr	160
Nature's Path								
Signature Tamari Flax	15	110	3	3	0	18	tr	280
New York Style								
Crispini Seeds & Spice	6	120	4	4	0	19	tr	190
Panetini Three Cheese	2	80	2	5	0	9	0	150
Panetini Original	2	80	2	4	0	10	0	90
Pita Chips Garlic	7	130	3	5	0	17	1	440
Pita Chips Natural Whole Wheat	7	120	3	5	0	17	3	350
Nonni's								
Panetini Roasted Garlic	5 (1 oz)	120	4	4	0	19	tr	300
Panetini Sun Dried Tomato Basil	5 (1 oz)	120	4	4	0	17	tr	170
Pepperidge Farm								
100 Calorie Pack Goldfish Cheddar	1 pkg	100	3	4	<5	14	1	170
100 Calorie Pack Goldfish Pretzel	1 pkg	100	2	2	0	18	tr	200
Goldfish Cinnamon Graham	1 pkg	210	3	8	5	32	1	220
Goldfish Pizza	55	140	3	5	0	20	tr	230
Goldfish w/ Whole Grain	55	140	4	5	<5	19	2	250
Snack Sticks Pumpernickel	15	120	3	2	0	24	2	410
Water Crackers	4	60	0	1	0	12	tr	90
Wheat Crisps Spicy Salsa	16	140	2	6	0	21	2	270
Peter Pan								
Peanut Butter Cheese	1 pkg	210	5	10	0	23	1	350
Peanut Butter Toast	1 pkg	210	5	11	0	23	1	280
Premium								
Saltine Fat Free	5 (0.5 oz)	60	1	0	0	12	0	170
Saltine Multigrain	5 (0.5 oz)	60	1	2	0	10	tr	170
Saltine Unsalted Tops	5	60	1	2	0	11	0	130
Saltines Low Sodium	0.5 oz	80	1	2	0	11	0	25
Saltines Original	0.5 oz	60	1	2	0	11	0	190
Ritz								
Crackers	0.5 oz	80	1	5	0	10	0	135
Reduced Fat	5 (0.5 oz)	70	1	2	0	11	0	150
Whole Wheat	0.5 oz	70	1	3	–	11	1	120

FOOD	PORTION	CALS	PROT	FAT	CHOL	CARB	FIBER	SOD
San-J								
Brown Rice Black Sesame	5	140	4	6	–	17	1	180
Brown Rice Sesame	5	130	3	5	–	19	1	170
Brown Rice Tamari	6	170	3	1	–	26	1	170
Sara Lee								
Cracked Pepper Trio	7	130	3	4	0	22	tr	35
English Water	7	130	3	4	0	22	tr	35
Harvest Vegetable	6	140	2	6	0	19	tr	350
Sociables								
Original	0.5 oz	70	1	4	0	9	0	140
South Beach								
Whole Wheat	1 pkg	100	2	4	0	16	3	250
Triscuit								
Deli-Style Rye	1 oz	120	3	5	0	19	3	150
Original	1 oz	120	3	5	0	19	3	180
Reduced Fat	1 oz	120	3	3	0	21	3	160
Utz								
Cheese Peanut Butter	6	200	4	10	<5	21	2	390
Vegetable Thins								
Original	1 oz	150	2	7	0	20	1	330
Wasa								
Crisp'N Light 7 Grain	3	60	2	0	0	13	2	95
Fiber Rye	1	30	1	1	0	7	2	50
Hearty Rye	1	45	1	0	0	11	2	70
Oats	1	60	2	1	0	11	2	95
Sourdough Rye	1	35	1	0	0	9	2	45
Westminster								
Oyster	1 pkg (0.5 oz)	66	1	2	0	11	0	60
Wheat Thins								
100% Whole Grain	1 oz	140	2	6	0	21	2	290
Low Sodium	1.1 oz	150	2	6	0	22	1	80
Original	1.1 oz	150	2	6	0	21	1	260
Reduced Fat	1 oz	130	3	4	0	21	1	260
Wheatsworth								
Crackers	5 (0.5 oz)	80	2	4	0	10	1	180
Wisecrackers								
Low Fat Roasted Garlic	10	110	3	2	0	20	tr	180

FOOD	PORTION	CALS	PROT	FAT	CHOL	CARB	FIBER	SOD
CRANBERRIES								
cranberry orange relish	¼ cup	118	tr	tr	0	31	2	1
cranberry sauce	¼ cup	109	tr	tr	0	27	1	20
dried	½ cup	85	tr	tr	0	23	2	1
dried organic	⅓ cup	120	0	1	0	29	2	0
fresh chopped	1 cup	13	tr	tr	0	3	1	1
fresh whole	1 cup	11	tr	tr	0	3	1	1
sauce	1 slice (2 oz)	86	tr	tr	0	22	1	17
De-Lite								
Dried Sweetened	1 oz	92	tr	tr	0	23	1	3
Earthbound Farm								
Organic Dried	⅓ cup	130	0	0	0	34	2	2
Eden								
Organic Dried	⅓ cup	140	0	1	0	33	2	20
Fool								
Cranberry Spread	1 tbsp	30	0	0	0	7	1	0
Frieda's								
Dried	⅓ cup (1.4 oz)	110	0	1	0	28	2	3
Good Sense								
Cranberries 'N More	¼ cup	170	5	10	0	15	2	0
Dried Sweetened	½ cup	130	0	0	0	31	4	0
Lollipop Tree								
Cranberry Curd	1 tbsp	50	tr	1	15	9	–	5
Mariani								
Dried Sweetened	⅓ cup	130	0	0	0	35	2	0
Newman's Own								
Organic Dried	¼ cup	130	0	0	0	34	2	0
Ocean Spray								
Craisins	⅓ cup	130	0	0	0	33	2	0
Sunsweet								
Dried	⅓ cup (1.5 oz)	140	0	0	0	35	2	0
CRANBERRY BEANS								
canned	½ cup	108	7	tr	0	20	8	432
dried cooked w/o salt	½ cup	120	8	tr	0	22	9	1
CRANBERRY JUICE								
cranberry juice cocktail low calorie w/ vitamin C	8 oz	46	tr	tr	0	11	0	7

FOOD	PORTION	CALS	PROT	FAT	CHOL	CARB	FIBER	SOD
cranberry juice cocktail w/ vitamin C	8 oz	137	0	tr	0	34	0	5
unsweetened	8 oz	116	1	tr	0	31	tr	5
Apple & Eve								
100% Juice	8 oz	130	0	0	0	32	–	25
Lakewood								
Organic	6 oz	50	1	0	0	12	1	4
Organic Light	6 oz	45	1	0	0	18	1	3
Langers								
Cranberry 100	8 oz	140	0	0	0	35	–	15
Northland								
100% Juice	8 oz	130	0	0	0	33	–	35
Ocean Spray								
White Cran Peach	8 oz	120	0	0	0	31	–	50
Old Orchard								
Cocktail	8 oz	140	0	0	0	34	–	30
SSips								
Cocktail	1 box (7 oz)	110	0	0	0	28	–	0
CRAYFISH								
cooked	3 oz	97	20	1	151	0	0	58
raw	3 oz	76	16	1	118	0	0	45
raw	8	24	5	tr	37	0	0	14
CREAM (see also WHIPPED TOPPINGS)								
clotted cream	2 tbsp (1 oz)	164	tr	18	48	1	0	18
creme fraiche	2 tbsp (1 oz)	100	1	11	40	1	0	10
half & half	1 cup (8.5 oz)	315	7	28	89	10	–	98
half & half	1 tbsp (0.5 oz)	20	tr	2	6	1	–	6
heavy whipping	1 tbsp (0.5 oz)	52	tr	6	21	tr	–	6
heavy whipping whipped	1 cup (4.1 oz)	411	5	44	163	7	–	89
light coffee	1 tbsp (0.5 oz)	29	tr	3	10	1	–	6
light coffee	1 cup (8.4 oz)	496	6	46	159	9	–	95
light whipping	1 tbsp (0.5 oz)	44	tr	5	17	tr	–	5

FOOD	PORTION	CALS	PROT	FAT	CHOL	CARB	FIBER	SOD
light whipping cream whipped	1 cup (4.2 oz)	345	5	37	132	7	–	82
Coffee-Mate								
Half & Half Fat Free	2 tbsp	20	tr	0	0	3	–	65
Hood								
Half & Half	2 tbsp	40	1	4	15	1	0	20
Light	1 tbsp	30	1	3	10	tr	0	10
Simply Smart Fat Free Half & Half	2 tbsp	15	tr	0	<5	2	0	30
Whipping Cream	1 tbsp	45	0	5	20	tr	0	5
Horizon Organic								
Half & Half	2 tbsp	35	1	3	10	1	0	15
Heavy Whipping	1 tbsp	50	0	5	20	0	0	10
Organic Valley								
Half & Half	2 tbsp (1 oz)	40	tr	4	10	1	0	10
CREAM CHEESE								
cream cheese	1 pkg (3 oz)	297	6	30	93	2	–	251
cream cheese	1 oz	99	2	10	31	1	–	84
Back To Nature								
Organic Cream Cheese	⅛ pkg (1 oz)	100	2	10	30	tr	0	90
Boar's Head								
Cream Cheese	2 tbsp (1 oz)	100	2	10	30	2	0	100
Connoisseur								
Wheel Mango Peach	2 tbsp	110	1	7	20	10	0	110
Wheel Wild Blueberry	2 tbsp	100	1	7	20	9	0	120
Crystal Farms								
Regular	1 oz	90	2	9	30	1	0	100
Tub	2 tbsp	100	2	9	25	2	0	135
Whipped	2 tbsp	70	1	7	20	1	0	80
Horizon Organic								
Reduced Fat	2 tbsp	70	2	7	25	2	0	100
Spreadable	2 tbsp	110	2	10	30	tr	0	90
Lifeway								
Lox & Onion	2 tbsp	80	2	8	25	1	0	80
Vegetable	2 tbsp	80	2	7	20	1	0	80
Whipped	2 tbsp	80	2	8	25	1	0	75
Organic Valley								
Cream Cheese	1 oz	100	2	10	35	1	0	105
Soft	2 tbsp	90	1	9	25	2	0	140

FOOD	PORTION	CALS	PROT	FAT	CHOL	CARB	FIBER	SOD
Philadelphia								
⅓ Less Fat	1 oz	70	2	6	20	tr	0	120
Fat Free	1 oz	30	4	0	5	2	0	200
Original	1 oz	100	2	9	40	1	0	105
Whipped	2 tbsp	60	1	6	20	1	0	90

CREAM CHEESE SUBSTITUTE
WholeSoy & Co.

FOOD	PORTION	CALS	PROT	FAT	CHOL	CARB	FIBER	SOD
Soy Cream Cheese Organic Original & Flavored	2 tbsp	70	tr	6	0	3	1	124

CREAM OF TARTAR

FOOD	PORTION	CALS	PROT	FAT	CHOL	CARB	FIBER	SOD
cream of tartar	1 tsp	8	0	0	0	2	0	2

CREPES

FOOD	PORTION	CALS	PROT	FAT	CHOL	CARB	FIBER	SOD
basic crepe unfilled	1 (7 in)	112	4	6	78	11	tr	142
Frieda's								
Ready-To-Use	1 (0.5 oz)	30	1	1	5	5	0	50

CROAKER

FOOD	PORTION	CALS	PROT	FAT	CHOL	CARB	FIBER	SOD
atlantic breaded & fried	3 oz	188	15	11	71	6	–	296
atlantic raw	3 oz	89	15	3	52	0	0	47

CROCODILE

FOOD	PORTION	CALS	PROT	FAT	CHOL	CARB	FIBER	SOD
cooked	3 oz	78	17	1	–	0	0	–

CROISSANT

FOOD	PORTION	CALS	PROT	FAT	CHOL	CARB	FIBER	SOD
apple	1 (2 oz)	145	4	5	–	21	1	156
cheese	1 (2 oz)	236	5	12	–	27	2	316
plain	1 (2 oz)	232	5	12	–	26	2	424
plain	1 mini (1 oz)	115	2	6	–	13	1	211
Sara Lee								
Croissant	1 (1.5 oz)	170	4	8	5	20	1	200
Petite	2 (2 oz)	230	6	11	5	26	1	260
TAKE-OUT								
w/ egg & cheese	1 (4.5 oz)	368	13	25	216	24	–	551
w/ egg cheese & bacon	1 (4.5 oz)	413	16	28	215	24	–	889
w/ egg cheese & ham	1 (5.3 oz)	474	19	34	213	24	–	1081
w/ egg cheese & sausage	1 (5.6 oz)	523	20	38	216	25	–	1115

CROUTONS

FOOD	PORTION	CALS	PROT	FAT	CHOL	CARB	FIBER	SOD
plain	1 cup (1 oz)	122	4	2	0	22	2	209
seasoned	1 cup (1.4 oz)	186	4	7	–	25	2	495

FOOD	PORTION	CALS	PROT	FAT	CHOL	CARB	FIBER	SOD
Cardini's								
Italian	2 tbsp	30	1	2	0	4	0	80
Edward & Sons								
Organic Lightly Salted	2 tbsp	30	tr	1	0	5	0	25
Fresh Gourmet								
Butter & Garlic	7 (7 g)	35	1	2	0	4	0	80
Cornbread Sweet Butter	½ cup (1 oz)	110	3	1	0	22	1	260
Country Ranch	6 (7 g)	35	1	2	0	4	–	75
Fat Free Garlic Caesar	12 (7 g)	30	1	0	0	5	0	45
Italian Seasoned	6 (7 g)	35	1	2	0	4	0	70
Organic Seasoned	5 (7 g)	30	1	2	0	4	0	70
Pepperidge Farm								
Whole Grain Seasoned	6	30	1	1	0	5	tr	70
Zesty Italian	6	30	tr	1	0	5	0	55
Rothbury Farms								
Seasoned	2 tbsp	30	1	1	0	5	0	100
CUCUMBER								
fresh peeled	1 med (7 oz)	24	1	tr	0	4	1	4
fresh sliced	1 cup	14	1	tr	0	3	1	2
fresh w/ peel sliced	½ cup	34	tr	tr	0	2	tr	1
Frieda's								
Japanese	⅔ cup	10	1	0	0	2	1	0
Seedless Hothouse	⅔ cup	110	1	0	0	2	1	0
TAKE-OUT								
cucumber & onion salad w/ vinegar	1 cup	52	1	tr	0	12	1	375
cucumber salad w/ oil & vinegar	1 cup	183	1	15	0	11	1	329
cucumber salad w/ sour cream dressing	1 cup	68	1	6	12	3	1	16
kimchee	½ cup (1.8 oz)	36	tr	2	0	4	tr	173
tzatziki	½ cup (3.4 oz)	72	2	6	5	4	1	197
CUMIN								
seed	1 tsp	8	tr	tr	0	1	tr	4

FOOD	PORTION	CALS	PROT	FAT	CHOL	CARB	FIBER	SOD
CURRANT JUICE								
black currant nectar	7 oz	110	tr	0	–	26	–	10
red currant nectar	7 oz	108	tr	tr	–	26	–	tr
CurrantC								
Black Currant Juice	8 oz	130	1	0	0	32	0	10
CURRANTS								
black fresh	½ cup	36	1	tr	0	9	–	1
zante dried	½ cup	204	3	tr	0	53	–	6
Sun-Maid								
Zante	¼ cup	130	1	0	0	31	2	10
CURRY								
curry powder	1 tsp	7	tr	tr	0	1	1	1
paste	1 tube (6 oz)	465	7	36	16	30	12	4394
A Taste Of Thai								
Curry Paste Green	1 tsp	15	0	2	0	1	1	200
Curry Paste Panang	1 tsp	25	0	2	0	2	0	170
Curry Paste Red	1 tsp	20	0	2	0	1	0	260
Curry Paste Yellow	1 tsp	30	0	3	0	1	1	135
Patak's								
Curry Paste Biryani	2 tbsp	180	1	16	0	6	3	890
Garam Masala Paste	2 tsp	130	1	12	0	4	0	1080
Tandoori Paste	2 tbsp	30	1	1	0	5	1	800
Vindaloo Paste	2 tbsp	160	1	16	0	4	0	1020
Spice Hunter								
Curry Seasoning Salt Free	¼ tsp	0	0	0	0	0	0	0
TAKE-OUT								
beef curry	1 cup	432	27	31	68	14	3	1293
chicken curry ½ breast	1 serv	160	15	9	45	6	1	624
chicken curry boneless	1 serv (6.2 oz)	219	20	12	62	8	2	857
chicken curry leg & thigh	1 serv	180	17	10	51	7	1	702
chickpea curry	1 serv (8.3 oz)	305	18	15	12	23	15	1206
lamb curry	1 cup	257	28	14	90	4	1	496
mixed vegetable curry	1 serv (7.7 oz)	398	4	33	–	22	–	–
pea & potato curry	1 serv (7 oz)	284	5	22	–	19	6	–
pork vindaloo curry	1 serv	620	–	47	–	3	–	–

FOOD	PORTION	CALS	PROT	FAT	CHOL	CARB	FIBER	SOD
potato	1 serv (6 oz)	292	4	16	–	36	4	–
sambhar dhal curry	1 serv (10 oz)	177	8	7	0	21	8	1314

CUSK
fillet baked	3 oz	106	23	1	50	0	0	38

CUSTARD
MIX
as prep w/ 2% milk	½ cup (4.7 oz)	148	7	4	74	24	–	200
as prep w/ whole milk	½ cup (4.7 oz)	163	6	5	–	23	–	–
flan as prep w/ 2% milk	½ cup (4.7 oz)	135	4	2	9	26	–	68
flan as prep w/ whole milk	½ cup (4.7 oz)	150	4	4	17	25	–	65

READY-TO-EAT
Kozy Shack
Flan	1 pkg (4 oz)	145	4	4	40	25	0	100

TAKE-OUT
baked	½ cup (5 oz)	148	7	7	123	15	–	109
flan	½ cup (5.4 oz)	220	7	6	140	35	–	86
flan de calabaza	1 piece (3.5 oz)	225	5	10	112	30	tr	342
flan de coco	1 piece (4.2 oz)	340	10	13	142	48	tr	160
tocino del cielo heaven's delight	1 cup	856	14	21	967	156	0	48
zabaione	½ cup (57.2 g)	135	3	5	213	13	0	9

CUTTLEFISH
steamed	3 oz	134	28	1	190	1	–	632

DANDELION GREENS
fresh cooked	½ cup	17	1	tr	0	3	–	23
raw chopped	½ cup	13	1	tr	0	3	–	21
Frieda's								
Dandelion Greens	2 cups	40	2	0	0	8	3	65

FOOD	PORTION	CALS	PROT	FAT	CHOL	CARB	FIBER	SOD
DANISH PASTRY								
READY-TO-EAT								
Entenmann's								
Danish Ring Walnut	⅙ ring (2 oz)	260	4	16	25	25	2	180
TAKE-OUT								
cheese	1 (2.5 oz)	266	6	16	11	26	1	320
cinnamon	1 (5 oz)	572	10	32	30	63	2	527
fruit	1 (5 oz)	527	8	27	162	68	3	503
lemon	1 (2.5 oz)	263	4	13	28	34	1	251
raisin nut	1 (2.3 oz)	280	5	16	30	30	1	236
DATES								
deglet noor dried	10	240	–	0	0		–	–
dried chopped	1 cup	489	4	1	0	131	–	5
dried whole	10	228	2	tr	0	61	–	2
jujube dried	1 oz	75	1	tr	–	19	2	2
jujube fresh	1 oz	30	tr	tr	0	7	–	1
jujube preserved in sugar	1 oz	91	tr	tr	–	22	–	2
medjool	2–3 (1.4 oz)	120	1	0	0	31	3	10
Bob's Red Mill								
Dried Crumbles	⅓ cup	130	1	0	0	33	4	15
Earthbound Farm								
Organic Dried	6 (1.4 oz)	120	1	0	0	31	3	0
Frieda's								
Medjool	2–3 (1.4 oz)	120	1	0	0	31	3	0
SunDate								
Fancy Medjool	3 (1.4 oz)	120	1	0	0	31	3	0
Sunsweet								
California Pitted	5–6 (1.4 oz)	120	1	0	0	30	3	0
DEER (see VENISON)								
DELI MEATS/COLD CUTS (see also BEEF, CHICKEN, HAM, MEAT SUBSTITUTES, TURKEY)								
barbecue loaf pork & beef	1 slice (0.8 oz)	40	4	2	9	1	0	307
beerwurst beef	1 slice (4 in x ⅛ in)	75	3	7	13	tr	–	214
beerwurst beef	2 oz	155	8	13	35	2	1	410
berliner pork & beef	1 slice (0.8 oz)	53	4	4	11	1	0	298

FOOD	PORTION	CALS	PROT	FAT	CHOL	CARB	FIBER	SOD
blood sausage	1 slice (0.9 oz)	95	4	9	30	tr	0	170
bologna beef	1 slice (1 oz)	88	3	8	16	1	0	302
bologna beef low fat	1 slice (1 oz)	57	3	4	12	1	0	330
bologna beef reduced sodium	1 slice (1 oz)	88	3	8	16	1	0	191
bologna beef & pork	1 slice (1 oz)	87	4	7	17	2	0	209
bologna beef & pork low fat	1 slice (1 oz)	64	3	5	11	1	0	310
braunschweiger pork	1 slice (1 oz)	92	4	8	50	1	0	325
dutch brand loaf pork & beef	1 slice (1.3 oz)	104	5	9	23	1	tr	401
headcheese pork	1 slice (1.6 oz)	71	6	5	31	0	0	374
honey loaf pork & beef	1 slice (1 oz)	35	4	1	10	1	0	370
lebanon bologna beef	2 slices (1 oz)	105	11	6	31	tr	0	783
mortadella beef & pork	1 slice (0.5 oz)	47	2	4	8	tr	0	187
olive loaf pork	2 slices (2 oz)	134	7	9	22	5	0	846
pastrami beef	1 slice (1 oz)	41	6	2	19	tr	tr	248
peppered loaf pork & beef	1 slice (1 oz)	41	5	2	13	1	0	426
pepperoni pork & beef	15 slices (1 oz)	135	6	12	34	1	tr	519
picnic loaf pork & beef	1 slice (1 oz)	65	4	5	11	1	0	326
salami cooked beef & pork	1 slice (0.8 oz)	58	3	5	15	1	0	245
salami hard pork	3 slices (0.9 oz)	14	6	8	27	1	0	543
salami hard pork & beef less sodium	1 slice (1 oz)	113	4	9	26	2	tr	177
sandwich spread pork & beef	¼ cup	141	5	10	23	7	tr	608
summer sausage thuringer cervelat	2 oz	203	10	17	41	2	0	728
Boar's Head								
Abruzzese Hot & Sweet	1 oz	100	8	8	25	tr	0	540
Bologna 25% Lowered Sodium	2 oz	150	8	13	30	0	0	410
Bologna Beef	2 oz	150	7	13	35	0	0	520

FOOD	PORTION	CALS	PROT	FAT	CHOL	CARB	FIBER	SOD
Bologna Garlic	2 oz	150	7	13	35	1	0	530
Bologna Lebanon	2 oz	100	11	5	40	3	0	680
Bologna Pork & Beef	2 oz	150	7	13	35	tr	0	530
Braunschweiger Lite	2 oz	120	9	8	50	1	0	450
Capocollo Hot & Sweet	1 oz	80	7	5	25	0	0	590
Dutch Loaf	2 oz	150	7	12	25	2	0	610
Liverwurst Smoked	2 oz	170	8	15	45	1	0	620
Mortadella	2 oz	160	9	14	30	0	0	560
Olive Loaf	2 oz	130	6	12	20	tr	0	630
Pastrami	2 oz	70	12	3	30	1	0	580
Pickle & Pepper Loaf	2 oz	150	6	13	30	2	0	500
Prosciutto	1 oz	60	8	3	15	0	0	750
Salami Beef	2 oz	120	10	9	25	0	0	470
Salami Cooked	2 oz	130	8	11	40	0	0	550
Salami Hard	1 oz	110	6	9	30	tr	0	490
Sopressata Hot & Sweet	1 oz	100	8	7	25	0	0	540
Spiced Ham	2 oz	120	7	10	30	1	0	570
Carl Buddig								
Beef	2 oz	90	10	5	–	1	–	–
Corned Beef	2 oz	90	10	5	–	1	–	–
Healthy Ones								
Pastrami 97% Fat Free	4 slices (2 oz)	60	10	2	25	3	0	450
Hebrew National								
Bologna Beef	1 slice (1 oz)	80	3	8	15	0	0	240
Bologna Lean Beef	4 slices (2 oz)	90	9	5	20	1	–	440
Salami Beef	3 slices (2 oz)	150	8	13	35	0	0	420
Salami Lean Beef	4 slices (2 oz)	90	9	5	25	1	–	480
Oscar Mayer								
Salami Beef	3 slices (1.8 oz)	150	8	13	40	1	0	640
Sara Lee								
Corned Beef	1 slice (2 oz)	50	8	2	25	1	0	600
Pastrami	2 slices (1.6 oz)	60	9	3	25	0	0	380
Salami Genoa	4 slices (1 oz)	110	6	10	35	1	0	390

FOOD	PORTION	CALS	PROT	FAT	CHOL	CARB	FIBER	SOD
Salami Hard (1 oz)	4 slices	120	6	11	40	0	0	410
Wellshire								
Salami Hard	1 oz	100	8	8	30	1	0	530
Salmi Genoa	1 oz	100	8	8	30	1	0	530
Sopressata Sliced	1 oz	100	8	8	30	1	0	530
DILL								
seed	1 tsp	6	tr	tr	0	1	tr	0
sprigs fresh	5 (0.3 oz)	0	tr	tr	0	tr	–	1
weed dry	1 tbsp	8	1	tr	0	2	tr	6

DINNER (see also ASIAN FOOD, PASTA DINNERS, POT PIES, SPANISH FOOD)

FOOD	PORTION	CALS	PROT	FAT	CHOL	CARB	FIBER	SOD
Banquet								
Turkey Meal	1 meal (9.25 oz)	290	15	13	35	28	6	1050
Birds Eye								
Voila! Pasta Primavera w/ Chicken	1⅔ cups	250	14	3	10	42	7	1130
Voila! Shrimp Scampi	1¾ cups	190	11	3	60	31	3	540
Voila! Southwestern Chicken	2 cups	250	14	6	30	32	2	640
Boston Market								
Glazed Rotisserie Chicken w/ Mashed Potatoes Gravy Vegetables	1 pkg (16 oz)	390	30	15	75	34	4	1740
Meatloaf w/ Mashed Potatoes & Gravy	1 pkg (16 oz)	880	23	55	100	55	3	2720
C&W								
Stir Fry Feast Pot Sticker + Sauce	2 cups	200	10	4	15	30	4	1200
Stir Fry Feast Ultimate + Sauce	1½ cups	190	11	5	30	25	3	1350
Campbell's								
Supper Bakes Cheesy Chicken w/ Pasta	⅙ pkg	170	6	4	5	28	1	840
Supper Bakes Garlic Chicken w/ Pasta	⅙ pkg	220	9	2	<5	42	2	760
Supper Bakes Savory Pork Chops w/ Herb Stuffing	⅙ box	160	5	2	<5	30	1	780
Supper Bakes Traditional Roast Chicken w/ Stuffing	⅙ pkg	160	5	3	<5	29	2	740

FOOD	PORTION	CALS	PROT	FAT	CHOL	CARB	FIBER	SOD
Contessa								
Beef Goulash not prep	1¾ cups	210	12	5	50	32	3	850
Chicken Cacciatore not prep	1¾ cups	230	14	7	35	24	6	810
Chicken Alfredo not prep	1¾ cups	330	15	18	70	28	2	660
Fantastic								
Ginger Shitake w/ Rice Noodles	1 pkg (7.4 oz)	340	8	10	0	58	4	690
Fillo Factory								
Organic Fillo Pie Eggplant & Red Pepper	1 serv (5 oz)	230	4	9	0	35	3	310
Glory								
Savory Singles Chicken & Dumplings	1 pkg	290	16	8	75	40	6	1400
Savory Singles Chicken Smoked Sausage & Rice Casserole	1 pkg	440	18	18	60	49	1	1390
Savory Singles Ham & Sausage Jambalaya	1 pkg	400	17	18	50	42	2	1320
Savory Singles Turkey & Gravy w/ Cornbread Stuffing	1 pkg	440	18	18	30	49	2	1380
Glutino								
Gluten Free Chicken Pomodoro w/ Brown Rice & Vegetables	1 pkg (9.1 oz)	190	11	3	15	33	3	910
Gluten Free Chicken Ranchero w/ Brown Rice	1 pkg (9.1 oz)	180	14	2	20	30	4	790
Golden Cuisine								
Beef Stew	1 pkg	350	31	10	61	32	9	508
Boneless Pork Patty	1 pkg	504	26	25	57	44	13	699
Breaded Baked Fish w/ Rice Pilaf	1 pkg	300	18	5	27	48	6	412
Chicken Cacciatore	1 pkg	417	24	10	48	56	10	352
Chicken & Noodles	1 pkg	331	26	8	54	39	8	523
Chicken Parmesan	1 pkg	430	18	19	30	47	14	574
Chicken w/ Marinara Sauce	1 pkg	329	28	8	44	37	15	590
Meatloaf Patty & Gravy	1 pkg	340	21	14	48	33	7	750
Mesquite Chicken	1 pkg	320	21	5	30	50	10	355
Pot Roast w/ Gravy	1 pkg	343	25	11	50	36	10	677

FOOD	PORTION	CALS	PROT	FAT	CHOL	CARB	FIBER	SOD
Salisbury Steak & Mushroom Sauce	1 pkg	350	18	10	38	47	7	676
Swedish Meatballs	1 pkg	440	20	26	48	32	9	835
Turkey Tetrazzini	1 pkg	304	33	6	58	29	11	454
Green Giant								
Create A Meal Stir Fry Sweet & Sour as prep	1 cup	280	2	7	54	36	3	528
Skillet Meal Chicken Teriyaki as prep	1½ cups	240	13	1	20	46	3	780
Healthy Choice								
Beef Merlot	1 pkg	240	17	8	40	25	6	600
Beef Pot Roast	1 pkg	320	19	9	45	39	6	550
Beef Stroganoff	1 pkg	320	20	9	65	39	6	580
Beef Teriyaki	1 pkg	310	16	7	40	44	5	600
Beef Tips Portabello	1 pkg	300	20	8	35	33	7	600
Blackened Chicken	1 pkg	300	20	6	35	36	5	600
Boneless Beef Ribs w/ Classic BBQ Sauce	1 pkg	360	22	9	55	47	8	580
Charbroiled Beef Patty	1 pkg	310	18	9	40	37	6	600
Cheesy Rice & Chicken	1 pkg	250	23	5	50	27	4	600
Chicken Carbonara	1 pkg	290	24	7	45	32	2	600
Chicken Margherita	1 pkg	340	25	8	50	42	6	600
Chicken Parmigiana	1 pkg	320	19	9	20	40	6	600
Chicken Breast & Vegetables	1 pkg	260	18	7	45	30	6	550
Chicken Broccoli Alfredo	1 pkg	300	25	7	50	34	2	530
Chicken Piccata	1 pkg	260	16	5	40	36	2	600
Chicken Teriyaki	1 pkg	270	16	6	40	37	6	600
Chicken Tuscany	1 pkg	340	24	9	40	39	4	600
Country Breaded Chicken	1 pkg	370	17	9	45	55	5	600
Country Glazed Chicken	1 pkg	230	17	5	45	28	3	600
Country Herb Chicken	1 pkg	280	18	6	40	37	5	600
Creamy Herb Roasted Chicken	1 pkg	240	18	5	60	29	5	580
Grilled Basil Chicken	1 pkg	330	23	9	40	37	5	600
Grilled Chicken Breast & Pasta	1 pkg	250	20	7	40	25	4	560
Grilled Chicken Breast w/ Mashed Potatoes	1 pkg	190	17	5	50	19	3	580
Grilled Chicken Caesar	1 pkg	300	23	8	35	33	5	580

FOOD	PORTION	CALS	PROT	FAT	CHOL	CARB	FIBER	SOD
Grilled Chicken Marinara	1 pkg	270	22	5	35	35	5	580
Grilled Steak w/ Roasted Garlic Sauce	1 pkg	220	16	7	35	22	5	600
Grilled Turkey Breast	1 pkg	250	18	5	35	31	5	600
Grilled Whiskey Steak	1 pkg	280	17	6	40	38	6	600
Herb Baked Fish	1 pkg	360	17	9	35	51	6	600
Homestyle Chicken & Pasta	1 pkg	250	21	6	40	28	5	570
Honey Glazed Chicken	1 pkg	320	18	6	40	46	6	580
Lemon Pepper Fish	1 pkg	280	13	5	20	46	4	580
Mandarin Chicken	1 pkg	250	18	4	40	36	4	520
Mesquite Chicken BBQ	1 pkg	300	18	5	45	44	5	480
Mixed Grills Chicken Honey BBQ w/ Dipping Sauce	1 pkg	380	24	7	25	53	8	580
Mixed Grills Chicken Honey Mustard w/ Dipping Sauce	1 pkg	360	24	7	25	49	10	600
Mixed Grills Chicken Teriyaki w/ Dipping Sauce	1 pkg	340	23	7	35	48	9	600
Mixed Grills Chicken Tomato Garlic w/ Dipping Sauce	1 pkg	370	25	7	30	50	10	600
Mixed Grills Steak BBQ Sauce	1 pkg	420	26	8	45	59	7	600
Mixed Grills Steak Teriyaki w/ Dipping Sauce	1 pkg	350	26	9	30	39	11	600
Mixed Grills Steak w/ Zesty Steak Sauce	1 pkg	350	24	8	40	44	8	600
Oriental Style Beef	1 pkg	310	22	9	35	33	5	580
Oriental Style Chicken	1 pkg	240	19	5	35	28	4	600
Oven Roasted Beef	1 pkg	280	22	7	60	33	5	600
Princess Chicken	1 pkg	310	19	7	60	41	5	590
Roast Turkey Breast	1 pkg	220	18	6	40	23	3	580
Roasted Chicken Breast	1 pkg	200	10	0	45	32	7	600
Roasted Chicken Chardonnay	1 pkg	290	22	8	40	32	4	600
Salisbury Steak	1 pkg	360	23	9	45	45	5	580
Salisbury Steak w/ Red Skin Mashed Potatoes	1 pkg	200	15	6	40	20	4	600
Sesame Chicken	1 pkg	260	17	6	35	34	4	580
Slow Roasted Turkey Breast w/ Mashed Potatoes	1 pkg	210	18	7	45	17	4	600

FOOD	PORTION	CALS	PROT	FAT	CHOL	CARB	FIBER	SOD
Sweet & Sour Chicken	1 pkg	340	15	7	25	54	3	580
Traditional Meatloaf	1 pkg	300	18	9	40	36	6	600
Traditional Turkey Breast	1 pkg	300	21	4	25	42	6	550
Tuna Casserole	1 pkg	270	21	7	30	31	5	600
Helen's Kitchen								
Indian Curry w/ Tofu Steaks & Rice	1 pkg (9 oz)	300	14	8	0	63	5	300
Ian's								
Chicken Finger Meal Allergen Free	1 pkg (7 oz)	368	17	9	40	56	3	420
Chicken Nugget Meal	1 pkg (8 oz)	440	18	14	50	50	2	320
Fish Stick Meal	1 pkg (8.4 oz)	480	17	11	25	79	4	480
Hamburger Meal	1 pkg (7 oz)	296	12	9	25	45	3	260
Pizza Meal	1 pkg (6.7 oz)	340	9	7	25	60	4	290
Popcorn Turkey Dog Meal Allergen Free	1 pkg (7 oz)	442	8	17	21	67	1	460
Kashi								
Black Bean Mango	1 pkg (10 oz)	340	8	8	0	58	7	430
Lemon Rosemary Chicken	1 pkg (10 oz)	330	17	9	15	45	5	640
Lime Cilantro Shrimp	1 pkg (10 oz)	250	12	8	0	33	6	690
Southwest Style Chicken	1 pkg (10 oz)	240	16	5	30	32	6	680
Sweet & Sour Chicken	1 pkg (10 oz)	320	18	4	35	55	6	380
Kid Cuisine								
All American Fried Chicken	1 meal	500	28	21	80	48	4	780
All Star Chicken Breast Nuggets	1 meal	460	18	19	25	50	8	830
Bug Safari Chicken Breast Nuggets	1 meal	450	17	16	25	58	6	990
Carnival Corn Dog	1 meal	430	10	12	30	68	7	810
Deep Sea Adventure Fish Sticks	1 meal	400	15	12	20	56	4	520
Fiesta Beef Taco Dippers	1 meal	370	11	16	18	44	4	594
Pop Star Popcorn Chicken	1 meal	410	12	10	15	67	6	840

FOOD	PORTION	CALS	PROT	FAT	CHOL	CARB	FIBER	SOD
Lean Cuisine								
Cafe Classics Baked Chicken Florentine	1 pkg (8 oz)	200	18	8	40	14	3	660
Cafe Classics Baked Lemon Pepper Fish	1 pkg (9 oz)	220	22	6	65	20	7	630
Cafe Classics Beef Peppercorn	1 pkg (8.75 oz)	220	14	7	25	25	3	690
Cafe Classics Beef Portabello	1 pkg (9 oz)	200	14	5	30	25	2	680
Cafe Classics Beef Pot Roast	1 pkg (9 oz)	190	12	6	25	23	2	690
Cafe Classics Bowl Creamy Basil Chicken	1 pkg (10.5 oz)	310	17	9	35	39	3	690
Cafe Classics Bowl Grilled Chicken Caesar	1 pkg (9 oz)	270	19	7	35	32	3	690
Cafe Classics Chicken Carbonara	1 pkg (9 oz)	280	18	7	30	33	2	690
Cafe Classics Chicken & Vegetables	1 pkg (10.5 oz)	240	20	5	30	29	2	640
Cafe Classics Chicken L'Orange	1 pkg (9 oz)	230	18	2	35	35	2	340
Cafe Classics Chicken Marsala	1 pkg (8.1 oz)	140	14	4	35	12	3	620
Cafe Classics Chicken Parmesan	1 pkg (10.9 oz)	280	22	5	40	36	3	510
Cafe Classics Chicken Tuscan	1 pkg (12 oz)	300	23	7	45	35	5	820
Cafe Classics Chicken w/ Almonds	1 pkg (8.5 oz)	260	18	4	30	38	3	620
Cafe Classics Chicken w/ Basil Cream Sauce	1 pkg (8.5 oz)	270	19	7	30	32	2	490
Cafe Classics Fiesta Grilled Chicken	1 pkg (9.5 oz)	250	19	6	40	31	3	580
Cafe Classics Garlic Beef & Broccoli	1 pkg (9 oz)	170	13	6	30	16	3	690
Cafe Classics Glazed Chicken	1 pkg (8.5 oz)	220	20	4	35	27	2	610
Cafe Classics Glazed Turkey Tenderloins	1 pkg (9 oz)	260	14	5	20	40	4	660

FOOD	PORTION	CALS	PROT	FAT	CHOL	CARB	FIBER	SOD
Cafe Classics Grilled Chicken	1 pkg (9.4 oz)	160	14	5	35	15	4	690
Cafe Classics Grilled Chicken w/ Teriyaki Glaze	1 pkg (10 oz)	270	19	3	40	42	0	660
Cafe Classics Herb Roasted Chicken	1 pkg (8 oz)	190	16	4	30	23	3	620
Cafe Classics Honey Dijon Grilled Chicken	1 pkg (8 oz)	220	17	4	50	22	2	640
Cafe Classics Honey Mustard Chicken	1 pkg (8 oz)	250	17	4	30	37	1	650
Cafe Classics Honey Roasted Pork	1 serv (9.5 oz)	230	18	9	50	18	5	580
Cafe Classics Mandarin Chicken	1 pkg (9 oz)	270	14	4	30	46	2	690
Cafe Classics Meatloaf w/ Gravy & Whipped Potatoes	1 pkg (9.4 oz)	280	20	9	45	29	3	580
Cafe Classics Orange Peel Chicken	1 pkg (12 oz)	390	15	9	25	63	3	850
Cafe Classics Oven Roasted Beef	1 pkg (9.25 oz)	210	16	8	35	18	2	690
Cafe Classics Roasted Garlic Chicken	1 pkg (8.8 oz)	200	17	8	40	14	2	690
Cafe Classics Roasted Turkey & Vegetables	1 pkg (8 oz)	150	15	5	25	12	3	650
Cafe Classics Roasted Turkey Breast	1 pkg (12 oz)	280	17	6	30	39	4	890
Cafe Classics Roasted Turkey Breast w/ Dressing	1 pkg (9.75 oz)	270	12	2	20	51	3	690
Cafe Classics Salisbury Steak	1 pkg (12.5 oz)	310	25	8	50	34	8	890
Cafe Classics Salisbury Steak w/ Mac & Cheese	1 pkg (9.5 oz)	280	25	8	50	26	3	670
Cafe Classics Sesame Chicken	1 pkg (9 oz)	330	15	8	20	49	2	690
Cafe Classics Southern Beef Tips	1 pkg (8.75 oz)	250	15	5	25	36	3	630
Cafe Classics Steak Tips Portabello	1 pkg (7.5 oz)	180	15	7	40	13	3	460

FOOD	PORTION	CALS	PROT	FAT	CHOL	CARB	FIBER	SOD
Cafe Classics Steak Tips Dijon	1 pkg (12 oz)	320	19	8	35	44	5	890
Cafe Classics Stuffed Cabbage	1 pkg (9.5 oz)	200	10	6	15	26	4	700
Cafe Classics Swedish Meatballs	1 pkg (9.1 oz)	290	22	8	50	33	2	640
Cafe Classics Sweet & Sour Chicken	1 pkg (10 oz)	290	14	3	25	52	1	680
Cafe Classics Three Cheese Chicken	1 pkg (8 oz)	230	21	10	45	14	2	520
Comfort Classics Baked Chicken	1 pkg (8.6 oz)	230	18	5	30	32	2	650
Dinnertime Selects Balsamic Glazed Chicken	1 pkg (12 oz)	400	20	8	40	61	4	890
Dinnertime Selects Chicken Florentine	1 pkg (13.25 oz)	420	28	8	45	59	6	840
Dinnertime Selects Chicken Portabello	1 pkg (12 oz)	370	22	6	40	58	3	810
Dinnertime Selects Lemon Garlic Shrimp	1 pkg (12 oz)	350	18	7	75	54	5	830
Skillet Beef Teriyaki & Rice	1 serv	190	9	3	15	32	2	550
Spa Cuisine Chicken Mediterranean	1 pkg (10.5 oz)	240	16	4	20	35	6	690
Spa Cuisine Chicken In Peanut Sauce	1 pkg (9 oz)	280	21	7	25	32	2	690
Spa Cuisine Chicken Pecan	1 pkg (9 oz)	260	18	6	30	34	4	570
Spa Cuisine Lemon Chicken	1 pkg (9 oz)	290	12	7	25	45	1	660
Spa Cuisine Lemongrass Chicken	1 pkg (9.4 oz)	240	18	6	30	29	4	660
Spa Cuisine Pork w/ Cherry Sauce	1 pkg (8.25 oz)	260	15	5	35	38	4	340
Spa Cuisine Rosemary Chicken	1 pkg (8.25 oz)	230	17	5	35	29	3	690
Spa Cuisine Salmon w/ Beef	1 pkg (9.5 oz)	360	17	8	30	31	5	680
Mon Cuisine								
Vegan Moroccan Couscous	1 pkg (10 oz)	280	20	4	0	46	10	440
Vegan Veal Schnitzel In Sauce	1 pkg (10 oz)	300	24	8	0	38	7	440

FOOD	PORTION	CALS	PROT	FAT	CHOL	CARB	FIBER	SOD
Vegetarian Stuffed Cabbage In Tomato Sauce	1 pkg (10 oz)	220	13	5	0	36	5	260
Organic Classics								
Chicken Marsala w/ Mashed Potatoes	1 pkg (9.5 oz)	330	14	16	60	31	3	530
Jamaican Style Jerk Chicken w/ Wehani Rice	1 pkg (9.5 oz)	270	16	7	40	37	4	620
Lemon Chicken w/ Wehani Rice	1 pkg (9.5 oz)	320	14	8	35	49	3	320
Pacific Foods								
Beef Steak Stew	1 cup	250	20	7	35	29	8	800
Chicken Stew	1 cup	200	12	5	40	25	2	750
Patak's								
Vegetable Curry w/ Rice Rice Creamy Coconut	1 pkg	400	6	18	10	54	5	990
Vegetable Curry w/ Rice Rich Tomato & Onion	1 pkg (10.5 oz)	290	6	6	0	53	5	900
Vegetable Curry w/ Rice Tangy Lemon & Cilantro	1 pkg	300	5	7	0	54	5	1020
Quorn								
Meat Free Simply Saute Indian	½ pkg	240	14	4	15	47	9	800
Meat Free Simply Saute Mexican	½ pkg	340	15	7	15	61	7	850
Meat Free Simply Saute Thai	½ pkg	240	14	9	15	34	8	660
Savvy Faire								
Baja Jack Scramble	1 pkg (8.2 oz)	370	24	25	50	12	2	1120
Braised Beef	1 pkg (9.4 oz)	320	30	18	60	15	3	1470
Herb Crusted Chicken	1 pkg (9.7 oz)	430	28	21	75	34	6	580
Seeds Of Change								
Chicken Teriyaki	1 pkg (10 oz)	300	19	4	30	47	4	770
Mushroom Wild Pilaf	1 pkg (11 oz)	350	13	16	45	40	5	800
Seven Grain Pilaf	1 pkg (11 oz)	390	15	14	20	52	10	500

FOOD	PORTION	CALS	PROT	FAT	CHOL	CARB	FIBER	SOD
Shady Brook								
Roasted Carved Turkey	1 pkg (18.6 oz)	550	24	18	55	72	4	2130
South Beach								
Beef & Broccoli & Asian Style Noodles	1 pkg	320	30	13	45	32	9	1050
Caprese Style Chicken w/ Cauliflower & Broccoli	1 pkg	250	35	8	95	12	3	1350
Cashew Chicken w/ Sugar Snap Peas	1 pkg	360	33	13	55	31	8	1120
Chicken Alfredo A La Roma	1 pkg	270	29	8	65	23	8	840
Chicken Basilico w/ Rotini	1 pkg	280	27	10	50	24	7	630
Chicken Santa Fe Style Rice & Beans	1 pkg (8.9 oz)	340	22	12	80	35	4	750
Garlic Herb Chicken w/ Green Beans Almondine	1 pkg	250	27	12	70	13	4	950
Garlic Parmesan Chicken w/ Penne	1 pkg	290	29	11	55	24	8	820
Garlic Sesame Beef w/ Cauliflower Sugar Snap Peas & Peppers	1 pkg	250	19	11	65	19	4	890
Kung Pao Chicken Breast Strips w/ Peppers & Broccoli	1 pkg	300	32	11	80	18	5	890
Meatloaf w/ Gravy	1 pkg (8.9 oz)	210	16	9	50	17	4	910
Orange Beef Slices & Brown Rice In Sauce w/ Broccoli & Carrots	1 pkg	260	22	8	55	27	4	940
Roasted Turkey	1 pkg (9.4 oz)	240	17	9	50	27	4	920
Savory Beef w/ Cheesy Broccoli	1 pkg	240	28	8	70	16	3	1060
Savory Pork w/ Pecans & Green Beans	1 pkg	260	25	13	65	13	4	990
Szechwan Pork & Asian Noodles In Sauce	1 pkg	270	24	8	40	32	9	880
Stouffer's								
Beef Stew	1 pkg (11 oz)	280	21	9	40	28	4	1000

FOOD	PORTION	CALS	PROT	FAT	CHOL	CARB	FIBER	SOD
Beef Stroganoff	1 pkg (9.75 oz)	380	22	17	70	34	2	990
Chicken A La King	1 pkg (11.5 oz)	360	18	12	35	44	0	800
Corner Bistro Bourbon Steak Tips	1 pkg (12 oz)	520	25	22	50	56	3	1000
Corner Bistro Sesame Chicken	1 pkg (12.63 oz)	510	22	15	75	72	5	1380
Country Fried Beef Steak	1 pkg (16 oz)	610	22	33	40	55	6	1330
Creamed Chipped Beef	½ pkg (5.5 oz)	140	9	7	35	9	0	590
Fish Filet	1 pkg (9 oz)	400	27	16	55	36	4	1050
Fried Chicken Breast	1 pkg (8.88 oz)	360	20	18	45	30	2	880
Green Pepper Steak	1 pkg (10.5 oz)	240	18	4	30	32	3	910
Grilled Lemon Pepper Chicken	1 pkg (9 oz)	240	19	8	40	24	4	670
Meatloaf	1 pkg (6 oz)	560	34	29	110	40	8	1180
Pork Cutlet	1 pkg (10 oz)	370	13	21	25	31	3	1110
Roast Pork	1 pkg (9.5 oz)	320	17	11	50	39	4	960
Roast Turkey Breast	1 pkg (16 oz)	390	21	13	40	48	6	1290
Salisbury Steak	1 pkg (16 oz)	470	29	24	65	34	6	1050
Stuffed Pepper	1 pkg (10 oz)	220	11	10	20	22	2	1000
Swedish Meatballs	1 pkg (11.5 oz)	560	32	27	100	47	3	1250
Swanson								
Chicken & Dumplings	1 cup	230	11	10	35	24	2	990
Chicken A La King	1 can	270	14	18	20	12	2	1370
Tamarind Tree								
Alu Chole	1 pkg (9.25 oz)	320	9	7	0	57	7	600
Channa Dal Masala	1 pkg (9.25 oz)	290	11	3	0	55	90	610

FOOD	PORTION	CALS	PROT	FAT	CHOL	CARB	FIBER	SOD
Dal Makhani	1 pkg (9.25 oz)	350	14	6	10	63	11	610
Navratan Korma	1 pkg (9.25 oz)	370	10	15	10	55	7	680
Palak Paneer	1 pkg (9.25 oz)	350	8	17	25	43	8	640
Saag Chole	1 pkg (9.25 oz)	330	12	9	0	53	9	750
Vegetable Jalfrazi	1 pkg (9.25 oz)	280	7	7	0	50	7	570
Taste Above								
Meatless Zesty BBQ w/ Veggie Beef & Rice	1 pkg (10 oz)	280	16	6	0	48	7	310
TastyBite								
Beans Marsala & Basmati Rice	1 pkg (12 oz)	426	14	8	0	75	13	600
Green Curry Vegetables & Jasmine Rice	1 pkg (12 oz)	320	6	10	0	52	2	530
Spinach Dal & Basmati Rice	1 pkg (12 oz)	372	12	9	0	62	8	640
Stir Fry Vegetables & Jasmine Rice	1 pkg (12 oz)	450	7	16	0	67	3	480
Vegetable Supreme & Basmati Rice	1 pkg (12 oz)	317	11	6	4	55	11	410
Yellow Curry Vegetables & Jasmine Rice	1 pkg (12 oz)	380	7	13	0	61	3	440
Yves								
Meatless Santa Fe Beef	1 pkg (10.5 oz)	360	15	9	0	57	5	750

DIP

FOOD	PORTION	CALS	PROT	FAT	CHOL	CARB	FIBER	SOD
spinach sour cream	¼ cup	155	2	15	13	4	1	166
Blue Bunny								
Incrediples	2 tbsp	30	2	1	–	4	0	230
Incrediples Taco Fiesta	2 tbsp	30	2	1	–	4	0	210
Spicy Buffalo	2 tbsp	30	2	1	–	4	0	270
Bravos!								
Salsa	2 tbsp	15	0	0	0	3	0	170
Salsa Con Queso	1 tbsp	25	0	2	0	3	0	180

FOOD	PORTION	CALS	PROT	FAT	CHOL	CARB	FIBER	SOD
Cabot								
Clam	2 tbsp	50	1	5	15	1	0	120
Cedarlane								
Organic Five Layer Mexican	2 tbsp	60	3	3	10	4	1	100
Eatsmart								
Flame Roasted Salsa Con Queso	2 tbsp	35	0	2	0	4	–	160
Garden Style Sweet Salsa	2 tbsp	20	0	0	0	5	–	95
Jalapeno & Lime Tres Bean	2 tbsp	25	1	0	0	5	–	150
Fritos								
Bean	2 tbsp	40	2	1	0	5	1	170
Chili Cheese	2 tbsp	45	1	3	<5	3	0	310
Hot Bean	2 tbsp	40	2	1	0	56	1	210
Jalapeno Cheddar Cheese	2 tbsp	50	1	4	5	4	0	300
Mild Cheddar	2 tbsp	60	1	4	5	3	0	330
Guiltless Gourmet								
Black Bean Mild	2 tbsp	30	2	0	0	5	2	115
Roasted Red Pepper Salsa	2 tbsp	15	0	0	0	2	0	130
Southwestern Grill Salsa	2 tbsp	15	0	0	0	2	0	115
Kraft								
Green Onion	2 tbsp	60	tr	5	0	3	0	170
LiteHouse								
Avocado	2 tbsp	140	1	15	15	2	0	210
Caramel Low Fat	1 tbsp	110	1	0	0	27	0	140
Caramel Original	2 tbsp	110	1	2	0	25	1	125
Dilly	2 tbsp	150	1	16	15	1	0	200
Fruit Dip Chocolate Yogurt	2 tbsp	110	1	6	0	14	0	95
Fruit Dip Vanilla Yogurt	2 tbsp	60	1	2	0	10	0	50
Lite Ranch Veggie	2 tbsp	70	1	7	10	3	0	125
Organic Ranch	2 tbsp	130	1	13	10	2	0	200
Marie's								
French Onion Roasted	2 tbsp	100	1	10	15	2	0	220
Guacamole	2 tbsp	40	1	3	5	3	1	140
Honey Vanilla Cream Fruit Dip	2 tbsp	60	1	5	15	5	0	20
Spinach Parmesan	2 tbsp	90	2	9	15	2	0	200
Marzetti								
Veggie Fat Free Ranch	2 tbsp	35	1	7	0	6	0	320
Veggie Dip Light Veggie	1 pkg (3.25 oz)	170	0	17	15	3	0	580

FOOD	PORTION	CALS	PROT	FAT	CHOL	CARB	FIBER	SOD
Phillips Seafood								
Crab & Spinach	2 tbsp	50	3	5	15	1	–	95
Maryland Crab	2 tbsp	70	3	6	30	1	–	95
Road's End Organics								
Nacho Cheese Gluten Free	2 tbsp	20	2	0	0	3	tr	110
Robert Rothchild Farm								
Artichoke	2 tbsp	60	2	5	<5	2	tr	65
Ruffles								
French Onion	¼ cup	200	7	15	0	9	2	100
Ranch	2 tbsp	60	1	5	<5	1	tr	240
Snyder's Of Hanover								
Three Bean	2 tbsp	25	1	0	0	5	1	150
Utz								
Jalapeno Cheddar	2 tbsp	260	0	4	0	2	0	260
Sour Cream & Onion	2 tbsp	60	1	5	20	2	0	250
Wise								
French Onion	2 tbsp	60	1	5	0	3	0	220
Nacho Cheese	2 tbsp	50	1	5	0	3	0	200
DOCK								
fresh cooked	3½ oz	20	2	1	0	3	–	3
raw chopped	½ cup	15	1	tr	0	2	–	3
DOUGHNUTS								
cake type unsugared	1 (1.6 oz)	198	2	11	18	23	1	257
chocolate glazed	1 (1.5 oz)	175	2	8	–	24	1	143
chocolate sugared	1 (1.5 oz)	175	2	8	–	24	1	143
chocolate coated	1 (1.5 oz)	204	2	13	–	21	1	185
creme filled	1 (3 oz)	307	6	21	20	26	–	262
french cruller glazed	1 (1.4 oz)	169	1	8	5	24	–	142
frosted	1 (1.5 oz)	204	2	13	–	21	1	185
honey bun	1 (2.1 oz)	242	4	14	4	27	1	205
jelly	1 (3 oz)	209	5	16	22	33	–	249
old fashioned	1 (1.6 oz)	198	2	11	18	23	1	257
sugared	1 (1.6 oz)	192	2	10	14	23	1	181
wheat glazed	1 (1.6 oz)	162	3	9	9	19	–	160
wheat sugared	1 (1.6 oz)	162	3	9	9	19	–	160
yeast glazed	1 (2.1 oz)	242	4	14	4	27	1	205
Entenmann's								
Crumb	1	260	2	12	10	36	tr	210
Frosted Devil's Food	1	310	2	19	10	36	2	170

FOOD	PORTION	CALS	PROT	FAT	CHOL	CARB	FIBER	SOD
Glazed	1	260	2	13	15	34	tr	230
Glazed Popems	4	220	2	10	0	30	0	170
Mini Frosted	1 (1 oz)	150	1	11	<5	13	tr	80
Plain Old Fashion	1	230	2	14	15	25	tr	240
Rich Chocolate Frosted	1	280	2	18	10	29	1	190
Super Bakery								
Daily Donut	1 (2.2 oz)	250	7	14	10	26	tr	280
Proballs Slam Powdered Baseballs	1 (1.3 oz)	130	3	6	5	17	0	160

DRINK MIXERS

FOOD	PORTION	CALS	PROT	FAT	CHOL	CARB	FIBER	SOD
whiskey sour mix not prep	1 pkg (0.6 oz)	64	tr	0	0	16	–	46
whiskey sour mix	2 oz	55	0	0	0	14	0	66
McIlhenny								
Bloody Mary Mix as prep	1 cup	70	2	0	0	15	2	1930

DRUM

FOOD	PORTION	CALS	PROT	FAT	CHOL	CARB	FIBER	SOD
freshwater fillet baked	5.4 oz	236	35	10	126	0	0	148
freshwater baked	3 oz	130	19	5	70	0	0	82

DUCK

FOOD	PORTION	CALS	PROT	FAT	CHOL	CARB	FIBER	SOD
w/ skin roasted	1 cup (4.9 oz)	472	27	40	118	0	0	83
w/ skin w/ bone leg roasted	3 oz	184	23	10	97	0	0	94
w/ skin w/o bone breast roasted	3 oz	172	21	9	116	0	0	71
w/o skin roasted	1 cup (4.9 oz)	281	33	16	125	0	0	91
w/o skin w/ bone leg braised	1 cup (6.1 oz)	310	51	10	183	0	0	188
w/o skin w/o bone breast broiled	1 cup (6.1 oz)	244	48	4	249	0	0	183
wild w/ skin raw	½ duck (9.5 oz)	571	47	41	216	0	0	152
wild w/o skin breast raw	½ breast (2.9 oz)	102	16	4	–	0	0	47

DUMPLING
Kahiki

FOOD	PORTION	CALS	PROT	FAT	CHOL	CARB	FIBER	SOD
Potstickers Chicken	5 (3.3 oz)	230	7	11	10	24	1	520
Samosas Coconut Curry Chicken	4 (2.8 oz)	170	8	3	15	26	1	520

FOOD	PORTION	CALS	PROT	FAT	CHOL	CARB	FIBER	SOD
Pepperidge Farm								
Apple	1	250	3	11	0	32	1	180
Peach	1	320	3	11	0	50	4	150
Traveling Chef								
Potstichers Chicken	5 pieces	285	13	7	20	42	1	840
+ Dipping Sauce	+ 1 tbsp sauce							
TAKE-OUT								
apple	1 (6.7 oz)	661	7	34	0	83	3	614
bread dumpling	1 lg	330	–	10	–	28	–	–
cherry	1 (2.7 oz)	238	3	12	0	31	1	216
cornmeal	1 (2.8 oz)	134	5	4	62	20	2	278
fried pork	1 (3.5 oz)	338	13	21	27	25	1	363
fried puerto rican style	1 med (1.1 oz)	117	2	7	0	11	tr	182
peach	1 (2.7 oz)	253	3	12	0	33	1	248
steamed meat	1 (1.3 oz)	41	4	1	18	4	tr	161
DURIAN								
fresh	3.5 oz	141	3	2	0	29	–	1
EEL								
fresh cooked	3 oz	200	20	13	137	0	0	55
fresh cooked	1 fillet (5.6 oz)	375	38	24	257	0	0	104
raw	3 oz	156	16	10	107	0	0	43
smoked	3.5 oz	330	19	28	–	0	0	–
EGG (see also EGG DISHES, EGG SUBSTITUTES)								
CHICKEN								
hard or soft cooked	1	77	6	5	211	1	0	139
pickled	1	72	6	5	198	1	0	131
poached	1	73	6	5	210	tr	0	147
scrambled plain	2	199	13	15	400	2	0	211
sunny side up	2	155	11	12	365	1	0	414
white cooked	1	17	4	tr	0	tr	0	106
yolk cooked	1	55	3	4	209	1	0	34
Crystal Farms								
In Shell Pasteurized	1	70	6	5	215	1	0	65
Peeled Hard Cooked	1	70	6	5	190	1	0	55
Davidson's								
Pasteurized Shell Eggs	1 lg	75	6	5	213	0	0	60

FOOD	PORTION	CALS	PROT	FAT	CHOL	CARB	FIBER	SOD
Egg-Land's Best								
Extra Large	1 (2 oz)	80	7	5	200	0	0	75
Large	1	70	6	4	180	0	0	65
Organic Brown	1	70	6	4	180	0	0	65
Eggology								
100% Organic Egg Whites	¼ cup	30	7	0	0	0	0	100
Gold Circle Farms								
Cage Free	1 large	70	6	5	215	tr	–	70
Horizon Organic								
Jumbo	1 (2.2 oz)	90	8	5	270	1	0	80
Land O Lakes								
Farm Fresh Brown Extra Large	1 (1.8 oz)	70	6	5	215	1	–	65
Organic Valley								
Egg Whites Pasteurized	¼ cup	25	5	0	0	1	0	90
Large Omega-3	1	70	7	5	225	tr	–	85
Pete And Gerry's								
Organic	1	70	6	5	250	1	–	65
Sunny Fresh								
Eggs ASAP!	2	140	11	10	380	1	0	110
OTHER POULTRY								
duck 100 year old	1 (1 oz)	49	4	3	173	1	–	154
duck cooked	1 (2.5 oz)	129	9	10	616	1	0	210
duck preserved hard core	1 (1.8 oz)	80	6	6	220	1	0	350
duck preserved soft core	1 (1.8 oz)	80	7	6	220	1	0	350
duck salted	1 (1 oz)	54	4	4	184	2	–	769
goose cooked	1 (5 oz)	265	20	19	1223	2	0	420
quail canned	1 (0.3 oz)	14	1	1	75	tr	0	47
quail cooked	1 (0.5 oz)	24	2	2	42	0	0	24
turkey raw	1 (2.8 oz)	135	11	9	737	1	0	119

EGG DISHES

FOOD	PORTION	CALS	PROT	FAT	CHOL	CARB	FIBER	SOD
Aunt Jemima								
Eggs & Sausage	1 pkg (6.2 oz)	370	14	27	335	16	2	750
Omelet Ham & Cheese	1 pkg (5.2 oz)	250	13	15	195	17	2	760
Cedarlane								
Zone Omelette Cheese	1 pkg (10.4 oz)	350	25	14	40	31	2	720

FOOD	PORTION	CALS	PROT	FAT	CHOL	CARB	FIBER	SOD
TAKE-OUT								
deviled	1 half	62	4	5	121	tr	0	94
eggs benedict	2	825	35	64	784	26	2	1654
omelet cheese	3 eggs	387	25	29	588	6	0	1134
omelet mushroom	3 eggs	251	18	17	511	6	1	796
omelet mushroom & onion	3 eggs	294	20	20	600	7	1	780
omelet plain	3 eggs	338	24	25	736	4	0	854
omelet spanish	3 eggs	496	23	38	626	17	3	876
omelet spinach	3 eggs	279	20	19	568	6	1	687
omelet western	3 eggs	355	24	23	537	6	tr	1007
salad	½ cup	353	10	34	344	2	0	402
scotch egg	1 (4.2 oz)	301	14	21	-	16	2	-
tortilla de amarillo omelet w/ plantain	3 eggs	536	16	35	467	43	3	1017
EGG ROLLS								
egg roll wrapper fresh	1	83	3	tr	3	16	–	162
Frieda's								
Egg Roll Wrappers	2 (1.6 oz)	130	5	1	0	28	1	250
Kahiki								
Chicken	1 (3 oz)	160	7	6	10	19	1	730
Chipotle Lime Chicken	1 (3 oz)	170	8	4	10	26	2	380
Lemongrass Chicken Stix	3 (2.6 oz)	100	7	2	20	13	tr	380
Pork & Shrimp	1 (3 oz)	140	8	4	30	20	1	630
Vegetable	1 (3 oz)	90	2	4	0	12	1	410
Lean Cuisine								
Cafe Classics Vegetable	1 pkg (9 oz)	310	7	5	5	60	3	640
Nasoya								
Egg Roll Wrapper	3	170	7	1	10	35	1	410
Pagoda								
Sweet & Sour Chicken	1 (2.7 oz)	170	6	6	5	25	2	260
Phillips								
Spring Rolls Crab & Shrimp w/ Sauce	3 (3.75 oz)	220	7	7	60	33	–	520
TAKE-OUT								
chicken	1 (3 oz)	140	7	4	15	20	4	510
lobster	1 (4.8 oz)	270	8	7	0	43	6	460
meat & shrimp	1 (4.8 oz)	320	10	12	10	41	4	470
pork & shrimp	1 (5 oz)	300	13	10	15	41	7	890
shrimp	1 (3 oz)	170	6	5	<5	24	5	420

FOOD	PORTION	CALS	PROT	FAT	CHOL	CARB	FIBER	SOD
spicy pork	1 (3 oz)	200	6	9	5	23	3	410
vegetable	1 (3 oz)	170	5	4	0	28	4	520

EGG SUBSTITUTES
Better'n Eggs
All Whites	¼ cup	30	6	0	0	1	0	100
Ham & Cheese	¼ cup	45	6	2	5	1	0	150
Original	¼ cup (2 oz)	30	6	0	0	1	0	115
Plus	¼ cup	35	6	0	0	1	0	115
Three Cheese	¼ cup	45	6	1	5	1	0	150

Bob's Red Mill
Egg White Dried	2 tsp	15	3	0	0	0	0	45
Vegetarian Egg Replacer	1 tbsp	30	3	1	0	2	1	20

Egg Beaters
Original	¼ cup	30	6	0	0	1	0	115

EggPro
Powder	1 tbsp	15	4	0	0	tr	0	55

Fantastic
Tofu Scrambler not prep	1 tbsp	35	1	0	0	7	1	260

Horizon Organic
Liquid Egg	¼ cup	35	6	0	0	1	0	100

Land O Lakes
Liquid Egg	¼ cup	30	6	0	0	1	0	115

Quick Eggs
Fat Free Cholesterol Free	¼ cup	30	6	0	0	1	0	115

EGGNOG
eggnog	1 qt	1368	39	76	596	138	–	553
eggnog	1 cup	342	10	19	149	34	–	138
eggnog flavor mix as prep w/ milk	9 oz	260	8	8	33	39	–	163

Farmland
Egg Nog	½ cup	180	4	8	50	23	0	150

Hood
Fat Free Sugar Free	1 cup	110	8	0	<5	18	0	210
Golden	½ cup	180	4	9	65	22	0	100
Light	½ cup	140	4	4	45	22	0	100

Horizon Organic
Lowfat	½ cup	140	6	3	45	22	0	135

Organic Valley
Ultra Pasteurized	½ cup	180	5	10	90	18	0	85

FOOD	PORTION	CALS	PROT	FAT	CHOL	CARB	FIBER	SOD
TAKE-OUT								
eggnog	1 cup	306	5	22	63	16	0	95
EGGPLANT								
cubed cooked w/ oil	1 cup	133	2	8	0	17	5	1000
pickled	½ cup	33	1	tr	0	7	2	1138
slices grilled	1 (2 oz)	36	tr	2	0	5	1	268
Cedarlane								
Eggplant Mediterranean	1 pkg (10 oz)	230	13	10	20	22	6	590
Celentano								
Eggplant Parmigiana	1 serv (7 oz)	330	9	22	25	26	5	480
Frieda's								
Chinese	⅔ cup (3 oz)	20	1	0	0	5	2	0
Japanese Nasu	⅔ cup (3 oz)	20	1	0	0	3	2	0
Peloponnese								
Baba Ganoush	2 tbsp	40	1	3	0	2	1	250
Sabra								
Baba Ghanoush	2 oz	50	3	6	0	4	1	125
Stonewall Kitchen								
Eggplant Spread	1 tbsp	25	0	1	–	4	–	90
TastyBite								
Punjab Eggplant	½ pkg (5 oz)	144	4	9	0	13	2	515
TAKE-OUT								
baba ghannouj	¼ cup	55	2	4	0	5	–	95
caponata	2 tbsp (1 oz)	30	1	2	0	3	–	115
iman bayildi eggplant w/ onion & tomato	1 serv (15.6 oz)	345	3	28	0	25	2	552
indian eggplant runi	1 serv	180	2	14	0	13	1	228
moussaka	1 serv (9 oz)	372	20	24	54	18	5	415
papoutsaki little shoes	1 serv (15.5 oz)	245	12	16	40	15	1	751
ELDERBERRIES								
fresh	1 cup	105	1	1	0	27	–	–

FOOD	PORTION	CALS	PROT	FAT	CHOL	CARB	FIBER	SOD
ELDERBERRY JUICE								
elderberry	7 oz	76	4	0	0	16	–	2
ELK								
eye of round roasted	3.5 oz	151	31	3	63	1	0	50
ground cooked	3.5 oz	143	29	3	70	0	0	56
ENERGY BARS (see also CEREAL BARS, NUTRITION SUPPLEMENTS)								
Activex								
Organic All Flavors	1 (1.6 oz)	200	8	12	0	17	2	75
All In One								
All Flavors	1 (1.8 oz)	180	15	5	<5	20	5	180
Amino Vital								
Fit Apple Pie	1 (1.76 oz)	150	8	2	–	26	2	135
Fit Chocolate Peanut	1 (1.76 oz)	190	7	8	–	25	2	130
Fit Toasted Nut Cranberry	1 (1.76 oz)	180	7	8	–	24	2	105
Attune								
Wellness Chocolate Crisp	1 (0.7 oz)	100	2	6	0	11	1	20
Wellness Cool Mint Chocolate	1 (0.7 oz)	100	2	6	0	11	1	20
Belly-bar								
Baby Needs Chocolate	1	170	8	6	0	22	2	280
Berry Nutty Cravings	1	170	8	4	0	26	2	70
Mellow Oat	1	180	8	5	0	26	2	70
Boomi Bar								
Almond Protein Plus	1	270	12	18	15	20	4	12
Cashew Almond Delicacy	1	260	8	17	0	23	1	55
Cranberry Apple	1	210	4	9	0	28	4	50
Merry Macadamia	1	220	3	14	0	26	3	25
Pistachio Pineapple	1	200	5	9	0	28	3	50
Bora Bora								
Organic Cranberry Crunch	1 (1.4 oz)	170	5	10	0	18	2	20
Organic Peanut Peanut	1 (1.4 oz)	230	6	17	0	10	2	10
Organic Sesame Raisin	1 (1.4 oz)	170	5	11	0	17	3	15
Clif								
Banana Nut Bread	1 (2.4 oz)	250	10	6	0	43	5	130
Builders Chocolate Mint	1 (2.4 oz)	270	20	8	0	31	4	230
Builders Peanut Butter	1 (2.4 oz)	270	20	8	0	30	4	310
Carrot Cake	1 (2.4 oz)	240	10	4	0	46	5	150
Chocolate Brownie	1 (2.4 oz)	240	10	5	0	45	5	150
Chocolate Chip	1 (2.4 oz)	250	10	5	0	45	5	150

FOOD	PORTION	CALS	PROT	FAT	CHOL	CARB	FIBER	SOD
Cool Mint Chocolate	1 (2.4 oz)	250	10	5	0	43	5	140
Crunchy Peanut Butter	1 (2.4 oz)	250	12	6	0	40	5	250
Mojo Mixed Nuts	1 (1.6 oz)	220	9	9	0	21	3	200
Mojo Mountain Mix	1 (1.6 oz)	200	8	8	0	24	2	260
Nectar Cinnamon Pecan	1 (1.6 oz)	170	2	9	0	26	6	0
Nectar Lemon Vanilla Cashew	1 (1.6 oz)	180	4	6	0	27	6	5
Oatmeal Raisin Walnut	1 (2.4 oz)	240	10	5	0	43	5	130
ZBar Peanut Butter	1 (1.3 oz)	140	3	5	0	20	3	170
Glucerna								
All Flavors	1 (0.7 oz)	80	4	3	0	12	tr	60
Gnu								
Flavor & Fiber Banana Walnut	1 (1.4 oz)	130	3	3	0	30	12	42
Flavor & Fiber Orange Cranberry	1 (1.4 oz)	130	4	3	0	31	12	31
Hooah!								
Chocolate Crisp	1 (2.29 oz)	280	10	9	<5	40	2	140
JojoBar								
Chocolate Cashew	1 (1.8 oz)	220	11	14	10	18	2	55
Peanut Butter & Jelly	1 (1.8 oz)	220	13	13	10	17	3	25
Kashi								
GoLean Chocolate Almond Toffee	1 (2.7 oz)	290	13	6	0	45	6	250
GoLean Cookies 'N Cream	1 (2.7 oz)	290	13	6	0	50	6	200
GoLean Malted Chocolate Chip	1 (2.7 oz)	290	13	6	0	49	6	200
GoLean Oatmeal Raisin Cookie	1 (2.7 oz)	280	13	5	0	49	6	140
GoLean Peanut Butter & Chocolate	1 (2.7 oz)	290	13	6	0	48	6	280
GoLean Crunchy Chocolate Peanut	1 (1.8 oz)	180	9	5	0	30	6	250
GoLean Roll Caramel Peanut	1 (1.9 oz)	200	12	5	0	29	6	210
GoLean Roll Fudge Sundae	1 (1.9 oz)	190	12	5	0	27	6	260
TLC Chewy Granola Cherry Dark Chocolate	1 (1.2 oz)	120	5	2	0	24	4	75

FOOD	PORTION	CALS	PROT	FAT	CHOL	CARB	FIBER	SOD
TLC Crunchy Granola Honey Toasted 7 Grain	1 (1.4 oz)	180	7	6	0	26	4	160
TLC Crunchy Granola Pumpkin Spice	1 (1.4 oz)	180	6	6	0	26	4	150
TLC Crunchy Granola Roasted Almond	1 (1.4 oz)	180	7	6	0	26	4	160
LaraBar								
Apple Pie	1	190	4	9	0	23	4	10
Banana Cookie	1	210	6	10	0	24	5	0
Cashew Cookie	1	230	5	13	0	23	3	0
Cherry Pie	1	190	5	9	0	24	4	0
Chocolate Coconut Chew	1	220	5	12	0	24	5	0
Ginger Snap	1	220	5	13	0	22	5	0
Jocolat	1 (1 oz)	110	2	6	0	14	3	0
Living Harvest								
Organic Hemp Protein Forbidden Fruit	1 (1.6 oz)	170	6	6	0	25	4	100
Luna								
Caramel Nut Brownie	1 (1.7 oz)	190	9	6	0	27	4	125
Chai Tea	1 (1.7 oz)	180	10	4	0	27	3	125
Dulce De Leche	1 (1.7 oz)	180	10	3	0	28	3	160
Iced Oatmeal Raisin	1 (1.7 oz)	180	10	4	0	28	3	170
Key Lime Pie	1 (1.7 oz)	180	10	4	0	29	2	80
LemonZest	1 (1.7 oz)	180	10	4	0	26	3	125
Nutz Over Chocolate	1 (1.7 oz)	180	10	5	0	24	3	200
Mommy Munchies								
Chocolate Mint	1 (1.8 oz)	180	12	7	5	32	5	35
Cinnamon Bun	1 (1.8 oz)	180	12	6	0	23	5	40
Mrs. May's								
Trio Blueberry	1 (1.2 oz)	170	5	12	0	15	2	45
Trio Tropical	1 (1.2 oz)	170	5	12	0	14	2	45
Nature's Path								
Optimum Blueberry Flax & Soy	1 (2 oz)	200	7	3	0	37	5	115
Optimum Cranberry Ginger & Soy	1 (2 oz)	200	6	3	0	37	5	140
Optimum Peanut Butter	1 (2 oz)	230	7	8	0	33	4	200
Optimum Pomegran Cherry	1 (2 oz)	230	4	5	0	39	4	140
Optimum ReBound	1 (2 oz)	190	10	4	0	33	4	140

FOOD	PORTION	CALS	PROT	FAT	CHOL	CARB	FIBER	SOD
Nutiva								
Organic Flax & Raisin	1 (1.4 oz)	200	7	15	0	15	4	0
Organic Flaxseed Flax Chocolate	1 (1.4 oz)	200	6	12	0	19	5	5
Original Organic Hempseed	1 (1.4 oz)	210	9	14	0	11	5	5
Odwalla								
Berries GoMega	1	220	5	5	0	41	5	230
Carrot	1	220	4	4	0	43	4	115
Choco-walla	1	240	5	6	0	42	5	80
Cranberry C Monster	1	220	4	3	0	44	3	85
Super Protein	1	230	16	5	0	31	4	160
Superfood	1	230	4	4	0	43	3	110
Oh Mama!								
Chocolate Peanut Butter	1 (1.8 oz)	190	9	6	0	26	3	170
Frosted White Lemon	1 (1.8 oz)	180	9	5	0	28	3	160
Frosted White Raspberry	1 (1.8 oz)	180	10	5	0	26	3	180
Perfect 10								
Bliss Apricot	1 (1.8 oz)	215	5	9	2	29	5	10
Bliss Cranberry	1 (1.8 oz)	215	4	12	2	26	4	10
Natural Apricot	1 (1.8 oz)	205	5	10	0	27	4	5
Natural Cranberry	1 (1.8 oz)	164	4	10	0	17	4	3
Natural Lemon	1 (1.8 oz)	210	5	12	0	24	5	5
PowerBar								
Harvest Apple Cinnamon Crisp	1 (2.3 oz)	240	7	4	0	45	4	80
Harvest Chunky Cherry Crunch	1 (2.3 oz)	240	7	4	0	45	4	45
Harvest Peanut Butter Chocolate Chip	1 (2.3 oz)	240	7	4	0	44	4	80
Harvest Strawberry Crunch	1 (2.3 oz)	230	7	4	0	45	4	100
Harvest Dipped Double Chocolate Crisp	1 (2.3 oz)	250	7	5	0	45	3	100
Harvest Dipped Oatmeal Raisin Cookie	1 (2.3 oz)	250	7	5	0	45	3	100
Harvest Dipped Toffee Chocolate Chip	1 (2.3 oz)	250	7	5	0	45	3	140
Performance Apple Cinnamon	1 (2.3 oz)	230	9	3	0	45	3	100
Performance Banana	1 (2.3 oz)	230	9	3	0	45	3	100

FOOD	PORTION	CALS	PROT	FAT	CHOL	CARB	FIBER	SOD
Performance Cappuccino	1 (2.3 oz)	230	10	2	0	45	3	110
Performance Chocolate	1 (2.3 oz)	230	10	2	0	45	3	95
Performance Chocolate Peanut Butter	1 (2.3 oz)	240	10	3	0	45	3	95
Performance Cookies & Cream	1 (2.3 oz)	240	79	4	0	45	2	120
Performance Malt Nut	1 (2.3 oz)	230	9	3	0	45	3	90
Performance Oatmeal Raisin	1 (2.3 oz)	230	10	3	0	45	3	110
Performance Peanut Butter	1 (2.3 oz)	230	10	4	0	45	3	120
Performance Strawberry Cream	1 (2.3 oz)	230	9	2	0	45	2	100
Performance Vanilla Crisp	1 (2.3 oz)	230	9	3	0	45	3	90
Performance Wild Berry	1 (2.3 oz)	230	9	3	0	45	3	95
Protein Plus Carb Select Chocolate	1 (2.5 oz)	260	22	7	5	30	1	190
Protein Plus Carb Select Chocolate Caramel Crunch	1 (2.6 oz)	270	20	11	5	32	2	170
Protein Plus Carb Select Chocolate Peanut Butter	1 (2.5 oz)	270	22	9	5	30	2	290
Protein Plus Carb Select Peanut Caramel	1 (2.6 oz)	270	20	11	5	32	1	290
Protein Plus Chocolate Fudge Brownie	1 (2.7 oz)	270	23	5	0	36	2	140
Protein Plus Chocolate Peanut Butter	1 (2.7 oz)	290	23	5	0	38	1	220
Protein Plus Cookies & Cream	1 (2.7 oz)	290	23	5	0	38	1	160
Protein Plus Vanilla Yogurt	1 (2.7 oz)	290	23	5	0	37	1	150
Triple Treat Caramel Peanut Crisp	1 (1.9 oz)	220	11	5	0	32	4	210
Triple Treat Caramel Peanut Fusion	1 (1.9 oz)	230	10	8	5	30	4	190
Triple Treat Chocolate Caramel Fusion	1 (1.9 oz)	230	10	8	0	30	4	150
Triple Treat Chocolate Peanut Butter Crisp	1 (1.9 oz)	220	11	5	0	32	4	180
Prana Bar								
Apricot Goji	1 (1.7 oz)	220	4	13	0	26	3	30

FOOD	PORTION	CALS	PROT	FAT	CHOL	CARB	FIBER	SOD
Coconut Acai	1 (1.7 oz)	220	4	13	0	26	3	35
Pear Ginseng	1 (1.7 oz)	220	5	15	0	21	4	30
Pria								
Carb Select Caramel Nut Brownie	1 (1.7 oz)	170	10	8	5	21	2	90
Carb Select Chocolate Mocha Crisp	1 (1.7 oz)	130	8	6	0	16	4	115
Carb Select Chocolate Peanut Butter Crisp	1 (1.7 oz)	130	8	6	0	16	4	140
Complete Nutrition Chocolate Mint Crisp	1 (1.6 oz)	170	11	6	0	22	5	190
Complete Nutrition Chocolate Peanut Butter Crisp	1 (1.6 oz)	170	11	6	0	22	5	200
Complete Nutrition French Vanilla Crisp	1 (1.6 oz)	170	11	5	0	22	5	190
Creme Carmel Crisp	1 (1 oz)	110	5	3	0	17	1	90
Double Chocolate Cookie	1 (1 oz)	110	5	3	0	16	1	100
French Vanilla Crisp	1 (1 oz)	110	5	3	–	17	1	85
Mint Chocolate Cookie	1 (1 oz)	110	5	4	0	15	1	90
Strawberry Shortcake	1 (1 oz)	110	5	3	0	16	1	80
PureFit								
Almond Crunch	1 (2 oz)	230	18	6	0	25	3	190
Peanut Butter Crunch	1 (2 oz)	240	18	7	0	26	2	200
Resource								
Mini Nutrition Bar	1	90	7	3	–	10	–	–
Simply Nutrilite								
Sweet & Salty	1 (1.6 oz)	170	4	6	0	27	4	310
Slim-Fast								
Classic Meal Bar Chocolate Cookie Dough	1	220	8	5	<5	36	2	160
Classic Meal Bar Milk Chocolate Peanut	1	220	8	5	<5	37	2	125
High Protein Granola Bar Chocolate Chip	1	190	15	6	<5	20	2	200
High Protein Granola Bar Peanut	1	200	15	7	0	21	2	200
Low Carb Breakfast Bar Apple Cobbler	1	180	14	6	<5	19	3	290

FOOD	PORTION	CALS	PROT	FAT	CHOL	CARB	FIBER	SOD
Low Carb Breakfast Bar Peanut Butter	1	190	15	8	<5	17	3	300
Low Carb Snack Bar Caramel Nut	1	120	2	5	<5	19	1	70
Low Carb Snack Bar Coconut Almond	1	120	6	5	<5	15	2	80
Low Carb Snack Bar Peanut Butter Crunch	1	120	1	5	<5	21	1	80
Optima Meal Bar Apple Crisp	1	180	8	3	0	29	3	108
Optima Meal Bar Caramel Crispy Peanut	1	220	8	6	<5	33	2	250
Optima Meal Bar Chewy Granola Trail Mix	1	210	8	5	<5	34	2	190
Optima Snack Bar Banana Nut Muffin	1	150	2	8	<5	18	1	200
Optima Snack Bar Blueberry Muffin	1	140	1	57	<5	22	1	170
Optima Snack Bar Chocolate Peanut Nougat	1	120	2	4	<5	20	1	70
Optima Snack Bar Oatmeal Raisin Cookie	1	120	2	4	0	19	1	115
Snickers Marathon								
Chewy Chocolate Peanut	1 (1.9 oz)	210	14	8	0	26	5	220
Solo GI								
Berry Bliss	1 (1.6 oz)	190	11	5	0	23	3	110
Chocolate Charger	1 (1.6 oz)	190	10	6	5	24	4	100
Mint Mania	1 (1.6 oz)	190	10	6	5	24	4	100
Peanut Power	1 (1.6 oz)	200	12	7	0	22	3	110
South Beach								
Energy Mix	1 pkg (1 oz)	160	6	13	0	8	2	45
SoyJoy								
Fruit & Soy Berry	1 (1.1. oz)	130	4	5	15	17	3	50
Fruit & Soy Mango Coconut	1 (1.1 oz)	140	4	6	20	16	3	45
Fruit & Soy Raisin Almond	1 (1.1 oz)	130	4	6	15	16	3	40
T.H.E. Bar								
Granola Raisin	1 (1.8 oz)	200	9	6	0	25	1	65
Think5								
Red Berry	1 (2.5)	240	4	4	0	48	3	140

FOOD	PORTION	CALS	PROT	FAT	CHOL	CARB	FIBER	SOD
Red Berry Chocolate Covered	1 (2.8 oz)	290	4	8	0	52	3	140
ThinkPink								
Blueberry Dark Chocolate	1 (2.1 oz)	240	20	8	0	26	2	80
Lemon Burst	1 (2.1 oz)	230	20	7	0	27	2	150
Peanut Butter Caramel	1 (2.1 oz)	230	20	8	5	26	1	280
White Chocolate Raspberry	1 (2.1 oz)	240	20	8	0	28	3	100
Zoe's								
Chocolate Delight	1 (1.7 oz)	190	8	7	0	27	5	70
Chocolate Peanut Butter Bliss	1 (1.7 oz)	200	8	8	0	26	5	70
Heavenly Apple	1	180	8	5	0	28	5	70
Peanut Butter Paradise	1 (1.7 oz)	190	8	6	0	27	5	70
ENERGY DRINKS								
1In3Trinity								
Energy Drink	1 can (8.4 oz)	10	0	0	0	3	0	0
Accelerade								
All Flavors	8 oz	80	4	0	0	16	0	110
Amino Vital								
Amino Acid Supplement All Flavors	8 oz	35	1	0	0	8	–	10
Pro Fruit Punch	8 oz	35	1	0	0	7	–	10
Pro Tropic Fruit	8 oz	40	1	0	0	7	–	10
Puredge All Flavors	8 oz	50	1	0	0	11	–	10
Arizona								
Diet Green Tea Energy Drinks	8 oz	10	0	0	0	3	–	10
Green Tea Energy Drink	8 oz	100	0	0	0	26	–	10
Pomegranate Lite	8 oz	70	0	0	0	18	–	10
B52								
Zero Sugar Citrus Berry	8 oz	10	0	0	0	1	–	190
Bally Blast								
Energy Drink	1 can (8.3 oz)	120	3	0	0	29	–	95
Sugar Free	1 can (8.3 oz)	10	0	0	0	3	–	10
Banzai								
Energy Drink	8 oz	120	1	0	0	30	–	210

FOOD	PORTION	CALS	PROT	FAT	CHOL	CARB	FIBER	SOD
Bawls								
Guarana	8 oz	90	0	0	0	25	–	30
Guaranexx Sugar Free	1 bottle (10 oz)	0	0	0	0	0	0	15
Beaver Buzz								
Citrus	1 can	140	0	0	0	36	–	20
Black Hole								
Blueberry	8 oz	100	1	0	0	27	–	15
Citrus	8 oz	110	1	0	0	29	–	40
Bloom								
All Flavors	1 can (10.5 oz)	100	tr	0	0	24	–	115
Blox								
Black Cherry	8 oz	86	0	0	0	25	–	38
Orange Rush	8 oz	103	0	0	0	25	–	40
Original	8 oz	105	0	0	0	26	–	40
Blu Fuel								
Energy Drink	1 can (10 oz)	133	0	0	0	33	–	11
BooKoo								
Energy Drink	8 oz	110	–	0	0	27	–	200
Shot All Flavors	1 can (5.57 oz)	80	–	0	0	19	–	150
Zero Carb	8 oz	0	0	0	0	0	0	200
Boost								
High Protein Vanilla	8 oz	240	15	6	10	33	0	170
Bossa Nova								
Acai Juice Mango	1 bottle (10 oz)	132	1	0	0	33	1	37
Acai Juice Original	1 bottle (10 oz)	138	2	1	–	34	1	70
Acai Juice Passion Fruit	1 bottle (10 oz)	132	1	1	–	33	1	37
Brain Toniq								
Functional Drink	1 can (8.4 oz)	80	0	0	0	20	–	0
C1.5								
Extreme	1 can (8.4 oz)	120	0	0	0	30	–	50

FOOD	PORTION	CALS	PROT	FAT	CHOL	CARB	FIBER	SOD
Caballo Negro								
Double Kick	8 oz	120	1	0	0	28	–	200
Energy Drink	1 can (8.4 oz)	120	1	0	0	29	–	–
Cascabel								
Energy Drink	1 can (8.4 oz)	110	1	0	0	28	–	10
Sugar Free	1 can (8.4 oz)	10	1	0	0	1	–	15
Cheetah								
Energy Drink	1 can (12 oz)	80	0	0	0	20	–	15
Cintron								
Citrus Mango	8 oz	110	tr	0	0	27	0	200
Citrus Mango Sugar Free	8 oz	0	tr	0	0	0	0	200
Coca-Cola								
Zero	8 oz	1	0	0	0	tr	0	28
Coolah								
Original	8 oz	120	0	0	0	31	–	40
Cytomax								
Sport Drinks All Flavors	1 bottle (20 oz)	130	0	0	0	33	tr	140
Defcon3								
Healthy Energy Soda	1 can (12 oz)	45	0	0	0	11	2	20
Defense								
Effervescent Supplement	1 can	150	0	0	0	39	–	48
Diablo								
Energy Drink	1 can (8.7 oz)	151	0	0	0	38	–	–
DNA Energy								
Low Carb Citrus	8 oz	0	0	0	0	0	–	96
Double Hit								
Maximum Energy Coffee Drink Sugar Free	1 can (12 oz)	0	0	0	0	0	0	65
Emu								
Energy Drink	1 bottle (8.4 oz)	170	tr	0	0	41	–	220
EQ Thirst Equalizer								
All Flavors	8 oz	60	0	0	0	15	–	15

FOOD	PORTION	CALS	PROT	FAT	CHOL	CARB	FIBER	SOD
Freedom								
Energy Drink	1 can (12 oz)	160	0	0	0	41	–	110
Full Throttle								
Energy Drink	8 oz	100	0	0	0	29	–	70
Fury	8 oz	110	0	0	0	29	–	85
Function								
Alternative Energy	8 oz	60	0	0	0	15	–	65
Brainiac Carambola Punch	8 oz	60	0	0	0	15	–	–
Urban Detox Citrus Prickly Pear	8 oz	60	0	0	0	17	–	48
Youth Trip Acai Grape	8 oz	60	0	0	0	15	–	10
Gatorade								
All Flavors	8 oz	50	0	0	0	14	–	110
Lemonade All Flavors	8 oz	50	0	0	0	14	–	110
Rain All Flavors	8 oz	50	0	0	0	14	–	110
Gleukos								
Preformance All Flavors	8 oz	70	0	0	0	17	0	40
Go Fast								
Energy Drink	1 can (8.4 oz)	90	0	0	0	23	–	65
Light	1 can (8.4 oz)	20	0	0	0	1	–	70
Sportsman's	1 can (8.4 oz)	90	0	0	0	23	–	65
Guaraviton								
Energy Drink	8 oz	98	0	0	0	20	–	–
Guayaki								
Organic Empower Mint	8 oz	38	0	0	0	9	tr	11
Organic Raspberry Revolution	8 oz	50	0	0	0	12	tr	11
Organic Unsweetened	8 oz	15	0	0	0	3	tr	11
Guru								
Energy Drink	1 can (8.3 oz)	100	0	0	0	25	–	110
Lite	1 can (8.3 oz)	5	0	0	0	1	–	110
Happy Bunny								
Spaz Juice	1 can (8.4 oz)	110	0	0	0	28	0	10
Her Energy								
Pink Lemonade	1 can (8.4 oz)	130	0	0	0	32	0	95
Pink Lemonade Sugar Free	1 can (8.4 oz)	0	0	0	0	0	0	95

FOOD	PORTION	CALS	PROT	FAT	CHOL	CARB	FIBER	SOD
Hiball								
All Flavors	1 bottle (10 oz)	10	1	0	0	0	0	0
Hooah!								
Soldier Fuel All Flavors	1 can (12 oz)	160	0	0	0	41	–	40
Hydrive								
All Flavors	1 bottle (11.2 oz)	25	0	0	0	5	–	135
Iron Energy								
All Flavors	8 oz	90	0	0	0	23	–	–
Jet Set								
Club Soda	1 can (12 oz)	0	0	0	0	0	0	105
Ginger Ale	1 can (12 oz)	150	0	0	0	37	0	25
Original	1 can (12 oz)	105	1	0	0	29	0	105
Tonic Water	1 can (12 oz)	150	0	0	0	37	0	150
Krank'd								
All Flavors	1 bottle (16 oz)	80	0	0	0	18	–	48
Liv Naturals								
All Flavors	8 oz	70	0	0	0	16	0	105
Lost								
Big Gun	6 oz	100	–	–	–	26	–	190
Five-O	8 oz	70	–	–	–	16	–	96
Perfect 10	8 oz	10	–	–	–	3	–	190
Marquis Platinum								
Vitality Drink	1 can	30	0	0	0	16	1	–
Mix1								
All Flavors	1 bottle (11 oz)	200	15	3	–	29	3	125
Monster								
Energy Assault	8 oz	100	–	–	–	26	–	180
Energy Drink	8 oz	100	–	–	–	26	–	100
Khaos Energy Juice	8 oz	90	–	–	–	21	–	24
Lo Carb	8 oz	10	–	–	–	3	–	180
Mr. Re								
Restorative	1 can (11 oz)	80	0	0	0	22	0	0
Nexcite								
Herbal Fizz	1 bottle	72	1	0	0	17	–	5
NOS								
High Performance	8 oz	110	1	0	0	28	–	115

FOOD	PORTION	CALS	PROT	FAT	CHOL	CARB	FIBER	SOD
Odwalla								
Berries GoMega	8 oz	160	3	2	0	34	5	15
Mo' Beta	8 oz	150	1	0	0	37	1	15
Super Protein Original	8 oz	190	10	1	0	35	1	180
Superfood	8 oz	130	1	1	0	30	0	10
Wellness	8 oz	150	2	1	0	33	1	35
Pickle Juice								
Dill	8 oz	0	0	0	0	1	–	820
Sport	8 oz	7	0	0	0	2	–	1640
Pimpjuice								
Energy Drink	1 can (8 oz)	140	0	0	0	35	–	5
PJ Tight	1 can (8 oz)	20	0	0	0	3	–	5
Power Trip								
Xtreme	1 can (10.5 oz)	140	1	0	0	35	–	200
Powerade								
Arctic Shatter	8 oz	64	0	0	0	17	–	53
Green Squall	8 oz	64	0	0	0	17	–	53
Jagged Ice	8 oz	65	0	0	0	17	–	53
NASCAR Grape	8 oz	64	0	0	0	17	–	53
Olympic Citrus	8 oz	63	0	0	0	17	–	53
Option All Flavors	8 oz	10	0	0	0	2	–	75
PowerBar								
Endurance Sport Drink	1 pkg (0.6 oz)	70	0	0	0	17	–	160
Performance Recovery Drink	1 pkg (0.8 oz)	90	3	0	0	20	–	250
Purity Organic								
Acerola Cherry	1 bottle	60	0	0	0	15	–	–
Pomegranate Blueberry	1 bottle	60	0	0	0	15	–	–
Pomegranate Raspberry	1 bottle	60	0	0	0	15	–	–
Rawlings EX2								
Sustained Energy	1 can (8.4 oz)	132	–	0	0	32	–	90
Red Eye								
Classic	1 bottle (12 oz)	208	0	0	0	50	–	0
Extreme	1 bottle (12 oz)	140	0	0	0	37	–	0
Gold	1 bottle (12 oz)	208	0	0	0	49	–	0

FOOD	PORTION	CALS	PROT	FAT	CHOL	CARB	FIBER	SOD
Passion	1 bottle (12 oz)	149	0	0	0	37	–	0
Platinum	1 bottle (12 oz)	149	0	0	0	37	–	0
Rehab								
Recovery Supplement	1 can (12 oz)	150	0	0	0	38	–	60
Resurrect								
Daily Detox & Anti-Hangover Elixir	1 can (12 oz)	5	0	0	0	2	–	45
Rip It								
Citrus X	8 oz	130	1	0	0	33	–	95
Citrus X Sugar Free	8 oz	0	1	0	0	0	0	95
Energy Fuel	8 oz	130	1	0	0	32	–	130
Energy Lite	8 oz	0	1	0	0	0	0	130
Rockstar								
Energy Cola	8 oz	120	0	0	0	30	–	35
Energy Drink	8 oz	140	0	0	0	31	–	40
Juiced	8 oz	90	0	0	0	22	0	15
Ronin								
Diet	1 can (16 oz)	15	0	0	0	2	–	370
Original	1 can (16 oz)	180	0	0	0	46	–	370
Rox								
Energy Drink	1 can	110	1	0	0	28	–	200
Zero	1 can	10	1	0	0	1	–	200
Rumba								
Energy Juice	8 oz	120	–	0	0	28	–	5
Simply Nutrilite								
Berry Antioxidant	1 can (8.4 oz)	120	1	0	0	29	0	15
Slim-Fast								
Classic Ready-To-Drink Creamy Milk Chocolate	1 can	220	10	3	5	40	5	220
Classic Ready-To-Drink French Vanilla	1 can	220	10	3	5	40	5	220
High Protein Ready-To-Drink All Flavors	1 can	190	15	5	10	23	5	200
Low Carb Diet Ready-To-Drink All Flavors	1 can	190	20	9	15	6	4	260

FOOD	PORTION	CALS	PROT	FAT	CHOL	CARB	FIBER	SOD
Snapple A Day								
Meal Replacement All Flavors	1 bottle (11.5 oz)	210	7	0	0	43	5	110
SoBe								
Lean Diet Citrus	8 oz	5	0	0	0	1	–	15
Sol Mate								
All Flavors	1 bottle	90	0	0	0	22	–	0
Source Burn								
2	8 oz	130	1	0	0	31	–	10
Energy Drink	8 oz	140	0	0	0	36	–	20
Sugar Free	8 oz	10	1	0	0	0	0	15
Speed Zone								
Energy Drink	1 can (8.4 oz)	110	0	0	0	28	–	210
Steaz								
Organic Fuel	8 oz	90	0	0	0	23	–	35
Stewie's								
Domination Serum	1 can (8.45 oz)	110	0	0	0	28	–	10
Mind Erase Elixir	1 can (8.45 oz)	100	0	0	0	28	–	10
Stinger								
All Flavors	1 can (8.4 oz)	130	0	0	0	34	0	55
Sugar Free All Flavors	1 can (8.4 oz)	0	0	0	0	0	0	55
Sum Poosie								
Energy Drink	1 bottle (12 oz)	170	0	0	0	44	–	45
Swing Juice								
Energy Drink	8 oz	60	0	0	0	15	–	0
Tantra								
Erotic	1 can (8.4 oz)	130	1	0	0	31	–	–
The Beast								
Energy Drink	1 can (8.3 oz)	120	1	0	0	28	–	240
Tornado								
Energy Drink	8 oz	110	1	0	0	30	–	130
Vault								
Energy Drink	8 oz	120	0	0	0	32	–	30

FOOD	PORTION	CALS	PROT	FAT	CHOL	CARB	FIBER	SOD
Who's Your Daddy								
Original	8 oz	110	0	0	0	29	–	50
Sugar Free	8 oz	0	0	0	0	0	0	50
Wide Open Performance								
Energy Drink	1 can (8.3 oz)	120	–	0	0	27	–	55
Xcyto								
Sugar Free	1 can (12.5 oz)	10	tr	0	0	2	0	35
XL								
Diet	1 can (8.8 oz)	10	0	0	0	3	–	200
Energy Drink	1 can (8.8 oz)	113	0	0	0	28	–	160
Xtazy								
All Flavors	1 can	160	0	0	0	40	–	50
Youth Juice								
Drink	2 oz	10	tr	0	0	3	1	5
ENGLISH MUFFIN								
READY-TO-EAT								
apple cinnamon	1	138	4	2	0	28	–	255
crumpets	1 (1.5 oz)	80	3	0	0	16	tr	270
granola	1	155	6	1	0	31	–	275
mixed grain	1	155	6	1	0	31	–	275
plain	1	134	4	1	0	26	–	265
plain toasted	1	133	4	1	0	26	–	262
raisin cinnamon	1	138	4	2	0	28	–	255
sourdough	1	134	4	1	0	26	–	265
wheat	1	127	5	1	0	26	–	218
whole wheat	1	134	6	1	0	27	4	420
Crystal Farms								
English Muffin	1	130	4	1	0	27	1	240
Food For Life								
7 Sprouted Grains	1	160	8	2	0	32	6	240
Ezekiel 4:9 Cinnamon Raisin	1	160	6	0	0	36	4	170
Ezekiel 4:9 Sprouted Grain	1	160	8	1	0	30	6	160
Genesis 1:29 Original	1	180	8	4	0	30	6	140
Pepperidge Farm								
100% Whole Wheat	1	140	6	2	0	26	3	210

FOOD	PORTION	CALS	PROT	FAT	CHOL	CARB	FIBER	SOD
Original	1	130	5	2	0	25	1	170
Rudi's Organic Bakery								
MultiGrain w/ Flax	1 (2 oz)	130	5	1	0	25	2	220
Whole Grain Wheat	1 (2 oz)	120	5	1	0	23	3	220
Sara Lee								
Heart Healthy Wheat w/ Honey	1	140	6	1	0	28	2	250
Original w/ Whole Grain	1	140	5	1	0	27	2	230
Thomas'								
100 Calories	1	100	4	1	0	24	5	220
Corn	1	150	5	1	0	29	2	260
Hearty Grains 100% Whole Wheat	1	120	6	1	0	23	3	190
Hearty Grains Honey Wheat	1	130	5	1	0	27	2	190
Light Multi-Grain	1	100	6	2	<5	24	8	170
Oatmeal & Honey	1	130	5	1	0	25	2	180
Original	1	120	4	1	0	25	1	200
Original Whole Grain	1	130	5	1	0	26	2	220
Raisin Cinnamon	1	140	4	1	0	29	1	170
Sandwich Size Original	1	190	7	2	0	38	2	280
Super Size Multi Grain	1	240	0	3	0	44	3	290
TAKE-OUT								
w/ butter	1 (2.2 oz)	189	5	6	13	30	–	386
w/ cheese & sausage	1 (4 oz)	393	15	24	59	29	–	1036
w/ egg cheese & canadian bacon	1 (4.8 oz)	289	17	13	234	28	2	729
w/ egg cheese & sausage	1 (5.8 oz)	487	22	31	274	31	–	1135
EPAZOTE								
fresh	1 tbsp (1 g)	tr	0	0	0	tr	tr	tr
fresh sprig	1 (2 g)	1	tr	tr	0	tr	tr	1
EPPAW								
raw	½ cup	75	2	1	0	16	–	6
FALAFEL								
Sabra								
Burger	1 (1.8 oz)	90	3	3	0	11	3	240
VeggieLand								
FalafelBurger	1 (4 oz)	190	9	6	0	26	8	285

FOOD	PORTION	CALS	PROT	FAT	CHOL	CARB	FIBER	SOD
TAKE-OUT								
falafel	1 (1.2 oz)	57	2	3	0	5	–	50
FAT (see also BUTTER, BUTTER SUBSTITUTES, MARGARINE, OIL)								
bacon grease	1 tbsp	116	0	13	12	0	0	19
beef shortening	1 tbsp	115	0	13	13	0	0	0
beef suet	1 oz	242	tr	27	19	0	0	2
chicken	1 cup	1846	0	205	174	0	0	–
chicken	1 tbsp	115	0	13	11	0	0	–
cocoa butter	1 tbsp	120	0	14	0	0	0	–
duck	1 tbsp (13 g)	115	0	13	13	0	0	0
goose	1 tbsp	115	0	13	13	0	0	–
goose	1 oz	257	0	29	–	0	0	–
lamb new zealand	1 oz	182	2	19	25	0	0	6
lard	1 cup (205 g)	1849	0	205	195	0	0	tr
lard	1 tbsp (13 g)	115	0	13	12	0	0	0
meat pan drippings	½ tbsp	124	0	14	14	0	0	76
nutmeg butter	1 tbsp	120	0	14	–	0	0	–
pork raw	1 oz	230	1	25	16	0	0	3
salt pork	1 cube (1 oz)	215	2	23	26	0	0	383
shortening	1 cup	1812	0	205	0	0	0	–
shortening	1 tbsp	113	0	13	0	0	0	–
turkey	1 tbsp	116	0	13	13	0	0	0
ucuhuba butter	1 tbsp	120	0	14	–	0	0	–
whale blubber	1 oz	244	tr	27	42	0	0	–
Crisco								
Shortening	1 tbsp	110	0	12	0	0	0	0
Nebraska Land								
Pork Fatback	½ oz	110	1	11	5	0	0	280
Smart Balance								
Shortening	1 tbsp	110	0	12	0	0	0	0
FEIJOA								
fresh	1 (1.75 oz)	25	1	tr	0	5	–	2
puree	1 cup	119	3	2	0	26	–	7
FENNEL								
fresh bulb	1 (8.2 oz)	73	3	tr	0	17	7	122
fresh sliced	1 cup	27	1	tr	0	6	3	45
leaves	1 oz	7	tr	tr	–	1	1	25

FOOD	PORTION	CALS	PROT	FAT	CHOL	CARB	FIBER	SOD
seed	1 tsp	7	tr	tr	0	1	1	2
stir fried	1 cup	85	2	6	0	9	3	669
Ocean Mist								
Fennel Sweet Anise Sliced Fresh	1 cup	27	1	1	0	6	3	45

FENUGREEK

FOOD	PORTION	CALS	PROT	FAT	CHOL	CARB	FIBER	SOD
seed	1 tsp	12	1	tr	0	2	1	2

FIBER

FOOD	PORTION	CALS	PROT	FAT	CHOL	CARB	FIBER	SOD
apple fiber	0.5 oz	40	1	1	0	15	7	–
Benefiber								
Supplement	1 pkg (4 g)	20	0	0	0	4	3	20
Metamucil								
Natural Fiber Regular Flavor	1 rounded tsp (7 g)	25	0	0	0	6	3	3
UniFiber								
Natural Fiber	1 pkg (4 g)	4	0	0	0	tr	3	–
Wellements								
Fiber-Psyll	1 scoop (0.5 oz)	55	0	0	0	14	12	0

FIDDLEHEAD FERNS

FOOD	PORTION	CALS	PROT	FAT	CHOL	CARB	FIBER	SOD
fresh	3.5 oz	34	5	tr	0	6	–	1

FIGS

FOOD	PORTION	CALS	PROT	FAT	CHOL	CARB	FIBER	SOD
canned in heavy syrup	3	75	tr	tr	0	19	–	1
canned in light syrup	3	58	tr	tr	0	15	–	1
canned water pack	3	42	tr	tr	0	11	–	1
dried california	½ cup (3.5 oz)	200	4	1	0	58	17	11
dried cooked	½ cup	140	2	1	0	16	–	6
dried whole	10	477	6	2	0	122	17	20
fresh	1 med	50	tr	tr	0	10	–	1
Blue Ribbon								
California Figs	1 pkg (1.5 oz)	120	1	0	0	28	5	0
Figamajigs								
Chocolate Covered Bar	1 bar (1.4 oz)	130	1	3	0	26	5	10
Chocolate Covered Bar w/ Almonds	1 bar (1.4 oz)	150	2	4	0	28	4	20

FOOD	PORTION	CALS	PROT	FAT	CHOL	CARB	FIBER	SOD
Trucco								
Kalamata	2	100	1	0	0	26	4	0
FIREWEED								
leaves chopped	1 cup (0.8 oz)	24	1	1	0	4	2	8

FISH (*see also individual names,* FISH SUBSTITUTES, SUSHI)
CANNED

FOOD	PORTION	CALS	PROT	FAT	CHOL	CARB	FIBER	SOD
Beach Cliff								
Fish Steaks In Louisiana Hot Sauce	1 can (3.7 oz)	160	19	7	75	2	0	480
Fish Steaks In Mustard Sauce	1 can (3.7 oz)	160	21	9	80	2	0	420
Fish Steaks In Soybean Oil	1 can (3.7 oz)	200	20	13	80	1	0	310
Fish Steaks w/ Hot Green Chilies	1 can (3.7 oz)	160	17	10	65	1	0	390
Fish Steaks w/ Jalapeno Peppers	1 can (3.7 oz)	130	20	14	80	1	0	240
Brunswick								
Fish Steaks In Louisiana Hot Sauce	1 can (3.7 oz)	160	19	7	75	2	0	480
Fish Steaks In Mustard Sauce	1 can (3.7 oz)	160	21	9	80	2	0	420
Fish Steaks In Soybean Oil	1 can (3.7 oz)	200	20	13	80	1	0	310
Fish Steaks In Spring Water	1 can (3.7 oz)	150	19	8	115	0	0	240
Fish Steaks w/ Hot Tabasco Peppers	1 can (3.7 oz)	220	20	14	80	1	0	240
Seafood Snacks Golden Smoked	1 can (3.2 oz)	170	19	11	55	0	0	270
Seafood Snacks In Lemon & Cracked Pepper	1 can (3.2 oz)	160	19	10	55	0	0	270
Seafood Snacks In Louisiana Hot Sauce	1 can (3.2 oz)	140	16	8	70	2	0	450
Seafood Snacks In Teriyaki Sauce	1 can (3.2 oz)	160	16	8	70	5	0	800
Seafood Snacks In Tomato & Basil Sauce	1 can (3.2 oz)	140	16	8	70	2	0	420

FOOD	PORTION	CALS	PROT	FAT	CHOL	CARB	FIBER	SOD
Seafood Snacks Kippered	1 can (3.2 oz)	160	18	9	55	0	0	490
Chicken Of The Sea								
Fish Steaks	½ can (2 oz)	70	9	3	50	1	1	430
FROZEN								
breaded fillet	1 (2 oz)	155	9	7	64	14	–	332
sticks	1 stick (1 oz)	76	4	3	31	7	–	163
Gorton's								
Classic Crispy Battered Fillets	2	230	6	10	25	22	5	650
Classic Crunchy Golden Fillets	2	140	9	12	36	23	–	500
Fillets Beer Battered	2 (3.6 oz)	250	8	17	20	17	1	600
Fillets Breaded Lemon Herb	2 (3.6 oz)	240	9	13	25	21	–	720
Fish Sticks Classic Breaded	6	290	10	18	25	19	1	340
Grilled Fillets Cajun Blackened	1 (3.8 oz)	100	17	3	60	1	0	330
Grilled Fillets Lemon Pepper	1 (3.7 oz)	100	17	3	70	1	0	290
Tenders Original Batter	3 pieces (3.6 oz)	230	8	12	20	23	2	660
Ian's								
Fillets	1 (3.4 oz)	260	14	8	20	32	2	410
Fish Stick Allergy Free	5 pieces	190	11	6	15	24	1	310
Fish Sticks	5 pieces	190	11	6	15	24	1	310
Van de Kamp's								
Battered Tenders	4 (4 oz)	210	9	10	20	22	1	700
Crisp & Healthy Breaded Fish Sticks	6 (3.6 oz)	140	9	1	25	24	1	380
Crunchy Fillets	2 (3.5 oz)	230	8	13	20	21	tr	440
Sticks	6 (4 oz)	260	11	13	30	26	1	410
TAKE-OUT								
fish cake	1 (4.7 oz)	166	18	7	–	6	–	–
jamaican brown fish stew	1 serv	426	48	22	84	9	2	419
kedgeree	5.6 oz	242	21	11	–	15	1	–
mousse	1 serv (3.5 oz)	185	13	14	–	3	tr	540
stew	1 cup (7.9 oz)	157	19	4	–	10	–	–
taramasalata	2 tbsp	124	1	14	10	1	–	182

FOOD	PORTION	CALS	PROT	FAT	CHOL	CARB	FIBER	SOD
FISH OIL								
cod liver	1 tbsp	123	0	14	78	0	0	0
herring	1 tbsp	123	0	14	104	0	0	0
menhaden	1 tbsp	123	0	14	71	0	0	0
salmon	1 tbsp	123	0	14	66	0	0	0
sardine	1 tbsp	123	0	14	97	0	0	0
shark	1 oz	270	0	29	–	0	0	–
whale beluga	1 oz	252	0	28	–	0	0	0
whale bowhead	1 oz	252	0	28	–	0	0	–
Cormega								
Omega-E Orange	1 pkg	20	–	2	8	0	0	–
Spectrum								
Cod Liver Oil w/ Lemon	1 tsp	40	0	5	25	0	0	0
FISH PASTE								
fish paste	2 tsp	15	1	1	–	tr	0	–
FLAXSEED								
Arrowhead Mills								
Organic	3 tbsp (1 oz)	140	6	9	0	9	7	0
Bob's Red Mill								
Flaxseed Meal	2 tbsp	60	3	5	0	4	4	0
Carringon Farms								
Organic Flax Paks	1 pkg (0.4 oz)	50	2	5	0	3	3	5
Hodgson Mill								
Milled	2 tbsp	60	3	5	0	4	4	0
FLOUNDER								
FRESH								
cooked	1 fillet (4.5 oz)	148	31	2	86	0	0	133
cooked	3 oz	99	21	1	58	0	0	89
FROZEN								
Mrs. Paul's								
Filets Lightly Breaded	1 (2.7 oz)	150	8	7	25	12	1	290
TAKE-OUT								
breaded & fried	3.2 oz	211	13	11	31	15	–	484
stuffed w/ crab	1 piece (7.6 oz)	332	43	11	160	14	1	903

FOOD	PORTION	CALS	PROT	FAT	CHOL	CARB	FIBER	SOD

FLOUR

FOOD	PORTION	CALS	PROT	FAT	CHOL	CARB	FIBER	SOD
arrowhead	1 cup	457	tr	tr	0	113	4	3
buckwheat whole groat	1 cup	402	15	4	0	85	12	13
corn masa	1 cup (4 oz)	416	11	4	0	87	11	6
cottonseed lowfat	1 oz	94	14	tr	0	10	–	10
peanut defatted	1 cup	196	31	tr	0	21	–	108
peanut lowfat	1 cup	257	20	13	0	19	–	0
potato	1 cup (6.3 oz)	628	14	1	0	143	–	61
rice brown	1 cup (5.5 oz)	574	11	4	0	121	7	13
rice white	1 cup (5.5 oz)	578	9	2	0	127	4	1
rye dark	1 cup (4.5 oz)	415	18	3	0	88	29	2
rye light	1 cup (3.6 oz)	374	9	1	0	82	15	2
rye medium	1 cup (3.6 oz)	361	10	2	0	79	15	3
sesame lowfat	1 oz	95	14	tr	0	10	–	11
triticale whole grain	1 cup (4.6 oz)	439	17	2	0	95	19	3
white all-purpose	1 cup (4.4 oz)	455	13	1	0	95	2	3
white bread	1 cup (4.8 oz)	495	16	2	0	99	3	3
white cake unsifted	1 cup (4.8 oz)	496	11	1	0	107	2	3
white self-rising	1 cup (4.4 oz)	443	12	1	0	93	3	1588
white unbleached	1 cup (4.4 oz)	455	13	1	0	95	3	3
whole wheat	1 cup (4.2 oz)	407	16	2	0	87	15	6
Arrowhead Mills								
Organic Barley	1/3 cup	95	3	1	0	19	4	0
Organic Brown Rice	1/3 cup	130	3	1	0	27	2	0
Organic Kamut	1/3 cup	130	5	1	0	25	4	0
Organic Oat	1/3 cup	120	4	3	0	21	3	0
Organic Rye	1/4 cup	110	3	1	0	24	4	0

FOOD	PORTION	CALS	PROT	FAT	CHOL	CARB	FIBER	SOD
Organic Spelt	⅓ cup	130	4	1	0	25	4	0
Organic Unbleached White	¼ cup	120	3	1	0	26	tr	0
Organic White Rice	⅓ cup	120	2	0	0	28	tr	0
Bob's Red Mill								
Brown Rice	¼ cup	140	3	1	0	31	1	5
Corn	¼ cup	160	2	1	0	22	4	2
Graham	¼ cup	120	5	1	0	21	3	1
Kamut Organic	¼ cup	94	3	1	0	21	3	0
Sorghum Sweet White Gluten Free	¼ cup	120	4	1	0	25	3	0
Spelt	¼ cup	120	4	1	0	22	41	1
Whole Wheat	¼ cup	110	4	1	0	23	4	0
Whole Wheat Hard White Organic	¼ cup	120	4	1	0	24	4	0
Domata Living Flour								
Gluten Free Casein Free	¼ cup	110	tr	0	0	26	tr	20
Heckers								
All Purpose Unbleached	¼ cup	100	3	0	0	22	tr	0
Hodgson Mill								
Best For Bread	¼ cup	100	4	0	0	22	1	5
Buckwheat	¼ cup	100	2	1	0	22	3	0
Oat Bran Flour	¼ cup	110	3	2	0	23	3	4
Kentucky Kernel								
Seasoned Flour	4 tsp	36	1	0	0	8	0	544
King Arthur								
All Purpose	¼ cup	110	4	0	0	22	tr	0
All Purpose Unbleached	¼ cup	110	4	0	0	22	1	0
Organic White Whole Wheat	¼ cup	100	4	1	0	18	3	0
Organic Whole Wheat	½ cup	110	4	1	0	23	4	0
Organic Artisan	¼ cup	110	3	0	0	23	tr	0
Self-Rising	¼ cup	120	2	0	0	27	1	440
White Whole Wheat	¼ cup	100	4	1	0	18	3	0
Whole Wheat	¼ cup	110	4	1	0	21	4	0
Lundberg								
Brown Rice	¼ cup	110	2	2	0	26	1	0
Manitoba Harvest								
Hemp Seed Flour	¼ cup	120	10	4	0	14	12	0

FOOD	PORTION	CALS	PROT	FAT	CHOL	CARB	FIBER	SOD
FOOD COLORS								
blue	1 tsp	0	0	0	0	0	0	86
orange	1 tsp	0	0	0	0	0	0	91
red	1 tsp	tr	0	0	0	tr	0	38
yellow	1 tsp	tr	tr	0	0	0	0	28
FRENCH BEANS								
dried cooked	1 cup	228	12	1	0	43	17	11
FRENCH FRIES (see POTATOES)								
FRENCH TOAST								
french toast frzn	1 slice (2 oz)	126	4	4	48	19	2	292
Aunt Jemima								
Cinnamon	2 slices (4 oz)	240	8	6	70	39	2	340
Whole Grain	2 slices (4 oz)	240	8	6	70	39	3	340
Eggo								
Toaster Sticks Original	2	220	5	6	20	36	1	530
Farm Rich								
Original Sticks	5 (4.2 oz)	330	6	15	0	42	2	490
Ian's								
Sticks	5 (3.2 oz)	250	6	9	5	38	6	330
TAKE-OUT								
plain	1 slice	151	7	7	75	16	–	311
sticks	5 (4.9 oz)	513	8	29	75	58	3	499
w/ butter	2 slices	356	10	19	116	36	–	513
FROG LEGS								
frog legs	3 oz	175	15	–	1	–	–	–
TAKE-OUT								
as prep w/ seasoned flour & fried	1 (0.8 oz)	70	4	5	12	15	–	–
FRUCTOSE								
Bob's Red Mill								
Fructose	1 tsp	15	0	0	0	4	0	0
Estee								
Fructose	1 tsp	15	0	0	0	4	0	0
Packet	1 pkg	10	0	0	0	3	0	0

FOOD	PORTION	CALS	PROT	FAT	CHOL	CARB	FIBER	SOD
FRUIT DRINKS (see also individual names, SMOOTHIES, YOGURT DRINKS)								
MIX								
Bio Fruit								
Mix	1 scoop (8 g)	42	–	1	0	5	1	–
Crystal Light								
LiveActive On The Go	1 pkg	10	0	0	0	3	3	20
Sugar Free All Flavors as prep	1 serv	5	0	0	0	0	0	0
Luna								
Dragonfruit Kiwi	1 pkg	50	0	0	0	13	0	30
Pomegranate Berry	1 pkg	50	0	0	0	13	0	30
South Beach								
Tide Me Over Strawberry Banana	1 pkg	30	3	0	0	6	5	20
Tide Me Over Tropical Breeze	1 pkg	30	3	0	0	6	5	25
Tang								
Orange Strawberry as prep	1 serv (8 oz)	110	0	0	0	27	0	10
Orange Pineapple as prep	1 serv (8 oz)	100	0	0	0	24	0	45
READY-TO-DRINK								
fruit punch	6 oz	87	tr	tr	0	22	–	41
After The Fall								
Banana Casablanca	8 oz	150	1	0	0	37	–	20
Mango Montage	8 oz	150	1	0	0	37	–	15
Apple & Eve								
100% Cranberry Apple Juice	8 oz	100	1	0	0	24	–	15
Mango Mangosteen	8 oz	120	0	0	0	30	–	15
Brazsoy								
Fruit Juice w/ Soy	8 oz	94	1	1	0	21	–	13
Capri Sun								
Fruit Punch	1 pkg (7 oz)	90	0	0	0	25		15
Crayons								
Kiwi Strawberry	1 bottle (12 oz)	130	0	0	0	45	4	15
Outrageous Orange Mango	1 bottle (12 oz)	140	0	0	0	45	4	15
Redder Than Ever Fruitpunch	1 bottle (12 oz)	130	0	0	0	45	4	15

FOOD	PORTION	CALS	PROT	FAT	CHOL	CARB	FIBER	SOD
Crystal Light								
Strawberry Kiwi Sugar Free	8 oz	5	0	0	0	0	0	15
Essn								
Sparkling Blood Orange & Cranberry	1 can (8.4 oz)	160	1	0	0	38	tr	15
Feel Good Drinks								
Spritz Cranberry & Lime No Sugar Added	1 bottle	159	tr	tr	–	36	–	–
Firefly								
Chill Out De-stress Drink	1 bottle (11.2 oz)	100	1	0	0	24	–	10
De-tox Morning After Drink	1 bottle (11.2 oz)	104	1	0	0	25	–	10
Five Alive								
Citrus	8 oz	120	0	0	0	30	–	15
Fizz Ed.								
Pomegranate Cherry	1 can (8.4 oz)	90	0	0	0	22	–	30
Frutzzo								
Organic 100% Juice Pomegranate Passionfruit	12 oz	140	0	0	0	34	0	10
Organic 100% Juice Pomegranate Acai	12 oz	140	0	0	0	35	0	10
Hawaiian Punch								
Bodacious Berry	8 oz	110	0	0	0	29	–	115
Fruit Juicy Red	8 oz	80	0	0	0	21	–	125
Green Berry Rush	8 oz	120	0	0	0	30	–	120
Mazin Melon Mix	8 oz	110	0	0	0	29	–	115
Tropical Vibe	8 oz	110	0	0	0	29	–	115
Wild Purple Smash	8 oz	110	0	0	0	29	–	115
Hog Wash								
All Flavors	10 oz	37	0	0	0	10	0	87
Hood								
Fruit Punch	1 cup	120	0	0	0	30	0	10
Juici								
Sparkling All Flavors	12 oz	105	0	0	0	28	–	60
Juicy Juice								
Harvest Surprise Orange Mango	8 oz	130	1	0	0	31	1	70
Harvest Surprise Tropical	8 oz	100	tr	0	0	24	1	70

FOOD	PORTION	CALS	PROT	FAT	CHOL	CARB	FIBER	SOD
Kagome								
Burgundy Berry Blossom	8 oz	100	0	0	0	23	0	110
Golden Peach Garden	8 oz	100	0	0	0	25	1	90
Orange Carrot Blossom	8 oz	100	1	0	0	24	1	60
Purple Roots & Fruits	8 oz	130	0	0	0	30	1	55
L&A								
Pineapple Coconut	8 oz	140	0	3	0	28	1	55
Lakewood								
Lean Green	6 oz	90	1	0	0	26	2	7
Organic Acai Amazon Berry	6 oz	95	2	3	0	21	3	24
Minute Maid								
Berry Kiwi	12 oz	160	0	0	0	43	–	110
Cranberry Grape	8 oz	150	0	0	0	39	–	20
Light Mango Tropical	8 oz	5	0	0	0	2	–	80
Light Orange Tangerine	8 oz	15	0	0	0	4	–	15
Orange Tangerine	8 oz	110	2	0	0	27	–	15
Pomegranate Blueberry 100% Juice	8 oz	120	0	1	0	31	–	20
Tropical Punch Chilled	8 oz	110	0	0	0	30	–	15
Naked Juice								
Berry Blast	8 oz	120	1	0	0	30	1	10
Blue Machine	8 oz	170	1	1	0	41	8	10
Green Machine	8 oz	130	1	0	0	33	1	15
Mango Acai	8 oz	190	2	3	0	38	3	90
Power C	8 oz	120	1	1	0	29	3	15
Protein Zone	8 oz	210	17	4	20	27	0	135
Red Machine	8 oz	160	2	3	0	32	4	15
Strawberry Banana C	8 oz	120	2	0	0	28	3	5
Very Berry	8 oz	130	2	0	0	30	1	0
Very Pro Berry	8 oz	190	14	1	15	30	1	110
Well Being	8 oz	140	1	0	0	32	0	5
Newman's Own								
Orange Mango Tango	8 oz	150	0	0	0	37	–	5
Noble								
Organic 100% Juice Orange Tangerine	8 oz	120	1	0	0	29	–	0
Northland								
Cranberry Blueberry	1 cup (8 oz)	140	0	0	0	34	–	35
NutraShake								
Fruit Punch Plus Fiber	1 pkg (8 oz)	120	0	0	0	29	10	8

FOOD	PORTION	CALS	PROT	FAT	CHOL	CARB	FIBER	SOD
Ocean Spray								
Ruby Tangerine	8 oz	120	0	0	0	31	–	65
Odwalla								
Quenchers AntioxiDance	8 oz	90	0	0	0	23	0	10
Quenchers B Berrier	8 oz	120	0	0	0	30	0	15
Old Orchard								
100% Juice Pomegranate Black Currant	8 oz	130	0	0	0	30	–	25
100% Juice Pomegranate Cherry	8 oz	140	0	0	0	34	–	15
Cocktail Apple Passion Mango	8 oz	120	0	0	0	29	–	15
Healthy Balance Apple Kiwi Strawberry	8 oz	30	0	0	0	6	–	9
Phat Phruit								
Peach Mango	8 oz	40	0	0	0	10	0	30
Pineapple Orange	8 oz	40	0	0	0	9	0	35
Sabor Latino								
Guava Mango Drink	1 box (7 oz)	110	0	0	0	29	–	15
Nectar Strawberry Banana + Calcium	8 oz	150	0	0	0	37	1	10
Pina Colada	8 oz	130	0	0	0	32	–	15
Snapple								
Cranberry Raspberry	8 oz	120	0	0	0	29	–	10
Diet Carrot Apple	8 oz	10	1	0	0	3	–	10
Diet Plum-A-Granate	8 oz	0	0	0	0	0	0	15
Go Bananas	8 oz	120	0	0	0	30	–	10
Kiwi Strawberry	8 oz	110	0	0	0	28	–	10
Snapricot Orange	8 oz	120	0	0	0	30	–	10
SSips								
Cherry Berry	1 box (7 oz)	110	0	0	0	26	–	10
Sun Shower								
100% Juice Nectarine Mango	8 oz	93	1	0	0	21	2	15
Sundia								
Tropical Medley	½ cup	70	1	0	0	18	2	10
Tree Ripe								
Organic Fruit Punch	8 oz	150	1	0	0	36	0	15
TreeTop								
Apple Grape No Sugar Added	8 oz	130	0	0	0	32	–	15

FOOD	PORTION	CALS	PROT	FAT	CHOL	CARB	FIBER	SOD
Tropicana								
Fruit Punch	1 cup	130	0	0	0	32	0	15
Light Fruit Punch	8 oz	10	0	0	0	3	0	5
Orange Tangerine Juice	8 oz	110	2	0	0	25	0	0
Orchard Berry	8 oz	110	1	0	0	27	0	25
Organic Orchard Medley	8 oz	120	0	0	0	29	0	25
Twister Berry Blast	8 oz	120	tr	0	0	29	0	10
Twister Citrus Spark	8 oz	120	0	0	0	30	0	10
Twister Fruit Fury	8 oz	120	tr	0	0	30	0	30
Twister Light Strawberry Spiral	8 oz	40	0	0	0	10	0	70
V8								
Light Peach Mango	8 oz	50	0	0	0	13	0	40
Splash Berry Blend	8 oz	70	0	0	0	18	0	50
Splash Diet Berry Blend	8 oz	10	0	0	0	3	0	35
Splash Mango Peach	8 oz	80	0	0	0	20	0	40
V-Fusion Pomegranate Blueberry	8 oz	100	0	0	0	25	0	60
Vrut								
Apple Carrot	1 box (8.45 oz)	120	1	0	0	29	–	50
Berry Veggie	1 box (8.45 oz)	110	1	0	0	27	–	25
Orange Veggie	1 box (8.45 oz)	110	1	1	0	26	–	20
Tropical Blend	1 box (8.45 oz)	110	1	0	0	27	–	20
Wadda Juice								
All Flavors	1 bottle (4 oz)	25	0	0	0	7	–	4
Walnut Acres								
Organic Orange Carrot	8 oz	110	0	0	0	27	–	30
Welch's								
White Grape Peach 100% Juice	8 oz	160	0	1	0	39	–	15

FRUIT MIXED *(see also individual names)*
CANNED

FOOD	PORTION	CALS	PROT	FAT	CHOL	CARB	FIBER	SOD
fruit cocktail in heavy syrup	½ cup	93	1	tr	0	24	–	7
fruit cocktail juice pack	½ cup	56	1	tr	0	15	–	4
fruit cocktail water pack	½ cup	40	1	tr	0	10	–	5

FOOD	PORTION	CALS	PROT	FAT	CHOL	CARB	FIBER	SOD
fruit salad in heavy syrup	½ cup	94	tr	tr	0	24	–	7
fruit salad in light syrup	½ cup	73	tr	tr	0	19	–	7
fruit salad juice pack	½ cup	62	1	tr	0	16	–	7
fruit salad water pack	½ cup	37	tr	tr	0	10	–	4
mixed fruit in heavy syrup	½ cup	92	tr	tr	0	24	–	5
tropical fruit salad in heavy syrup	½ cup	110	1	tr	0	29	–	3
Del Monte								
Carb Clever Fruit Cocktail	½ cup	40	0	0	0	11	tr	10
Fruit Cocktail In 100% Juice	½ cup	60	0	0	0	15	1	10
Fruit Cocktail In Extra Light Syrup	½ cup	60	0	0	0	15	1	10
Fruit Cocktail In Heavy Syrup	½ cup	100	0	0	0	24	1	10
Fruit Naturals Tropical Medley	½ cup	70	tr	0	0	18	tr	5
Orchard Select Premium Mixed	½ cup	80	tr	0	0	20	tr	10
SunFresh Citrus Salad	½ cup	80	0	0	0	20	0	20
Dole								
Tropical Fruit Salad	½ cup	80	tr	0	0	20	1	10
Liberty Gold								
Fruit Cocktail In Heavy Syrup	½ cup	90	0	0	0	23	1	15
DRIED								
mixed	11 oz pkg	712	7	1	0	188	–	52
Goodniks								
Fruit Medley	¼ cup	110	1	2	0	24	2	30
Mariani								
Berries 'N Cherries	¼ cup	140	tr	0	0	38	2	0
Sun-Maid								
Mixed	¼ cup	100	1	0	0	25	3	60
Sunsweet								
Berry Blend	¼ cup (1.4 oz)	120	1	0	0	32	3	5
Orchard Mix	¼ cup (1.4 oz)	100	1	0	0	25	3	60
Tropical Mix	⅓ cup	150	0	0	0	33	2	30
FROZEN								
mixed fruit sweetened	1 cup	245	4	tr	0	61	–	8

FOOD	PORTION	CALS	PROT	FAT	CHOL	CARB	FIBER	SOD
FRUIT SNACKS								
fruit leather	1 bar (0.8 oz)	81	tr	1	0	18	–	18
fruit leather pieces	1 oz	97	tr	2	0	22	–	114
fruit leather pieces	1 pkg (0.9 oz)	92	tr	2	0	21	–	109
fruit leather rolls	1 sm (0.5 oz)	49	tr	tr	0	12	–	8
fruit leather rolls	1 lg (0.7 oz)	73	tr	1	0	18	–	13
Bare Fruit								
Bananas & Cherries	1 pkg (0.6 oz)	55	2	1	0	12	2	0
Funky Monkey								
Bananamon	1 pkg (1 oz)	110	1	0	0	27	3	2
Carnaval Mix	1 pkg (1 oz)	110	1	0	0	26	2	5
Jivealime	1 pkg (1 oz)	110	1	0	0	27	2	1
Purple Funk	1 pkg (1 oz)	120	1	1	0	26	3	1
Peeled Snacks								
Fruit & Nuts FigSated	⅓ cup	150	3	6	0	20	3	60
Fruit & Nuts Plu-what?	⅓ cup	150	3	6	0	22	3	50
Sharkies								
Organic Energy Fruit Chews All Flavors	1 pkg (1.8 oz)	170	0	0	0	42	1	125
Stretch Island								
Fruit Leather Bountiful Blueberry	1 pkg (0.5 oz)	45	0	0	0	12	1	0
Fruit Leather Harvest Grape	1 pkg (0.5 oz)	45	0	0	0	12	1	0
Fruit Leather Truly Tropical	1 pkg (0.5 oz)	45	0	0	0	11	1	0
Fruit Leathers Mango Sunrise	1 pkg (0.5 oz)	45	0	0	0	11	1	0
Organic Smooshed Fruit Apple	1 piece (0.4 oz)	40	0	0	0	10	1	0
Organic Smooshed Fruit Strawberry	1 piece (0.4 oz)	40	0	0	0	10	tr	0
Tropicana								
Fruit Wise Bars All Flavors	1 bar (1.4 oz)	140	0	0	0	36	2	10
Fruit Wise Strips All Flavors	1 strip (0.7 oz)	70	0	0	0	17	1	0
Welch's								
White Grape Peach	20 pieces	110	1	0	0	24	–	20

FOOD	PORTION	CALS	PROT	FAT	CHOL	CARB	FIBER	SOD
GARLIC								
clove	1	4	tr	tr	0	1	tr	1
fresh chopped	1 tbsp	18	1	tr	0	4	tr	2
powder	1 tsp	9	tr	tr	0	2	tr	1
Dorot								
Crushed Cubes frzn	1 cube (4 g)	7	tr	tr	0	1	tr	31
Frieda's								
Elephant	1 tbsp	5	0	0	0	1	0	0
Vinegar Marinated	1 oz	30	1	0	0	7	0	140
GEFILTE FISH								
sweet	1 piece (1.5 oz)	35	4	1	12	3	–	220
Mrs. Adler's								
Pike'n Whitefish	1 piece (1.8 oz)	50	6	1	15	4	0	330
GELATIN								
READY-TO-EAT								
Del Monte								
Mandarin Orange In Lite Orange Gel	1 pkg (4.5 oz)	60	0	0	0	14	0	40
Mixed Fruit In Cherry Gel	1 pkg (4.5 oz)	90	0	0	0	23	0	40
Peaches In Peach Gel	1 pkg (4.5 oz)	90	0	0	0	22	0	40
Peaches In Raspberry Gel	1 pkg (4.5 oz)	90	0	0	0	23	0	40
Peaches In Lite Strawberry Banana Gel	1 pkg (4.5 oz)	60	0	0	0	14	0	40
Hunt's								
Snack Pack Juicy Gels Raspberry Mixed Berry	1 serv (3.5 oz)	100	0	0	0	24	0	40
Snack Pack Juicy Gels Strawberry	1 serv (3.5 oz)	100	0	0	0	24	0	40
Snack Pack Juicy Gels Strawberry Orange	1 serv (3.5 oz)	100	0	0	0	24	0	40
Snack Pack Tropical Punch	1 serv (3.5 oz)	100	0	0	0	24	0	40
Jell-O								
Sugar Free Tropical Berry	1 serv (3.2 oz)	10	1	0	0	0	0	45
Kozy Shack								
Gel Treats Cherry	1 pkg (4 oz)	85	0	0	0	22	1	7

FOOD	PORTION	CALS	PROT	FAT	CHOL	CARB	FIBER	SOD
Gel Treats Lemon Lime	1 pkg (4 oz)	85	0	0	0	22	1	7
Gel Treats Orange	1 pkg (4 oz)	85	0	0	0	22	1	7
Gel Treats Strawberry	1 pkg (4 oz)	85	0	0	0	22	1	7
Gel Treats Sugar Free Orange	1 pkg (4 oz)	11	0	0	0	2	1	9
Gel Treats Sugar Free Strawberry	1 pkg (4 oz)	11	0	0	0	2	1	9

GIBLETS

FOOD	PORTION	CALS	PROT	FAT	CHOL	CARB	FIBER	SOD
capon simmered	1 cup (5 oz)	238	38	8	629	0	0	80
chicken fried	1 cup (5 oz)	402	47	20	647	6	0	164
chicken simmered	1 cup (5 oz)	289	30	17	419	1	0	93
turkey simmered	1 cup (5 oz)	243	39	7	606	3	–	85

GINGER

FOOD	PORTION	CALS	PROT	FAT	CHOL	CARB	FIBER	SOD
ground	1 tsp	6	tr	tr	0	1	tr	1
pickled	0.5 oz	5	tr	0	0	1	tr	52
preserved	1.5 oz	34	0	0	0	8	1	8
root fresh	5 slices	9	tr	tr	0	2	tr	1
root fresh sliced	¼ cup	19	tr	tr	0	4	1	3
Eden								
Pickled w/ Shiso Leaves	1 tbsp	20	0	0	0	4	tr	100
Frieda's								
Crystallized	9 pieces (1.1 oz)	100	0	0	0	26	0	10
Galanga Thai Ginger	⅔ cup	60	1	1	0	13	2	10

GINKGO NUTS

FOOD	PORTION	CALS	PROT	FAT	CHOL	CARB	FIBER	SOD
canned	1 oz	32	1	tr	0	6	–	87
dried	1 oz	99	3	tr	0	21	–	4
raw	1 oz	52	1	tr	0	11	–	1

GINSENG

FOOD	PORTION	CALS	PROT	FAT	CHOL	CARB	FIBER	SOD
dried	1 oz	90	5	tr	–	20	2	16
fresh	1 oz	28	1	tr	–	6	tr	5

GIZZARDS

FOOD	PORTION	CALS	PROT	FAT	CHOL	CARB	FIBER	SOD
chicken simmered	1 cup (5 oz)	212	44	4	536	0	0	81
turkey simmered	1 (3 oz)	103	18	3	171	tr	0	56

GNOCCHI

FOOD	PORTION	CALS	PROT	FAT	CHOL	CARB	FIBER	SOD
Vantia								
Gnocchi Whole Wheat	¾ cup	210	5	1	0	46	4	630

FOOD	PORTION	CALS	PROT	FAT	CHOL	CARB	FIBER	SOD
GOAT								
roasted	3 oz	122	23	3	64	0	0	73
GOJI BERRIES								
dried	1 oz	106	2	3	0	19	2	–
Navitas Naturals								
Dried	1 oz	90	4	0	0	18	1	140
Sunfood								
Organic	1 oz	90	4	0	0	18	3	105
Superfood Snacks								
Organic Chocolate Goji Treats	3 pieces (1.4 oz)	150	4	4	5	24	7	55
GOJI JUICE								
Gojilania								
Organic	8 oz	110	5	0	0	23	0	110
GOOSE								
w/ skin roasted	½ goose (1.7 lbs)	2362	195	170	708	0	0	543
w/ skin roasted	6.6 oz	574	47	41	172	0	0	132
w/o skin roasted	½ goose (1.3 lbs)	1406	171	75	569	0	0	447
w/o skin roasted	5 oz	340	41	18	138	0	0	108
GOOSEBERRIES								
canned in light syrup	½ cup	93	1	tr	0	24	–	3
fresh	1 cup	67	1	1	0	15	–	1
Navitas Naturals								
Cape Gooseberry Dried	1 oz	80	2	0	0	17	3	25
GRAPE JUICE								
bottled unsweetened	1 cup	154	1	tr	0	38	tr	8
Apple & Eve								
Vintage Concord	8 oz	150	0	0	0	40	–	15
Cascadian Farm								
Organic frzn as prep	8 oz	150	0	0	0	38	–	5
Juicy Juice								
Harvest Surprise	8 oz	120	1	0	0	28	0	80
Lakewood								
Organic Concord	6 oz	105	1	0	0	25	1	5

FOOD	PORTION	CALS	PROT	FAT	CHOL	CARB	FIBER	SOD
Langers								
Plus 100% Juice	8 oz	160	0	0	0	40	–	15
White Grape Plus 100% Juice	8 oz	160	0	0	0	40	–	15
Newman's Own								
Gorilla Grape	8 oz	140	0	0	0	34	–	140
Old Orchard								
100% Juice White	8 oz	160	0	0	0	38	–	20
Tang								
Drink Mix as prep	1 serv (8 oz)	110	0	0	0	28	0	10
Tree Ripe								
Organic 100% Juice	6 oz	120	1	0	0	28	0	10
Tropicana								
Grape	1 bottle (14 oz)	270	tr	0	0	67	0	25
Walnut Acres								
Organic	8 oz	120	0	0	0	31	0	0
Welch's								
100% Juice	8 oz	170	0	0	0	42	–	20
100% White	8 oz	160	0	0	0	39	–	20
Light White Grape	8 oz	70	0	0	0	18	–	80
GRAPE LEAVES								
canned	1 (4 g)	3	tr	tr	0	tr	–	114
fresh raw	1 (3 g)	3	tr	tr	0	1	tr	0
Sabra								
Stuffed Meatless	1	45	2	1	0	8	1	65
TAKE-OUT								
dolmas w/ beef & rice	1 (0.7 oz)	50	2	4	5	2	1	14
dolmas w/ lamb & rice	1 (0.7 oz)	56	2	4	5	3	1	14
dolmas w/ rice	1 (2 oz)	92	1	6	0	8	2	93
GRAPEFRUIT								
CANNED								
juice pack	½ cup	46	1	tr	0	11	–	9
unsweetened	1 cup	93	1	tr	0	22	–	3
water pack	½ cup	44	1	tr	0	11	–	2
Del Monte								
Fruit Naturals Red	½ cup	60	0	0	0	16	tr	15
SunFresh Red	½ cup	80	1	0	0	19	2	10

FOOD	PORTION	CALS	PROT	FAT	CHOL	CARB	FIBER	SOD
SunFresh White In Real Fruit Juice	½ cup	45	1	0	0	9	2	15
FRESH								
pink	½	37	1	tr	0	9	1	0
pink sections	1 cup	69	1	tr	0	18	1	1
red	½	37	1	tr	0	9	–	0
red sections	1 cup	69	1	tr	0	18	–	1
white	½	39	1	tr	0	10	1	0
white sections	1 cup	76	2	tr	0	19	1	0
Ocean Spray								
Sweet Ruby	½ med	60	1	0	0	16	6	0
Sunkist								
Fresh	½ med	60	1	0	0	16	6	0
Oroblanco	½	100	1	1	0	22	4	0
GRAPEFRUIT JUICE								
fresh	1 cup	96	1	tr	0	23	–	2
frzn as prep	1 cup	102	1	tr	0	24	–	2
frzn not prep	6 oz	302	4	1	0	72	–	6
sweetened	1 cup	116	1	tr	0	28	–	4
Apple & Eve								
Ruby Red	8 oz	130	0	0	0	32	–	10
Crystal Light								
Sunrise Sunrise Ruby Red as prep	1 serv (8 oz)	5	0	0	0	0	0	0
Izze								
Sparkling Grapefruit	8 oz	160	2	0	0	37	–	10
Minute Maid								
Frozen + Calcium	8 oz	100	0	0	0	25	–	0
Ruby Red	8 oz	130	0	0	0	34	–	20
Odwalla								
100% Juice	8 oz	90	2	0	0	20	0	5
Sundia								
Ruby	½ cup	70	1	0	0	18	1	0
Tao Tea								
Grapefruit Lemon Fusion	8 oz	72	0	0	0	18	–	26
Tropicana								
Sweet	8 oz	130	1	0	0	31	0	20
GRAPES								
seedless red or green	20	69	1	tr	0	18	1	2

FOOD	PORTION	CALS	PROT	FAT	CHOL	CARB	FIBER	SOD
seedless red or green	1 cup	110	1	tr	0	29	1	3
thompson seedless in heavy syrup	½ cup	93	1	tr	0	25	1	6
thompson seedless water pack	½ cup	49	1	tr	0	13	1	7
with seeds red or green	20	80	1	tr	0	21	1	2
with seeds red or green	1 cup	106	1	tr	0	28	1	3
Earthbound Farm								
Organic Black	1½ cups	190	1	1	0	24	1	0
Frieda's								
Champagne	½ cup (3 oz)	50	1	0	0	15	1	0

GRAVY
CANNED

FOOD	PORTION	CALS	PROT	FAT	CHOL	CARB	FIBER	SOD
beef	1 cup	124	9	6	7	11	–	1305
beef	1 can (10 oz)	155	11	7	9	14	–	1630
chicken	1 cup	189	5	14	5	13	–	1375
mushroom	1 cup	120	3	6	0	13	–	1259
turkey	1 cup	122	6	5	5	12	–	–
Boston Market								
Roasted Chicken	¼ cup	25	0	2	<5	3	–	280
Campbell's								
Au Jus	¼ cup	5	1	0	0	0	0	230
Chicken	¼ cup	40	0	3	5	3	0	260
Fat Free Beef	¼ cup	15	1	0	0	3	0	300
Fat Free Turkey	¼ cup	20	1	0	0	4	0	290
Mushroom	¼ cup	20	0	1	<5	3	0	280
Franco-American								
Fat Free Slow Roast Chicken	¼ cup	20	tr	0	0	4	0	250
Slow Roast Chicken	¼ cup	20	1	1	<5	3	0	240
Heinz								
Home Style Classic Chicken	¼ cup	25	0	1	0	4	0	340
HomeStyle Roasted Turkey	¼ cup	25	1	1	<5	3	0	290
Pacific Foods								
Natural Mushroom	¼ cup	20	1	0	0	4	1	270
Natural Turkey	¼ cup	25	1	1	–	4	0	230
FROZEN								
Tofurky								
Giblet & Mushroom	2 tbsp	30	2	1	0	3	1	210

FOOD	PORTION	CALS	PROT	FAT	CHOL	CARB	FIBER	SOD
MIX								
au jus as prep w/ water	1 cup	32	1	1	1	4	–	964
brown as prep w/ water	1 cup	75	2	2	2	13	–	1076
chicken as prep	1 cup	83	3	2	3	14	–	1133
mushroom as prep	1 cup	70	2	1	1	14	–	1402
onion as prep w/ water	1 cup	77	2	1	tr	16	–	1013
pork as prep	1 cup	76	2	2	3	13	–	1235
turkey as prep	1 cup	87	3	2	3	15	–	1498
Bournvita								
Extract	2 heaping tsp	34	1	1	–	7	–	–
Bovril								
Extract	1 heaping tsp	9	2	0	–	tr	0	–
Knorr								
Au Jus Instant as prep	2 oz	10	tr	0	0	2	–	470
Beef Instant as prep	2 oz	20	1	1	0	3	–	330
Brown Instant as prep	2 oz	25	1	0	0	6	–	410
Brown Low Sodium Instant as prep	2 oz	25	1	tr	0	5	–	115
Chicken Instant as prep	2 oz	25	tr	tr	0	5	–	395
Chicken Low Sodium Instant as prep	2 oz	25	1	1	5	4	–	120
Leahey Gardens								
No Beef Brown Gluten Free	¼ cup	9	tr	tr	0	3	–	114
No Chicken Golden	¼ cup	18	tr	2	0	3	–	275
Marmite								
Extract	1 heaping tsp	9	2	0	–	tr	–	–
Road's End Organics								
Savory Herb Cholesterol Free Gluten Free	¼ cup	25	tr	0	0	5	0	210
TAKE-OUT								
au jus	1 cup	62	1	6	6	1	tr	290
giblet gravy	¼ cup	45	3	3	23	3	tr	313

GREAT NORTHERN BEANS

FOOD	PORTION	CALS	PROT	FAT	CHOL	CARB	FIBER	SOD
canned	1 cup	299	19	1	0	55	13	11
dried cooked	1 cup	209	15	1	0	37	12	4
Eden								
Organic	½ cup	110	5	1	0	20	8	45

FOOD	PORTION	CALS	PROT	FAT	CHOL	CARB	FIBER	SOD
DRIED								
HamBeens								
Great Northerns as prep	½ cup	120	7	1	0	22	11	63
GREEN BEANS								
CANNED								
drained	1 cup	27	2	tr	0	6	3	354
Allens								
Italian Cut	½ cup	30	2	0	0	5	2	370
Del Monte								
Cut	½ cup	20	1	0	0	4	2	390
Cut w/ Potatoes & Ham Flavor	½ cup	30	1	0	0	6	tr	330
French Style	½ cup	20	1	0	0	4	2	390
Fresh Cut Italian	½ cup	30	1	0	0	6	3	390
Whole	½ cup	20	1	0	0	4	2	390
Gertie's Finest								
Pickled	1 oz	15	1	0	0	3	1	160
Green Giant								
50% Less Sodium Cut	½ cup	20	1	0	0	4	1	200
Tillen Farms								
Crispy Dilly Beans Pickled	¼ cup	15	1	0	0	3	0	250
FRESH								
cooked w/o salt	1 cup	44	2	tr	0	10	4	1
raw	1 cup	34	2	tr	0	8	4	7
raw whole beans	10	17	1	tr	0	4	2	3
Frieda's								
Purple Wax	⅔ cup	25	2	0	0	6	3	5
GreenLine								
Fresh Trimmed	3 oz	25	1	0	0	5	2	0
FROZEN								
cooked	1 cup	38	2	tr	0	9	4	12
Birds Eye								
Steamfresh Cut	½ cup	30	1	0	0	5	2	0
C&W								
French Cut	1 cup	30	1	0	0	5	2	0
Cascadian Farm								
Organic Petite Whole	1 cup	25	1	0	0	5	2	90
Green Giant								
Green Bean Casserole	⅔ cup	110	2	8	0	8	1	460

FOOD	PORTION	CALS	PROT	FAT	CHOL	CARB	FIBER	SOD
Pictsweet								
Cut	⅔ cup	30	1	0	0	5	2	0
TAKE-OUT								
casserole w/ mushroom sauce	1 cup	108	3	6	2	11	3	525
pickled	½ cup	19	1	tr	0	4	2	160

GREENS
Ready Pac

Microwave Leafy Greens as prep	½ cup	15	2	0	0	2	2	100

GROUNDCHERRIES

fresh	½ cup	37	1	tr	0	8	–	–

GROUPER

cooked	3 oz	100	21	1	40	0	0	45
cooked	1 fillet (7.1 oz)	238	50	3	95	0	0	107
raw	3 oz	78	16	1	31	0	0	45

GUAR GUM
Bob's Red Mill

Guar Gum	1 tbsp	20	0	0	0	6	6	2

GUAVA

fresh	1	45	1	1	0	11	–	2
guava sauce	½ cup	43	tr	tr	0	11	–	4
Frieda's								
Fresh	1 (3 oz)	45	4	1	0	10	5	0

GUAVA JUICE
Apple & Eve

Nectar	5 oz	130	0	0	0	32	–	35
Sabor Latino								
Nectar + Calcium	8 oz	160	0	0	0	39	–	20

GUINEA HEN

w/ skin raw	½ hen (12.1 oz)	545	81	22	–	0	0	–
w/o skin raw	½ hen (9.3 oz)	292	55	7	166	0	0	–

FOOD	PORTION	CALS	PROT	FAT	CHOL	CARB	FIBER	SOD
HADDOCK								
fresh broiled	4 oz	127	27	1	84	0	0	99
roe raw	1 oz	37	7	tr	103	tr	–	–
smoked	1 oz	33	7	tr	22	0	0	216
Van de Kamp's								
Battered Fillets	2 (3.6 oz)	210	9	11	20	21	2	580
TAKE-OUT								
breaded & fried	4 oz	229	23	10	88	10	1	528
HALIBUT								
atlantic & pacific cooked	3 oz	119	23	2	35	0	0	59
atlantic & pacific cooked	½ fillet (5.6 oz)	223	42	5	65	0	0	110
atlantic & pacific raw	3 oz	93	18	2	27	0	0	46
greenland baked	3 oz	203	16	15	50	0	0	87
greenland baked	5.6 oz	380	29	28	94	0	0	163
FROZEN								
Van de Kamp's								
Battered Fillets	3 (4 oz)	230	10	11	25	22	0	630
HALVA (see SESAME)								
HAM								
boneless extra lean roasted	3 oz	123	18	5	45	1	0	1023
boneless roasted	3 oz	151	19	8	50	0	0	1275
canned extra lean roasted	3 oz	116	18	4	26	tr	0	965
canned lean roasted	3 oz	142	18	7	35	tr	0	908
center slice lean & fat roasted	3 oz	173	17	11	46	tr	0	1179
deviled	¼ cup	188	7	17	35	1	0	724
ham salad spread	2 tbsp	65	3	5	11	3	0	274
patty grilled	1 patty (2 oz)	205	8	19	43	1	0	638
prosciutto	4 slices (1.3 oz)	72	10	3	26	tr	0	992
sliced	3 slices (2.9 oz)	137	14	7	48	3	1	1095
sliced extra lean	3 slices (2.2 oz)	69	11	2	30	2	0	697
westphalian smoked	1 oz	105	5	10	–	0	0	398
whole roasted	3 oz	207	18	14	53	0	0	1009

FOOD	PORTION	CALS	PROT	FAT	CHOL	CARB	FIBER	SOD
Boar's Head								
Black Forest Smoked	2 oz	60	10	1	30	2	0	580
Deluxe	2 oz	60	9	1	25	2	0	590
Deluxe 42% Lowered Sodium	2 oz	60	10	1	25	2	0	460
Fresh Seasoned	2 oz	90	14	3	35	1	0	310
Maple Glazed Honey	2 oz	60	10	1	20	3	0	570
Pepper	2 oz	60	10	1	20	2	0	610
Rosemary & Sundried Tomato	2 oz	70	10	3	10	2	0	590
Virginia Smoked	2 oz	60	9	1	25	2	0	590
Carl Buddig								
Ham Sliced	2 oz	85	10	5	–	1	–	–
Honey Ham Sliced	2 oz	90	10	5	–	2	–	–
Healthy Ones								
Honey 97% Fat Free	7 slices (2 oz)	90	9	2	20	2	–	410
Organic Prairie								
Hardwood Smoked Bone In Spiral Sliced	3 oz	110	19	3	40	tr	0	940
Oscar Mayer								
Ham Brown Sugar Thin Sliced	⅓ pkg (2 oz)	70	10	2	25	4	–	830
Lunchables Ham Bagels	1 pkg	410	16	10	40	64	2	890
Virginia Shaved	2 oz	50	9	1	25	1	0	570
Sara Lee								
Bavarian Oven Roasted Honey	2 oz	70	9	4	40	2	0	560
Brown Sugar	2 oz	70	10	3	20	5	0	600
Homestyle Baked	2 oz	60	10	2	25	2	0	600
Virignia Baked	4 slices (1.8 oz)	60	10	2	20	2	0	550
Tyson								
Glazed Ham Maple & Brown Sugar	1 serv (5 oz)	180	17	5	60	18	0	780
Honey Ham	2 slices (1.6 oz)	50	9	2	25	1	0	740
TAKE-OUT								
croquette	1 (2.2 oz)	149	9	9	18	8	tr	532
salad	½ cup	287	16	23	237	5	tr	671
spam musubi	1 serv (6 oz)	253	6	6	14	42	1	283
thick slice fried	1 (2.2 oz)	140	13	9	33	tr	0	756

FOOD	PORTION	CALS	PROT	FAT	CHOL	CARB	FIBER	SOD
HAMBURGER								
Ian's								
Mini	2 (4.6 oz)	360	23	12	25	42	1	450
Mini Cheeseburger	2 (5 oz)	420	25	17	65	42	1	540
Kid Cuisine								
Cheeseburger Builder	1 meal	390	14	11	20	58	2	600
Lean Pockets								
Cheeseburger	1 (4.5 oz)	280	12	7	20	42	3	810
Oscar Meyer								
Lunchables All-Star Burgers	1 pkg	420	14	14	35	60	1	980
Quaker Maid								
Pure Beef Patties	1 (4 oz)	240	19	18	50	0	0	40
Wellshire								
Beef	1 (4 oz)	260	20	12	60	0	0	60
Turkey Burgers	1 (4 oz)	200	13	2	30	0	0	25
TAKE-OUT								
cheeseburger + condiments	1 reg (4.5 oz)	347	17	17	46	28	1	644
double hamburger + condiments	1 reg (5.8 oz)	384	23	19	66	30	2	809
single patty + condiments	1 reg (4 oz)	299	15	11	33	35	2	589
HAMBURGER SUBSTITUTES (*see also* MEAT SUBSTITUTES)								
Boca								
American Flame Grilled	1 (2.5 oz)	90	14	3	5	4	3	280
Cheeseburger	1 (2.5 oz)	100	12	5	5	5	3	360
Grilled Vegetable	1 (2.5 oz)	70	12	1	0	6	4	300
Ground Burger	1 serv (2 oz)	60	13	1	0	6	3	270
Original	1 (2.5 oz)	70	13	1	0	6	4	280
Original Vegan	1 (2.5 oz)	70	13	1	0	6	4	280
Fantastic								
Natures Burger Mix not prep	¼ cup	170	8	3	0	30	5	320
Tofu Burger Mix not prep	3 tbsp	80	3	3	0	13	1	400
Gardenburger								
Black Bean Chipotle	1 (2.5 oz)	80	5	3	0	13	5	250
Flamed Grilled	1 (2.5 oz)	90	11	4	0	5	4	420
GardenVegan	1 (2.5 oz)	100	10	1	0	12	3	230
Original	1 (2.5 oz)	100	5	4	5	14	5	420
Portabella	1 (2.5 oz)	90	5	3	0	15	5	360

FOOD	PORTION	CALS	PROT	FAT	CHOL	CARB	FIBER	SOD
Lightlife								
Light Burgers	1 (3 oz)	120	16	2	0	11	3	500
Smart Menu Burger	1	80	4	1	0	14	2	360
Morningstar Farms								
Classic Burger	1 (2.2 oz)	150	14	7	0	10	3	340
Garden Veggie Patties	1 (2.4 oz)	100	10	3	0	9	4	350
Okara Pattie	1 (2.2 oz)	120	12	5	0	6	3	300
Vegan Burger	1 (2.5 oz)	100	13	2	0	8	5	460
Tofurky								
SuperBurgers Original	1 (3.5 oz)	120	10	2	0	16	2	390
VeggieLand								
Veggie Burger Original	1 (3.5 oz)	132	13	4	0	12	7	330
Veggie Burger Peppadew	1 (5 oz)	210	15	5	0	28	4	430
WildWood								
Organic Original Burgers Tofu-Veggie	1 (3.2 oz)	180	12	13	0	8	1	330
HAZELNUTS								
dried blanched	1 oz	191	4	19	0	5	–	1
dried unblanched	1 oz	179	4	18	0	4	–	1
dry roasted unblanched	1 oz	188	3	19	0	5	–	1
oil roasted unblanched	1 oz	187	4	18	0	5	2	1
Kettle								
Butter Creamy Unsalted	2 tbsp	180	4	17	0	5	3	0
Love'n Bake								
Hazelnut Praline	2 tbsp	170	3	12	0	13	2	0
HEART								
beef simmered	3 oz	140	24	4	180	tr	0	50
chicken cooked	1 (3 g)	5	1	tr	6	0	0	11
chicken diced simmered	½ cup	134	19	6	175	tr	0	35
lamb braised	3 oz	157	21	7	212	2	0	54
pork braised	1 (4.5 oz)	191	30	7	285	1	0	45
turkey simmered	½ cup	94	16	3	133	tr	0	65
veal braised	3 oz	158	25	6	150	tr	0	49
HEARTS OF PALM								
canned	1 (1.2 oz)	9	1	tr	0	2	1	141
canned	½ cup	20	2	tr	0	3	2	311
Del Monte								
Hearts Of Palm	2–3 pieces	20	2	0	0	3	2	450

FOOD	PORTION	CALS	PROT	FAT	CHOL	CARB	FIBER	SOD
Native Forest								
Organic	1 oz	15	1	0	0	2	1	125
HEMP								
Living Harvest								
Organic Hemp Nuts	2 tbsp (1 oz)	170	10	12	0	5	0	0
Organic Protein Powder	2 scoops (1 oz)	110	14	3	0	9	1	0
Manitoba Harvest								
Hemp Seed Butter	2 tbsp	160	11	10	0	7	1	10
Protein Powder	2 scoops (1 oz)	134	15	6	0	5	4	15
Shelled Seed	2 tbsp	160	11	10	0	7	1	10
Nutiva								
Organic Protein Powder	2 scoops (1 oz)	120	11	3	0	14	14	15
Shelled Hempseed	2 tbsp	110	6	8	0	2	1	0
HERBAL TEA (see TEA/HERBAL TEA)								
HERBS/SPICES (see also individual names)								
cajun seasoning	1 tbsp	19	1	1	–	3	1	5
chinese five spice	1 tsp	7	0	tr	–	2	tr	1
garam masala	1 tsp	8	tr	tr	0	1	–	2
poultry seasoning	1 tsp	5	tr	tr	0	1	tr	tr
pumpkin pie spice	1 tsp	6	tr	tr	0	1	tr	1
A Taste Of Thai								
Chicken & Rice Seasoning	¼ pkg (6 g)	15	0	0	0	3	0	740
Chef Paul Prudhomme's								
Magic Blackened Redfish	¼ tsp	0	0	0	0	0	0	95
Magic Fajita	¼ tsp	0	0	0	0	0	0	70
Magic Pork & Veal	¼ tsp	0	0	0	0	0	0	130
Magic Poultry	¼ tsp	0	0	0	0	0	0	105
Cut N Clean								
Greens Seasoning	1½ tsp	20	1	0	0	5	tr	240
Eden								
Shake Furikake	½ tsp	5	0	0	0	1	1	25
Emeril's								
Asian Essence	½ tsp	0	0	0	0	0	0	155
Bayou Blast!	½ tsp	0	0	0	0	0	0	296
Chicken Rub	½ tsp	0	0	0	0	0	0	80

FOOD	PORTION	CALS	PROT	FAT	CHOL	CARB	FIBER	SOD
Original Essence	½ tsp	0	0	0	0	0	0	271
Steak Rub	½ tsp	0	0	0	0	0	0	220
Mrs. Dash								
Grilling Blend Chicken	¼ tsp	0	0	0	0	0	0	0
Grilling Blend Steak	¼ tsp	0	0	0	0	0	0	0
Original Blend	¼ tsp	0	0	0	0	0	0	0
Tomato Basil Garlic	¼ tsp	0	0	0	0	0	0	0
Nueva Cocina								
Picadillo	2 tsp	15	0	0	0	3	–	220
Taco Fresco	2 tsp	15	tr	0	0	3	–	230
Ortega								
Burrito Seasoning	1½ tsp	20	0	0	0	3	tr	230
Fajita Seasoning	1½ tsp	20	0	0	0	3	–	430
Taco Seasoning	1 tbsp	20	0	0	0	4	–	430
Spice Hunter								
All Purpose Blend	¼ tsp	0	0	0	0	0	0	0
Greek Seasoning Salt Free	¼ tsp	0	0	0	0	0	0	0
HERRING								
atlantic baked	4 oz	230	26	13	87	0	0	130
dried salted	1 fillet (1.4 oz)	161	18	9	61	0	0	680
pickled	1 oz	74	4	5	4	3	0	247
pickled in cream sauce	1 oz	72	3	5	5	2	0	200
roe	1 tbsp	39	6	2	105	tr	0	25
smoked kippered	1 oz	620	7	4	23	0	0	260
Beach Cliff								
Kippered Snacks	1 can (4 oz)	220	19	16	135	0	0	490
TAKE-OUT								
breaded fried	1 serv (4 oz)	225	15	14	67	9	1	432
HIBISCUS								
flowers dried sweetened	⅓ cup	100	0	0	0	23	2	15
HICKORY NUTS								
dried	1 oz	187	4	18	0	5	–	0
HOMINY								
CANNED								
white	1 cup (5.6 oz)	482	2	1	0	23	4	336

FOOD	PORTION	CALS	PROT	FAT	CHOL	CARB	FIBER	SOD
HONEY								
honey	1 cup (11.9 oz)	1031	1	0	0	279	–	12
honey	1 tbsp (0.7 oz)	64	tr	0	0	17	–	1
orange blossom	1 tbsp	60	0	0	0	17	0	0
wild honey	1 tbsp	60	0	0	0	17	–	0
Dutch Gold								
Clover	1 tbsp	60	0	0	0	17	0	0
Frieda's								
Honeycomb	½ cup (3 oz)	260	0	0	0	70	0	0
HONEYDEW								
balls frzn	1 cup (8 oz)	83	1	tr	0	21	2	41
fresh cut up	1 cup	61	1	tr	0	15	1	31
fresh wedge	⅛ melon (4.5 oz)	45	1	tr	0	11	1	22
whole fresh	1 (35 oz)	360	5	1	0	91	8	180
HORSE								
roasted	3 oz	149	24	5	58	0	0	47
HORSERADISH								
sauce	1 tbsp	7	tr	tr	0	2	1	47
wasabi root raw	1 (5.9 oz)	184	8	1	0	40	13	29
wasabi root raw sliced	½ cup (2.3 oz)	71	3	tr	0	15	5	11
Boar's Head								
Horseradish	1 tsp (5 g)	0	0	0	0	0	0	30
Horseradish Sauce Pub Style	1 tsp	15	0	2	5	1	0	15
Horseradish & Beets	1 tsp	0	0	0	0	0	0	30
Robert Rothchild Farm								
Sauce	1 tsp	20	0	2	<5	1	0	30
Sara Lee								
Horseradish Sauce	1 tbsp	20	0	2	0	0	0	45
HOT CHOCOLATE								
mix as prep w/ water	7 oz	103	3	1	–	23	–	149
mix w/ equal as prep w/ water	7 oz	48	4	tr	–	9	–	173

FOOD	PORTION	CALS	PROT	FAT	CHOL	CARB	FIBER	SOD
Country Choice Naturals								
Irish Chocolate Mint Cocoa	1 pkg	100	3	0	0	23	tr	160
Royal Chocolate Cocoa	1 pkg	100	3	0	0	23	tr	160
Soy Cocoa Royal Chocolate	1 pkg	100	2	1	0	23	1	130
Nestle								
Hot Cocoa Carb Select Fat Free	1 pkg	25	1	0	0	5	tr	150
Hot Cocoa Milk Chocolate	1 pkg (1 oz)	80	tr	3	0	15	tr	180
Swiss Miss								
Hot Cocoa Milk Chocolate Fat Free	1 pkg	50	3	0	0	10	tr	200
Milk Chocolate	1 pkg	120	1	3	0	23	1	170
Milk Chocolate w/ Marshmallows	1 pkg	120	1	3	tr	23	tr	150
TAKE-OUT								
hot cocoa	1 cup	218	9	9	33	26	–	123
mexican hot chocolate	1 cup	173	10	6	18	20	1	150
HOT DOG								
beef	1 (1.5 oz)	149	5	13	24	2	0	513
beef & pork	1 (1.5 oz)	137	5	12	23	1	1	504
beef low fat	1 (2 oz)	133	7	11	23	1	0	593
chicken	1 (1.5 oz)	116	6	9	45	3	0	617
fat free	1 (2 oz)	62	7	1	23	6	0	455
low fat	1 (2 oz)	88	6	6	25	3	0	716
low sodium	1 (2 oz)	180	7	16	35	1	0	177
pork and beef cheese smokie	1 (1.5 oz)	141	6	12	29	1	0	465
turkey	1 (1.5 oz)	102	6	8	48	1	0	642
Ball Park								
Franks	1 (2 oz)	180	6	16	40	3	0	560
Franks Beef	1 (2 oz)	180	6	16	35	3	0	550
Franks Bun Size	1 (2 oz)	180	6	16	40	3	0	560
Franks Smoked White Turkey	1 (1.8 oz)	45	6	0	10	5	0	420
Franks Fat Free	1 (1.8 oz)	40	5	0	10	4	0	420
Franks Lite	1 (1.8 oz)	100	6	7	25	3	0	460
Franks Singles Cheese	1 (1.6 oz)	150	5	13	30	2	0	460
Grillmaster Hearty Beef	1	250	9	23	50	3	0	780
Grillmaster Smokehouse	1	210	9	24	50	3	0	790

FOOD	PORTION	CALS	PROT	FAT	CHOL	CARB	FIBER	SOD
Boar's Head								
Beef	1 (2 oz)	160	7	14	30	1	0	440
Beef Lite	1 (1.6 oz)	90	7	6	25	0	0	270
Beef Cocktail	5 (2 oz)	170	8	15	30	0	0	430
Pork & Beef	1 (2 oz)	150	7	14	25	0	0	460
Dietz & Watson								
New York Style Beef	1 (2.3 oz)	130	8	15	35	2	0	560
Healthy Choice								
Beef Low Fat	1 (1.8 oz)	70	6	3	15	7	0	440
Healthy Ones								
Beef	1 (1.8 oz)	70	6	3	20	7	0	430
Franks	1 (1.8 oz)	70	6	3	20	6	0	430
Hebrew National								
97% Fat Free Beef	1 (1.7 oz)	45	6	2	15	3	0	400
Beef	1 (1.7 oz)	150	6	14	30	1	0	370
Cocktail Franks	5 (2 oz)	180	7	16	40	1	0	450
Dinner Frank	1 (4 oz)	350	13	32	70	1	0	990
Franks In A Blanket	5 (2.8 oz)	290	9	24	40	8	1	690
Reduced Fat Beef	1 (1.7 oz)	120	6	10	25	0	0	360
Ian's								
Popcorn Turkey Corn Dog	5 pieces (3 oz)	237	6	13	20	25	0	340
Johnsonville								
Stadium Beef	1 (2.7 oz)	240	9	22	50	2	–	760
Organic Prairie								
Beef Uncured	1 (1.5 oz)	120	5	11	25	0	0	360
Chicken Uncured	1 (1.5 oz)	100	7	6	35	1	0	480
Pork Uncured	1 (1.5 oz)	130	5	12	25	0	0	390
Turkey Uncured	1 (1.5 oz)	80	8	6	25	1	0	480
Oscar Mayer								
Beef	1 (1.6 oz)	140	5	13	30	1	0	460
Beef Light	1 (1.6 oz)	90	5	6	20	2	–	500
Cheese Dogs	1 (1.6 oz)	140	5	13	35	1	0	540
Corn Dogs	1	210	6	12	25	21	1	590
Smokies	1 (1.8 oz)	150	6	13	30	1	0	500
State Fair								
Corn Dogs	1 (2.67 oz)	180	4	12	15	18	1	560
Wellshire								
Beef Premium	1 (2 oz)	110	8	9	30	0	0	300
Cheese Franks	1 (2 oz)	110	8	9	30	0	0	300

FOOD	PORTION	CALS	PROT	FAT	CHOL	CARB	FIBER	SOD
Chicken Franks	1 (1.6 oz)	70	8	8	30	1	0	320
Turkey Franks	1 (1.6 oz)	110	10	6	30	1	0	330
TAKE-OUT								
corndog	1	460	17	19	79	56	–	972
w/ bun chili	1	297	14	13	51	31	–	480
w/ bun plain	1	242	10	15	44	18	–	671

HOT DOG SUBSTITUTES
Lightlife

FOOD	PORTION	CALS	PROT	FAT	CHOL	CARB	FIBER	SOD
Smart Dogs	1	45	9	0	0	2	1	320
Smart Franks	1 (2 oz)	110	12	5	0	5	0	470
Tofu Pups	1 (1.5 oz)	60	8	3	0	2	1	300
Loma Linda								
Big Franks	1 (1.8 oz)	110	11	6	0	3	2	220
Big Franks Low Fat Vegan	1 (1.8 oz)	80	12	3	0	3	2	240
Morningstar Farms								
Corn Dog Veggie	1 (2.5 oz)	170	8	6	0	22	3	530
Quorn								
Meat-Free Dogs	1 (1.5 oz)	70	5	4	5	3	2	250
Yves								
Meatless Hot Dog	1	50	10	1	0	2	0	400
Tofu Dogs	1	45	8	1	0	2	0	300

HUMMUS
Athenos

FOOD	PORTION	CALS	PROT	FAT	CHOL	CARB	FIBER	SOD
Original	2 tbsp	80	2	5	0	5	1	180
Roasted Garlic	2 tbsp	80	2	5	0	5	1	200
Roasted Red Pepper	2 tbsp	80	2	6	0	5	1	130
Guiltless Gourmet								
Roasted Garlic	2 tbsp	35	1	2	0	4	1	115
Sabra								
Homus	2 oz	110	5	5	0	12	3	75
Homus Spicy	½ cup	171	6	4	0	27	5	242
Tribe								
40 Spices	2 tbsp	50	1	4	0	3	1	140
French Onion	2 tbsp	50	1	4	0	4	1	120
Organic Classic	2 tbsp	50	2	4	0	4	1	100
Roasted Eggplant	2 tbsp	35	1	3	0	3	1	150
Scallion	2 tbsp	50	1	4	0	4	1	125
Zesty Lemon	2 tbsp	50	1	3	0	4	1	130

FOOD	PORTION	CALS	PROT	FAT	CHOL	CARB	FIBER	SOD
Wholesome Valley								
Organic Classic	2 tbsp (1 oz)	60	2	4	0	5	1	115
Wild Garden								
Hummus Dip	2 tbsp	35	2	2	0	4	1	70
WildWood								
Organic Low Fat	2 tbsp	50	2	2	0	6	1	130
Organic Mid-Eastern	2 tbsp	65	2	4	0	6	1	120
TAKE-OUT								
hummus	⅓ cup	140	4	7	0	17	–	200

HYACINTH BEANS

| dried cooked | 1 cup | 228 | 16 | 1 | 0 | 40 | – | 13 |

ICE CREAM AND FROZEN DESSERTS

(*see also* ICES AND ICE POPS, SHERBET, YOGURT FROZEN)

FOOD	PORTION	CALS	PROT	FAT	CHOL	CARB	FIBER	SOD
chocolate	½ cup (4 fl oz)	143	3	7	22	19	–	50
dixie cup chocolate	1 (3.5 fl oz)	125	2	6	20	16	–	44
dixie cup strawberry	1 (3.5 fl oz)	112	2	5	17	16	–	35
dixie cup vanilla	1 (3.5 fl oz)	116	2	6	25	14	–	46
freeze dried ice cream chocolate strawberry & vanilla	1 pkg (0.75 oz)	158	2	5	1	24	1	97
strawberry	½ cup (4 fl oz)	127	2	6	19	18	–	40
vanilla	½ cup (4 fl oz)	132	2	7	29	16	–	53
vanilla soft serve	½ cup	111	4	2	10	19	–	62
Blue Bunny								
Bar Candy Center Crunch	1 (3.2 oz)	370	3	29	20	28	1	75
Bar English Toffee	1 (1.4 oz)	130	1	9	15	12	0	40
Bar Homemade Vanilla	1 (2.3 oz)	190	3	13	20	16	0	50
Bar Orange Dream	1 (2.1 oz)	80	1	2	5	16	0	35
Bar Strawberry Sundae Crunch	1 (2.2 oz)	170	2	9	15	20	0	55
Blendz Peanut Butter Cup	1 (4.4 oz)	270	5	11	25	40	tr	160
Caramel Sundae Bite Size	4 bars (3.1 oz)	340	4	23	25	30	1	75
Chocolate	½ cup	130	2	7	25	17	0	55
Cone Bunny Tracks	1 (4.8 oz)	420	7	21	35	51	2	180

FOOD	PORTION	CALS	PROT	FAT	CHOL	CARB	FIBER	SOD
Cone The Champ Chocolate Lovers	1 (3.5 oz)	300	5	15	40	38	1	130
Cone Vanilla Nutty Sundae	1 (3 oz)	250	5	11	10	34	1	120
Cups Vanilla & Chocolate	1 (1.7 oz)	100	2	5	20	13	0	50
Mint Chip	½ cup	140	2	7	25	17	0	55
Neapolitan	½ cup	130	2	6	25	16	0	50
Orange Dream	½ cup	130	2	5	20	19	0	45
Premium All Natural Vanilla	½ cup	160	3	9	55	16	0	50
Premium Bunny Tracks	½ cup	190	4	11	25	21	tr	95
Premium Butter Pecan	½ cup	150	3	9	25	15	0	70
Premium Cookies & Cream	½ cup	150	3	8	25	19	0	75
Premium Double Strawberry	½ cup	140	2	6	25	20	0	40
Premium Exquisite Mint	½ cup	170	3	8	25	22	0	65
Premium Rocky Road	½ cup	150	3	7	20	21	0	90
Premium Toasted Almond Fudge	½ cup	160	3	9	25	18	tr	55
Sandwich Big Vanilla	1 (3.7 oz)	260	4	10	35	39	0	160
Sandwich Chips Galore	1 (3.4 oz)	310	3	16	35	40	1	170
Strawberry	½ cup	120	2	6	25	17	0	50
Breyers								
Bar Light Creamy Vanilla Chocolate Coated	1	160	3	8	5	21	3	45
Bubbies								
Mochi Mango	1 piece (1.3 oz)	110	1	4	15	18	0	15
Butterfinger								
Bar	1 (1.9 oz)	210	2	15	15	17	0	50
Celestial Seasonings								
Tea Dreams Cinnamon Apple Spice	½ cup	140	0	6	0	24	1	55
Tea Dreams Vanilla Ginger Spice Chai	½ cup	140	0	6	0	24	1	70
Tea Dreams Bars Chocolate Caramel Chai	1 (2.7 oz)	240	tr	15	0	28	2	65
Dove								
Beyond Vanilla	½ cup	240	4	15	50	23	0	60
Give In To Mint	½ cup	300	4	18	45	30	1	75
Irresistibly Raspberry	½ cup	240	3	13	30	29	1	40

FOOD	PORTION	CALS	PROT	FAT	CHOL	CARB	FIBER	SOD
Milk Chocolate w/ Almonds	1 bar (3.3 oz)	340	6	23	35	28	1	135
Milk Chocolate w/ Vanilla Ice Cream	1 bar (3.3 oz)	330	4	21	40	31	1	60
Miniatures Milk Chocolate w/ Vanilla Ice Cream	5 pieces (3.1 oz)	300	4	20	30	30	1	55
Triple Chocolate	1 bar (2.8 oz)	200	4	18	25	28	3	40
Unconditional Chocolate	½ cup	290	4	17	40	31	2	65
Vanilla w/ A Chocolate Soul	½ cup	290	4	18	45	29	1	75
Edy's								
Carb Benefit Butter Pecan	½ cup	170	2	12	30	13	6	55
Carb Benefit Chocolate	½ cup	150	2	10	30	13	7	35
Carb Benefit Chocolate Chip	½ cup	160	2	11	30	14	6	30
Carb Benefit Mint Chocolate Chip	½ cup	160	2	11	30	14	6	30
Carb Benefit Vanilla Bean	½ cup	140	3	9	30	13	6	30
Dibs Chocolate	26 pieces	420	4	32	30	28	–	75
Dibs Mint	26 pieces	420	3	32	25	29	–	65
Dibs Vanilla	26 pieces	420	3	32	25	29	–	65
Grand Andes Cool Mint	½ cup	170	2	9	25	19	–	40
Grand Butter Pecan	½ cup	170	3	10	25	16	–	95
Grand Chocolate	½ cup	150	3	8	25	17	–	35
Grand Chocolate Caramel Swirl	½ cup	170	2	9	25	19	–	45
Grand Chocolate Chip	½ cup	160	2	8	20	19	–	40
Grand Chocolate Fudge Mousse	½ cup	160	2	8	25	20	–	45
Grand Chocolate Fudge Sundae	½ cup	170	3	9	20	20	–	50
Grand Coffee	½ cup	140	2	8	25	15	–	40
Grand Cookie Dough	½ cup	180	3	9	25	21	–	55
Grand Cookies'N Cream	½ cup	160	3	8	25	19	–	50
Grand Double Fudge Brownie	½ cup	170	3	9	25	20	–	45
Grand Dulce De Leche	½ cup	150	2	7	25	20	–	50
Grand Espresso Chip	½ cup	150	2	8	25	17	–	50
Grand French Vanilla	½ cup	160	2	9	50	16	–	35
Grand Fudge Tracks	½ cup	180	3	11	25	18	–	60

FOOD	PORTION	CALS	PROT	FAT	CHOL	CARB	FIBER	SOD
Grand Ice Cream Sandwich	½ cup	150	3	7	25	19	–	75
Grand Mint Chocolate Chips	½ cup	170	3	9	25	18	–	45
Grand Peanut Butter Cup	½ cup	180	3	10	20	19	–	75
Grand Real Strawberry	½ cup	130	2	6	20	16	–	30
Grand Rocky Road	½ cup	170	3	10	30	19	–	35
Grand Spumoni	½ cup	150	3	8	25	16	–	40
Grand Toffee Bar Crunch	½ cup	170	2	9	25	19	–	65
Grand Toll House Cookie Swirl	½ cup	170	2	9	25	21	–	60
Grand Turtle Sundae	½ cup	160	3	9	25	18	–	50
Grand Ultimate Caramel Cup	½ cup	170	2	8	20	22	–	55
Grand Vanilla	½ cup	140	2	8	25	15	–	35
Neapolitan	½ cup	140	2	7	25	16	–	35
Slow Churned Light Butter Pecan	½ cup	120	3	5	20	16	–	80
Slow Churned Light Caramel Delight	½ cup	120	3	4	20	19	–	50
Slow Churned Light Chocolate	½ cup	110	3	4	20	16	–	45
Slow Churned Light Chocolate Chip	½ cup	120	3	5	20	17	–	50
Slow Churned Light Chocolate Fudge Chunk	½ cup	120	3	5	20	18	–	50
Slow Churned Light Coffee	½ cup	105	3	4	20	15	–	45
Slow Churned Light Cookie Dough	½ cup	130	3	5	20	20	–	60
Slow Churned Light Cookies 'N Cream	½ cup	120	3	4	20	18	–	60
Slow Churned Light French Silk	½ cup	130	3	5	20	20	–	70
Slow Churned Light French Vanilla	½ cup	100	3	4	30	15	–	45
Slow Churned Light Fudge Tracks	½ cup	120	3	5	20	18	–	50
Slow Churned Light Mint Chocolate Chips	½ cup	120	3	5	20	17	–	50
Slow Churned Light Mocha Almond Fudge	½ cup	120	3	5	20	16	–	45

FOOD	PORTION	CALS	PROT	FAT	CHOL	CARB	FIBER	SOD
Slow Churned Light Neapolitan	½ cup	100	3	3	20	15	–	40
Slow Churned Light Rocky Road	½ cup	120	3	4	20	17	–	40
Slow Churned Light Strawberry	½ cup	110	2	3	15	18	–	40
Slow Churned Light Vanilla	½ cup	100	3	4	20	15	–	45
Slow Churned No Sugar Added Butter Pecan	½ cup	120	3	5	10	15	–	65
Slow Churned No Sugar Added Chocolate	½ cup	95	3	3	10	14	–	50
Slow Churned No Sugar Added Cookie Dough	½ cup	110	3	4	15	16	–	60
Slow Churned No Sugar Added Fat Free Chocolate Fudge	½ cup	100	4	0	0	22	–	60
Slow Churned No Sugar Added Fat Free Raspberry Vanilla Swirl	½ cup	90	3	0	0	19	–	50
Slow Churned No Sugar Added Fat Free Vanilla	½ cup	90	3	0	0	20	–	50
Slow Churned No Sugar Added Fat Free Vanilla Chocolate Swirl	½ cup	100	4	0	0	20	–	50
Slow Churned No Sugar Added Fudge Tracks	½ cup	110	3	4	10	16	–	55
Slow Churned No Sugar Added Mint Chocolate Chips	½ cup	110	3	5	10	15	–	45
Slow Churned No Sugar Added Neapolitan	½ cup	95	3	3	10	14	–	45
Slow Churned No Sugar Added Triple Chocolate	½ cup	110	3	4	10	17	–	55
Slow Churned No Sugar Added Vanilla	½ cup	90	3	3	10	13	–	45
Eskimo Pie								
Milk Chocolate	1 bar (1.8 oz)	160	2	11	20	12	0	35

FOOD	PORTION	CALS	PROT	FAT	CHOL	CARB	FIBER	SOD
Fat Boy								
Casco Nut Sundae On A Stick	1 (3 oz)	310	7	24	15	21	2	40
Casco Nut Sundae On A Stick Cherry Cordial	1 (3 oz)	300	3	22	15	26	1	45
Sandwich Chocolate	1 (3 oz)	210	4	9	20	31	1	150
Sandwich Egg Nog	1 (3 oz)	220	4	10	35	31	tr	160
Sandwich Jr. Vanilla	1 (1.6 oz)	120	2	5	15	17	0	25
Sandwich Vanilla	1 (3 oz)	220	4	10	20	30	1	160
Glace De Vino								
Chocolate Amarreto Cream Sherry	½ cup	180	2	7	20	21	0	50
Raspberry Merlot Cheesecake	½ cup	180	2	7	20	22	0	50
GoodBody								
Chocolate Banana	1 bar (3.5 oz)	120	7	1	0	25	4	170
Chocolate Double Dutch	1 bar (3.5 oz)	130	7	1	0	26	4	160
Chocolate Peanut Butter	1 bar (3.5 oz)	180	10	7	0	26	5	220
Vanilla & Raspberry Sorbet	1 bar (3.5 oz)	120	7	0	0	25	4	90
Vanilla & Strawberry Sorbet	1 bar (3.5 oz)	120	7	0	0	25	4	90
Vanilla & Tropical Sorbet	1 bar (3.5 oz)	120	7	0	0	25	4	90
Green & Black's								
Organic Chocolate Covered Chocolate	1 bar (3.5 oz)	214	4	14	–	19	2	tr
Organic Chocolate Covered Vanilla	1 bar (3.5 oz)	233	4	16	–	19	2	tr
Hawaiian Punch								
Cream Surfers	1 bar	90	1	2	5	16	0	35
Healthy Choice								
Bar Sorbet & Cream	1	100	1	1	5	20	tr	40
Brownie Bliss	½ cup	130	4	2	10	24	1	70
Butter Pecan Crunch	½ cup	100	2	2	10	18	2	65
Cappuccino Chocolate Chunk	½ cup	120	3	2	10	20	tr	70

FOOD	PORTION	CALS	PROT	FAT	CHOL	CARB	FIBER	SOD
Caramel Fudge Brownie	½ cup	120	3	2	10	21	1	70
Cherry Chocolate Mambo	½ cup	130	2	2	10	23	1	70
Chocolate Chocolate Chunk	½ cup	120	3	2	5	21	1	60
Cookies 'N Cream	½ cup	120	3	2	5	21	tr	90
Crazy Caramel	½ cup	120	2	2	10	23	tr	70
Double Karma	½ cup	140	2	2	10	28	tr	90
French Silk	½ cup	120	2	2	5	24	2	50
Happy Together	½ cup	150	3	2	10	29	1	70
Jumpin' Java	½ cup	130	3	2	10	25	tr	75
Low Fat Bar Fudge	1	90	3	1	5	13	0	60
Low Fat Bar Mocha Fudge	1	90	2	2	5	17	2	50
Low Fat Bar Strawberry & Cream	1	90	2	2	5	17	tr	45
Mint Chocolate Chip	½ cup	120	3	2	10	20	tr	70
No Sugar Added Chocolate Fudge Brownie	½ cup	120	3	2	5	21	1	60
No Sugar Added Coffee Almond Fudge	½ cup	110	3	2	5	20	1	55
No Sugar Added Mint Chocolate Chip	½ cup	110	3	2	10	18	1	50
No Sugar Added Vanilla	½ cup	100	3	2	10	17	1	55
Peanut Butter Cup	½ cup	120	3	2	5	21	tr	70
Praline & Caramel	½ cup	120	2	2	10	23	tr	80
Rocky Road	½ cup	130	3	2	5	25	tr	60
Sandwich Caramel	1	140	2	3	5	27	tr	120
Sandwich Fudge Swirl	1	140	2	3	5	27	tr	150
Sandwich Vanilla	1	130	2	3	5	24	tr	150
Turtle Fudge Cake	½ cup	130	2	2	10	23	tr	70
Vanilla	½ cup	110	3	2	10	19	tr	90
Vanilla Bean	½ cup	120	3	2	10	21	tr	60
Vanilla Caramel Fudge	½ cup	140	2	2	10	28	tr	90
Hershey's								
French Vanilla	½ cup	170	3	10	70	17	0	90
Neapolitan	½ cup	160	3	9	35	18	tr	60
Hood								
Butterscotch Blast	½ cup	160	2	7	25	20	0	60
Chocolate	½ cup	140	2	7	25	17	0	45
Chocolate Eclair	1 bar (2.2 oz)	150	1	10	5	14	0	45
Cookie Dough Delight	½ cup	160	2	8	25	20	0	60

FOOD	PORTION	CALS	PROT	FAT	CHOL	CARB	FIBER	SOD
Creamy Coffee	½ cup	140	2	7	30	16	0	50
Fat Free Chocolate Passion	½ cup	100	3	0	0	22	0	70
Fat Free Very Vanilla	½ cup	100	2	0	0	23	0	70
Fudge Twister	½ cup	150	2	7	25	20	0	50
Grasshopper Pie	½ cup	160	2	7	25	22	0	70
Hoodsie Cups	1 (1.7 oz)	100	2	5	20	12	0	35
Light Butter Pecan	½ cup	140	3	6	10	18	0	100
Light Creamy Vanilla	½ cup	110	2	3	10	18	0	60
Low Fat No Sugar Added Vanilla Dream	½ cup	90	3	2	5	20	3	70
Maple Walnut	½ cup	160	3	9	25	17	0	45
No Sugar Added Chocolate Chip	½ cup	100	3	3	5	21	3	65
Nutty Royale	1 cone (2.5 oz)	220	4	12	15	26	tr	75
Orange Cream	1 bar (2.2 oz)	90	1	2	5	19	0	40
Sandwich Vanilla	1	180	3	6	20	29	tr	120
Sandwich Vanilla Light	1 (2.2 oz)	160	3	3	10	29	tr	125
Sandwich Vanilla Lowfat	1 (2.8 oz)	80	2	2	<5	15	2	70
Spumoni	½ cup	140	2	7	25	17	0	50
Klondike								
Slim-A-Bear 98% Fat Free Sandwich Vanilla	1	130	3	2	5	29	3	95
M&M's								
Cone	1 (2.8 oz)	250	3	12	20	33	1	100
Sandwich	1 (3 oz)	260	3	12	30	34	0	170
Vanilla Fudge	½ cup	180	2	10	15	20	0	55
Natural Choice								
Organic Double Chocolate	½ cup	230	3	14	35	25	0	65
Organic Strawberry	½ cup	210	2	13	35	22	0	65
Organic Vanilla	½ cup	220	2	14	35	22	0	70
No Pudge!								
Giant Cone Cookies & Cream Low Fat	1	140	4	3	<5	29	3	130
Giant Cone Fudgy Brownie Low Fat	1	140	4	3	<5	32	4	115
Giant Cone Vanilla No Sugar Added	1	110	7	4	<5	22	5	55
Giant Sandwich Vanilla & Chocolate No Sugar Added	1	130	8	5	<5	22	6	110

FOOD	PORTION	CALS	PROT	FAT	CHOL	CARB	FIBER	SOD
Giant Strawberry Shortcake 98% Fat Free	1 bar	90	3	1	<5	20	4	85
Rice Dream								
Bar Vanilla Nutty	1 (3.3 oz)	320	5	24	0	27	2	65
Bar Vanilla w/ Chocolate Coating	1 (3 oz)	230	1	15	0	24	tr	70
Carob Almond	½ cup	180	0	10	0	26	2	70
Frozen Pie Chocolate	1 (3.4 oz)	330	3	19	0	40	2	50
Mint Carob Chip	½ cup	170	1	8	0	25	0	85
Strawberry	½ cup	160	0	8	0	25	2	70
Skinny Cow								
Bar Vanilla Strawberry Sorbet Swirl	1	110	4	1	3	22	0	50
Cone Chocolate w/ Fudge	1	150	4	3	4	28	3	95
Cone Vanilla & Caramel	1	150	4	3	4	29	3	85
Fudge Bar	1	100	4	1	3	22	4	45
Sandwich Chocolate Peanut Butter	1	150	4	2	5	30	5	95
Sandwich Strawberry Shortcake	1	140	4	2	3	30	3	120
Sandwich Vanilla	1	140	3	2	1	30	3	90
Sandwich Vanilla No Sugar Added	1	140	3	2	15	30	3	120
Soy Dream								
Butter Pecan	½ cup	140	1	9	0	17	tr	130
Sandwich Lil' Dreamers Chocolate	1 (1.4 oz)	100	1	5	0	15	tr	60
Vanilla	½ cup	140	1	7	0	18	tr	140
Tofutti								
Cuties Vanilla	1 (1.4 oz)	120	2	5	0	17	0	121
Turkey Hill								
Carb IQ Vanilla Bean	½ cup	110	2	8	30	15	5	30
Twix								
Ice Cream	½ cup	160	2	8	20	21	0	60
Ice Cream Bar	1 (1.6 oz)	170	2	10	10	19	0	50
Weight Watchers								
English Toffee Crunch	1 bar	110	1	6	<5	13	2	40
Smart Ones Giant Sundae	1 serv (8 oz)	150	5	1	5	39	7	130
TAKE-OUT								
cone vanilla light soft serve	1 (4.6 oz)	164	4	6	28	24	–	92

FOOD	PORTION	CALS	PROT	FAT	CHOL	CARB	FIBER	SOD
gelato chocolate hazelnut	½ cup (5.3 oz)	370	9	29	92	26	2	49
gelato vanilla	½ cup (3 oz)	211	3	15	151	18	0	78
sundae caramel	1 (5.4 oz)	303	7	9	25	49	–	195
sundae hot fudge	1 (5.4 oz)	284	6	9	21	48	–	182
sundae strawberry	1 (5.4 oz)	269	6	8	21	45	–	92

ICE CREAM CONES AND CUPS

FOOD	PORTION	CALS	PROT	FAT	CHOL	CARB	FIBER	SOD
brown sugar cone	1 (10 g)	40	1	tr	0	8	tr	32
wafer cone	1	17	tr	tr	0	3	tr	6
waffle cone	1 lg	121	2	2	0	23	1	41

ICE CREAM TOPPINGS

FOOD	PORTION	CALS	PROT	FAT	CHOL	CARB	FIBER	SOD
butterscotch	2 tbsp (1.4 oz)	103	1	tr	–	27	–	143
caramel	2 tbsp (1.4 oz)	103	1	tr	–	27	–	143
marshmallow cream	1 jar (7 oz)	615	3	tr	0	157	–	90
marshmallow cream	1 oz	88	1	tr	0	23	–	13
nuts in syrup	2 tbsp	184	2	9	0	24	1	17
pineapple	1 cup (11.5 oz)	861	1	–	0	226	–	214
pineapple	2 tbsp (1.5 oz)	106	tr	0	0	28	–	26
strawberry	1 cup (11.5 oz)	863	1	1	0	225	–	73
strawberry	2 tbsp (1.5 oz)	107	tr	tr	0	28	–	9
Lollipop Tree								
Hot Fudge Sauce	1 tbsp	80	tr	5	15	8	tr	20
Maple Walnut Cream	2 tbsp	190	1	12	30	22	0	35
Sanders								
Butterscotch Caramel	2 tbsp	90	0	4	10	15	0	95
Smucker's								
Butterscotch Caramel	2 tbsp	130	1	1	<5	30	tr	70
Dove Dark Chocolate	2 tbsp	140	tr	5	0	22	1	80
Dove Milk Chocolate	2 tbsp	130	2	4	0	21	1	75
Dulce De Leche Milk Caramel Spread	2 tbsp	110	2	2	10	23	–	45
Hot Fudge	2 tbsp	140	2	4	0	22	tr	70

FOOD	PORTION	CALS	PROT	FAT	CHOL	CARB	FIBER	SOD
Hot Fudge Sugar Free Fat Free	2 tbsp	90	1	0	0	23	1	30
Magic Shell Caramel	2 tbsp	220	2	18	5	14	0	30
Magic Shell Chocolate	2 tbsp	210	1	17	0	16	1	20
Magic Shell Chocolate Fudge	2 tbsp	120	1	14	0	19	1	50
Magic Shell Turtle Delight	2 tbsp	210	1	16	0	17	1	20
Magic Shell Twix	2 tbsp	210	1	15	0	18	1	35

ICED TEA
MIX
A La Source
FOOD	PORTION	CALS	PROT	FAT	CHOL	CARB	FIBER	SOD
Organic as prep	8 oz	90	0	0	0	23	–	0
Organic Green Tea as prep	8 oz	90	0	0	0	23	–	0
Organic Herbal Tea Red Rooibos	8 oz	80	0	0	0	20	–	5

Celestial Seasonings
Blueberry Ice	1 cup	0	0	0	0	0	0	0

Crystal Light
On The Go All Flavors as prep	1 serv	5	0	0	0	0	0	0
Sugar Free All Flavors as prep	1 serv	5	0	0	0	0	0	0

Lipton
FOOD	PORTION	CALS	PROT	FAT	CHOL	CARB	FIBER	SOD
Chailatta Chocolate as prep	8 oz	120	3	2	<5	21	–	180
Chailatta Hazelnut as prep	8 oz	120	3	2	<5	21	–	200
Chailatta Original as prep	8 oz	120	3	2	<5	21	–	180
Chialatta Vanilla as prep	8 oz	120	3	2	<5	21	–	200
Decaffeinated Lemon Unsweetened as prep	1 serv	0	0	0	0	0	0	0
Decaffeinated Lemon as prep	1 serv	70	0	0	0	18	–	0
Diet Lemon as prep	1 serv	5	0	0	0	1	–	5
Diet Peach as prep	1 serv	5	0	0	0	1	–	5
Diet Raspberry as prep	1 serv	5	0	0	0	1	–	0
Green Tea as prep	1 serv	70	0	0	0	18	–	5
Lemon Sweetened as prep	1 serv	70	0	0	0	18	–	0
Sweetened All Fruit Flavors as prep	1 serv	80	0	0	0	19	–	0
To Go w/ Honey & Lemon	1 pkg	0	0	0	0	0	0	0

FOOD	PORTION	CALS	PROT	FAT	CHOL	CARB	FIBER	SOD
To Go w/ Lemon	1 pkg	0	0	0	0	0	0	0
To Go w/ Mandarin & Mango	1 pkg	0	0	0	0	tr	–	0
Unsweetened as prep	1 serv	0	0	0	0	0	0	0
Nestea								
Lemon Liquid Concentrate as prep	8 oz	80	0	0	0	19	–	0
Peach Liquid Concentrate as prep	8 oz	90	0	0	0	21	–	0
Sugar Free w/ Lemon	2 tsp	5	0	0	0	2	–	0
Sweetened w/ Lemon	1⅓ tbsp	60	0	0	0	15	–	0
Unsweetened w/ Lemon	2 tsp	5	0	0	0	1	–	0
READY-TO-DRINK								
Anteadote								
All Flavors	8 oz	0	0	0	0	0	0	40
Arizona								
Green Tea w/ Ginseng & Honey	8 oz	70	0	0	0	18	0	20
Lemon	8 oz	90	0	0	0	25	0	20
Bina								
Lemon	8 oz	70	0	0	0	17	–	25
Peach	8 oz	114	0	0	0	29	–	0
Bolthouse Farms								
Perfectly Protein Vanilla Chai Tea w/ Soy	8 oz	160	10	3	0	25	0	60
Bombilla & Gourd								
Organic Eco Teas All Flavors	8 oz	40	0	0	0	11	–	0
Brazil Gourmet								
Nectar Tea All Flavors	8 oz	90	0	0	0	23	0	10
Nectar Tea Light Mango Passion	8 oz	60	0	0	0	17	0	10
C+Swiss								
Hemp Ice Tea	1 can (8.4 oz)	90	0	0	0	23	–	<10
Cafe Sepia								
Matcha Latte	1 can (8.6 oz)	130	3	3	10	23	1	50
Crystal Light								
Sugar Free Lemon	8 oz	5	0	0	0	0	0	15

FOOD	PORTION	CALS	PROT	FAT	CHOL	CARB	FIBER	SOD
Delta Blues								
Spearmint Tea Punch	8 oz	90	0	0	0	21	0	0
Enviga								
All Flavors	1 can (12 oz)	5	0	0	0	0	0	35
Fuze								
Slender Energy All Flavors	8 oz	20	0	0	0	5	–	4
Glaceau Vitamin Water								
Vital-T	8 oz	50	0	0	0	13	–	0
Hood								
Iced Tea	1 cup	100	0	0	0	25	0	10
Inko's								
White Tea All Flavors	1 bottle (16 oz)	56	0	0	0	14	–	tr
White Tea Honeysuckle	1 bottle	0	0	0	0	0	0	tr
Ito En								
Apricot	8 oz	60	0	0	0	15	0	20
Green Tea Apple	8 oz	70	0	0	0	18	0	20
Mango	8 oz	50	0	0	0	15	0	20
Shencho Shot	1 can (6.4 oz)	0	0	0	0	0	0	20
White Tea Grape	8 oz	60	0	0	0	15	0	15
Joe Tea								
All Flavors	8 oz	100	0	0	0	25	–	10
Kalahari								
Rooibos Red Tea All Flavors	8 oz	50	0	0	0	13	–	0
Kombucha								
Wonder Drink Asian Pear Ginger	1 bottle (8.5 oz)	60	0	0	0	16	–	0
Wonder Drink Rooibus Red Peach	1 bottle (8.5 oz)	60	0	0	0	15	–	10
Lipton								
Diet Green Tea w/ Citrus	8 oz	0	0	0	0	0	0	70
Diet Lemon	8 oz	0	0	0	0	0	0	60
Diet Sweet	8 oz	0	0	0	0	0	0	0
Extra Sweet	8 oz	100	0	0	0	24	–	5
Green Tea w/ Citrus	8 oz	80	0	0	0	21	–	70
Green Tea w/ Honey	8 oz	70	0	0	0	19	–	0
Lemon	8 oz	90	0	0	0	21	–	0
Original Sweetened	8 oz	70	0	0	0	18	–	5
Original Unsweetened	8 oz	0	0	0	0	0	0	0
Peach	8 oz	110	0	0	0	26	–	0

FOOD	PORTION	CALS	PROT	FAT	CHOL	CARB	FIBER	SOD
Raspberry	8 oz	110	0	0	0	26	–	0
Nestea								
Green Tea Peach	1 bottle (20 oz)	220	0	0	0	57	–	75
Green Tea Diet Peach	8 oz	0	0	0	0	0	0	30
Lemon	1 bottle (20 oz)	210	0	0	0	56	–	75
Lemon Diet	8 oz	0	0	0	0	0	–	30
Sweetened	8 oz	60	0	0	0	17	–	25
Sweetened Green Tea	8 oz	80	0	0	0	20	–	0
Sweetened Diet Green Tea	8 oz	0	0	0	0	0	0	0
Old Orchard								
Green Tea w/ Lemon & Honey	8 oz	45	0	0	0	12	0	9
Green Tea w/ Pomegranate	8 oz	45	0	0	0	12	0	9
Pacific Foods								
Organic Lemon	8 oz	70	0	0	0	17	0	10
Organic Peach	8 oz	70	0	0	0	17	0	10
Organic Raspberry	8 oz	70	0	0	0	18	0	10
Organic Sweetened Black Tea	8 oz	60	0	0	0	16	0	10
Organic Unsweetened Green Tea	8 oz	0	0	0	0	0	0	10
Pixie								
Black Tea Mate Lemon Ginger	8 oz	35	0	0	0	8	0	15
Yerba Mate Authentic	8 oz	30	0	0	0	7	0	5
POM								
Light Tea Pomegranate Hibiscus Green	8 oz	35	0	0	0	16	0	0
Light Tea Pomegranate Orange Blossom	8 oz	35	0	0	0	14	0	0
Light Tea Pomegranate Wildberry White	8 oz	35	0	0	0	16	0	5
Snapple								
Diet Lemonade Ice Tea	8 oz	10	0	0	0	2	–	15
Just Plain Tea	8 oz	0	0	0	0	0	0	10
Lemonade Ice Tea	8 oz	110	0	0	0	28	–	10
Lime Green Tea	8 oz	100	0	0	0	25	–	10

FOOD	PORTION	CALS	PROT	FAT	CHOL	CARB	FIBER	SOD
Mint	8 oz	110	0	0	0	27	–	10
Peach	8 oz	100	0	0	0	26	–	10
SoBe								
Lean Diet Green Tea	8 oz	0	0	0	0	1	–	5
Lean Diet Peach Tea	8 oz	5	0	0	0	1	–	15
Solebury Home								
Organic All Flavors	8 oz	33	0	0	0	8	–	0
Sri Lankan								
Apple	8 oz	70	0	0	0	17	0	15
Lemon	8 oz	60	0	0	0	15	0	20
SSips								
Diet Green Tea w/ Honey & Ginseng	1 box (7 oz)	0	0	0	0	0	0	10
Green Tea w/ Honey & Ginseng	1 box (7 oz)	60	0	0	0	15	–	10
Lemon	8 oz	100	0	0	0	24	0	10
Tao Tea								
Grapefruit Green Tea	8 oz	71	0	0	0	18	–	64
Lemon Green Tea	8 oz	67	0	0	0	17	–	44
True Brew								
Green Tea	8 oz	64	0	0	0	16	0	–
Sweet Tea	8 oz	76	0	0	0	19	0	–
VidaTea								
All Flavors	1 can	90	0	0	0	24	–	–
VitaZest								
Green Tea Vitamin Enriched	8 oz	0	0	0	0	0	0	0
Weil For Tea								
Gyokuro	1 can (8.6 oz)	0	0	0	0	0	0	30
Turmeric	1 can (8.6 oz)	0	0	0	0	0	0	15

ICES AND ICE POPS

FOOD	PORTION	CALS	PROT	FAT	CHOL	CARB	FIBER	SOD
Blue Bunny								
Bar Big Fudge	1 (2.7 oz)	110	3	2	5	21	0	75
Chill Cups Double Lemon	1 (4 oz)	100	0	0	0	26	0	20
FrozFruit Creamy Coconut	1 bar (3 oz)	150	1	10	25	14	tr	20
Frozfruit Strawberries & Cream	1 bar (4 oz)	190	tr	5	20	27	tr	25
Pop Banana	1 (1.9 oz)	35	0	0	0	9	0	5
Pop Jolly Rancher	1 (4 oz)	120	0	0	0	24	0	30

FOOD	PORTION	CALS	PROT	FAT	CHOL	CARB	FIBER	SOD
Pop Root Beer	1 (1.9 oz)	40	0	0	0	10	0	10
The Original Bomb	1 (1.8 oz)	50	0	0	0	11	0	5
Breeze Freeze								
100% Fruit Juice	1 (8 oz)	54	0	0	0	13	0	24
Fruit Granita	1 (8 oz)	120	1	0	0	28	tr	15
Edy's								
Sherbet Berry Rainbow	½ cup	130	1	2	5	29	–	35
Sherbet Key Lime	½ cup	130	1	2	0	28	–	35
Sherbet Orange Cream	½ cup	120	2	2	10	23	–	40
Sherbet Raspberry	½ cup	130	1	1	4	28	–	35
Sherbet Swiss Orange	½ cup	150	1	3	5	30	–	40
Sherbet Tropical Rainbow	½ cup	130	1	1	0	29	–	35
Whole Fruit Creamy Coconut	1 bar	120	3	3	0	21	–	40
Whole Fruit Lemonade	1 bar	80	0	0	0	20	–	0
Whole Fruit Lime	1 bar	80	0	0	0	20	–	0
Whole Fruit Orange & Cream	1 bar	80	1	2	5	16	–	30
Whole Fruit Peach	½ cup	90	0	0	0	23	–	0
Whole Fruit Strawberry	1 bar	80	0	0	0	21	–	0
Whole Fruit Tangerine	1 bar	80	0	0	0	20	–	0
Whole Fruit Tropical	1 bar	100	0	0	0	26	–	0
Whole Fruit Wild Berry	1 bar	80	0	0	0	21	–	0
Hawaiian Punch								
Arctic Surfers	1 pop	50	0	0	0	12	0	5
Hendrie's								
Citrus N' Berry Stix	1 (1.9 oz)	15	0	0	0	3	0	5
Fudge Stix Fat Free	1 bar (1.8 oz)	70	1	0	0	14	0	60
Hood								
Hoodsie Pop	1 (3.3 oz)	60	0	0	0	16	0	5
Luigi's								
Italian Ice Cherry	1 (6 oz)	130	0	0	0	32	tr	15
Italian Ice Lemon Strawberry	1 (6 oz)	120	0	0	0	31	tr	10
Italian Ice No Sugar Added Lemon	1 (6 oz)	60	0	0	0	20	0	10
Italian Ice Pina Colada	1 (6 oz)	130	0	0	0	33	0	40
Swirl Blue Ribbon Lemonade	1 (6 oz)	150	0	0	0	39	0	10

FOOD	PORTION	CALS	PROT	FAT	CHOL	CARB	FIBER	SOD
Minute Maid								
Fruit And Cream Swirl	1 tube (3 oz)	90	0	3	10	16	–	25
Fruit Bars	1 bar	60	0	0	0	15	–	15
Mr. J								
All Flavors	1 bar (2.25 oz)	50	tr	tr	–	12	–	5
Natural Choice								
Organic Vegan Fruit Bars Coconut	1 (2.75 oz)	90	0	4	0	16	1	10
Organic Vegan Fruit Bars Pink Lemonade	1 (2.75 oz)	50	0	0	0	13	0	5
Organic Vegan Grape	1 (2.75 oz)	50	0	0	0	13	0	5
Organic Vegan Sorbet Blueberry	½ cup	110	0	0	0	29	tr	10
Organic Vegan Sorbet Lemon	½ cup	110	0	0	0	30	0	15
Organic Vegan Sorbet Mango	½ cup	110	0	0	0	29	1	10
PickleSickle								
Pop	1 (2 oz)	3	0	0	0	1	0	245
The Power Of Fruit								
Original Fruit Bar	1 (1.75 oz)	28	tr	tr	0	7	1	1
Tropicana								
Fruit Juice Bar Orange	1	45	0	0	0	11	0	0
Fruit Juice Bar Raspberry	1	45	0	0	0	11	0	0
Strawberry	1	45	0	0	0	11	0	0
Wawona								
Peach	1 pop	78	1	tr	0	19	1	7
Strawberry	1 pop	77	1	tr	0	18	1	9
JACKFRUIT								
fresh	3.5 oz	70	1	tr	0	4	–	2
JALAPENO (see PEPPERS)								
JAM/JELLY/PRESERVES								
all flavors jam	1 pkg (0.5 oz)	34	tr	0	0	9	tr	–
all flavors jam	1 tbsp (0.7 oz)	48	tr	0	0	13	tr	–

FOOD	PORTION	CALS	PROT	FAT	CHOL	CARB	FIBER	SOD
all flavors jelly	1 pkg (0.5 oz)	38	tr	0	0	10	tr	–
all flavors jelly	1 tbsp (0.7 oz)	52	tr	0	0	14	tr	–
all flavors preserve	1 pkg (0.5 oz)	34	tr	0	0	9	tr	–
all flavors preserve	1 tbsp (0.7 oz)	48	tr	0	0	13	tr	–
apple butter	1 tbsp (0.6 oz)	33	0	0	0	9	–	0
orange marmalade	1 tbsp (0.7 oz)	49	tr	0	0	13	–	11
orange marmalade	1 pkg (0.5 oz)	34	0	0	0	9	–	8
strawberry jam	1 tbsp (0.7 oz)	48	tr	0	0	13	tr	8
Cascadian Farm								
Organic Fruit Spread Blackberry	1 tbsp	45	0	0	0	11	–	0
Organic Fruit Spread Raspberry	1 tbsp	45	0	0	0	11	–	0
Organic Sweet Orange Marmalade	1 tbsp	45	0	0	0	11	–	0
Eden								
Organic Apple Butter	1 tbsp	20	0	0	0	4	1	0
Organic Butter Apple Cherry	1 tbsp	25	0	0	0	6	tr	0
Organic Cherry Butter	1 tbsp	35	0	0	0	9	1	0
El Angel								
Strawberry Marmalade	1 tbsp	25	tr	0	0	6	0	1
Lollipop Tree								
Butter Cranberry Pear	1 tbsp	25	0	0	0	6	–	0
Butter Pumpkin Maple Pecan	1 tbsp	30	0	0	0	7	tr	0
Jam Raspberry Peach	1 tbsp	50	0	0	0	13	–	0
Jam Triple Cherry	1 tbsp	50	0	0	0	13	–	0
Jelly Hot Pepper	1 tbsp	60	0	1	0	16	–	0
Jelly Wasabi Lime Pepper	1 tbsp	60	0	0	0	16	0	0
Matouk's								
Guava Jam	1 tbsp	50	0	0	0	13	–	0
Mango Jam	1 tbsp	50	0	0	0	12	–	0

FOOD	PORTION	CALS	PROT	FAT	CHOL	CARB	FIBER	SOD
Polaner								
All Fruit Apricot	1 tbsp	40	0	0	0	10	–	0
All Fruit Grape	1 tbsp	40	0	0	0	10	–	0
All Fruit Pineapple	1 tbsp	40	0	0	0	10	–	0
All Fruit Raspberry Seedless	1 tbsp	40	0	0	0	10	–	0
Robert Rothchild Farm								
Preserves Cherry Acai	1 tbsp	35	0	0	0	9	0	0
Smucker's								
Cider Apple Butter	1 tbsp	45	0	0	0	11	–	10
Jam Concord Grape	1 tbsp	50	0	0	0	13	–	0
Jam Red Plum	1 tbsp	50	0	0	0	13	–	5
Jam Seedless Red Raspberry	1 tbsp	50	0	0	0	13	–	0
Jam Seedless Strawberry	1 tbsp	50	0	0	0	13	–	0
Jelly Apple	2 tbsp	50	0	0	0	13	–	0
Jelly Concord Grape	1 tbsp	50	0	0	0	13	–	5
Jelly Currant	1 tbsp	50	0	0	0	13	–	5
Jelly Elderberry	1 tbsp	50	0	0	0	13	–	0
Jelly Guava	1 tbsp	50	0	0	0	13	–	0
Jelly Mixed Fruit	2 tbsp	50	0	0	0	13	–	0
Low Sugar All Flavors	1 tbsp	25	0	0	0	6	–	0
Preserves All Flavors	1 tbsp	50	0	0	0	13	–	0
Simply Fruit All Flavors	1 tbsp	40	0	0	0	10	–	0
Sugar Free All Flavors	1 tbsp	10	0	0	0	5	–	0

JAPANESE FOOD (see ASIAN FOOD, SUSHI)

JELLY (see JAM/JELLY/PRESERVES)

JERKY (see MEAT STICKS)

JICAMA

FOOD	PORTION	CALS	PROT	FAT	CHOL	CARB	FIBER	SOD
fresh	1 sm (12.8 oz)	139	3	tr	0	32	18	15
raw sliced	1 cup	46	1	tr	0	11	6	5
Frieda's								
Jicama	¾ cup	35	1	0	0	7	1	5

JUJUBE

FOOD	PORTION	CALS	PROT	FAT	CHOL	CARB	FIBER	SOD
dried	1 oz	82	1	tr	0	21	–	3

JUTE

FOOD	PORTION	CALS	PROT	FAT	CHOL	CARB	FIBER	SOD
cooked	1 cup	32	3	tr	0	6	2	10

FOOD	PORTION	CALS	PROT	FAT	CHOL	CARB	FIBER	SOD
KALE								
chopped cooked w/o salt	1 cup	36	2	1	0	7	3	30
fresh cooked w/ fat	1 cup	69	2	4	0	7	2	339
scotch chopped cooked w/o salt	1 cup	36	2	1	0	7	2	58
Glory								
Fresh Greens	1 serv (2.8 oz)	40	3	1	0	8	2	35
Seasoned canned	½ cup	35	2	1	0	5	1	490
KANGAROO								
kangaroo	3 oz	120	24	2	56	–	–	–
KEFIR								
kefir	8 oz	98	8	2	10	12	0	257
Lifeway								
Greek Style	8 oz	202	7	14	55	12	0	120
Nonfat All Fruit Flavors	8 oz	188	14	0	5	33	3	125
Nonfat Plain	8 oz	116	14	0	5	15	3	120
Organic Helios All Fruit Flavors	8 oz	160	8	4	15	26	2	85
Organic Helios Plain	8 oz	120	8	4	15	12	2	85
Organic Lowfat All Fruit Flavors	8 oz	160	14	2	10	25	3	125
Organic Lowfat Plain	8 oz	110	14	2	10	12	3	125
Original	8 oz	162	8	8	30	15	3	125
Probugs All Flavors	1 bottle	130	9	5	19	15	2	78
Slim6 All Flavors	8 oz	110	14	2	10	8	2	125
KETCHUP								
banana	1 tsp	10	0	0	0	2	0	75
ketchup	1 pkg (0.2 oz)	6	tr	tr	0	2	tr	71
ketchup	1 tbsp	15	tr	tr	0	4	0	167
low sodium	1 tbsp	15	tr	tr	0	4	0	3
Del Monte								
Ketchup	1 tbsp	15	0	0	0	4	0	190
Estee								
No Sugar Added	1 tbsp	15	0	0	0	5	0	190
Heinz								
Ketchup	1 tbsp	15	0	0	0	4	0	190
Organic	1 tbsp	20	0	0	0	5	0	190

FOOD	PORTION	CALS	PROT	FAT	CHOL	CARB	FIBER	SOD
Hunt's								
Ketchup	1 tbsp	15	0	0	0	4	0	180
No Salt Added	1 tbsp	20	0	0	0	4	0	0
Squeeze	1 tbsp	15	0	0	0	4	0	180
Muir Glen								
Organic	1 tbsp	20	0	0	0	4	0	230
Wholemato								
Organic Agave	1 tbsp	15	0	0	0	3	0	230
KIDNEY								
beef simmered	3 oz	134	23	4	609	0	0	80
lamb braised	3 oz	116	20	3	480	1	0	128
pork braised	3 oz	128	22	4	408	0	0	68
veal braised	3 oz	139	22	5	672	0	0	94
KIDNEY BEANS								
canned	½ cup	108	7	1	0	19	6	379
dried cooked w/o salt	½ cup	112	8	tr	0	20	6	1
Bush's								
Light Red	½ cup	110	7	0	0	20	7	260
Eden								
Chili Beans	½ cup	130	9	0	0	21	7	250
Organic	½ cup	100	8	0	0	18	10	15
Organic Cannellini	½ cup	100	6	1	0	17	5	40
Organic Refried	½ cup	80	7	1	–	15	6	180
Goya								
Dark	½ cup	90	7	1	0	18	7	380
Progresso								
Red	½ cup	110	8	0	0	20	6	340
Rienzi								
Cannellini	½ cup	80	6	0	0	18	7	390
Red	½ cup	90	5	1	0	18	7	380
KIWI								
fresh	1 med (2.6 oz)	46	1	tr	0	11	2	2
fresh	1 lg (3.2 oz)	56	1	tr	0	13	3	3
Zespri								
Gold	2 med	80	2	1	0	20	2	0
Green	2 med	100	2	2	0	24	4	0

FOOD	PORTION	CALS	PROT	FAT	CHOL	CARB	FIBER	SOD
KIWI JUICE								
Auna								
Kiwifruit Juice	1 bottle (12 oz)	120	0	0	0	33	4	25
KNISH								
TAKE-OUT								
cheese	1 (2.1 oz)	205	6	12	56	19	1	268
meat	1 (1.8 oz)	174	7	11	53	13	1	202
potato	1 lg (7 oz)	332	8	12	72	49	1	470
potato	1 (2.1 oz)	212	5	12	59	21	1	210
KOHLRABI								
raw sliced	1 cup	36	2	tr	0	8	4	27
sliced cooked w/o salt	1 cup	48	3	tr	0	11	2	35
Frieda's								
Kohlrabi	⅔ cup	25	1	0	0	5	3	15
TAKE-OUT								
creamed	1 cup	150	5	9	6	14	1	555
KRILL								
fresh	1 oz	22	3	1	–	tr	0	119
KUMQUATS								
canned in syrup	1	13	tr	tr	0	3	1	1
fresh	1	13	tr	tr	0	3	1	2
KUZU								
Eden								
Root Starch	1 tbsp	30	0	0	0	8	–	0
LAMB								
cubed lean & fat braised	4 oz	253	38	10	122	0	0	79
cubed lean broiled	4 oz	211	32	8	102	0	0	86
ground broiled	4 oz	321	28	22	110	0	0	92
leg roasted	4 oz	213	19	15	74	0	0	182
loin chop lean & fat broiled	1 chop (4 oz)	222	17	16	72	0	0	278
rib chop lean & fat broiled	1 chop (1.6 oz)	165	10	14	46	0	0	109
rib roast baked	4 oz	386	25	31	109	0	0	84
shank lean & fat braised	4 oz	360	42	20	157	0	0	107

FOOD	PORTION	CALS	PROT	FAT	CHOL	CARB	FIBER	SOD
shoulder chop lean & fat cooked	1 chop (5.5 oz)	274	22	20	91	0	0	388
shoulder w/ bone braised	4 oz	231	19	17	77	0	0	192

LAMB DISHES
TAKE-OUT

moroccan pilaf w/ bulgur	1 serv	327	–	13	54	–	–	303
moussaka	4 in sq (16 oz)	659	35	43	96	32	8	737
stew w/ potatoes & vegetables	1 cup	260	22	6	58	29	4	728

LAMBSQUARTERS

chopped cooked w/ salt	1 cup	58	6	1	0	9	4	477

LEEKS

chopped cooked w/o salt	¼ cup	8	tr	tr	0	2	tr	3
cooked	1 (4.4 oz)	38	1	tr	0	9	1	12
freeze dried	1 tbsp	1	tr	0	0	tr	0	0
Frieda's								
Fresh	1 cup	50	1	0	0	12	2	15

LEMON

fresh	1 med (4 oz)	22	1	tr	0	12	5	3
peel	1 tsp	1	tr	0	0	tr	tr	0
peel	1 tbsp	3	tr	tr	0	1	1	0
wedge	1 (7 g)	2	tr	tr	0	1	tr	0
Sunkist								
Fresh	1 (2 oz)	15	0	0	0	5	tr	0
True Lemon								
Crystallized Lemon	1 pkg (1 g)	0	0	0	0	tr	–	0

LEMON CURD

lemon curd made w/ egg	2 tsp	29	tr	1	–	4	0	–
Lollipop Tree								
Lemon Curd	1 tbsp	50	1	2	20	8	–	10
Robert Rothchild Farm								
Lemon Curd & Tart Filling	1 tbsp	50	0	2	10	8	0	5

LEMON EXTRACT

lemon extract	½ tsp	12	0	tr	0	0	0	0

LEMON GRASS

fresh	1 tbsp	5	tr	tr	0	1	–	0

FOOD	PORTION	CALS	PROT	FAT	CHOL	CARB	FIBER	SOD
LEMON JUICE								
bottled	1 oz	6	1	tr	0	2	tr	6
bottled	1 tbsp	3	tr	tr	0	1	tr	3
fresh	1 oz	8	tr	0	0	3	tr	0
from 1 lemon	1.6 oz	12	tr	0	0	4	tr	0
from wedge	6 g	1	tr	0	0	1	0	0
Essn								
Sparkling Meyer Lemon Juice	1 can (8.4 oz)	170	1	0	0	41	–	20
Izze								
Sparkling Lemon	8 oz	150	1	0	0	36	–	15
LEMONADE								
MIX								
A La Source								
Organic as prep	8 oz	110	0	0	0	28	–	0
Country Time								
Lemonade as prep	8 oz	60	0	0	0	16	–	25
Pink as prep	8 oz	60	0	0	0	16	–	25
Raspberry as prep	8 oz	80	0	0	0	19	–	0
Strawberry as prep	8 oz	80	0	0	0	20	–	0
Crystal Light								
Lemonade as prep	1 serv	5	0	0	0	0	0	35
On The Go as prep	1 pkg	5	0	0	0	0	0	35
Pink as prep	1 serv	5	0	0	0	0	0	0
READY-TO-DRINK								
Adina								
Hibiscus Lemon Bissap	8 oz	80	0	0	0	28	–	15
Apple & Eve								
Organic	8 oz	130	0	0	0	32	–	5
Crystal Light								
Sugar Free	8 oz	5	0	0	0	0	0	10
Honest Ade								
Cranberry	8 oz	50	0	0	0	13	–	5
Hood								
Lemonade	1 cup	110	0	0	0	28	0	5
Minute Maid								
Chilled	8 oz	100	0	0	0	28	–	80
Lemonade	1 can (12 oz)	150	0	0	0	42	–	50
Light	8 oz	15	0	0	0	4	–	15

FOOD	PORTION	CALS	PROT	FAT	CHOL	CARB	FIBER	SOD
Naked Juice								
Just Made	8 oz	110	1	0	0	28	0	15
Nesbitt's								
Honey	1 bottle (12 oz)	180	0	0	0	44	–	120
Newman's Own								
Pink Virgin	8 oz	110	0	0	0	27	–	40
Roadside Virgin	8 oz	110	0	0	0	27	–	40
Virgin Lemon Aided	8 oz	110	0	0	0	27	–	40
Odwalla								
PomaGrand	8 oz	110	0	0	0	28	0	10
Pure Squeezed	8 oz	120	0	0	0	30	0	10
Santa Cruz								
Organic	1 can	160	0	0	0	40	–	15
Organic Raspberry	1 can	120	0	0	0	29	–	0
Simply								
Lemonade	8 oz	120	0	0	0	30	–	15
Snapple								
Lemonade	8 oz	110	0	0	0	28	–	50
Super Sour	8 oz	130	0	0	0	33	–	50
SSips								
Lemonade	8 oz	110	0	0	0	27	0	5
Sweet Leaf								
Lemonade Stand All Flavors	8 oz	95	tr	0	0	25	–	0
Tropicana								
Light	1 cup	10	0	0	0	2	0	5
Orchard Style	8 oz	120	0	0	0	31	0	20
Twister Strawberry	8 oz	140	tr	0	0	35	0	20
Uncle Matt's								
Organic	8 oz	120	tr	0	0	30	0	10
LENTILS								
dried cooked	1 cup	230	18	1	0	40	16	4
Eden								
Organic Green w/ Onion & Bay Leaf	½ cup	90	8	0	0	13	4	210
Sabra								
Dardara	2 oz	40	1	2	0	5	1	200
TastyBite								
Jodhpur Lentils	½ pkg (5 oz)	106	6	4	0	12	7	664

FOOD	PORTION	CALS	PROT	FAT	CHOL	CARB	FIBER	SOD
Madras Lentils	½ pkg (5 oz)	127	6	5	3	14	5	455
TAKE-OUT								
lentil loaf	1 slice (1.6 oz)	83	4	4	0	10	3	40
middle eastern lentil salad	1 serv (4.5 oz)	158	–	3	0	–	–	382
yemiser selatta ethiopian lentil salad	1 serv (3 oz)	115	4	7	0	11	2	536
LETTUCE (see also SALAD)								
arugula	6 leaves (0.4 oz)	3	tr	tr	0	tr	tr	3
arugula shredded	1 cup	5	1	tr	0	1	tr	5
boston	1 head (5.7 oz)	21	2	tr	0	4	2	8
boston chopped	6 leaves	7	1	tr	0	1	1	3
cornsalad field salad	1 cup (1.9 oz)	7	1	tr	0	1	1	2
iceberg	1 lg head (26.5 oz)	106	7	1	0	22	9	76
iceberg	6 med leaves	7	tr	tr	0	1	1	5
iceberg shredded	1 cup	10	1	tr	0	2	1	7
looseleaf outer leaves	6 (5 oz)	22	2	tr	0	4	2	40
looseleaf shredded	1 cup	5	tr	tr	0	1	1	10
red leaf	6 leaves (3.6 oz)	16	1	tr	0	2	1	26
red leaf shredded	1 cup	4	tr	tr	0	1	tr	7
romaine	3 leaves (3 oz)	14	1	tr	0	3	2	7
romaine heart	6 leaves (1.3 oz)	6	tr	tr	0	1	1	3
romaine shredded	1 cup	8	1	tr	0	2	1	4
Andy Boy								
Romaine Hearts	6 leaves (3 oz)	20	1	1	0	3	1	0
Dole								
Classic Romaine	1½ cups (3 oz)	15	1	0	0	4	1	10
Shredded	1½ cups (3 oz)	15	1	0	0	3	1	10

FOOD	PORTION	CALS	PROT	FAT	CHOL	CARB	FIBER	SOD
Earthbound Farm								
Organic Baby Romaine Salad	2 cups	15	1	0	0	2	1	50
Frieda's								
Limestone	⅔ cup	10	1	0	0	2	1	10
Green Giant								
Hearts Of Romaine	6 leaves (3 oz)	14	1	0	0	3	2	5
Mann's								
Romaine Hearts	6 leaves (3 oz)	15	1	1	0	3	1	5
Ocean Mist								
Butter Leaf Shredded	1 cup (2 oz)	7	1	0	0	1	1	3
Green Or Green Leaf Shredded	1 cup (1.3 oz)	5	0	0	0	1	0	10
Iceberg	⅙ head (3 oz)	15	1	0	0	3	1	10
Romaine Hearts	6 leaves	20	1	1	0	3	1	0
River Ranch								
Romaine Chopped	1½ cups	10	1	0	0	3	1	5
Romaine Hearts	1½ cups	10	1	0	0	2	1	5
LILY ROOT								
dried	1 oz	89	2	1	–	21	tr	25
fresh	1 oz	32	1	tr	–	8	tr	3
LIMA BEANS								
CANNED								
lima beans	½ cup	95	6	tr	0	18	6	405
Allens								
Medium Green	½ cup	140	9	1	0	26	7	270
Del Monte								
Green	½ cup	80	4	0	0	15	4	390
Hanover								
Butter Beans In Sauce	½ cup	100	7	0	0	18	5	390
DRIED								
cooked	½ cup	150	6	tr	0	20	5	14
FROZEN								
C&W								
Baby	½ cup	110	6	0	0	20	5	240

FOOD	PORTION	CALS	PROT	FAT	CHOL	CARB	FIBER	SOD
Green Giant								
Baby & Butter Sauce as prep	⅔ cup	100	5	2	<5	18	5	420
LIME								
fresh	1 (2.4 oz)	20	tr	tr	0	7	1	1
wedge	1 (8 g)	2	tr	tr	0	1	tr	0
Sunkist								
Fresh	1 (2 oz)	20	0	0	0	7	2	1
LIME JUICE								
bottled	1 oz	6	tr	tr	0	2	tr	5
fresh	1 oz	8	tr	tr	0	3	tr	1
from 1 lime	1.1 oz	11	tr	tr	0	4	tr	1
Adina								
Lime Mint Mojita	8 oz	70	0	0	0	19	–	0
Honest Ade								
Limeade	8 oz	50	0	0	0	13	–	5
Minute Maid								
Light Limeade	8 oz	15	0	0	0	4	–	15
Newman's Own								
Virgin Limeade	8 oz	140	0	0	0	34	–	35
Sabor Latino								
Limeade	8 oz	160	0	0	0	39	–	5
Simply								
Limeade	8 oz	120	0	0	0	31	–	15
LING								
blue raw	3.5 oz	83	17	1	–	0	0	–
fresh baked	3 oz	95	21	1	–	0	0	147
fresh fillet baked	5.3 oz	168	37	1	–	0	0	261
LINGCOD								
baked	3 oz	93	19	1	57	0	0	64
fillet baked	5.3 oz	164	34	2	101	0	0	114
LIQUOR/LIQUEUR (see also BEER AND ALE, CHAMPAGNE, MALT, WINE)								
7&7	1 serv	178	0	0	0	19	0	21
alabama slammer	1 serv	103	tr	tr	0	7	tr	tr
amaretto sour	1 serv	295	2	tr	0	57	4	98
angel's kiss	1 serv	85	tr	1	5	5	0	4
anisette	1 oz	111	–	0	0	11	0	–

FOOD	PORTION	CALS	PROT	FAT	CHOL	CARB	FIBER	SOD
antifreeze	1 serv	177	1	tr	0	31	tr	2
apricot brandy	1 oz	96	–	0	0	9	0	–
apricot sour	1 serv	164	tr	tr	0	8	tr	5
aquavit	1 oz	65	0	0	–	0	0	–
b 52	1 serv	247	1	4	0	25	0	24
b&b	1 serv	75	0	0	0	0	0	tr
bahama breeze	1 serv	70	tr	tr	0	9	tr	2
bahama mama	1 serv	153	1	tr	0	23	tr	2
bailey's & amaretto	1 serv	184	1	5	0	16	0	29
banana colada	1 serv	376	2	1	0	64	3	4
bay breeze	1 serv	173	1	tr	0	18	tr	2
bend me over	1 serv	242	1	tr	0	32	tr	33
benedictine	1 oz	104	–	0	0	11	0	–
betsy ross	1 serv	206	tr	0	0	5	0	3
black devil	1 serv	220	tr	tr	0	1	tr	43
black russian	1 serv	184	0	tr	0	12	0	3
bloody mary	1 serv	150	1	tr	0	5	1	332
blue whale	1 serv	222	tr	tr	0	23	0	63
bourbon & soda	1 serv (4 oz)	105	0	0	0	0	0	16
bourbon sour	1 serv	166	tr	tr	0	8	tr	5
brandy alexander	1 serv	266	1	6	20	12	0	17
brandy sour	1 serv	164	tr	tr	0	8	tr	5
bushwacker	1 serv	286	tr	5	0	27	tr	23
coffee liqueur	1 serv (1.5 oz)	175	tr	tr	0	24	0	4
cognac	1 oz	67	0	0	0	tr	0	–
cosmopolitan martini	1 serv	126	tr	tr	0	7	tr	1
creme de menthe	1 serv (1.5 oz)	186	0	tr	0	21	0	3
curacao liqueur	1 oz	81	–	0	0	9	0	–
daiquiri	1 serv (2 oz)	112	tr	tr	0	4	tr	3
daiquiri banana	1 serv	277	1	tr	0	32	1	7
dark & stormy	1 serv	64	0	0	0	0	0	tr
doctor pepper	1 serv	95	0	0	0	12	0	1
frozen daiquiri	1 serv	393	–	2	–	–	–	–
frozen daiquiri pineapple	1 serv	186	1	tr	0	28	2	3
frozen tequila screwdriver	1 serv	159	1	tr	0	17	1	2
fuzzy navel	1 serv	247	1	tr	0	10	tr	2
gimlet vodka	1 serv	150	tr	tr	0	6	1	3

FOOD	PORTION	CALS	PROT	FAT	CHOL	CARB	FIBER	SOD
gin	1 serv (1.5 oz)	110	0	0	0	0	0	1
gin & tonic	1 serv (7.5 oz)	171	0	.0	0	16	–	10
gin ricky	1 serv	114	tr	tr	0	1	tr	38
grasshopper	1 serv	275	1	5	15	26	0	13
happy hawaiian	1 serv	434	2	8	0	60	tr	50
harvey wallbanger	1 serv	198	1	tr	0	16	tr	2
head banger	1 serv	165	0	0	0	4	0	tr
hot buttered rum	1 serv	219	tr	4	10	15	4	48
hot toddy	1 serv	188	tr	1	0	13	5	9
hurricane	1 serv	205	tr	tr	0	19	tr	2
kamikaze	1 serv	136	0	0	0	2	0	2
long island iced tea	1 serv	292	tr	tr	0	7	0	33
lynchburg lemonade	1 serv	465	tr	tr	0	85	1	38
mai tai	1 serv	165	tr	tr	0	17	tr	51
manhattan	1 serv	171	tr	tr	0	3	tr	9
margarita	1 serv	173	0	0	0	11	0	3
margarita strawberry	1 serv	106	tr	tr	0	11	1	1
martini	1 serv (3 oz)	206	tr	0	0	2	0	3
martini apple	1 serv	147	tr	tr	0	4	tr	2
martini rum	1 serv	131	tr	0	0	tr	tr	1
mellow yellow	1 serv	95	0	0	0	4	0	0
mexican grasshopper	1 serv	638	1	19	66	52	0	29
mint julep	1 serv	136	tr	tr	0	17	tr	3
mississippi mud	1 serv	496	3	12	45	46	0	46
mudslide	1 serv	566	2	10	0	46	0	65
narragansett	1 serv	168	0	0	0	2	0	5
nutcracker	1 serv	730	2	10	0	64	0	65
old fashioned	1 serv	223	tr	tr	0	4	tr	5
orange crush	1 serv	461	0	tr	0	65	tr	5
pain killer	1 serv	277	1	tr	0	20	tr	5
peppermint pattie	1 serv	344	tr	tr	0	37	0	7
pina colada	1 serv (4.5 oz)	245	1	3	0	32	tr	8
planter's cocktail	1 serv	105	tr	0	0	3	tr	1
planter's punch	1 serv	233	2	tr	0	34	4	33
presbyterian	1 serv	170	tr	0	0	8	tr	26
purple passion	1 serv	215	tr	tr	0	22	0	14

FOOD	PORTION	CALS	PROT	FAT	CHOL	CARB	FIBER	SOD
rob roy	1 serv	171	tr	0	0	3	tr	13
rum	1 serv (1.5 oz)	97	0	0	0	0	0	0
rum boogie	1 serv	134	tr	tr	0	12	tr	3
rum cola	1 serv	209	tr	tr	0	21	tr	8
rum highball	1 serv	170	0	0	0	11	0	9
rum punch	1 serv	448	1	1	0	88	1	12
rusty nail	1 serv	159	0	0	0	6	0	tr
sake	1 serv (1 oz)	39	tr	0	0	1	0	1
salty dog	1 serv	210	1	tr	0	19	tr	3
scotch & soda	1 serv	104	tr	0	0	tr	tr	38
screwdriver rum	1 serv	166	1	tr	0	16	tr	2
sea breeze	1 serv	207	tr	tr	0	19	tr	3
sex on the beach	1 serv	190	tr	tr	0	18	tr	2
singapore sling	1 serv (4 oz)	115	–	–	–	–	–	–
slippery nipple	1 serv	142	tr	2	0	11	0	16
sloe gin fizz	1 serv (2.5 oz)	132	0	0	0	4	0	1
snake bite	1 serv	362	0	0	0	22	0	7
sour rum	1 serv	156	tr	tr	0	8	tr	5
swizzle rum	1 serv	187	0	0	0	15	0	44
tequila gimlet	1 serv	150	tr	tr	0	6	1	3
tequila sour	1 serv	156	tr	tr	0	8	tr	5
tequila stinger	1 serv	221	0	tr	0	14	0	2
tequila sunrise	1 serv (6.8 oz)	232	1	tr	0	24	0	120
tom collins	1 serv (7.5 oz)	121	tr	0	0	3	–	39
vermouth cassis	1 serv	97	tr	tr	0	5	tr	54
vodka	1 serv (1.5 oz)	97	0	0	0	0	0	0
vodka sour	1 serv	138	tr	tr	0	3	tr	1
vodka stinger	1 serv	378	0	tr	0	28	0	4
whiskey	1 serv (1.5 oz)	105	0	0	0	tr	0	0
whiskey sour	1 serv (3.5 oz)	162	tr	tr	0	14	0	65
white russian	1 serv	290	tr	8	31	17	0	12
zombie	1 serv	235	tr	tr	0	10	tr	5

FOOD	PORTION	CALS	PROT	FAT	CHOL	CARB	FIBER	SOD
LIVER (see also PATÉ)								
beef braised	1 slice (2.4 oz)	130	20	4	269	3	0	54
beef pan-fried	1 slice (2.8 oz)	142	21	4	309	4	0	62
chicken fried	3 oz	146	22	5	479	1	0	78
chicken simmered	3 oz	142	21	6	479	1	0	65
lamb braised	3 oz	187	26	7	426	2	0	48
lamb fried	3 oz	202	22	11	419	3	0	105
moose braised	3 oz	132	21	4	331	3	–	60
pork braised	3 oz	140	22	4	302	3	0	42
turkey simmered	1 liver (2.9 oz)	227	17	17	322	1	0	46
veal braised	1 slice (2.8 oz)	154	23	5	409	3	0	62
veal pan fried	1 slice (2.4 oz)	129	18	4	325	3	0	57
Organic Prairie								
Beef	2 oz	80	11	2	155	2	0	40
TAKE-OUT								
calves liver w/ onions	1 serv (5 oz)	177	24	4	335	10	1	390
LLAMA								
llama	3 oz	120	22	3	60	–	–	–
LOBSTER								
northern cooked	1 cup	142	30	1	104	2	–	551
northern cooked	3 oz	83	17	1	61	1	–	323
northern raw	1 lobster (5.3 oz)	136	28	1	143	1	–	–
northern raw	3 oz	77	77	1	81	tr	–	–
spiny steamed	1 (5.7 oz)	233	43	3	146	5	–	370
spiny steamed	3 oz	122	22	2	76	3	–	193
Phillips Seafood								
Lobster Cake	1 (3 oz)	230	16	15	75	7	–	310
TAKE-OUT								
newburg	1 cup	485	46	27	455	13	–	127
LOGANBERRIES								
frzn	1 cup	80	2	tr	0	19	–	1

FOOD	PORTION	CALS	PROT	FAT	CHOL	CARB	FIBER	SOD
LONGANS								
fresh	1	2	tr	0	0	tr	–	0
LOQUATS								
fresh	1	5	tr	tr	0	1	–	0
LOTUS								
root raw sliced	10 slices	45	2	tr	0	14	–	33
root sliced cooked	10 slices	59	1	tr	0	14	–	40
seeds dried	1 oz	94	4	1	0	18	–	1
Eden								
Dried Sliced	5 slices (0.3 oz)	35	1	0	0	8	2	25
Frieda's								
Lotus Root Fresh	1 cup	50	2	0	0	15	4	35
LOX (see SALMON)								
LUPINES								
dried cooked	1 cup	197	26	5	0	16	–	7
LYCHEES								
fresh	1	6	tr	tr	0	2	–	0
Frieda's								
Fresh	6 to 8 (3.5 oz)	60	1	0	0	14	1	0
MACA ROOT								
Navitas Naturals								
Raw Powder	1 tsp (5 g)	20	1	0	0	4	1	0
MACADAMIA NUTS								
dry roasted w/ salt	11 nuts (1 oz)	200	2	22	0	4	1	80
oil roasted	1 oz	204	2	22	0	4	–	3
Hawaiian Host								
White Choco	3 pieces (1.4 oz)	230	1	15	0	22	0	40
Mauna Loa								
Maui Onion & Garlic	1 pkg (1.2 oz)	230	2	23	0	5	3	190
Milk Chocolate Coated	3 pieces	230	3	16	5	18	1	30

FOOD	PORTION	CALS	PROT	FAT	CHOL	CARB	FIBER	SOD
MACE								
ground	1 tsp	8	tr	1	0	1	tr	1
MACKEREL								
CANNED								
jack	1 can (12.7 oz)	563	84	23	285	0	0	1368
jack	1 cup	296	44	12	150	0	0	720
Brunswick								
Jack In Water	2 oz	100	13	5	50	5	0	80
Chicken Of The Sea								
Jack In Tomato Sauce	¼ cup	70	10	3	45	2	0	250
Jack In Water	⅓ cup	90	13	4	55	0	0	280
Orleans								
Jack	¼ cup	90	13	4	55	0	0	280
DRIED								
Eden								
Bonito Flakes	2 tbsp	5	1	0	1	0	0	4
FRESH								
atlantic cooked	3 oz	223	20	15	64	0	0	71
atlantic raw	3 oz	174	16	12	60	0	0	76
jack baked	3 oz	171	22	9	51	0	0	94
jack fillet baked	6.2 oz	354	45	18	106	0	0	194
king baked	3 oz	114	22	2	58	0	0	172
king fillet baked	5.4 oz	207	40	4	105	0	0	312
pacific baked	3 oz	171	22	9	51	0	0	94
pacific fillet baked	6.2 oz	354	45	18	106	0	0	194
spanish cooked	1 fillet (5.1 oz)	230	34	9	107	0	0	96
spanish cooked	3 oz	134	20	5	62	0	0	56
spanish raw	3 oz	118	16	5	65	0	0	50
SMOKED								
atlantic	3.5 oz	296	19	24	93	0	0	384
MAHI MAHI								
fresh baked	4 oz	192	18	13	49	1	0	464
Phillips Seafood								
Coconut Mahi Mahi w/ Sauce	3 pieces	290	14	13	65	31	–	580
MALANGA								
dasheen mashed	1 cup	226	3	tr	0	53	8	743

FOOD	PORTION	CALS	PROT	FAT	CHOL	CARB	FIBER	SOD
dasheen pieces boiled	1 cup	212	3	tr	0	50	8	694
pieces fried	1 cup	304	1	11	0	52	8	442
root raw	1 (10.7 oz)	299	5	1	0	72	5	64
Frieda's								
Malanga	⅔ cup	90	1	0	0	23	2	10

MALT

FOOD	PORTION	CALS	PROT	FAT	CHOL	CARB	FIBER	SOD
malt liquor	1 bottle (12 oz)	148	1	0	0	13	tr	14
nonalcoholic	1 bottle (12 oz)	133	1	tr	0	29	0	47

MALTED MILK

FOOD	PORTION	CALS	PROT	FAT	CHOL	CARB	FIBER	SOD
chocolate as prep w/ milk	1 cup	179	8	5	16	27	1	136
chocolate flavor powder	3 heaping tsp (0.7 oz)	79	1	1	0	18	1	53
natural flavor as prep w/ milk	1 cup	186	9	6	21	24	tr	181
natural flavor powder	3 heaping tsp (0.7 oz)	87	2	2	7	16	tr	104

MAMMY-APPLE

FOOD	PORTION	CALS	PROT	FAT	CHOL	CARB	FIBER	SOD
fresh	1	431	4	4	0	106	–	127

MANGO

FOOD	PORTION	CALS	PROT	FAT	CHOL	CARB	FIBER	SOD
fresh	1	135	1	1	0	35	–	4
C&W								
Chunks	¾ cup	90	tr	0	0	24	3	0
Peeled Snacks								
Fruit Picks Go-Mango-Man-Go	1 pkg (1.4 oz)	120	2	0	0	28	2	0
Sunsweet								
Philippine dried	6 pieces (1.5 oz)	130	1	0	0	30	2	220
Thailand dried	⅓ cup (1.4 oz)	140	0	0	0	34	1	20

MANGO JUICE

Naked Juice

FOOD	PORTION	CALS	PROT	FAT	CHOL	CARB	FIBER	SOD
Mighty Mango	8 oz	120	1	0	0	30	0	15
Old Orchard								
Nectar Cocktail	8 oz	120	0	0	0	30	–	15

FOOD	PORTION	CALS	PROT	FAT	CHOL	CARB	FIBER	SOD
MANGOSTEEN								
canned in syrup	1 cup	143	1	1	0	35	4	14
MARGARINE								
squeeze	1 tsp	34	tr	4	0	0	0	37
stick corn	1 stick (4 oz)	815	1	91	0	1	–	1070
stick corn	1 tsp	34	0	4	0	0	0	44
tub corn	1 tsp	34	0	4	0	0	0	51
tub diet	1 tsp	17	0	2	0	0	0	46
Benecol								
Spread Light	1 tbsp	50	0	5	0	0	0	110
Spread Regular	1 tbsp	70	0	8	0	0	0	110
Blue Bonnet								
Light Stick	1 tbsp	50	0	5	0	0	0	80
Soft Spread	1 tbsp	60	0	7	0	0	0	125
Soft Spread Light	1 tbsp	40	0	5	0	0	0	90
Stick	1 tbsp	80	0	9	0	0	0	110
Brummel & Brown								
Creamy Fruit Spread Strawberry	1 tbsp	50	0	4	0	3	–	45
Spread w/ Yogurt	1 tbsp	45	0	5	0	0	0	90
Crystal Farms								
60/40 Margarine Butter	1 tbsp	100	0	11	5	0	0	90
Margarine	1 tbsp	100	0	11	0	0	0	95
Fleischmann's								
Soft Spread Light	1 tbsp	40	0	5	0	0	0	90
Soft Spread Original	1 tbsp	70	0	8	0	0	0	75
Soft Spread Unsalted	1 tbsp	70	0	8	0	0	0	0
Soft Spread w/ Olive Oil	1 tbsp	70	0	8	0	0	0	95
I Can't Believe Its Not Butter								
Regular Stick	1 tbsp	90	0	10	0	0	0	95
Soft Fat Free	1 tbsp	5	0	0	0	0	0	90
Soft Light	1 tbsp	50	0	5	0	0	0	85
Soft Regular	1 tbsp	80	0	9	0	0	0	90
Soft w/ Calcium	1 tbsp	50	0	5	0	0	0	90
Spray	5 sprays	0	0	0	0	0	0	15
Squeeze	1 tbsp	60	0	7	0	0	0	85
Stick Light	1 tbsp	50	0	6	0	0	0	85
Parkay								
Light Spread	1 tbsp	50	0	5	0	0	0	130

FOOD	PORTION	CALS	PROT	FAT	CHOL	CARB	FIBER	SOD
Original Spread	1 tbsp	60	0	7	0	0	0	100
Original Stick	1 tbsp	90	0	10	0	0	0	105
Spray	5 sprays	0	0	0	0	0	0	5
Spread + Calcium	1 tbsp	45	0	5	0	0	0	115
Squeeze	1 tbsp	70	0	8	0	0	0	110
Stick Light	1 tbsp	50	0	5	0	0	0	75
Promise								
Buttery Spread	1 tbsp	80	0	8	0	0	0	85
Stick	1 tbsp	90	0	10	0	0	0	65
Smart Balance								
37% Light	1 tbsp	45	0	5	0	0	0	90
67% Light	1 tbsp	80	0	9	0	0	0	90
Omega Plus w/ Flax Oil	1 tbsp	80	0	9	0	0	0	85
Spectrum								
Essential Omega	1 tbsp	80	0	10	0	0	0	55
Spread	1 tbsp	88	0	10	0	0	0	55
MARINADE (*see* SAUCE)								
MARJORAM								
dried	1 tsp	2	tr	tr	0	tr	tr	0
MARLIN								
raw	3 oz	110	20	3	–	0	0	–
MARSHMALLOW								
marshmallow	1 reg (0.3 oz)	23	tr	0	0	6	–	3
marshmallow	1 cup (1.6 oz)	146	1	tr	0	37	–	22
MATZO								
brie	1 piece (0.5 oz)	54	1	3	21	5	tr	47
egg	1 (1 oz)	109	3	1	23	22	1	6
matzo ball	1 med (1.2 oz)	48	2	2	36	6	tr	12
plain	1 (1 oz)	111	3	tr	0	23	1	1
whole wheat	1 (1 oz)	98	4	tr	0	22	3	1
Horowitz Margareten								
Egg	1 (1.2 oz)	130	3	1	15	28	1	10

FOOD	PORTION	CALS	PROT	FAT	CHOL	CARB	FIBER	SOD
Manischewitz								
Dark Chocolate Coated Egg	½ (1.5 oz)	90	4	5	25	31	2	5
Egg	1 (1.2 oz)	120	3	1	15	28	1	5
Egg & Onion	1 (1 oz)	100	3	1	10	23	2	200
Matzo Ball Mix	2 tbsp	50	1	0	0	11	1	700
Thin Unsalted	1 (0.8 oz)	90	2	0	0	20	0	0
Streit's								
Egg	1 (1.1 oz)	120	3	1	20	25	1	5
Egg & Onion	1 (1 oz)	100	3	1	5	23	1	20
MAYONNAISE								
diet	1 tbsp	36	tr	3	4	3	0	78
imitation	1 tbsp	35	tr	3	4	2	0	75
mayonnaise	1 tbsp	99	tr	11	5	1	0	78
Cains								
All Natural	1 tbsp	100	0	11	5	0	0	75
Light	1 tbsp	50	0	5	5	2	0	130
Hellman's								
Light	1 tbsp	45	0	5	5	tr	–	120
Real	1 tbsp	90	0	10	5	0	0	90
Real Canola No Cholesterol	1 tbsp	90	0	10	5	0	0	90
Reduced Fat	1 tbsp	20	0	2	0	2	–	125
Hollywood								
Canola	1 tbsp	100	0	11	5	0	0	100
Safflower	1 tbsp	100	0	11	5	0	0	100
Kraft								
Mayo	1 tbsp	90	0	10	<5	0	0	70
Miracle Whip								
Free	1 tbsp	15	0	0	0	3	–	125
Light	1 tbsp	25	0	2	0	3	0	140
Original	1 tbsp	40	0	3	5	2	0	125
Nasoya								
Fat Free Nayonaise	1 tbsp	10	tr	0	0	2	0	100
Nayonaise	1 tbsp	35	tr	4	0	1	0	115
Smart Balance								
Omega	1 tbsp	120	0	14	0	0	0	0
Omega Plus	1 tbsp	50	0	5	5	2	–	125
MEAT STICKS								
beef jerky	1 piece (0.7 oz)	82	7	5	10	2	tr	443

FOOD	PORTION	CALS	PROT	FAT	CHOL	CARB	FIBER	SOD
pork jerky	1 strip (0.5 oz)	62	5	4	7	2	tr	332
venison jerky	1 strip (0.5 oz)	55	5	3	18	2	0	414
Jack Link's								
Beef Jerky Teriyaki	1 oz	80	14	1	20	5	0	600
Organic Prairie								
Beef Jerky	1 oz	75	9	2	25	5	0	420
Pemmican								
Homestyle Tender All Flavors	1 oz	80	12	2	35	3	1	720
Kippered Beef Original	1 pkg (1 oz)	60	10	1	25	2	0	730
Kippered Beef Peppered	1 pkg (1 oz)	60	10	1	25	2	0	740
Kippered Beef Sweet & Hot	1 pkg (1 oz)	70	10	1	15	6	0	810
Kippered Beef Teriyaki	1 pkg (1 oz)	60	10	1	20	2	0	870
Long Lasting Hot & Spicy	1 oz	60	12	1	10	4	0	340
Long Lasting Original	1 oz	60	12	1	10	5	0	530
Long Lasting Peppered	1 oz	60	12	1	10	4	0	340
Long Lasting Teriyaki	1 oz	70	12	1	10	6	0	310
Premium Cut Beef Jerky	1 oz	80	13	1	35	4	1	610
Premium Cut Turkey Peppered	1 oz	70	10	1	25	5	0	670
Premium Cut Turkey Sweet Smoked	1 oz	70	10	1	25	5	0	700
Shredded Beef Jerky All Flavors	¼ cup	80	12	2	35	3	1	720
Steak Tips All Flavors	1 oz	70	9	2	20	5	0	510
Slim Jim								
Beef Jerky	7 pieces	130	11	8	35	3	0	770
Beef Jerky Hickory Smoked	1 oz	80	12	2	30	4	0	470
Classic Handipack	1 box	210	8	19	50	3	tr	610
Giant Caddy Pepperoni	1 pkg	150	6	13	35	3	0	450
Twin Pack Cheese & Pepperoni	1 pkg	150	9	12	40	2	1	620
Tanka								
Natural Buffalo Cranberry Bar	1 (1 oz)	70	7	2	17	7	1	360
Natural Buffalo Cranberry Bite	1 (0.5 oz)	35	4	1	9	3	0	180

FOOD	PORTION	CALS	PROT	FAT	CHOL	CARB	FIBER	SOD
Tofurky								
Jurky Original	4 pieces (1 oz)	100	12	2	–	9	1	260
Wellshire								
Matt's Select Pepperoni	1 stick (0.9 oz)	90	5	7	20	1	0	420
Tom Tom Snack Hot n' Spicy Turkey	1 stick (0.8 oz)	50	5	3	20	1	0	210

MEAT SUBSTITUTES (*see also* BACON SUBSTITUTES, CANADIAN BACON SUBSTITUTES, CHICKEN SUBSTITUTES, HAMBURGER SUBSTITUTES, SAUSAGE SUBSTITUTES, TURKEY SUBSTITUTES)

FOOD	PORTION	CALS	PROT	FAT	CHOL	CARB	FIBER	SOD
Fantastic								
Sloppy Joe Mix not prep	¼ cup	70	10	1	0	11	3	450
Taco Filling not prep	¼ cup	80	11	1	0	10	4	430
Gardenburger								
BBQ Riblets w/ Sauce	1 serv (5 oz)	240	17	5	0	33	5	580
Helen's Kitchen								
Garden Steak Tofu Steak	1 (3 oz)	150	12	2	0	14	3	190
Lightlife								
Balogna	4 slices (2 oz)	60	15	0	0	0	2	370
Gimme Lean Ground Beef	1 serv (2 oz)	50	8	0	0	4	2	270
Smart BBQ	¼ cup	70	6	0	0	13	1	380
Smart Cutlet Salisbury Steak	1 (4.5 oz)	130	17	1	0	13	6	570
Smart Deli Country Ham	4 slices (2 oz)	90	16	0	0	5	1	400
Smart Deli Pastrami Style	4 slices (2 oz)	60	13	0	0	1	0	400
Smart Deli Pepperoni Style	13 slices (1 oz)	45	8	0	0	3	1	300
Smart Ground Original	⅓ cup (1.9 oz)	80	11	1	0	7	3	280
Smart Ground Taco Burrito	⅓ cup (2 oz)	70	10	0	0	5	4	210
Smart Menu Crumbles	⅓ cup	80	11	1	0	7	3	330
Smart Menu Meatless Meatballs	5	160	19	7	0	6	2	630
Smart Menu Steak Strips	1 serv (3 oz)	80	15	0	0	5	5	580

FOOD	PORTION	CALS	PROT	FAT	CHOL	CARB	FIBER	SOD
Smart Tex Mex	¼ cup	50	6	0	0	6	2	170
Loma Linda								
Dinner Cuts	2 slices (3.2 oz)	90	18	1	0	4	2	500
Swiss Steak	1 piece (3.2 oz)	130	9	6	0	9	3	430
Morningstar Farms								
Meal Starters Steak Strips	12 pieces (3 oz)	140	23	3	0	5	1	720
Quorn								
Grounds	⅔ cup (3 oz)	80	13	3	0	5	4	220
VeggieLand								
Crumbles Beef	½ cup	70	13	0	0	5	–	200
Veg-T-Balls	3 (3 oz)	113	11	3	0	9	5	285
Viana								
Cowgirl Veggie Steaks	1 (3.7 oz)	260	29	14	0	6	4	890
Veggie Cevapcici	4 pieces (2.8 oz)	240	23	14	0	5	3	680
Veggie Gyros	24 strips (3 oz)	220	26	11	0	5	2	1050
Veggie Kebab	½ cup	210	18	14	0	3	2	810
Worthington								
Bolono	3 slices (2 oz)	80	11	3	0	3	2	660
Choplets	2 slices (3.2 oz)	90	18	1	0	4	2	500
Corned Beef Vegetarian	3 slices (2 oz)	140	10	9	0	5	0	460
Dinner Roast	1 slice (3 oz)	180	14	11	0	6	3	580
Multigrain Cutlets	2 slices (3.2 oz)	100	17	1	0	5	3	290
Prime Steaks	1 piece (3.2 oz)	120	9	6	0	7	1	440
Vegetable Skallops	½ cup (3 oz)	90	17	1	0	4	3	390
Wham	2 slices (2 oz)	110	10	7	0	3	0	400

FOOD	PORTION	CALS	PROT	FAT	CHOL	CARB	FIBER	SOD
Yves								
Meatless Beef Skewers	1 (2.8 oz)	100	14	1	0	10	3	400
Meatless Bologna	4 slices	60	14	3	0	2	0	460
Meatless Pepperoni	6 slices	90	14	1	0	4	0	390
Meatless Ground Round Original	1/3 cup	60	10	1	0	5	2	270
MEATBALL SUBSTITUTES								
meatless	2 (1.3 oz)	71	8	3	0	3	2	198
Gardenburger								
Mama Mia Meatballs	6 (3 oz)	110	12	5	0	7	4	400
Loma Linda								
Tender Rounds	6 (2.8 oz)	120	13	5	0	6	1	340
MEATBALLS								
beef	1 med (1 oz)	74	7	5	25	0	0	111
beef	1 lg (1.5 oz)	111	11	7	37	0	0	167
beef cocktail	1 (0.2 oz)	18	2	1	6	0	0	28
turkey	1 med (1 oz)	47	6	2	24	2	tr	128
Honeysuckle White								
Turkey Italian Style frzn	3 (3 oz)	190	17	10	65	6	1	600
Ian's								
Italian	3 (2.2 oz)	145	16	4	70	10	1	250
Mama Lucia								
Homestyle	4	207	14	20	50	8	1	610
Italian Style	4	280	11	23	50	8	0	640
Sausage Beef	8	220	14	17	50	3	1	690
Organic Classics								
Italian Beef	3 (3 oz)	180	17	11	50	5	1	430
Shady Brook								
Italian Beef	3 oz	260	15	20	55	5	1	510
Turkey Meatballs Appetizer Size + Sweet & Sour Sauce	6 + 2 tbsp sauce	235	17	10	65	17	tr	770
Turkey Meatballs Italian Style	3 (3 oz)	190	17	10	65	6	tr	600
Tyson								
Italian Style Chicken	6 (3 oz)	180	13	11	45	6	2	610
TAKE-OUT								
albondigas w/ sauce	3 + sauce (5.3 oz)	372	21	27	102	11	1	1194

FOOD	PORTION	CALS	PROT	FAT	CHOL	CARB	FIBER	SOD
porcupine + tomato sauce	3 + sauce	160	11	7	34	14	1	591
swedish w/ cream sauce	3 + sauce (4.7 oz)	215	17	12	86	9	tr	678
sweet & sour	3 + sauce (4.5 oz)	188	15	11	67	8	1	609

MELON

sprite	1 (10.6 oz)	110	1	0	0	29	1	190
Frieda's								
Camouflage	1 cup (5 oz)	50	1	0	0	13	1	15
SpriteMelon	1 (10.5 oz)	115	0	0	0	29	2	190
Temptation	1/10 melon (4.7 oz)	55	1	0	0	14	1	45

MEXICAN FOOD (see SALSA, SPANISH FOOD, TORTILLA)

MILK
CANNED

condensed sweetened	1 oz	123	3	3	13	21	–	49
condensed sweetened	1 cup	982	24	27	104	166	–	389
evaporated	½ cup	169	9	10	37	13	–	122
evaporated skim	½ cup	99	10	tr	5	14	–	147
Carnation								
Evaporated	2 tbsp	40	2	2	10	3	–	30
Evaporated Lowfat 2%	2 tbsp	25	2	1	5	3	–	35
Meyenberg								
Evaporated Goat Milk	8 oz	145	8	8	27	10	–	112
DRIED								
buttermilk	1 tbsp	25	2	tr	5	3	–	34
nonfat instantized	1 pkg (3.2 oz)	244	32	tr	12	47	–	499
Alba								
Instant Non-Fat as prep	1 cup	80	8	0	0	11	0	120
Bob's Red Mill								
Buttermilk Sweet Cream as prep	8 oz	60	5	1	10	7	0	85
Non Fat as prep	8 oz	80	7	0	0	11	0	110
Carnation								
Instant Nonfat as prep	1 cup	80	8	0	<5	12	0	125
Meyenberg								
Instant Goat Milk as prep	1 cup	142	8	7	25	11	–	115

FOOD	PORTION	CALS	PROT	FAT	CHOL	CARB	FIBER	SOD
Organic Valley								
Buttermilk	3 tbsp	110	10	1	0	16	0	45
Nonfat	3 tbsp	90	9	0	0	13	0	130
REFRIGERATED								
1%	1 cup	102	8	3	10	12	–	123
1%	1 qt	409	32	10	39	47	–	493
2%	1 cup	121	8	5	18	12	–	122
2%	1 qt	485	33	19	73	47	–	487
buffalo	7 oz	224	8	16	–	10	–	80
buttermilk	1 cup	99	8	2	9	12	–	257
buttermilk	1 qt	396	32	9	34	47	–	1028
camel	7 oz	160	10	8	–	10	–	60
donkey	7 oz	86	4	2	–	12	–	–
goat	1 cup	168	9	10	28	11	–	122
goat	1 qt	672	35	40	111	43	–	486
human	1 cup	171	3	11	34	17	–	42
indian buffalo	1 cup	236	9	17	46	13	–	127
low sodium	1 cup	149	8	4	33	11	–	6
mare	7 oz	98	4	4	–	12	–	–
nonfat	1 cup	86	8	tr	4	12	–	125
sheep	1 cup	264	15	17	–	13	–	108
whole	1 cup	150	8	8	33	11	–	120
Active Lifestyle								
Fat Free w/ Plant Sterols	8 oz	90	8	0	<0	13	0	125
Borden								
Fat Free Skim	1 cup	80	8	0	5	12	0	125
Farmland								
Buttermilk	8 oz	160	12	4	20	19	0	190
Fat Free	8 oz	80	8	0	5	12	0	130
Special Request 1% Plus Omega-3	8 oz	130	11	3	10	17	0	170
Special Request Skim Plus	8 oz	110	11	0	5	17	0	170
Special Request Skim Plus 100% Lactose Free	8 oz	110	11	0	5	17	0	170
Whole	8 oz	160	12	4	20	19	0	190
Hood								
1%	1 cup	110	8	3	15	13	0	125
2%	1 cup	130	8	5	20	13	0	125
Buttermilk Fat Free	1 cup	90	9	0	<5	13	0	220

FOOD	PORTION	CALS	PROT	FAT	CHOL	CARB	FIBER	SOD
Calorie Countdown 2%	8 oz	90	8	5	20	3	0	160
Calorie Countdown Fat Free	8 oz	45	8	0	0	3	0	160
Fat Free	1 cup	80	8	0	<5	13	0	125
Simply Smart 0% Fat	1 cup	90	10	0	<5	13	0	130
Simply Smart 1% Fat	1 cup	120	10	3	15	13	0	130
Whole	1 cup	150	8	8	35	12	0	125
Horizon Organic								
Fat Free	8 oz	90	9	0	<5	12	0	130
Lactaid								
1% Lowfat	1 cup	110	8	3	10	13	0	125
2% Reduced Fat	1 cup	130	8	5	20	12	0	125
Calcium Fortified	1 cup	80	8	0	<5	13	0	125
Fat Free	1 cup	90	8	0	<5	13	0	125
Whole	1 cup	150	8	8	35	12	0	125
Meyenberg								
Goat Milk	8 oz	142	8	7	25	11	–	115
Goat Milk Low Fat	8 oz	89	7	2	8	9	–	100
Organic Valley								
Fat Free	1 cup	90	8	0	5	13	0	125
Lactose Free Fat Free	1 cup	90	8	0	0	14	0	130
Whole Nonhomogenized	1 cup	150	8	8	35	12	0	125
SunMilk								
Heart Healthy 1% Sunflower Oil	8 oz	120	11	2	<5	15	0	160
Heart Healthy 2% Sunflower Oil	8 oz	120	10	3	<5	15	0	150
Tuscan								
Whole	8 oz	150	8	8	35	12	0	120
Welsh Farms								
Fat Free	8 oz	80	8	0	5	12	0	130
SHELF-STABLE								
Parmalat								
2% Reduced Fat	8 oz	130	8	5	20	12	0	130
Fat Free	8 oz	80	8	0	5	12	0	130
Lactose Free 2% Reduced Fat	8 oz	130	8	5	20	12	0	130

MILK DRINKS

FOOD	PORTION	CALS	PROT	FAT	CHOL	CARB	FIBER	SOD
chocolate milk	1 cup	208	8	8	30	26	–	149

FOOD	PORTION	CALS	PROT	FAT	CHOL	CARB	FIBER	SOD
chocolate milk	1 qt	833	32	34	122	103	–	596
chocolate milk 1%	1 cup	158	8	3	7	26	–	152
chocolate milk 2%	1 cup	179	8	5	17	26	–	150
Bravo!								
Blenders Creamy Double Chocolate	1 bottle (11 oz)	180	17	4	20	19	2	350
Blenders Creamy French Vanilla	1 bottle (11 oz)	160	17	4	20	20	2	260
CocoaVia								
Indulgence Rich Chocolate	1 bottle (5.65 oz)	150	6	3	5	28	3	135
Dove								
Bravo! Dark Chocolate	1 bottle	310	8	16	60	37	2	140
Bravo! Milk Chocolate	1 bottle	310	8	16	60	36	1	105
Farmland								
Really Really Good! Chocolate Milk	8 oz	160	8	3	10	25	0	150
Hood								
Calorie Countdown Chocolate 2%	8 oz	90	8	5	15	5	1	300
Chocolate Lowfat	1 cup	170	9	3	15	28	tr	170
Chocolate Milk	1 cup	230	9	9	35	31	tr	170
Coffee Lowfat Milk	1 cup	170	8	3	15	28	0	125
Horizon Organic								
Lowfat Chocolate Milk	8 oz	170	8	3	15	27	tr	140
Strawberry	8 oz	200	8	5	20	31	0	130
Lifeway								
La Fruta All Flavors	8 oz	180	8	2	10	33	0	125
Nesquik								
Chocolate as prep w/ lowfat milk	1 cup	210	tr	5	18	30	1	144
Chocolate No Sugar as prep w/ lowfat milk	1 cup	130	1	1	3	18	1	85
Double Chocolate as prep w/ lowfat milk	1 cup	210	1	5	18	30	1	80
Ready-To-Drink Banana	1 cup	200	7	5	20	30	0	120
Ready-To-Drink Chocolate	1 cup	200	8	5	15	32	tr	150
Ready-To-Drink Double Chocolate	1 cup	200	8	5	15	30	tr	170

FOOD	PORTION	CALS	PROT	FAT	CHOL	CARB	FIBER	SOD
Ready-To-Drink Fat Free Chocolate	1 cup	160	8	0	0	32	tr	150
Ready-To-Drink Strawberry	1 cup	200	8	5	15	33	tr	120
Ready-To-Drink Very Vanilla	1 cup	200	8	5	15	30	tr	120
Strawberry as prep w/ lowfat milk	1 cup	210	0	4	18	33	0	120
Vanilla as prep w/ lowfat milk	1 cup	210	0	4	18	33	0	120
Organic Valley								
Buttermilk Lowfat 1%	1 cup	100	8	3	15	12	0	250
Parmalat								
Chocolate Milk 2% Reduced Fat	1 cup	190	8	5	20	28	1	130
Quaker								
Chocolate	8 oz	140	5	5	16	18	3	180
Strawberry	8 oz	130	4	5	17	18	tr	180
Sipahh								
Straw Banana	1 straw	15	0	0	0	3	–	0
Straw Cookies and Cream	1 straw	15	0	0	0	3	–	0
MILK SUBSTITUTES								
imitation milk	1 cup	150	4	8	tr	15	–	191
imitation milk	1 qt	600	17	33	2	60	–	764
soy milk	1 cup	79	7	5	0	4	–	30
8th Continent								
Soymilk Chocolate	8 oz	140	7	3	0	23	1	180
Soymilk Original	8 oz	80	7	3	0	8	0	160
Soymilk Vanilla	8 oz	100	7	3	0	11	0	170
Soymilk Fat Free Original	8 oz	60	6	0	0	8	0	160
Soymilk Fat Free Vanilla	8 oz	70	6	0	0	11	0	160
Soymilk Light Chocolate	8 oz	90	7	2	0	13	tr	190
Soymilk Light Original	8 oz	50	7	2	0	2	0	170
Soymilk Light Vanilla	8 oz	60	7	1	0	5	0	190
Almond Breeze								
Chocolate	8 oz	115	1	3	0	22	1	152
Original	8 oz	57	1	3	0	8	1	148
Original Unsweetened	8 oz	40	1	3	0	2	1	150
Vanilla	8 oz	91	1	3	0	16	1	150

FOOD	PORTION	CALS	PROT	FAT	CHOL	CARB	FIBER	SOD
Brazsoy								
Condensed Soy Milk	1 serv (0.7 oz)	54	1	1	0	10	0	11
Soy Cream	1 tbsp (0.5 oz)	27	0	3	0	0	0	15
DariFree								
Fat Free as prep	8 oz	70	0	0	0	20	0	120
Fat Free Chocolate as prep	8 oz	110	0	0	5	27	tr	125
EdenBlend								
Organic	8 oz	120	7	3	0	18	tr	90
Edensoy								
Organic Carob	8 oz	170	7	4	0	28	tr	95
Organic Chocolate	8 oz	180	8	4	0	28	tr	105
Organic Original	8 oz	140	11	5	0	14	tr	105
Organic Original Unsweetened	8 oz	120	12	6	0	5	tr	5
Organic Original Light	8 oz	100	5	2	0	15	0	90
Organic Vanilla	8 oz	150	7	3	0	24	tr	85
Organic Light Vanilla	8 oz	110	4	1	0	22	0	110
Lifeway								
SoyTreat All Flavors	8 oz	160	7	4	0	23	0	2
Living Harvest								
Hempmilk Original	1 cup	130	4	3	0	20	1	120
Hempmilk Vanilla	1 cup	130	4	3	0	20	1	120
Lundberg								
Organic Drink Rice Original	8 oz	120	1	3	0	22	tr	85
Manitoba Harvest								
Hemp Bliss Chocolate	8 oz	160	5	7	0	17	1	120
Hemp Bliss Original	1 cup	110	5	7	0	7	1	95
Hemp Bliss Vanilla	8 oz	150	5	7	0	14	1	120
Odwalla								
Soy Smart Chai	8 oz	150	6	4	–	22	–	30
Soy Smart Vanilla	8 oz	120	6	4	–	15	–	55
Soymilk Plain	8 oz	110	7	4	0	12	3	65
Soymilk Vanilla Being	8 oz	100	4	3	0	13	3	65
Organic Valley								
Soy Original	1 cup	100	7	3	0	11	3	95
Soy Unsweetened	1 cup	80	7	4	0	3	1	110

FOOD	PORTION	CALS	PROT	FAT	CHOL	CARB	FIBER	SOD
Pacific Foods								
Almond Low Fat Original	1 cup	70	2	3	0	11	1	105
Almond Low Fat Vanilla	1 cup	100	2	3	0	15	1	105
Multi Grain Low Fat Original	1 cup	160	5	2	0	30	1	80
Oat Organic Low Fat Original	1 cup	130	4	3	0	24	2	110
Oat Organic Low Fat Vanilla	1 cup	130	4	3	0	24	2	110
Rice Low Fat Plain	1 cup	130	1	2	0	27	0	75
Rice Low Fat Vanilla	1 cup	130	1	2	0	27	0	75
Soy Organic Unsweetened Original	1 cup	90	9	5	0	4	2	15
Soy Select Low Fat Plain	1 cup	70	5	3	0	9	tr	115
Soy Select Low Fat Vanilla	1 cup	80	5	3	0	11	tr	115
Soy Ultra	1 cup	130	10	4	0	14	1	150
Soy Ultra Plain	1 cup	120	10	4	0	12	1	150
Rice Dream								
Carob	8 oz	150	1	3	0	30	tr	80
Heartwise Vanilla	8 oz	140	1	2	0	30	3	80
Horchata	8 oz	130	7	4	0	16	2	150
Original	8 oz	120	1	3	0	24	0	100
Original Enriched	8 oz	120	1	3	0	23	0	100
Vanilla Enriched	8 oz	130	1	3	0	26	0	105
Sno*e								
Tofu as prep	8 oz	80	2	5	0	20	0	130
Tofu Low Fat as prep	8 oz	70	2	3	0	10	0	135
Soy Dream								
Classic Vanilla	8 oz	140	7	4	0	18	2	135
Original Enriched	8 oz	100	7	4	0	8	2	135
Vitasoy								
Classic Original	8 oz	120	8	5	0	11	1	160
Creamy Original	8 oz	110	7	4	0	11	1	160
Green Tea Soymilk	8 oz	120	7	4	0	13	1	180
Light Original	8 oz	60	4	2	0	7	0	110
Light Vanilla	8 oz	70	4	2	0	10	0	120
Original Unsweetened	8 oz	80	7	4	0	5	tr	140
WildWood								
Organic Soymilk Plain	8 oz	100	7	4	0	8	1	80

FOOD	PORTION	CALS	PROT	FAT	CHOL	CARB	FIBER	SOD
Organic Soymilk Unsweetened	8 oz	72	7	4	0	3	1	70

MILKFISH (AWA)

FOOD	PORTION	CALS	PROT	FAT	CHOL	CARB	FIBER	SOD
baked	3 oz	162	22	7	57	0	0	–

MILKSHAKE

FOOD	PORTION	CALS	PROT	FAT	CHOL	CARB	FIBER	SOD
chocolate	1 serv (10 oz)	393	9	14	42	60	2	156
malted milk shake	1 serv (10 oz)	402	9	14	51	62	1	201
vanilla	1 serv (10 oz)	379	8	13	48	60	1	133
Ben & Jerry's								
Cherry Garcia	1 bottle (8 oz)	320	6	12	40	47	–	130
Chocolate Fudge Brownie	1 bottle (8 oz)	340	6	12	40	51	–	105
Chunky Monkey	1 bottle (8 oz)	330	5	10	35	54	–	180
Buffy's Cool Cow								
Chocolate	1 pkg (8 oz)	150	9	3	5	23	tr	135
Vanilla	1 pkg (8 oz)	150	9	3	5	24	0	135
Nesquik								
Ready-To-Drink Chocolate	1 cup	170	8	5	15	26	tr	180

MILLET

FOOD	PORTION	CALS	PROT	FAT	CHOL	CARB	FIBER	SOD
cooked	1 cup (6.1 oz)	207	6	2	0	41	2	3
Arrowhead Mills								
Organic Hulled not prep	¼ cup	150	4	2	0	33	1	0

MINERAL WATER (see WATER)

MISO

FOOD	PORTION	CALS	PROT	FAT	CHOL	CARB	FIBER	SOD
dried	1 oz	86	7	3	–	10	1	2130
miso	½ cup	284	16	8	0	39	7	5036
Eden								
Hacho	1 tbsp	40	3	2	0	4	tr	680
Organic Genmai	1 tbsp	25	2	1	0	3	2	780
Organic Mugi	1 tbsp	25	2	1	0	4	tr	640
Organic Shiro	1 tbsp	30	1	1	0	6	tr	330
Tekka	1 tsp	5	tr	0	0	tr	0	70

FOOD	PORTION	CALS	PROT	FAT	CHOL	CARB	FIBER	SOD
MOLASSES								
blackstrap	1 tbsp (0.7 oz)	47	0	0	0	12	–	11
blackstrap	1 cup (11.5 oz)	771	0	tr	0	199	–	180
molasses	1 tbsp (0.7 oz)	53	0	0	0	14	–	7
molasses	1 cup (11.5 oz)	873	0	1	0	226	–	120
Grandma's								
Robust	1 tbsp	60	0	0	0	15	–	15
MONKFISH								
baked	3 oz	82	16	2	27	0	0	20
MOOSE								
roasted	4 oz	142	31	1	83	0	0	73
MOTH BEANS								
dried cooked	1 cup	207	14	1	0	37	–	17
MOUSSE								
TAKE-OUT								
chocolate	½ cup	454	8	32	283	32	1	77
fish timbale	1 cup	329	22	25	210	3	0	394
MUFFIN								
MIX								
blueberry	1 (1.75 oz)	149	3	4	23	24	–	219
corn	1 (1.75 oz)	160	4	5	31	25	–	397
wheat bran as prep	1 (1.75 oz)	138	5	5	34	23	–	233
Glory								
Golden Sweet Corn as prep	1	170	2	5	36	27	1	360
Jiffy								
Apple Cinnamon as prep	1	190	2	7	33	28	1	300
Banana Nut as prep	1	180	2	7	27	25	2	300
Blueberry as prep	1	190	2	7	36	28	1	288
Bran w/ Dates as prep	1	170	2	6	36	26	3	240
Corn as prep	1	180	2	6	30	30	1	320
Raspberry as prep	1	180	2	7	42	26	1	336
King Arthur								
Cranberry Orange Whole Grain not prep	¼ cup	180	4	1	0	41	3	130

FOOD	PORTION	CALS	PROT	FAT	CHOL	CARB	FIBER	SOD
Miracle Maize								
Country Style as prep	1	155	3	6	15	22	1	360
Sweet as prep	1	180	3	6	15	29	1	312
Miracle Muffins								
Banana w/ Splenda as prep	1	86	9	3	0	12	7	130
READY-TO-EAT								
blueberry	1 (2 oz)	158	3	4	17	27	2	255
oat bran wheat free	1 (2 oz)	154	4	4	0	28	4	224
toaster type blueberry	1	103	2	3	–	18	–	158
toaster type corn	1	114	2	4	–	19	–	142
toaster type wheat bran w/ raisins	1 (1.3 oz)	106	2	3	–	19	–	178
Fred's Incredible Muffins								
All Flavors	1 (2.5 oz)	100	8	3	55	26	–	400
Hostess								
100 Calorie Pack Mini Banana Streusel	1 pkg (1.2 oz)	100	2	4	10	19	4	120
100 Calorie Pack Mini Blueberry Streusel	1 pkg (1.2 oz)	100	2	3	10	20	4	120
VitaMuffin								
AppleBerryBran	1 (2 oz)	100	3	0	0	25	5	140
BlueBran	1 (2 oz)	100	3	0	0	24	4	360
CranBran	1 (2 oz)	100	3	0	0	24	4	360
Sugar Free Low Carb Banana Nut	1 (2 oz)	90	5	2	0	24	7	270
VitaTops Dark Chocolate Pomegranate	1 (2 oz)	100	3	2	0	21	6	140
VitaTops Deep Chocolate	1 (2 oz)	100	4	2	0	25	6	230
VitaTops Golden Corn	1 (2 oz)	100	4	1	0	25	6	135
VitaTops MultiBran	1 (2 oz)	100	4	1	0	22	5	140
TAKE-OUT								
corn	1 lg (2.5 oz)	214	5	7	31	32	2	371
raisin bran lowfat	1 (4 oz)	270	5	1	0	61	5	560
MULBERRIES								
fresh	1 cup	61	2	1	0	14	–	14
Navitas Naturals								
Dried	1 oz	91	3	0	0	21	3	25
MULLET								
striped cooked	3 oz	127	21	4	54	0	0	61
striped raw	3 oz	99	16	3	42	0	0	55

FOOD	PORTION	CALS	PROT	FAT	CHOL	CARB	FIBER	SOD
MUNG BEANS								
dried cooked	1 cup	213	14	1	0	39	–	4
MUNGO BEANS								
dried cooked	1 cup	190	14	1	1	33	–	13
MUSHROOMS								
CANNED								
caps	8 (1.6 oz)	12	1	tr	0	2	1	200
caps pickled	6 (0.8 oz)	5	1	tr	0	1	tr	53
chanterelle	3.5 oz	12	1	1	0	tr	6	165
pickled	1 cup	33	4	tr	0	5	1	351
pieces	½ cup	20	1	tr	0	2	1	332
straw	1 cup	58	7	1	0	8	5	699
Green Giant								
Pieces & Stems	½ cup	25	2	0	0	4	1	440
Sunny Dell								
Portabella Sliced	½ cup	20	1	0	0	4	2	460
DRIED								
chanterelle	1 oz	25	5	tr	0	tr	17	9
shiitake	1 (3.6 g)	11	tr	tr	0	3	tr	0
tree ear	½ cup (0.4 oz)	36	1	tr	0	10	–	8
wood ear mok yee	½ cup (0.4 oz)	25	2	tr	–	8	4	6
Eden								
Maitake Sliced	10 pieces (0.3 oz)	35	2	0	0	7	4	0
Shitake	3 (0.4 oz)	35	2	0	0	7	5	0
Shitake Sliced	3 pieces (0.3 oz)	35	2	0	0	7	5	0
Frieda's								
Chanterelle	2 pieces (4 g)	15	1	0	0	2	1	0
Wood Ear	3 pieces (4 g)	15	1	0	0	2	1	0
FRESH								
brown italian or crimini sliced	1 cup	19	2	tr	0	3	tr	4
brown italian or crimini whole	1 (0.7 oz)	5	1	tr	0	1	tr	1
chanterelle	3.5 oz	11	2	tr	0	tr	6	3
enoki raw	1 lg (5 g)	2	tr	tr	0	tr	tr	0

FOOD	PORTION	CALS	PROT	FAT	CHOL	CARB	FIBER	SOD
enoki sliced	1 cup	29	2	tr	0	5	2	2
enoki whole	1 cup	28	2	tr	0	5	2	2
maitake diced	1 cup	26	1	tr	0	5	2	1
maitake whole	1 (6.6 g)	2	tr	tr	0	tr	tr	0
morel	3.5 oz	9	2	tr	0	0	7	2
oyster	1 sm (0.5 oz)	5	1	tr	0	1	tr	3
oyster sliced	1 cup	30	3	tr	0	6	2	15
portabella raw	1 cap (3 oz)	22	2	tr	0	4	1	5
portabella sliced grilled	1 cup (4.2 oz)	42	5	1	0	6	3	12
raw sliced	½ cup	8	1	tr	0	1	tr	2
shiitake cooked	4 (2.5 oz)	40	1	tr	0	10	2	3
shiitake pieces cooked	1 cup	81	2	tr	0	21	3	6
white	1 (0.6 oz)	4	1	tr	0	1	tr	1
white sliced cooked	1 cup	28	4	tr	0	4	2	13
Frieda's								
Enoki	¼ pkg (1 oz)	10	1	0	0	2	1	0
Golden Gourmet								
Beech Brown	4 oz	20	3	1	0	7	–	1
Beech White	4 oz	13	3	1	0	6	–	1
King Trumpet	4 oz	20	3	0	0	7	–	2
Maitake	4 oz	20	3	1	0	8	–	1
FROZEN								
Alexia								
Mushroom Bites	1 serv (2 oz)	110	3	4	0	16	1	280
Farm Rich								
Breaded	5 (3 oz)	120	3	2	0	23	1	430
TAKE-OUT								
battered fried	1 lg (0.6 oz)	39	1	3	1	3	tr	29
creamed	1 cup	171	6	11	7	15	3	853
stuffed	1 (0.8 oz)	67	3	4	3	6	1	142

MUSKRAT

FOOD	PORTION	CALS	PROT	FAT	CHOL	CARB	FIBER	SOD
roasted	3 oz	199	26	10	–	0	0	81

MUSSELS

FOOD	PORTION	CALS	PROT	FAT	CHOL	CARB	FIBER	SOD
blue raw	3 oz	73	10	2	24	3	–	243
blue raw	1 cup	129	18	3	42	6	–	429
fresh blue cooked	3 oz	147	20	4	48	6	–	313

FOOD	PORTION	CALS	PROT	FAT	CHOL	CARB	FIBER	SOD
MUSTARD								
dry mustard	1 tsp	15	1	1	0	1	–	tr
hot chinese	1 tsp	3	tr	tr	0	tr	tr	56
organic yellow	1 tsp	5	0	0	0	0	0	70
seed	1 tsp	15	1	1	0	1	1	0
yellow prepared	1 tbsp	3	tr	tr	0	tr	tr	57
Annie's Naturals								
Organic Horseradish Mustard	1 tsp	5	0	0	0	1	–	90
Boar's Head								
Delicatessen Style	1 tsp (5 g)	0	0	0	0	0	0	40
Honey	1 tsp (5 g)	10	0	0	0	2	0	25
Bone Suckin'								
Fat Free Gluten Free	1 tbsp	25	0	0	0	5	0	95
D'Oni								
Bold As Love Honey Habanero	1 tsp	5	0	0	0	2	–	45
Eden								
Organic Brown	1 tsp	0	0	0	0	tr	0	80
Yellow	1 tsp	0	0	0	0	0	0	80
Emeril's								
Horseradish	1 tbsp	5	0	0	0	0	0	60
Smooth Honey	1 tbsp	10	0	0	0	1	–	25
French's								
Classic Yellow	1 tsp	0	0	0	0	0	0	55
Honey	1 tsp	10	0	0	0	1	–	30
Honey Dijon	1 tsp	10	0	0	0	1	–	40
Horseradish	1 tsp	5	0	0	0	0	0	80
Spicy Brown	1 tsp	5	0	0	0	0	0	80
Gulden's								
Spicy Brown	1 tsp	5	0	0	0	0	0	50
Hebrew National								
Deli	1 tsp	4	0	0	0	0	0	65
Hellman's								
Deli	1 tsp	5	0	0	0	tr	0	55
Dijonnaise	1 tsp	5	0	0	0	1	0	70
Honey Mustard	1 tsp	10	0	0	0	2	0	25
Kosciusko								
Spicy Brown	1 tsp	0	0	0	0	0	0	60

FOOD	PORTION	CALS	PROT	FAT	CHOL	CARB	FIBER	SOD
Robert Rothchild Farm								
Champagne Garlic	1 tsp	6	0	0	0	1	0	120
Sara Lee								
Country Honey	1 tbsp	10	0	0	0	2	0	25
Cranberry Honey	1 tbsp	10	0	0	0	2	0	25
School House Kitchen								
Sweet Smooth Hot	1 tsp	15	0	1	0	1	0	10
MUSTARD GREENS								
fresh chopped cooked	½ cup	11	2	tr	0	1	–	11
fresh raw chopped	½ cup	7	1	tr	0	1	–	7
frozen chopped cooked	½ cup	14	2	tr	0	2	–	19
Allen's								
Seasoned Southern Style	½ cup	30	2	0	0	5	2	530
Glory								
Seasoned canned	½ cup	35	2	0	0	3	1	490
NATTO								
natto	½ cup	187	16	10	0	13	–	6
NAVY BEANS								
CANNED								
navy	1 cup	296	20	1	0	54	–	1173
Eden								
Organic	½ cup	110	7	0	0	20	7	15
DRIED								
cooked	1 cup	259	16	1	0	48	–	2
NECTARINE								
fresh	1	67	1	1	0	16	2	0
Sunsweet								
Dried	3 pieces (1.4 oz)	100	1	0	0	25	3	60
NECTARINE JUICE								
Sun Shower								
100% Juice	8 oz	93	1	0	0	21	2	15
NEUFCHATEL								
neufchatel	1 oz	74	3	7	22	1	–	113
neufchatel	1 pkg (3 oz)	221	8	20	65	3	–	339

FOOD	PORTION	CALS	PROT	FAT	CHOL	CARB	FIBER	SOD
Back To Nature								
Organic	⅛ pkg (1 oz)	70	3	6	20	tr	0	120
Organic Valley								
Soft	2 tbsp	70	2	6	20	2	0	140

NONI JUICE
Lakewood
Noni Pure Juice	2 oz	8	0	0	0	2	0	5

NOODLE DISHES (see PASTA DINNERS)

NOODLES
FOOD	PORTION	CALS	PROT	FAT	CHOL	CARB	FIBER	SOD
cellophane	1 cup	492	tr	tr	0	121	–	14
chow mein	1 cup (1.6 oz)	237	4	14	0	25	2	189
egg	1 cup (38 g)	145	5	2	36	27	–	8
egg cooked	1 cup (5.6 oz)	213	8	2	53	40	2	11
japanese soba cooked	1 cup (4 oz)	113	6	tr	0	24	–	68
japanese somen cooked	1 cup (6.2 oz)	231	7	tr	0	48	–	283
korean acorn noodles not prep	2 oz	195	7	tr	–	41	tr	–
rice cooked	1 cup (6.2 oz)	192	2	tr	0	44	2	33
spinach/egg cooked	1 cup (5.6 oz)	211	8	3	53	39	4	19
A Taste Of Thai								
Rice Wide	2 oz	200	3	0	0	46	2	20
Annie Chun's								
Chow Mein	2 oz	200	8	1	0	39	3	350
Noddle Express Spicy Szechuan	½ pkg	170	4	3	0	29	1	470
Noodle Bowl Teriyaki	1 pkg	310	9	3	0	60	2	800
Noodle Express Chinese Chow Mein	½ pkg	160	5	4	0	27	1	510
Noodle Express Singapore Curry	½ pkg	160	4	3	0	28	2	550
Noodle Express Teriyaki	½ pkg	160	5	2	0	31	1	510

FOOD	PORTION	CALS	PROT	FAT	CHOL	CARB	FIBER	SOD
Noodle Express Thai Peanut	½ pkg	200	6	7	0	29	1	300
Rice	2 oz	210	2	0	0	50	0	75
Rice Pad Thai	2 oz	210	2	0	0	50	0	75
Azumaya								
Asian Style Thin Cut	1 cup	210	8	1	0	43	2	400
Catelli								
Egg	3 oz	317	13	3	–	60	–	15
Hodgson Mill								
Egg Whole Wheat not prep	2 oz	190	10	2	30	34	4	20
Light 'N Fluffy								
Egg Extra Wide cooked	1½ cups	210	8	3	70	40	2	15
Manischewitz								
Egg Medium	1¼ cups	220	8	3	65	40	2	15
Nasoya								
Chinese	1 cup	210	8	1	0	43	2	400
Japanese	1 cup	210	8	1	0	43	2	410
Spinach	1 cup	210	8	1	0	42	2	370
No Yolks								
Extra Broad	2 oz	210	8	1	0	41	3	30

NUTMEG

FOOD	PORTION	CALS	PROT	FAT	CHOL	CARB	FIBER	SOD
ground	1 tsp	12	tr	1	0	1	1	0

NUTRITION SUPPLEMENTS (see also CEREAL BARS, ENERGY BARS, ENERGY DRINKS)

FOOD	PORTION	CALS	PROT	FAT	CHOL	CARB	FIBER	SOD
Amino Vital								
Jel All Flavors	1 pkg (4.9 oz)	70	0	0	0	17	1	115
Boost								
Breeze	8 oz	160	8	0	0	31	–	50
Diabetic	8 oz	250	14	12	–	20	3	180
Clif								
Shot Energy Gel All Flavors	1 pkg (1.1 oz)	100	0	0	0	25	0	40
DiabetiTrim								
Shake French Vanilla	1 pkg	90	14	1	5	10	4	200
Ensure								
Shake Creamy Milk Chocolate	1 bottle (8 oz)	250	9	6	5	40	1	190
Shake Strawberries & Cream	1 bottle (8 oz)	250	9	6	5	40	0	200

FOOD	PORTION	CALS	PROT	FAT	CHOL	CARB	FIBER	SOD
Glucerna								
Shake Creamy Chocolate Delight	1 bottle (8 oz)	200	10	7	<5	27	5	210
Shake Homemade Vanilla	1 bottle (8 oz)	200	10	7	<5	26	5	210
Jelly Belly								
Sport Beans Berry Blue	1 pkg (1 oz)	100	0	0	0	25	0	80
Joint Juice								
Tropical Fruit	1 can (8 oz)	30	0	0	0	6	–	30
PowerBar								
Powergel All Flavors	1 pkg (1.4 oz)	120	0	2	0	26	–	45
Pria								
Complete Shake Creamy Milk Chocolate	1 pkg (11.6 oz)	170	13	5	10	21	7	250
Resource								
Beneprotein Protein Powder	1 scoop	25	6	0	0	0	0	–
Optisource High Protein Drink	1 box (4 oz)	100	12	3	<5	6	0	70
Slim-Fast								
Optima Ready-To-Drink Creamy Milk Chocolate	1 can (11 oz)	190	10	6	5	25	5	200
Optima Shake Mix Chocolate Royale as prep w/ fat free milk	1 serv	190	10	5	5	29	4	240
Optima Shake Mix French Vanilla as prep w/ fat free milk	1 serv	200	10	4	5	30	4	240
Vitasoy								
Weight Management Meal All Flavors	1 bottle (10 oz)	200	10	1	0	39	8	100
NUTS MIXED (see also individual names)								
dry roasted w/ peanuts salted	¼ cup	203	6	18	0	9	3	229
dry roasted w/ peanuts w/o salt	¼ cup	203	6	18	0	9	3	4
oil roasted w/o peanuts salted	¼ cup	221	6	20	0	8	2	110

FOOD	PORTION	CALS	PROT	FAT	CHOL	CARB	FIBER	SOD
oil roasted w/o peanuts w/o salt	¼ cup	221	6	20	0	8	2	4
Estee								
Chocolate Covered Fruit & Nut Mix Fructose Sweetened	¼ cup	210	6	12	<5	19	2	45
Good Sense								
Deluxe Mix	¼ cup	180	7	13	0	8	2	45
Organic Trails								
Tamari Roasted Nuts & Seeds	¼ cup	190	7	15	0	10	5	130
Peanut Better								
Mixed Nut Butter Creamy & Crunchy	2 tbsp	190	8	17	0	5	3	135
Planters								
NUT-rition Energy Mix	¼ cup	180	5	14	0	10	3	95
NUT-rition Heart Healthy Mix	1 (0.9 oz)	170	6	16	0	5	3	40

OCA
Frieda's

FOOD	PORTION	CALS	PROT	FAT	CHOL	CARB	FIBER	SOD
Oca	½ cup	70	2	0	0	15	1	5

OCTOPUS

FOOD	PORTION	CALS	PROT	FAT	CHOL	CARB	FIBER	SOD
dried boiled	3 oz	144	26	2	84	4	0	695
fresh steamed	3 oz	139	25	2	81	4	0	111
smoked	1 oz	40	7	1	23	1	0	111
TAKE-OUT								
ensalada de pulpo	1 cup	299	17	21	52	10	2	232

OHELOBERRIES

FOOD	PORTION	CALS	PROT	FAT	CHOL	CARB	FIBER	SOD
fresh	1 cup	39	1	tr	0	10	–	2

OIL

FOOD	PORTION	CALS	PROT	FAT	CHOL	CARB	FIBER	SOD
almond	1 cup	1927	0	218	0	0	0	–
almond	1 tbsp	120	0	14	0	0	0	–
apricot kernel	1 cup	1927	0	218	0	0	0	–
apricot kernel	1 tbsp	120	0	14	0	0	0	–
avocado	1 cup	1927	0	218	0	0	0	–
avocado	1 tbsp	124	0	14	0	0	0	–
babassu palm	1 tbsp	120	0	14	0	0	0	–
butter oil	1 tbsp	112	tr	13	33	0	0	–

FOOD	PORTION	CALS	PROT	FAT	CHOL	CARB	FIBER	SOD
butter oil	1 cup	1795	1	204	524	0	0	–
canola	1 cup	1927	0	218	0	0	0	–
canola	1 tbsp	124	0	14	0	0	0	–
coconut	1 tbsp	117	0	14	0	0	0	0
corn	1 cup	1927	0	218	0	0	0	–
corn	1 tbsp	120	0	14	0	0	0	–
cottonseed	1 tbsp	120	0	14	0	0	0	–
cottonseed	1 cup	1927	0	218	0	0	0	–
cupu assu	1 tbsp	120	0	14	0	0	0	–
garlic oil	1 tbsp	150	0	17	0	0	0	0
grapeseed	1 tbsp	120	0	14	0	0	0	0
hazelnut	1 cup	1927	0	218	0	0	0	–
hazelnut	1 tbsp	120	0	14	0	0	0	–
mustard	1 cup	1927	0	218	0	0	0	–
mustard	1 tbsp	124	0	14	0	0	0	–
oat	1 tbsp	120	0	14	0	0	0	–
olive	1 tbsp	119	0	14	0	0	0	0
olive	1 cup	1909	0	216	0	0	0	tr
palm	1 cup	1927	0	218	0	0	0	–
palm	1 tbsp	120	0	14	0	0	0	–
palm kernel	1 cup	1879	0	218	0	0	0	–
palm kernel	1 tbsp	117	0	14	0	0	0	–
peanut	1 tbsp	119	0	14	0	0	0	tr
peanut	1 cup	1909	0	216	0	0	0	tr
peppermint	1 tsp	42	–	4	0	0	0	–
poppyseed	1 tbsp	120	0	14	0	0	0	–
pumpkin seed	1 oz	217	0	29	–	0	0	–
rice bran	1 tbsp	120	0	14	0	0	0	–
safflower	1 tbsp	120	0	14	0	0	0	–
safflower	1 cup	1927	0	218	0	0	0	–
sesame	1 tbsp	120	0	14	0	0	0	–
sheanut	1 tbsp	120	0	14	0	0	0	–
soybean	1 cup	1927	0	218	0	0	0	tr
soybean	1 tbsp	120	0	14	0	0	0	0
sunflower	1 cup	1927	0	218	0	0	0	–
sunflower	1 tbsp	120	0	14	0	0	0	–
teaseed	1 tbsp	120	0	14	0	0	0	–
tomatoseed	1 tbsp	120	0	14	0	0	0	–
vegetable	1 tbsp	120	0	14	0	0	0	–
vegetable	1 cup	1927	0	218	0	0	0	–

FOOD	PORTION	CALS	PROT	FAT	CHOL	CARB	FIBER	SOD
walnut	1 cup	1927	0	218	0	0	0	–
walnut	1 tbsp	120	0	14	0	0	0	–
wheat germ	1 tbsp	120	0	14	0	0	0	–
Asoyia								
Soybean Ultra Low Lin	1 tbsp	129	0	14	0	0	0	–
Botticelli								
Olive	1 tbsp	120	0	14	0	0	0	0
Carapelli								
Grapeseed	1 tbsp	120	0	14	0	0	0	0
Olive Extra Virgin	1 tbsp	120	0	14	0	0	0	0
Consorzio								
Dipping Oil	1 tbsp	120	0	14	0	0	0	0
Olive Basil	1 tbsp	120	0	14	0	0	0	0
Olive Roasted Pepper	1 tbsp	120	0	14	0	0	0	250
Organic Extra Virgin Olive Meyer Lemon	1 tbsp	120	0	14	0	0	0	0
Eden								
Olive Extra Virgin	1 tbsp	120	0	14	0	0	0	0
Organic Safflower	1 tbsp	120	0	14	0	0	0	0
Organic Soybean	1 tbsp	120	0	14	0	0	0	0
Toasted Sesame	1 tbsp	120	0	14	0	0	0	0
Enova								
Oil	1 tbsp	120	0	14	0	0	0	0
Hollywood								
Canola Enriched	1 tbsp	120	0	14	0	0	0	0
Peanut Enriched Gold	1 tbsp	120	0	14	0	0	0	0
Safflower Expeller Pressed	1 tbsp	120	0	14	0	0	0	0
House Of Tsang								
Mongolian Fire	1 tsp	45	0	5	0	0	0	0
Wok Oil	1 tbsp	130	0	14	0	0	0	0
Iowa Natural								
Soybean 1% Linolenic	1 tbsp	129	0	14	0	0	0	–
Kinloch Plantation								
100% Virgin Pecan	1 tbsp	130	0	14	0	0	0	0
Living Harvest								
Organic Hemp Oil	2 tbsp	250	0	28	0	0	0	0
Manitoba Harvest								
Hemp Seed Oil	1 tbsp	126	0	14	0	0	0	0
Mazola								
Corn	1 tbsp	120	0	14	0	0	0	0

FOOD	PORTION	CALS	PROT	FAT	CHOL	CARB	FIBER	SOD
No Stick Spray	⅓ sec spray	0	0	0	0	0	0	0
Pure Cooking Spray Canola All Flavors	¼ sec spray	0	0	0	0	0	0	0
Right Blend	1 tbsp	120	0	14	0	0	0	0
Vegetable	1 tbsp	120	0	14	0	0	0	0
Nutiva								
Organic Coconut Extra Virgin	1 tbsp	120	0	14	0	0	0	0
Organic Hemp Cold Pressed	1 tbsp	120	0	14	0	0	0	0
Nutrium								
Soybean Low Linolenic	1 tbsp	129	0	14	0	0	0	–
Olivo								
Spray Olive Oil 100% Extra Virgin	⅓ sec spray	0	0	0	0	0	0	0
Orville Redenbacher's								
Popping & Topping	1 tbsp	120	0	14	0	0	0	0
Pacifica Culinaria								
Avocado	1 tbsp	120	0	14	0	1	–	0
Avocado Blood Orange	1 tbsp	120	0	14	0	1	–	0
Pam								
Cooking Spray All Types	⅓ sec spray	0	0	0	0	0	0	0
Organic Canola	⅓ sec spray	0	0	0	0	0	0	0
Pompeian								
Olive	1 tbsp	130	–	14	0	–	–	–
Robert Rothchild Farm								
Basil Infused	1 tbsp	120	0	14	0	0	0	0
Smart Balance								
Omega Oil	1 tbsp	120	0	14	0	0	0	0
Spectrum								
Almond	1 tbsp	120	0	14	0	0	0	0
Apricot Kernel	1 tbsp	120	0	14	0	0	0	0
Avocado	1 tbsp	120	0	14	0	0	0	0
Canola Organic	1 tbsp	120	0	14	0	0	0	0
Coconut Organic	1 tbsp	120	0	14	0	0	0	0
Corn	1 tbsp	120	0	14	2	0	0	0
Grapeseed	1 tbsp	120	0	14	1	0	0	0
Hazelnut Toasted Organic	1 tbsp	120	0	14	0	0	0	0
Mediterranean Olive Organic	1 tbsp	120	0	14	0	0	0	0

FOOD	PORTION	CALS	PROT	FAT	CHOL	CARB	FIBER	SOD
Peanut	1 tbsp	120	0	14	0	0	0	0
Pumpkin Seed Organic	1 tbsp	120	0	14	0	0	0	0
Sesame Organic	1 tbsp	120	0	14	0	0	0	0
Sesame Toasted Organic	1 tbsp	120	0	14	0	0	0	0
Soy Organic	1 tbsp	120	0	14	0	0	0	0
Sunflower Organic	1 tbsp	120	0	14	0	0	0	0
Walnut	1 tbsp	120	0	14	0	0	0	0
Walnut Organic	1 tbsp	120	0	14	0	0	0	0
Vistive								
Soybean Low Linolenic	1 tbsp	129	0	14	0	0	0	–

OKRA
CANNED
pickled	6 pods (2.3 oz)	18	1	tr	0	4	2	150
Glory								
Cut	½ cup	25	2	0	0	6	2	0
McIlhenny								
Spicy Pickled	1 oz	10	0	0	0	2	1	270
FRESH								
cooked w/ salt	8 pods	19	2	tr	0	4	2	205
luffa chinese okra cooked	1 cup	39	3	tr	0	8	4	422
sliced cooked w/ salt	½ cup	18	2	tr	0	4	2	193
FROZEN								
McKenzie's								
Breaded Okra	1 serv (2.8 oz)	90	3	1	0	17	–	350
Cut	1 serv (3 oz)	25	1	0	0	5	3	35
TAKE-OUT								
batter dipped fried	10 pieces (2.6 oz)	142	2	10	2	12	2	100

OLIVES
green	4 med	15	tr	2	0	tr	tr	312
green	3 extra lg	15	tr	2	0	tr	tr	312
green olive tapenade	1 tbsp	25	0	3	0	1	0	210
ripe	1 sm	4	tr	tr	0	tr	tr	28
ripe	1 lg	5	tr	tr	0	tr	tr	38
ripe	1 jumbo	7	tr	1	0	tr	–	75
ripe	1 colossal	12	tr	1	0	1	–	136
spanish stuffed	5 (0.5 oz)	15	0	1	0	1	0	320

FOOD	PORTION	CALS	PROT	FAT	CHOL	CARB	FIBER	SOD
Peloponnese								
Amfissa	3	45	0	5	0	1	0	200
Ionian Green	3	25	0	3	0	1	0	250
Kalamata Pitted	5	45	0	5	0	1	0	210
Kalamata Spread	1 tsp	15	0	2	0	0	0	160
Stonewall Kitchen								
Mixed Olive Spread	1 tbsp	35	0	2	–	5	–	150
ONION								
CANNED								
cocktail	½ cup	41	2	tr	0	9	2	257
Boar's Head								
Sweet Vidalia In Sauce	1 tbsp	10	0	0	0	2	0	15
French's								
Original French Fried	2 tbsp	45	0	4	0	3	0	60
DRIED								
flakes	1 tbsp	17	tr	tr	0	4	1	1
powder	1 tsp	7	tr	tr	0	2	tr	1
shallots	1 tbsp	3	tr	0	0	1	–	1
Bob's Red Mill								
Minced	1 tbsp	40	1	1	0	8	1	4
FRESH								
cooked w/o salt	1 sm (2 oz)	26	1	tr	0	6	1	2
cooked w/o salt	1 med (3.3 oz)	41	1	tr	0	10	1	3
cooked w/o salt	1 lg (4.5 oz)	56	2	tr	0	13	2	4
cooked w/o salt chopped	1 tbsp	7	tr	tr	0	2	tr	0
raw chopped	1 tbsp	4	tr	tr	0	1	tr	0
raw chopped	½ cup	32	1	tr	0	7	1	3
raw slice	1 (0.5 oz)	6	tr	tr	0	1	tr	1
raw sliced	½ cup	23	1	tr	0	5	1	2
scallions raw	1 med (0.5 oz)	5	tr	tr	0	1	tr	2
scallions raw chopped	¼ cup	8	tr	tr	0	2	1	4
shallots raw chopped	¼ cup	29	1	tr	0	7	–	5
sweet whole raw	1 (11.6 oz)	106	3	tr	0	25	3	26
whole raw	1 sm (2.5 oz)	28	1	tr	0	7	1	3
whole raw	1 med (4 oz)	44	1	tr	0	10	2	4
whole raw	1 lg (5.3 oz)	60	2	tr	0	14	3	6

FOOD	PORTION	CALS	PROT	FAT	CHOL	CARB	FIBER	SOD
Antioch Farms								
Vidalia	1 med	60	1	0	0	14	3	10
Arrowfarms								
Cipoline	2 (1.1 oz)	20	3	0	0	4	5	6
Blue Ribbon								
Yellow	1 med (5.2 oz)	60	2	0	0	14	3	5
Christopher Ranch								
Shallots	1 (1 oz)	20	0	0	0	4	1	6
Earthbound Farm								
Organic Green Onions	¼ cup	10	0	0	0	2	1	5
Organic Red	1 med (5.2 oz)	60	2	0	0	14	3	5
Frieda's								
Cipolline	3 (3 oz)	30	1	0	0	7	2	0
Maui	⅓ cup (1.1 oz)	10	0	0	0	3	1	0
Pearl	⅔ cup (3 oz)	30	1	0	0	7	2	0
Shallots	1 tbsp (1 oz)	20	1	0	0	5	0	0
Nature's Harvest								
Onion	1 med (5.2 oz)	60	2	0	0	14	3	5
Ocean Mist								
Green Onions Chopped	¼ cup	10	0	0	0	2	1	5
OsoSweet								
Onion	1 med (5 oz)	60	2	0	0	14	3	5
FROZEN								
Alexia								
Onion Rings	6 (3 oz)	230	4	12	0	28	4	230
C&W								
Petite Whole	⅔ cup (3 oz)	30	0	0	0	6	tr	10
Farm Rich								
Petals Breaded + Sauce	10 (3 oz)	200	2	12	5	22	1	700
Ian's								
Rings & Strings	5–9 pieces (2.5 oz)	152	2	7	0	16	1	180
TAKE-OUT								
creamed	1 cup	187	5	9	7	22	2	306

FOOD	PORTION	CALS	PROT	FAT	CHOL	CARB	FIBER	SOD
fried	½ cup	57	tr	5	0	3	1	5
rings breaded & fried	8 to 9 (3 oz)	276	4	16	14	31	–	430

OPOSSUM

| roasted | 3 oz | 188 | 26 | 9 | – | 0 | 0 | – |

ORANGE
CANNED
Del Monte

| SunFresh Mandarin | ½ cup | 80 | 0 | 0 | 0 | 19 | tr | 15 |

FRESH

california navel	1	65	1	tr	0	16	3	1
california valencia	1	59	1	tr	0	14	3	0
florida	1	69	1	tr	0	17	4	1
peel	1 tbsp	6	tr	tr	0	2	–	0
sections	1 cup	85	2	tr	0	21	4	0

Frieda's

Cara Cara	1 med (5 oz)	70	1	0	0	16	3	0
Mandarin Delite	1 cup (5 oz)	60	0	0	0	16	3	0
Mandarin Page	1 cup (5 oz)	60	0	0	0	12	3	0
Mandarin Pixie	1 cup (5 oz)	60	0	0	0	16	3	0
Mandarin Satsuma	1 (5 oz)	60	1	0	0	16	3	0
Melogold	½ (6 oz)	50	0	0	0	13	2	0
Seville	1 (3 oz)	40	1	0	0	10	2	0

Sunkist

Cara Cara Navel	1 med	80	1	0	0	21	7	0
Minneola Tangelo	1 (3.8 oz)	70	1	0	0	13	2	0
Moro	1 (5.4 oz)	70	1	0	0	16	3	0
Orange	1 med	80	1	0	0	21	7	0
Satsuma Mandarin	1 (3.8 oz)	50	1	0	0	11	2	0

ORANGE JUICE

canned	1 cup	104	1	tr	0	25	–	6
chilled	1 cup	110	2	1	0	25	–	2
fresh	1 cup	111	2	tr	0	26	–	2
frzn as prep	1 cup	112	2	tr	0	27	1	2
frzn not prep	6 oz	339	5	tr	0	81	2	7
mandarin orange	7 oz	94	2	tr	–	20	–	–
orange drink	6 oz	94	0	0	0	24	–	31

FOOD	PORTION	CALS	PROT	FAT	CHOL	CARB	FIBER	SOD
After The Fall								
24 Karrot Orange	8 oz	120	1	0	0	28	–	55
Bright & Early								
Orange Drink	8 oz	110	0	0	0	30	–	20
Crystal Light								
Sunrise Sunrise Sugar Free Mix as prep	1 serv	5	0	0	0	0	0	0
Dole								
100% Juice	8 oz	110	1	0	0	27	–	15
Florida's Natural								
Calcium & Vitamin D	8 oz	110	2	0	0	26	0	0
Hood								
100% Juice	1 cup	120	0	0	0	30	0	20
Italian Volcano								
Blood Orange Organic	1 serv (6.75 oz)	84	1	0	0	21	1	30
Minute Maid								
Country Style	8 oz	110	2	0	0	27	–	15
Heart Wise	8 oz	110	2	0	0	27	–	20
Kids+	8 oz	110	2	0	0	27	–	20
Light	8 oz	50	0	0	0	13	–	15
Original	8 oz	110	2	0	0	27	–	15
Plus Calcium	8 oz	110	2	0	0	27	–	15
W/ Extra Vitamin C & E Plus Zinc	8 oz	110	2	0	0	27	–	15
Mr. J								
100% Juice Calcium Fortified	1 pkg (4 oz)	60	0	0	0	19	–	–
Naked Juice								
Just OJ	8 oz	110	2	0	0	25	0	0
NutraBalance								
Fortified	1 pkg (4 oz)	60	1	0	0	17	4	25
Odwalla								
100% Juice	8 oz	110	1	0	0	25	0	15
Organic Valley								
W/ Calcium	1 cup	110	2	0	0	26	0	0
Simply								
Orange Calcium Fortified	8 oz	110	2	0	0	26	–	0
Orange Original	8 oz	110	2	0	0	26	–	0
Snapple								
Orangeade	8 oz	120	0	0	0	29	–	10

FOOD	PORTION	CALS	PROT	FAT	CHOL	CARB	FIBER	SOD
SSips								
Orangeade	8 oz	120	0	0	0	31	–	10
Tang								
Orange Drink as prep	1 serv	90	0	0	0	23	0	35
Sugar Free Orange as prep	1 serv (8 oz)	5	0	0	0	0	0	0
Tree Ripe								
100% Juice + Calcium & Vitamins	8 oz	120	1	0	0	29	0	0
Organic 100% Juice	6 oz	90	0	0	0	22	0	10
Tropicana								
Antioxidant Advantage	8 oz	110	2	0	0	26	0	0
Calcium + Vitamin D	8 oz	110	2	0	0	26	0	0
Fiber	8 oz	120	2	0	0	29	3	0
Healthy Heart	8 oz	120	2	0	0	26	0	0
Healthy Kids	8 oz	110	2	0	0	26	0	0
Light 'n Healthy w/ Calcium	8 oz	50	tr	0	0	13	0	10
Light 'n Healthy w/ Pulp	8 oz	50	tr	0	0	13	0	10
No Pulp	8 oz	110	2	0	0	26	0	0
Orangeade	8 oz	111	0	0	0	33	0	0
Organic	8 oz	120	1	0	0	28	0	25
Uncle Matt's								
Organic 100% Juice Pulp Free	8 oz	110	2	0	0	26	0	10
Organic 100% Juice w/ Pulp	8 oz	110	2	0	0	26	0	10
Welsh Farms								
Juice	8 oz	110	0	0	0	27	–	–
TAKE-OUT								
orange julius	1 serv (24 oz)	443	2	tr	0	118	1	10

OREGANO

crumbled	1 tsp	3	tr	tr	0	1	tr	0
ground	1 tsp	6	tr	tr	0	1	1	0

ORGAN MEATS (see BRAINS, GIBLETS, GIZZARD, HEART, KIDNEY, LIVER, SWEETBREADS)

OSTRICH

cooked	3 oz	120	22	3	74	–	–	57

OYSTERS

canned eastern	1 cup	112	11	4	89	6	0	181

FOOD	PORTION	CALS	PROT	FAT	CHOL	CARB	FIBER	SOD
eastern baked	6 med	47	4	1	22	4	0	96
eastern raw	6 med	50	4	1	21	5	0	150
eastern sauteed	6 med	76	5	5	36	3	0	342
smoked	6	33	3	1	26	2	0	259
Brunswick								
Smoked	1 can (3 oz)	140	11	8	23	7	1	230
Bumble Bee								
Smoked	¼ cup	120	10	7	35	6	0	210
Whole	¼ cup	70	7	3	45	3	0	140
Chicken Of The Sea								
Smoked In Oil	1 can (3.75 oz)	140	10	8	45	8	–	280
Smoked In Water	1 can (3.75 oz)	120	12	3	55	10	0	400
Smoked Teriyaki	1 can (3.75 oz)	120	12	3	55	12	1	470
Whole	½ can (2 oz)	80	7	3	35	6	0	220
TAKE-OUT								
breaded & fried	6	368	13	18	108	40	–	677
fritter	1 (1.4 oz)	121	4	6	36	12	tr	276
oysters rockefeller	1 cup	302	18	17	90	22	4	1113
stew	1 cup	208	11	13	78	11	0	892
PANCAKE/WAFFLE SYRUP								
lite	¼ cup	98	0	0	0	27	0	120
pancake syrup	1 pkg (2 oz)	156	0	tr	0	41	0	36
pancake syrup	¼ cup	209	0	tr	0	55	0	48
Eggo								
Lite	¼ cup	110	0	0	0	27	–	180
Original	¼ cup	240	0	0	0	60	–	35
Estee								
Maple	¼ cup	30	tr	0	0	7	–	–
Hungry Jack								
Lite	¼ cup	100	0	0	0	24	0	180
Original	¼ cup	210	0	0	0	52	0	140
Karo								
Pancake Syrup	¼ cup	240	0	0	0	63	–	85
Log Cabin								
Lite	¼ cup	100	0	0	0	25	–	130

FOOD	PORTION	CALS	PROT	FAT	CHOL	CARB	FIBER	SOD
Mrs. Butterworth's								
Lite	¼ cup	100	0	0	0	25	–	130
Smucker's								
Breakfast Syrup Sugar Free	¼ cup	30	0	0	0	8	–	60
Stonewall Kitchen								
Maine Maple	¼ cup	210	0	0	0	54	0	5
PANCAKES								
FROZEN								
Aunt Jemima								
Buttermilk	3 (3 oz)	210	6	4	20	40	2	600
Buttermilk Low Fat	3 (3 oz)	210	6	4	20	40	2	560
Whole Grain	3 (3 oz)	230	7	6	20	38	3	480
Eggo								
Buttermilk	3	280	6	9	15	44	1	580
Minis	11	260	5	8	10	42	1	550
Golden								
Potato Latkes	1 (1.3 oz)	70	2	3	<5	10	1	190
Ian's								
Blueberry	1 (1.3 oz)	100	3	2	<5	19	1	150
Pancake	1 (1.3 oz)	100	3	2	<5	19	1	150
Inland Valley								
Potato	1 (2 oz)	120	2	8	20	12	2	310
McCain								
Homestyle BabyCakes	4 pieces (2.6 oz)	150	1	9	0	17	2	440
Ratner's								
Potato Latkes	2 (3 oz)	160	3	7	0	23	1	530
MIX								
Arrowhead Mills								
Gluten Free Pancake & Waffle as prep	2 (5 in)	240	11	6	57	42	0	312
Don's Chuck Wagon								
Buckwheat Mix	⅓ cup	160	5	1	0	33	1	457
Hodgson Mill								
Buckwheat not prep	⅓ cup	140	5	1	0	28	3	290
Whole Wheat Buttermilk not prep	⅓ cup	120	4	1	0	28	4	321

FOOD	PORTION	CALS	PROT	FAT	CHOL	CARB	FIBER	SOD
Hungry Jack								
Buttermilk Pancake & Waffle not prep	⅓ cup	150	4	2	–	31	tr	550
Easy Pack Blueberry not prep	½ cup	200	5	3	–	40	1	640
Pancake & Waffle Extra Light & Fluffy not prep	⅓ cup	150	4	2	–	30	tr	600
Potato not prep	2 tbsp	70	2	0	–	15	1	360
King Arthur								
Multi-Grain Buttermilk not prep	6 tbsp	160	7	2	5	31	5	180
TAKE-OUT								
buckwheat	1 (7 in)	142	5	5	45	19	2	366
plain	1 (7 in)	183	4	3	7	35	1	407
potato	1 (1.3 oz)	70	2	4	26	8	1	151
w/ butter & syrup	2 (8.1 oz)	520	8	14	58	91	–	1104
whole wheat	1 (7 in)	183	6	8	47	23	3	489

PANCREAS (*see* SWEETBREAD)

PANINI (*see* SANDWICHES)

PAPAYA

FOOD	PORTION	CALS	PROT	FAT	CHOL	CARB	FIBER	SOD
fresh	1	117	2	tr	0	30	–	8
fresh cubed	1 cup	54	1	tr	0	14	–	4
Del Monte								
In Extra Light Syrup w/ Passion Fruit Puree	½ cup	70	1	0	0	17	1	5
Frieda's								
Mexican	1 cup (5 oz)	50	1	0	0	14	3	0

PAPAYA JUICE

FOOD	PORTION	CALS	PROT	FAT	CHOL	CARB	FIBER	SOD
nectar	1 cup	142	tr	tr	0	36	–	14
Lakewood								
Red	8 oz	80	1	0	0	20	2	6
Yellow	8 oz	105	2	0	0	26	2	5
Langers								
Papaya Delight 100% Juice	8 oz	130	1	0	0	32	1	10
Old Orchard								
Nectar Cocktail	8 oz	120	0	0	0	30	–	15

FOOD	PORTION	CALS	PROT	FAT	CHOL	CARB	FIBER	SOD
PAPRIKA								
dried	1 tsp	1	tr	tr	0	tr	tr	2
Bob's Red Mill								
Hungarian	½ tsp	11	0	0	0	2	1	0
PARSLEY								
dried	1 tbsp	4	tr	tr	0	1	1	7
freeze dried	1 tbsp	1	tr	tr	0	tr	tr	2
fresh chopped	1 tbsp	1	tr	tr	0	tr	tr	2
fresh sprigs	5 (1.8 oz)	18	1	tr	0	3	2	28
Dorot								
Chopped Cubes frzn	1 cube (4 g)	5	tr	tr	0	tr	tr	17
Frieda's								
Parsley Root	⅔ cup	10	2	1	0	2	1	70
PARSNIPS								
fresh cooked	1 (5.6 oz)	130	2	tr	0	31	–	17
fresh sliced cooked	½ cup	63	1	tr	0	15	–	8
raw sliced	½ cup	50	1	tr	0	12	–	7
Frieda's								
Sliced	1 cup	100	2	0	0	24	7	10
PASSION FRUIT								
purple fresh	1	18	tr	tr	0	4	–	5
PASSION FRUIT JUICE								
purple	1 cup	126	1	tr	0	34	–	–
yellow	1 cup	149	2	tr	0	36	–	15
PASTA (see also NOODLES, PASTA DINNERS, PASTA SALAD)								
DRY								
corn cooked	1 cup (4.9 oz)	176	4	1	0	39	7	0
elbows	1 cup	389	13	2	0	78	–	8
elbows cooked	1 cup (4.9 oz)	197	7	1	0	40	2	1
shells small cooked	1 cup (4 oz)	162	5	1	0	33	2	1
spaghetti cooked	1 cup (4.9 oz)	197	7	1	0	40	2	1
spinach spaghetti cooked	1 cup (4.9 oz)	182	6	1	0	37	–	20
spirals cooked	1 cup (4.7 oz)	189	6	tr	0	38	2	1

FOOD	PORTION	CALS	PROT	FAT	CHOL	CARB	FIBER	SOD
vegetable cooked	1 cup (4.7 oz)	172	6	tr	0	36	6	8
whole wheat all shapes cooked	1 cup	174	7	tr	0	37	4	4
Annie Chun's								
Soba Noodles	2 oz	200	8	1	0	39	3	390
Barilla								
Pastina	2 oz	210	8	2	65	40	2	20
Penne	1 cup (2 oz)	200	7	1	0	42	2	0
Plus Penne	2 oz	200	10	1	0	38	4	25
Plus Rotini not prep	2 oz	210	10	2	0	38	4	25
Catelli								
All Shapes	3 oz	301	10	1	–	63	–	3
Bistro Cracked Black Pepper Fettucine	¼ pkg	320	00	1	0	65	2	110
Bistro Italian Herb Fettuccine	¼ pkg	310	11	2	0	64	3	5
Bistro Lemon Pepper Linguine	¼ pkg	320	00	2	0	64	3	268
Bistro Rainbows	3 oz	320	11	1	0	66	2	5
Bistro Spinach Lasagne	3 oz	320	00	2	0	64	3	35
Bistro Sun Dried Tomato & Basil Spaghettini	¼ pkg	320	11	2	0	65	3	10
Bistro Vegetable Fusilli	3 oz	320	11	1	0	65	2	10
Healthy Harvest Flax Omega-3	3 oz	290	11	3	0	60	6	0
Healthy Harvest Multigrain	3 oz	310	11	2	0	60	6	0
Healthy Harvest Organic Whole Wheat	3 oz	320	11	2	0	64	3	0
Healthy Harvest Whole Wheat All Shapes	3 oz	310	12	2	0	62	5	0
DeBoles								
Angel Hair Rice Pasta	¼ pkg (2 oz)	210	4	1	0	46	tr	15
Elbow Corn Pasta Wheat Free	⅙ pkg (2 oz)	200	4	2	0	43	5	15
Fettuccine	¼ pkg (2 oz)	210	7	1	0	41	1	0

FOOD	PORTION	CALS	PROT	FAT	CHOL	CARB	FIBER	SOD
Organic Angel Hair Whole Wheat	¼ pkg (2 oz)	210	7	2	0	42	5	10
Organic Eggless Ribbon	1 cup (2 oz)	210	7	1	0	43	1	5
Organic Fettucine Spinach	¼ pkg (2 oz)	210	7	1	0	43	3	20
Organic Lasagna	¼ pkg (2.5 oz)	260	9	1	0	54	1	5
Organic Rigatoni Whole Wheat	1 cup (2 oz)	210	7	2	0	42	5	10
Rigatoni	¼ pkg (2 oz)	210	7	1	0	41	1	0
DeCecco								
Spaghetti w/ Spinach	⅛ pkg (2 oz)	200	7	1	0	41	2	0
Dreamfields								
Lasagna not prep	2 pieces (2 oz)	190	7	1	0	42	5	15
Rotini not prep	⅔ cup (2 oz)	190	7	1	0	42	5	15
Eden								
Bifun Pasta not prep	2 oz	200	5	1	5	44	0	5
Harusame Pasta not prep	2 oz	190	0	0	0	47	0	5
Kudzu	2 oz	200	0	0	0	48	2	0
Organic Gemelli Spelt & Buckwheat not prep	½ cup (2 oz)	210	6	2	0	41	4	15
Organic Ribbons Artichoki not prep	½ cup (2 oz)	210	9	2	0	40	2	10
Organic Rigatoni Kamut & Buckwheat not prep	½ cup (2 oz)	200	9	2	0	39	5	10
Organic Spaghetti 100% Whole Wheat not prep	2 oz	210	10	2	0	40	6	0
Organic Spirals Flax Rice not prep	½ cup (2 oz)	200	9	2	0	40	4	10
Organic Spirals Rye not prep	½ cup (2 oz)	200	6	0	0	44	8	10
Organic Spirals Spinach not prep	½ cup (2 oz)	210	8	1	0	41	5	30
Organic Udon not prep	¼ pkg	200	6	2	0	38	3	80
Organic Udon Spelt not prep	¼ pkg	200	8	1	0	39	2	75

FOOD	PORTION	CALS	PROT	FAT	CHOL	CARB	FIBER	SOD
Organic Vegetable Alphabets not prep	½ cup (2 oz)	210	9	2	0	40	4	20
Organic Vegetable Shells not prep	½ cup (2 oz)	210	9	2	0	40	4	20
Organic Ziti Rigati Spelt not prep	½ cup (2 oz)	210	7	2	0	41	5	10
Soba Japanese 100% Buckwheat not prep	2 oz	200	6	1	0	43	3	5
Soba Japanese Lotus Root not prep	2 oz	190	9	1	0	37	4	470
Soba Japanese Mugwort not prep	2 oz	190	8	1	0	37	2	550
Soba Japanese Wild Yam not prep	2 oz	190	9	1	0	37	2	510
Udon Japanese Brown Rice not prep	2 oz	190	8	1	0	38	2	510
Udon Japanese not prep	2 oz	190	8	2	0	37	3	660
Food For Life								
Ezekiel 4:9 Sprouted Grain	2 oz	210	9	2	0	39	7	10
Hodgson Mill								
Lasagne Whole Wheat not prep	2 oz	190	9	1	0	41	6	10
Organic Fettuccine Whole Wheat w/ Milled Flax Seed not prep	2 oz	200	9	2	0	40	6	10
Pasta Ribbons Whole Wheat not prep	2 oz	190	10	1	0	34	5	15
Spaghetti Whole Wheat not prep	2 oz	190	9	1	0	41	6	10
Veggie Bows not prep	2 oz	200	8	1	0	41	1	15
Wagon Wheels Veggie not prep	2 oz	200	8	1	0	41	1	15
LifeStream								
Organic All Shapes	2 oz	208	9	4	0	36	8	15
Lundberg								
Organic Spaghetti Brown Rice	2 oz	210	4	2	0	44	3	5
Maddy's								
Gluten Free not prep	4 oz	310	5	2	0	66	2	120

FOOD	PORTION	CALS	PROT	FAT	CHOL	CARB	FIBER	SOD
Mueller's								
Elbow Macaroni not prep	½ cup	210	7	1	0	41	2	0
Multi Grain Rotini not prep	1 cup (2 oz)	190	8	2	0	40	5	15
Notta Pasta								
Rice Pasta All Shapes	2 oz	200	3	0	0	48	2	20
Rice Select								
Orzo Original not prep	⅓ cup	210	7	1	0	42	–	0
Ronzoni								
Healthy Harvest Multigrain Spaghetti	⅐ pkg (2 oz)	190	7	2	0	40	5	0
Healthy Harvest Whole Wheat Blend Spaghetti	⅐ pkg (2 oz)	180	6	1	0	42	6	0
Lasagne	2½ pieces (2 oz)	210	7	1	0	42	2	0
Smart Pasta not prep	2 oz	180	6	1	0	43	8	5
San Giorgio								
Elbows not prep	½ cup	210	7	1	0	42	2	0
FRESH								
cooked	2 oz	75	3	1	33	14	–	3
spinach cooked	2 oz	74	3	1	19	14	–	3
REFRIGERATED								
Buitoni								
Angel Hair	1¼ cups	230	10	3	50	43	2	20
Fettuccine	1¼ cups	240	10	3	55	45	2	20
Fettuccine Spinach	1¼ cups	260	12	3	75	45	2	110
Linguine	1¼ cups	240	10	3	55	45	2	20
Ravioletti Three Cheese	1 cup	270	12	6	35	43	2	330
Ravioli Doublestuffed Mozzarella & Herb	1½ cups	340	16	12	55	43	3	620
Ravioli Four Cheese 100% Whole Wheat	1¼ cups	320	16	10	65	42	5	690
Ravioli Chicken & Roasted Garlic	1¼ cups	340	14	11	50	47	2	550
Ravioli Chicken Parmesan	1¼ cups	310	14	8	55	45	2	620
Ravioli Classic Beef	1¼ cups	340	15	10	60	48	2	530
Ravioli Garden Vegetable	1 cup	250	11	5	40	39	2	500
Ravioli Light Four Cheese	1¼ cups	230	12	4	35	37	2	390
Tortellini Herb Chicken	1 cup	340	13	9	40	52	2	410
Tortellini Mixed Cheese	1 cup	320	15	7	60	50	3	500
Tortellini Spinach Cheese	1 cup	320	15	7	55	49	3	510
Tortellini Three Cheese	1 cup	320	15	7	40	50	3	480

FOOD	PORTION	CALS	PROT	FAT	CHOL	CARB	FIBER	SOD
Tortelloni Cheese & Roasted Garlic	1 cup	270	12	8	35	37	2	360
Tortelloni Chicken & Prosciutto	1 cup	320	14	9	40	46	2	630
Tortelloni Mozzarella & Herb	1 cup	330	14	9	40	47	2	450
Tortelloni Mozzarella & Pepperoni	1 cup	330	15	10	45	45	2	440
Tortelloni Portabello Mushroom & Cheese	1 cup	290	10	6	25	49	3	430
Tortelloni Sun Dried Tomato	1 cup	310	12	9	25	46	3	340
Tortelloni Sweet Italian Sausage	1 cup	330	13	9	35	48	3	280
Pasta Prima								
Ravioli Spinach & Mozzarella	1 cup	200	9	5	27	29	4	390
Ravioli Sun Dried Tomato & Mozzarella	1 cup	200	9	5	27	29	3	290

PASTA DINNERS (see also PASTA SALAD)
CANNED

FOOD	PORTION	CALS	PROT	FAT	CHOL	CARB	FIBER	SOD
Annie's Homegrown								
Organic All Stars	1 cup	150	4	1	0	31	tr	680
Organic BernieOs	1 cup	150	4	1	0	31	tr	680
Organic Cheesy Ravioli	1 cup	180	6	4	5	31	3	730
Organic P'sghetti Loops	1 cup	190	9	4	0	29	2	650
Chef Boyardee								
99% Fat Free Beef Ravioli	1 cup	170	7	2	10	33	2	880
Beef Ravioli	1 cup	240	8	8	15	35	3	900
Beefaroni	1 cup	260	10	10	25	33	3	990
Mini Ravioli	1 cup	250	8	9	15	35	3	950
Spaghetti & Meat Balls	1 cup	270	11	10	20	32	2	900
SpaghettiOs								
A to Z's w/ Meatballs	1 cup	260	11	9	20	33	3	990
A to Z's w/ Sliced Franks	1 cup	230	9	6	20	32	2	990
Mini Beef Ravioli In Meat Sauce	1 cup	260	11	5	10	43	5	1060
Pasta	1 cup	180	6	1	5	37	3	630
Plus Calcium	1 cup	170	6	1	5	35	3	620

FOOD	PORTION	CALS	PROT	FAT	CHOL	CARB	FIBER	SOD
FROZEN								
Bertolli								
Meatballs Pomodoro & Penne	1 serv (12 oz)	600	27	31	50	54	6	1370
Boca								
Lasagna Meatless	1 pkg (9.4 oz)	290	21	5	15	42	5	880
Cedarlane								
Zone Chicken & Vegetables Pasta & Ginger	1 pkg (10 oz)	340	24	12	140	35	3	650
Zone Lasagna Vegetable	1 pkg (10.9 oz)	310	24	12	15	33	5	910
Celentano								
Cheese Ravioli	4 (4.3 oz)	230	11	4	30	36	2	290
Contessa								
Ravioli Portobello	6 (6.7 oz)	360	14	17	65	39	2	640
Glory								
Macaroni & Cheese	1 pkg	480	21	23	90	47	1	1300
Glutino								
Gluten Free Duo Mushroom Penne	1 pgk (10.5 oz)	380	8	6	5	73	5	720
Gluten Free Macaroni & Cheese	1 pkg (8.8 oz)	430	19	20	45	44	2	1430
Gluten Free Penne Alfredo	1 pkg (9.1 oz)	340	15	8	50	48	3	830
Golden Cuisine								
Cheese Manicotti	1 pkg	360	21	12	50	43	6	773
Spaghetti & Meatballs	1 pkg	490	22	22	33	51	12	800
Tuna Casserole	1 pkg	386	25	8	41	53	8	700
Green Giant								
Skillet Meal Chicken & Cheesy Pasta as prep	1 ¼ cups	270	15	6	33	42	4	740
Healthy Choice								
Breaded Chicken Breast w/ Mac & Cheese	1 pkg	290	24	5	40	35	3	600
Creamy Garlic Shrimp w/ Bow Tie Pasta	1 pkg (11.5 oz)	280	13	5	25	44	5	600
Fettuccini Alfredo	1 pkg	280	12	7	15	40	3	600
Fettuccini Alfredo Chicken	1 pkg	290	24	7	45	32	3	570
Lasagna Bake	1 pkg	270	13	7	20	38	4	600

FOOD	PORTION	CALS	PROT	FAT	CHOL	CARB	FIBER	SOD
Macaroni & Cheese	1 pkg	290	12	7	15	44	5	600
Manicotti	1 pkg	280	14	5	45	44	4	600
Rigatoni w/ Broccoli & Chicken	1 pkg	270	22	7	40	29	5	600
Spaghetti w/ Meat Sauce	1 pkg	310	16	6	25	48	7	600
Stuffed Pasta Shells	1 pkg	290	17	6	20	40	5	470
Helen's Kitchen								
Farfalle & Basil Pasta w/ Tofu Steaks	1 pkg (9 oz)	320	20	11	30	70	5	370
Kashi								
Chicken Pasta Pomodoro	1 pkg (10 oz)	280	19	6	25	38	6	470
Kid Cuisine								
Cheese Blaster Mac & Cheese	1 meal	380	12	11	16	58	5	930
Twist & Twirl Spaghetti w/ Mini Meatballs	1 meal	460	16	14	19	66	6	600
Lean Cuisine								
Cafe Classics Bow Tie Pasta & Chicken	1 pkg (9.5 oz)	240	16	5	45	33	3	670
Cafe Classics Bowl Three Cheese Stuffed Ragatoni	1 pkg (10 oz)	260	12	7	20	38	4	690
Cafe Classics Cheese Lasagna w/ Chicken Breast Scallopini	1 pkg (10 oz)	290	18	8	30	36	3	610
Cafe Classics Four Cheese Cannelloni	1 pkg (9.1 oz)	260	18	7	20	30	3	690
Cafe Classics Grilled Chicken & Penne Pasta	1 pkg (12 oz)	320	19	5	40	52	4	560
Cafe Classics Jumbo Rigatoni w/ Meatballs	1 pkg (15.4 oz)	400	24	8	40	58	6	890
Cafe Classics Lasagna w/ Meat Sauce	1 pkg (10.5 oz)	310	19	7	30	43	4	650
Cafe Classics Macaroni & Cheese	1 pkg (10 oz)	300	16	7	20	43	1	650
Cafe Classics Macaroni & Beef	1 pkg (9.5 oz)	270	16	5	20	39	3	600
Cafe Classics Penne Pasta w/ Tomato Basil Sauce	1 pkg (10 oz)	270	9	3	0	51	5	390

FOOD	PORTION	CALS	PROT	FAT	CHOL	CARB	FIBER	SOD
Cafe Classics Roasted Chicken w/ Lemon Pepper Fettuccini	1 pkg (8.1 oz)	250	16	6	30	32	2	670
Cafe Classics Shrimp & Angel Hair Pasta	1 pkg (10 oz)	240	14	5	50	35	2	640
Cafe Classics Spaghetti w/ Meat Sauce	1 pkg (11.5 oz)	280	13	4	15	48	3	580
Cafe Classics Spaghetti w/ Meatballs	1 pkg (9.5 oz)	270	17	5	25	38	3	590
Dinnertime Selects Chicken Fettuccini	1 pkg (12 oz)	360	20	7	45	54	4	700
One Dish Favorites Alfredo Pasta w/ Chicken & Broccoli	1 pkg (10 oz)	270	17	6	40	38	3	690
One Dish Favorites Angel Hair Pasta Marinara	1 pkg (10 oz)	260	8	4	5	48	4	690
One Dish Favorites Cheese Ravioli	1 pkg (8.5 oz)	250	10	6	35	38	3	590
One Dish Favorites Chicken Fettuccini	1 pkg (9.25 oz)	280	22	7	35	33	2	690
One Dish Favorites Lasagna Cheese Florentine Bake	1 pkg (10 oz)	270	19	6	25	35	3	690
One Dish Favorites Lasagna Chicken Florentine	1 pkg (10 oz)	270	19	6	25	35	3	690
One Dish Favorites Lasagna Classic Five Cheese	1 pkg (11.5 oz)	330	18	7	25	48	4	690
Skillet Chicken Alfredo	1 serv	180	12	4	25	25	3	490
Marie Callender's								
Meat Lasagna	1 cup	240	14	9	45	24	2	950
Michelina's								
Lasagna w/ Meat Sauce	1 pkg (9 oz)	340	14	12	35	40	3	740
Milton's								
Lasagna Vegetable w/ Multi-Grain Pasta	1 cup (8 oz)	340	17	16	60	30	5	950
Mon Cuisine								
Vegetarian Spaghetti & Meatballs	1 pkg (10 oz)	360	29	4	0	54	9	440
Organic Classics								
Cajun Chicken Tetrazzine w/ Penne Pasta	1 pkg (10 oz)	370	25	10	55	43	3	490

FOOD	PORTION	CALS	PROT	FAT	CHOL	CARB	FIBER	SOD
Chicken Cacciatore w/ Penne Pasta	1 pkg (10 oz)	270	20	4	40	37	3	390
Macaroni & Meat Sauce	1 pkg (10 oz)	340	16	9	20	49	3	580
Savvy Faire								
Lasagna Florentine	1 pkg (9.2 oz)	300	19	19	5	14	5	970
Seeds Of Change								
Chicken Fettuccine Alfredo	1 pkg (10 oz)	340	23	10	50	40	3	670
Lasagna Creamy Spinach	1 pkg (11 oz)	370	19	16	35	36	7	750
Lasagne Vegetable	1 pkg (11 oz)	310	16	9	20	41	5	1020
Penne Marinara	1 pkg (11 oz)	290	13	7	10	44	5	680
South Beach								
Penne & Chicken In Roasted Red Pepper Sauce w/ Broccoli	1 pkg	290	24	13	50	26	8	1120
Stouffer's								
Cheesy Spaghetti Bake	1 pkg (12 oz)	460	21	24	120	39	4	950
Chicken Parmigiana	1 pkg (13.13 oz)	460	18	18	35	56	4	1060
Escalloped Chicken & Noodles	1 pkg (8 oz)	330	14	18	35	28	2	910
Homestyle Chicken & Noodles	1 pkg (12 oz)	340	25	12	65	33	3	950
Italian Sausage Stuffed Rigatoni	1 pkg (9.13 oz)	380	18	14	60	46	2	880
Lasagna Vegetable	1 pkg (10.5 oz)	390	17	18	25	40	4	730
Lasagna Bake w/ Meat Sauce	1 pkg (11.5 oz)	380	18	13	40	47	5	1080
Macaroni & Cheese	1 cup (6 oz)	350	15	17	25	34	2	920
Macaroni & Beef	1 pkg (11.5 oz)	330	19	11	40	38	4	920
Manicotti Cheese	1 pkg (9 oz)	360	18	14	70	41	2	920

FOOD	PORTION	CALS	PROT	FAT	CHOL	CARB	FIBER	SOD
Shrimp Scampi	1 pkg (14 oz)	410	21	11	80	57	6	990
Tuna Noodle Casserole	1 pkg (10 oz)	350	18	15	40	35	2	930
Turkey Tettrazini	1 pkg (10 oz)	380	19	20	60	32	1	970
Taste Above								
Meatless Thai Peanut Coconut Sauce w/ Veggie Chicken & Vermicelli	1 pkg (10 oz)	320	26	19	0	22	8	300
Meatless Tuscan Marinara Sauce w/ Veggie Chicken & Penne Pasta	1 pkg (10 oz)	320	26	19	0	22	8	300
Weight Watchers								
Smart Ones Lasagna w/ Meat Sauce	1 pkg (10.5 oz)	300	17	6	25	43	5	780
Yves								
Meatless Lasagna	1 pkg (10.5 oz)	300	17	3	0	51	4	650
MIX								
A Taste Of Thai								
Coconut Ginger	1 cup	280	5	7	0	5	1	680
Pad Thai For Two	½ pkg	345	5	1	0	89	4	395
Peanut Noodles as prep	1 cup	330	7	10	0	53	1	490
Red Curry Noodles as prep	1 cup	280	4	8	5	51	2	820
Annie's Homegrown								
Gluten Free Rice Pasta & Cheddar as prep	1 cup	330	9	5	10	60	0	510
Organic Shells & Real Aged Wisconsin Cheddar as prep	1 cup	370	10	15	39	48	2	540
Organic Whole Wheat Shells & Cheddar as prep	1 cup	360	11	15	42	48	5	530
Organic Skillet Meals Beef Stroganoff as prep	1 cup	320	5	13	51	16	1	520
Organic Skillet Meals Cheddar & Herb Chicken as prep	1 cup	310	7	7	75	30	1	330
Organic Skillet Meals Cheese Lasagna as prep	1 cup	280	5	9	36	25	1	580

FOOD	PORTION	CALS	PROT	FAT	CHOL	CARB	FIBER	SOD
Organic Skillet Meals Cheeseburger Macaroni as prep	1 cup	350	6	13	51	27	1	500
Organic Skillet Meals Chicken Fettucine as prep	1 cup	330	6	8	84	27	1	340
Organic Skillet Meals Creamy Tuna Spirals as prep	1 cup	260	7	7	30	30	1	440
Shells & Real Aged Wisconsin Cheddar as prep	1 cup	290	10	5	10	51	1	550
Shells & White Cheddar as prep	1 cup	290	10	5	10	51	1	550
Back To Nature								
Alfredo & Gemelli as prep	1 cup	340	7	11	30	48	1	590
Macaroni & Cheese as prep	1 cup	320	6	10	24	48	1	640
White Cheddar & Spirals as prep	1 cup	330	7	12	30	48	1	640
Carapelli								
Penne Alfredo as prep	1 cup	240	9	1	5	47	4	960
Spirals Creamy Tomato as prep	1 cup	240	9	1	0	49	4	900
DeBoles								
Organic Macaroni & Cheese Whole Wheat as prep	1 cup	410	11	14	42	60	9	384
Pasta & Cheese as prep	1 cup	420	10	15	51	60	6	384
Rice Shells & Cheddar as prep	½ cup	260	3	8	24	57	1	216
Knorr								
Pasta & Sauce Jalapeno Jack as prep	1 cup	230	8	3	3	45	2	504
Pasta Sides w/ Whole Grains Alfredo as prep	⅔ cup	300	10	11	15	42	4	864
Kraft								
Bistro Deluxe Sundried Tomato Parmesan as prep	1 cup	300	12	10	30	40	3	890
Pasta Roni								
Angel Hair w/ Herbs as prep	1 cup	310	9	13	5	41	2	820

FOOD	PORTION	CALS	PROT	FAT	CHOL	CARB	FIBER	SOD
Chicken as prep	1 cup	300	9	12	5	39	2	1060
Chicken Quesadilla as prep	1 cup	310	10	13	5	40	2	860
Fettuccine Alfredo as prep	1 cup	450	11	25	5	47	2	1140
Nature's Way Mushrooms In Cream Sauce as prep	1 cup	280	9	10	5	39	2	710
Sour Cream & Chives as prep	1 cup	310	8	15	5	38	2	880
Stroganoff as prep	1 cup	350	12	14	10	47	2	970
Road's End Organics								
Mac & Cheese Dairy Free Gluten Free as prep	1 cup	310	8	1	0	63	5	310
Shells & Cheese as prep	1 cup	330	14	1	0	66	7	408
REFRIGERATED								
Country Crock								
Elbow Macaroni & Cheese	1 cup	380	15	17	0	40	1	990
SHELF-STABLE								
TastyBite								
Peanut Sauce w/ Noodles	1 pkg (10 oz)	530	17	19	0	104	12	595
TAKE-OUT								
bami goreng indonesian noodle dish	1 cup	170	5	3	0	25	4	500
lasagna meatless	1 piece (9 oz)	356	19	11	38	46	3	896
lasagna w/ meat	1 piece (8 oz)	362	22	14	56	37	3	838
lasagna w/ vegetbles	1 serv (9 oz)	315	17	10	33	41	4	776
macaroni & cheese w/ ham	1 cup	542	21	33	61	41	3	1375
manicotti cheese filled marinara sauce	1 (5 oz)	229	13	10	83	22	1	615
manicotti cheese filled w/ meat sauce	1 (5 oz)	239	14	11	86	20	3	612
pasta w/ pesto sauce	1 cup	370	10	25	10	27	2	178
ravioli cheese & spinach filled w/ cream sauce	1 cup	362	15	17	160	38	2	962
ravioli meat filled w/ marinara sauce	1 cup	372	22	16	168	36	3	1488
ravioli cheese w/ tomato sauce	1 cup	335	14	14	158	38	2	1570
rigatoni w/ sausage sauce	¾ cup	260	10	12	59	28	3	106

FOOD	PORTION	CALS	PROT	FAT	CHOL	CARB	FIBER	SOD
spaghetti w/ red clam sauce	1 cup	285	13	8	17	41	3	280
spaghetti w/ sauce & meatballs	2 cups	670	34	26	114	80	12	1820
spaghetti w/ white clam sauce	1 cup	456	25	20	50	43	3	461
tortellini cheese w/ tomato sauce	1 cup	332	14	14	158	38	2	1560
tortellini meat filled w/ marinara sauce	1 cup	281	14	10	90	33	2	1294
tortillini spinach filled w/ marinara sauce	1 cup	238	10	8	72	32	2	1190

PASTA SALAD
MIX
Dole

FOOD	PORTION	CALS	PROT	FAT	CHOL	CARB	FIBER	SOD
Veggie Pasta Salads Broccoli Ranch	1½ cups	230	5	13	5	25	2	490
Veggie Pasta Salads Cheddar Bacon Ranch	1½ cups	370	10	22	25	35	3	470
Veggie Pasta Salads Garden Vegetable	1½ cups	240	5	14	0	25	2	390
Veggie Pasta Salads Italian Herb	1½ cups	270	8	12	5	33	2	330

TAKE-OUT

FOOD	PORTION	CALS	PROT	FAT	CHOL	CARB	FIBER	SOD
pasta salad w/ crab vegetables mayonnaise	1 cup	317	10	16	32	33	2	866
tortellini salad cheese filled w/ vinaigrette dressing	1 cup	333	12	18	144	30	1	1070

PATÉ

FOOD	PORTION	CALS	PROT	FAT	CHOL	CARB	FIBER	SOD
chicken liver canned	1 tbsp	26	2	2	51	1	0	50
duck paté	1 oz	96	4	8	–	1	–	–
fish paté	1 oz	76	3	7	–	1	–	286
liver w/ truffle	1 serv (2 oz)	183	6	16	59	4	–	452
mushroom anchovy paté	1 can (2.25 oz)	130	2	11	5	7	1	400
paté de foie gras smoked canned	1 tbsp	60	1	6	20	1	0	91
pork paté	1 oz	107	3	10	51	1	0	189
pork paté en croute	1 oz	91	3	7	32	3	tr	214

FOOD	PORTION	CALS	PROT	FAT	CHOL	CARB	FIBER	SOD
rabbit paté	1 oz	66	5	5	21	1	–	97
shrimp	1 can (2.25 oz)	140	6	10	25	7	0	450

PEACH
CANNED
FOOD	PORTION	CALS	PROT	FAT	CHOL	CARB	FIBER	SOD
halves in heavy syrup	1 half	60	tr	tr	0	16	–	5
halves in light syrup	1 half	44	tr	tr	0	12	–	4
halves juice pack	1 half	34	tr	tr	0	9	–	3
halves water pack	1 half	18	tr	tr	0	5	–	3
peachsauce	½ cup	120	tr	0	0	32	1	0
spiced in heavy syrup	1 cup	180	1	tr	0	49	–	9
spiced in heavy syrup	1 fruit	66	tr	tr	0	18	–	3
Del Monte								
Carb Clever Sliced	½ cup	30	1	0	0	7	1	10
Freestone Lite Slices	½ cup	60	0	0	0	14	1	10
Freestone Sliced	½ cup	100	0	0	0	24	1	10
Fruit Naturals Chunks	½ cup	70	tr	0	0	17	tr	10
Halves In Heavy Syrup	½ cup	100	0	0	0	24	1	10
Orchard Select Sliced Cling	½ cup	80	tr	0	0	22	tr	10
Sliced In 100% Juice	½ cup	60	0	0	0	15	1	10
Sliced Light Syrup Raspberry Flavor	½ cup	80	tr	0	0	20	tr	10
Liberty Gold								
Sliced Cling In Heavy Syrup	½ cup	100	1	0	0	24	1	10
S&W								
Slices Lightly Sweetened Juice	½ cup	80	1	0	0	19	1	20
Yellow Cling In Heavy Syrup	½ cup	100	0	0	0	24	1	10
DRIED								
halves	10	311	5	1	0	80	11	9
halves	1 cup	383	6	1	0	98	13	12
halves cooked w/ sugar	½ cup	139	1	tr	0	36	–	3
halves cooked w/o sugar	½ cup	99	1	tr	0	25	–	3
Crispy Green								
Crispy Peaches	1 pkg (0.36 oz)	38	0	0	0	9	tr	0
Mrs. May's								
Fruit Chips	1 pkg	35	0	0	0	8	1	0

FOOD	PORTION	CALS	PROT	FAT	CHOL	CARB	FIBER	SOD
FRESH								
peach	1	37	1	tr	0	10	1	0
sliced	1 cup	73	1	tr	0	19	–	1
FROZEN								
slices sweetened	1 cup	235	2	tr	0	60	–	16
C&W								
Ultimate Sliced	¾ cup	50	1	0	0	13	2	0
PEACH JUICE								
nectar	1 cup	134	1	tr	0	35	–	17
After The Fall								
Georgia Peach	8 oz	130	1	0	0	31	–	15
Froose								
Playful Peach	1 box (4.2 oz)	80	1	0	0	19	3	15
PEANUT BUTTER								
chunky	1 cup	1520	62	129	0	56	17	1255
chunky	2 tbsp	188	8	16	0	7	2	156
chunky w/o salt	2 tbsp	188	8	16	0	7	2	5
chunky w/o salt	1 cup	1520	62	129	0	56	17	44
smooth	1 cup	1517	63	128	0	53	15	1234
smooth	2 tbsp	188	8	16	0	7	2	153
smooth w/o salt	2 tbsp	188	8	16	0	7	2	5
smooth w/o salt	1 cup	1517	63	129	0	53	15	44
Arrowhead Mills								
Organic Creamy	2 tbsp	190	8	17	0	6	2	0
Organic Honey Sweetened Creamy	2 tbsp	190	7	16	0	7	2	100
Organic Natural Crunchy	2 tbsp	190	8	17	0	6	2	0
Cream-Nut								
Natural	2 tbsp	190	8	16	0	6	2	35
Estee								
Creamy Low Sodium	2 tbsp	180	7	16	0	6	2	0
Jif								
Creamy	2 tbsp	190	8	16	0	7	2	150
Creamy To Go	1 pkg (2.25 oz)	270	15	32	0	15	4	270
Extra Crunchy	2 tbsp	190	8	16	0	7	2	130
Peanut Butter & Honey	2 tbsp	190	6	15	0	11	2	120
Reduced Fat Creamy	2 tbsp	190	8	12	0	15	2	250

FOOD	PORTION	CALS	PROT	FAT	CHOL	CARB	FIBER	SOD
Reduced Fat Crunchy	2 tbsp	190	8	12	0	15	2	220
Simply	2 tbsp	190	8	16	0	6	2	65
Kettle								
Organic Unsalted	2 tbsp	170	7	14	0	5	2	0
Peanut Better								
Cinnamon Currant	2 tbsp	180	7	14	0	9	3	0
Deep Chocolate	2 tbsp	170	6	13	0	11	2	5
Hickory Smoked	2 tbsp	190	9	16	0	5	3	135
Onion Parsley	2 tbsp	180	8	15	0	6	3	115
Peanut Praline	2 tbsp	180	8	15	0	8	3	0
Rosemary Garlic	2 tbsp	180	8	15	0	7	3	85
Spicy Southwestern	2 tbsp	190	8	17	0	5	3	100
Sweet Molasses	2 tbsp	180	8	14	0	8	2	0
Thai Ginger & Red Pepper	2 tbsp	180	8	15	0	7	3	110
Vanilla Cranberry	2 tbsp	170	7	13	0	9	2	0
Reese's								
Creamy	2 tbsp	200	7	15	0	8	2	140
Smart Balance								
Chunky Omega	2 tbsp	200	7	17	0	6	2	110
Smucker's								
Goober All Flavors	3 tbsp	240	7	13	0	24	2	140
Natural Chunky	2 tbsp	210	8	16	0	6	2	120
Natural Creamy	2 tbsp	210	8	16	0	6	2	120
Natural Honey	2 tbsp	200	7	16	0	9	2	30
Natural No Salt Added Creamy	2 tbsp	210	7	16	0	7	2	0
Natural Reduced Fat Creamy	2 tbsp	200	9	12	0	12	2	120
Teddies								
Old Fashioned	2 tbsp	190	8	16	0	7	3	125
PEANUTS								
chocolate coated	¼ cup	193	5	12	3	18	2	15
cooked w/ salt	½ cup	286	12	20	0	19	8	676
dry roasted w/ salt	28 nuts (1 oz)	164	7	14	0	6	1	230
dry roasted w/o salt	28 (1 oz)	164	7	14	0	6	2	2
dry roasted w/o salt	¼ cup	214	9	18	0	8	3	2
honey roasted	¼ cup	191	8	16	0	8	3	95
milk chocolate coated	1	21	1	1	0	2	tr	2

FOOD	PORTION	CALS	PROT	FAT	CHOL	CARB	FIBER	SOD
sugar coated	¼ cup	203	6	13	0	18	2	61
yogurt coated	¼ cup	230	6	16	0	18	2	24
A Taste Of Thai								
Spicy Peanut Bake	¼ pkg	45	1	2	0	7	1	198
Brach's								
Double Dippers Chocolate Covered	15 pieces	210	4	12	10	23	2	65
Estee								
Chocolate Coated Fructose Sweetened	¼ cup	170	5	9	<5	23	1	45
Frito Lay								
Salted	1 oz	160	7	14	0	6	2	170
Salted w/ Shells	½ cup	160	7	14	0	6	2	170
Nuts Are Good								
Buffalo	1 oz	120	3	6	0	16	2	180
Pina Colada	1 oz	130	3	7	0	16	1	0
Raspberry	1 oz	130	3	7	0	16	1	0
Vanilla Rum	1 oz	130	3	7	0	17	1	0
Planters								
Cocktail	1 oz	170	7	14	0	6	2	115
Dry Roasted	1 oz	170	8	14	0	5	2	190
Sunfood								
Organic Wild Jungle	1 oz	174	7	14	0	5	2	5

PEAR
CANNED

FOOD	PORTION	CALS	PROT	FAT	CHOL	CARB	FIBER	SOD
halves in heavy syrup	1 cup	188	1	tr	0	49	–	13
halves in heavy syrup	1 half	68	tr	tr	0	15	–	4
halves in light syrup	1 half	45	tr	tr	0	12	–	4
halves juice pack	1 cup	123	1	tr	0	32	–	10
halves water pack	1 half	22	tr	tr	0	6	–	41
Del Monte								
Carb Clever Sliced	½ cup	40	0	0	0	10	1	10
Halves In 100% Juice	½ cup	60	0	0	0	15	1	10
Halves In Light Syrup	½ cup	60	0	0	0	15	1	10
Orchard Select Sliced Bartlett	½ cup	80	tr	0	0	20	2	10
S&W								
Halves In Lightly Sweetened Juice	½ cup	80	0	0	0	21	2	10

FOOD	PORTION	CALS	PROT	FAT	CHOL	CARB	FIBER	SOD
DRIED								
halves	10	459	3	1	0	122	–	10
halves	1 cup	472	3	1	0	125	–	10
halves cooked w/ sugar	½ cup	196	1	tr	0	52	–	4
halves cooked w/o sugar	½ cup	163	tr	tr	0	43	–	4
Bare Fruit								
Organic	1 pkg (0.6 oz)	46	1	0	0	12	2	0
FRESH								
asian	1 (4.3 oz)	51	1	tr	0	13	–	0
pear	1	98	1	1	0	25	4	1
sliced w/ skin	1 cup	97	1	1	0	25	4	1
PEAR JUICE								
nectar	1 cup	149	tr	tr	0	39	–	9
Froose								
Perfect Pear	1 box (4.2 oz)	80	0	0	0	18	3	15
Izze								
Sparkling Pear	8 oz	130	1	0	0	33	–	15
Langers								
Kid's 100% Juice	4 oz	60	0	0	0	14	–	0
PEAS								
CANNED								
green	½ cup	59	4	tr	0	11	–	186
green low sodium	½ cup	59	4	tr	0	11	–	2
Del Monte								
Sweet	½ cup	60	3	0	0	13	4	390
Sweet No Salt Added	½ cup	60	3	0	0	11	4	10
Sweet Very Young Small	½ cup	60	3	0	0	10	4	360
Green Giant								
50% Less Sodium Young Tender Sweet	½ cup	60	4	0	0	11	3	200
Young Tender Sweet	½ cup	60	4	0	0	12	3	400
Le Sueur								
50% Less Sodium Young Tender	½ cup	60	4	0	0	11	3	190
Libby's								
No Salt No Sugar Added	½ cup	70	4	1	0	10	3	15

FOOD	PORTION	CALS	PROT	FAT	CHOL	CARB	FIBER	SOD
Tillen Farms								
Crispy Snapper Pickled	¼ cup	15	1	0	0	3	1	230
DRIED								
split cooked	1 cup	231	16	1	0	41	–	4
Arrowhead Mills								
Organic Green Split not prep	¼ cup	160	12	1	0	24	4	10
HamPeas								
Green Split Peas as prep	½ cup	120	8	1	0	21	4	63
Snapea Crisps								
Baked Original	22 (1 oz)	70	5	8	0	14	2	125
FRESH								
green cooked	½ cup	67	4	tr	0	13	–	2
green raw	½ cup	58	4	tr	0	11	–	3
snap peas cooked	½ cup	34	3	tr	0	6	2	3
snap peas raw	½ cup	30	2	tr	0	5	2	3
Frieda's								
Snow Peas	1 cup	35	2	0	0	6	2	0
Sugar Snap	⅔ cup (3 oz)	35	2	0	0	6	2	0
Mann's								
Snow Peas	1 serv (3 oz)	35	2	0	0	6	2	0
River Ranch								
Sugar Snap	1½ cups	35	2	0	0	6	2	0
FROZEN								
green cooked	½ cup	63	4	tr	0	11	–	70
snap peas cooked	½ cup	42	3	tr	0	7	–	4
Birds Eye								
Steamfresh Garlic Baby Peas & Mushrooms	¾ cup	80	4	2	0	12	3	340
Steamfresh Sweet Peas	⅓ cup	70	5	0	0	12	4	0
C&W								
Alfredo	½ cup	110	6	5	15	11	4	380
Early Harvest Petite No Salt Added	⅔ cup	70	4	0	0	12	4	0
Sugar Snap	⅔ cup	40	2	0	0	7	2	0
Green Giant								
Early June No Sauce	⅔ cup	50	5	1	0	11	4	95
Pictsweet								
Green Peas	⅔ cup	70	5	0	0	12	4	200

FOOD	PORTION	CALS	PROT	FAT	CHOL	CARB	FIBER	SOD
SHELF-STABLE								
TastyBite								
Agra Peas & Greens	½ pkg (5 oz)	138	4	10	3	9	4	417
PECANS								
candied	1 oz	190	tr	17	0	10	5	75
dry roasted	1 oz	187	2	18	0	6	–	0
dry roasted salted	1 oz	187	2	18	0	6	–	260
halves dry roasted w/ salt	20 (1 oz)	200	3	21	0	4	3	110
halves dried	1 cup	721	8	73	0	20	7	1
oil roasted	1 oz	195	2	20	0	5	–	0
oil roasted salted	1 oz	195	2	20	0	5	–	252
Emerald								
Glazed Pecan Pie	¼ cup	150	1	11	0	12	1	110
PECTIN								
liquid	1 oz	3	0	0	0	1	1	0
powder	1 pkg (1.75 oz)	162	0	tr	0	45	4	100
PEPEAO								
dried	¼ cup	18	tr	tr	0	5	–	4
raw sliced	1 cup	25	tr	tr	0	7	–	9
PEPPER								
black	1 tsp	5	tr	tr	0	1	1	1
cayenne	1 tsp	6	tr	tr	0	1	1	1
white	1 tsp	7	tr	tr	0	2	1	0
Emeril's								
Kicked Up Red Sauce	1 tsp	0	0	0	0	0	0	140
PEPPERMINT								
fresh chopped	2 tbsp	2	tr	tr	0	tr	tr	1
PEPPERS								
CANNED								
chili green	1 cup (5.5 oz)	29	1	tr	0	6	2	552
chili green hot chopped	½ cup	17	1	tr	0	4	–	–
chili pepper paste	1 tbsp	6	tr	1	–	1	1	1445
chili red hot	1 (2.6 oz)	18	1	tr	0	4	–	–
chili red hot chopped	½ cup	17	1	tr	0	4	–	–

FOOD	PORTION	CALS	PROT	FAT	CHOL	CARB	FIBER	SOD
green halves	½ cup	13	1	tr	0	3	–	958
jalapeno chopped	½ cup	17	1	tr	0	3	–	995
red halves	½ cup	13	1	tr	0	3	–	958
B&G								
Cherry Hot	1 (1 oz)	10	0	0	0	2	–	310
Cherry Sweet	1 (1 oz)	10	0	0	0	2	–	310
Hot Pepper Rings	7 pieces (1 oz)	0	0	0	0	1	–	310
Pepperoncini	3 pieces (1 oz)	10	0	0	0	2	–	330
Roasted w/ Balsamic Vinegar	½ piece (1 oz)	10	0	0	0	2	–	70
Sweet Fried	1 oz	25	0	2	–	2	1	160
Gertie's Finest								
Piquillo	1 oz	10	1	0	0	2	tr	134
Las Palmas								
Diced Green Chiles	2 tbsp	5	0	0	0	1	1	110
Jalapenos Sliced	3 tbsp	10	tr	0	0	2	0	210
Pace								
Green Chiles Diced	2 tbsp	10	0	0	0	2	tr	100
Tillen Farms								
Bell Peppers Pickled Sweet	¼ cup	25	0	0	0	6	0	0
DRIED								
ancho	1 (0.6 oz)	48	2	1	0	9	4	7
ancho	1 tsp	3	tr	tr	0	1	tr	0
casabel	1 tsp	3	tr	tr	0	1	tr	–
chipotle smoked	1 tsp	3	tr	tr	0	1	tr	–
green	1 tbsp	1	tr	tr	0	tr	–	1
guajillo	1 tsp	3	tr	tr	0	1	tr	–
mulato	1 tsp	3	tr	tr	0	1	tr	–
pasilla	1 (7 g)	24	1	1	0	4	2	6
pasilla	1 tsp	3	tr	tr	0	1	tr	1
red	1 tbsp	1	tr	tr	0	tr	–	1
Frieda's								
California Chili	2 tbsp	15	0	0	0	2	0	15
FRESH								
banana	1 cup (4.4 oz)	33	2	1	0	7	4	16
banana	1 (4 in) (1.2 oz)	9	1	tr	0	2	1	4

FOOD	PORTION	CALS	PROT	FAT	CHOL	CARB	FIBER	SOD
chili green hot	1	18	1	tr	0	4	–	3
chili green hot chopped	½ cup	30	2	tr	0	7	–	5
chili red chopped	½ cup	30	2	tr	0	7	–	5
chili red hot	1 (1.6 oz)	18	1	tr	0	4	–	3
green	1 (2.6 oz)	20	1	tr	0	5	1	1
green chopped	½ cup	13	tr	tr	0	3	1	1
green chopped cooked	½ cup	19	1	tr	0	5	–	1
green cooked	1 (2.6 oz)	20	1	tr	0	5	–	1
habanero	1 tsp	9	1	tr	0	2	1	2
hungarian	1 (0.9 oz)	8	tr	tr	0	2	0	tr
jalapeno	1 (0.5 oz)	4	tr	tr	0	1	tr	tr
jalapeno sliced	1 cup (3.2 oz)	27	1	1	0	5	3	1
red	1 (2.6 oz)	20	1	tr	0	5	1	1
red chopped	½ cup	13	tr	tr	0	3	1	1
red chopped cooked	½ cup	19	1	tr	0	5	–	1
red cooked	1 (2.6 oz)	20	1	tr	0	5	–	1
serrano	1 (6 g)	2	tr	tr	0	tr	tr	1
serrano chopped	1 cup (3.7 oz)	34	2	tr	0	7	4	11
yellow	1 (6.5 oz)	50	2	tr	0	12	–	3
yellow	10 strips	14	1	tr	0	3	–	1
Frieda's								
Peppadew	⅓ cup	40	0	0	0	32	3	80
FROZEN								
green chopped	1 oz	6	tr	tr	0	1	–	1
red chopped	1 oz	6	tr	tr	0	1	–	1
C&W								
Strips	¾ cup	25	1	0	0	4	1	10
Roast Works								
Flame Roasted Red	1 serv (3 oz)	45	1	1	0	7	3	320
PERCH								
FRESH								
cooked	3 oz	99	21	1	98	0	0	67
cooked	1 fillet (1.6 oz)	54	11	1	53	0	0	36
ocean perch atlantic cooked	1 fillet (1.8 oz)	60	12	1	27	0	0	48

FOOD	PORTION	CALS	PROT	FAT	CHOL	CARB	FIBER	SOD
ocean perch atlantic cooked	3 oz	103	20	2	46	0	0	82
ocean perch atlantic raw	3 oz	80	16	1	36	0	0	64
raw	3 oz	77	16	1	76	0	0	52
red raw	3.5 oz	114	18	4	–	0	0	80

PERSIMMONS

FOOD	PORTION	CALS	PROT	FAT	CHOL	CARB	FIBER	SOD
dried japanese	1 (1.2 oz)	93	tr	tr	0	25	5	1
fresh	1 (6 oz)	118	1	tr	0	31	6	2

Frieda's

FOOD	PORTION	CALS	PROT	FAT	CHOL	CARB	FIBER	SOD
Dried Fuyu	⅓ cup (1.4 oz)	140	1	0	0	35	3	10

PHEASANT

FOOD	PORTION	CALS	PROT	FAT	CHOL	CARB	FIBER	SOD
breast cooked	½ breast (4.5 oz)	312	41	15	113	0	0	260
leg cooked	1 (2.6 oz)	184	24	9	67	0	0	154

PHYLLO

FOOD	PORTION	CALS	PROT	FAT	CHOL	CARB	FIBER	SOD
sheet	1 (0.7 oz)	57	1	1	0	10	tr	92

Ekizian

FOOD	PORTION	CALS	PROT	FAT	CHOL	CARB	FIBER	SOD
Sheets	¼ lb	433	12	9	62	76	–	287

Fillo Factory

FOOD	PORTION	CALS	PROT	FAT	CHOL	CARB	FIBER	SOD
Kataifi Shredded Fillo	1 (2 oz)	180	5	2	0	35	4	140
Organic	2 sheets (1.5 oz)	130	4	1	0	27	1	160
Organic Whole Wheat	2 sheets (1.8 oz)	140	4	1	0	30	2	200
Shells Large	1 (0.7 oz)	80	2	2	0	13	0	55

PICANTE (see SALSA)

PICKLES

FOOD	PORTION	CALS	PROT	FAT	CHOL	CARB	FIBER	SOD
bread & butter	6 slices	39	tr	tr	0	9	1	323
dill	1 lg (4.7 oz)	24	1	tr	0	6	2	1731
dill low sodium	1 med (2.3 oz)	12	tr	tr	0	3	1	12
dill sliced	6 slices	7	tr	tr	0	2	1	497
sweet gherkin	1 (1.2 oz)	41	tr	tr	0	11	tr	329
tsukemono japanese pickles sliced	¼ cup	10	tr	tr	0	2	1	180

FOOD	PORTION	CALS	PROT	FAT	CHOL	CARB	FIBER	SOD
B&G								
Bread & Butter	3 slices (1 oz)	25	0	0	0	6	–	190
Kosher Dill	⅓ pickle (1 oz)	0	0	0	0	0	0	200
Kosher Dill No Salt	½ pickle (1 oz)	10	0	0	0	2	–	0
Sour	½ pickle (1 oz)	0	0	0	0	0	0	270
Sweet Gerkins	1 (1 oz)	35	0	0	0	9	–	115
Claussen								
Kosher Dills Whole	½ (1 oz)	5	0	0	0	1	0	330
Del Monte								
Dill Halves	1 piece (1 oz)	5	0	0	0	1	1	370
Hamburger Dill Chips	1 serv (1 oz)	0	0	0	0	0	0	370
Sweet	1 serv (1 oz)	40	0	0	0	10	tr	210
Sweet Gerkins	1 serv (1 oz)	40	0	0	0	10	tr	210
Tiny Kosher Dill	1 serv (1 oz)	5	0	0	0	1	tr	240
Hebrew National								
Dill	1	23	1	0	0	4	–	1570

PIE (see also PIE CRUST, PIE FILLING)
FROZEN
Edwards

FOOD	PORTION	CALS	PROT	FAT	CHOL	CARB	FIBER	SOD
Pie Slices Chocolate Creme	1 slice (2.7 oz)	290	3	17	10	30	tr	200
Pie Slices Key Lime	1 slice (3.2 oz)	330	4	16	35	42	0	250
Pie Slices Oreo Cream	1 slice (2.6 oz)	290	3	17	10	32	1	220
Mrs. Smith's								
Bake & Serve No Sugar Added Apple	1 slice (4.6 oz)	310	3	16	0	40	4	430
Blueberry Crumb	1 slice (4.2 oz)	320	3	14	0	48	2	280
Cherry	1 slice (4.6 oz)	330	3	16	0	44	1	280
Cinnabon Apple Crumb	1 slice (4.6 oz)	350	3	16	0	49	2	340

FOOD	PORTION	CALS	PROT	FAT	CHOL	CARB	FIBER	SOD
Classic Cream Key Lime	1 slice (4.2 oz)	410	5	19	15	56	1	200
Coconut Custard	1 slice (4.4 oz)	300	6	17	65	31	1	260
Deep Dish Berry Burst	1 slice (4.2 oz)	340	3	15	0	51	3	240
Dutch Apple Crumb	1 slice (4.6 oz)	370	3	17	0	52	2	250
Pumpkin Custard	1 slice (4.6 oz)	300	5	15	40	38	2	280
Soda Shoppe Boston Cream	1 slice (2.7 oz)	220	2	9	30	32	0	160
Soda Shoppe Chocolate Cream	1 slice (4.6 oz)	350	4	17	15	47	1	270
Soda Shoppe Lemon Meringue	1 slice (4.2 oz)	300	3	10	40	51	0	190
Sara Lee								
Apple	1 slice (4.6 oz)	340	3	16	0	46	1	310
Cherry	1 slice (4.6 oz)	320	4	14	0	44	0	260
Coconut Cream	1 slice (4.8 oz)	330	3	19	5	42	2	190
Dulce de Leche Caramel Swirl	1 slice (4.4 oz)	400	7	26	5	37	2	100
French Silk	1 slice (4.8 oz)	340	4	21	10	51	2	230
Key West Lime	1 slice (4.2 oz)	400	7	25	5	41	2	95
Lemon Meringue	1 slice (5 oz)	220	1	5	0	41	1	160
Mince	1 slice (4.6 oz)	370	3	15	0	55	2	400
Pumpkin	1 slice (4.6 oz)	260	4	11	30	37	2	460
Southern Pecan	1 slice (4.2 oz)	520	5	24	45	70	3	480
Southern Sweet Potato	1 slice (4.6 oz)	280	4	10	35	45	2	420

FOOD	PORTION	CALS	PROT	FAT	CHOL	CARB	FIBER	SOD
READY-TO-EAT								
Entenmann's								
Peach Raspberry Melba	⅛ pie (2.6 oz)	250	2	9	10	40	tr	160
SNACK								
Lifestream								
Pie Oh-My Apple	1 (3.5 oz)	280	3	11	0	43	2	240
Pie Oh-My Pineapple	1 (3.5 oz)	280	3	11	0	45	2	400
TAKE-OUT								
apple	⅛ of 9 in pie (5.4 oz)	411	4	19	0	58	3	327
banana cream	⅛ of 9 in pie (5.2 oz)	398	7	20	75	49	–	355
blueberry	⅛ of 9 in pie (5.2 oz)	360	4	18	0	49	–	272
butterscotch	⅛ of 9 in pie (4.5 oz)	355	6	18	78	42	–	335
cherry	⅛ of 9 in pie (6.3 oz)	486	5	22	0	69	–	343
chocolate creme	1 slice (4 oz)	344	3	22	6	38	–	153
coconut creme	⅛ of 9 in pie (4.7 oz)	396	6	21	77	46	–	356
coconut custard	⅙ of 8 in pie (3.6 oz)	271	6	14	36	32	–	348
custard	⅛ of 9 in pie (4.5 oz)	262	7	11	87	34	2	256
key lime	1 slice (5 oz)	420	4	14	25	71	tr	210
lemon meringue	1 slice (4.5 oz)	303	2	10	51	53	1	165
mince	⅛ of 9 in pie (5.8 oz)	477	18	18	0	79	–	419
pecan	1 slice (4 oz)	452	5	21	36	65	4	480
pumpkin	1 slice (3.8 oz)	229	4	10	22	30	3	308
vanilla cream	⅛ of 9 in pie (4.4 oz)	350	6	18	78	41	–	327

FOOD	PORTION	CALS	PROT	FAT	CHOL	CARB	FIBER	SOD
PIE CRUST								
FROZEN								
baked	1/8 of 9 in pie	113	1	7	0	11	tr	142
baked	9 in crust	884	8	56	0	85	2	1113
puff pastry shell	1 (1.4 oz)	223	3	15	0	18	1	101
tart shell	1 (1 oz)	149	1	10	0	14	tr	188
Mrs. Smith's								
Deep Dish Shell	1 slice (1 oz)	130	2	7	0	14	0	110
Pepperidge Farm								
Puff Pastry Sheets	1/6 sheet	170	3	11	0	14	tr	200
Puff Pastry Shell	1	190	4	13	0	16	tr	230
MIX								
Jiffy								
Pie Crust Mix	1/2 crust	180	2	10	<5	19	tr	250
READY-TO-EAT								
chocolate crumb	1/8 of 9 in pie	132	1	8	0	14	tr	175
chocolate crumb	1 (9 in crust)	1063	11	65	2	114	3	1411
graham cracker	1 (9 in crust)	1037	9	52	0	137	3	1199
graham cracker	1/8 of 9 in pie	109	1	5	0	14	tr	126
graham cracker dessert shell	1 (1.1 oz)	148	1	7	0	20	tr	171
Nilla Wafers								
Pie Crust	1/6 (1 oz)	140	1	8	5	18	0	85
PIE FILLING								
apple	1 can (21 oz)	599	1	1	0	156	6	259
apple	1/6 can (2.6 oz)	74	tr	tr	0	19	1	32
cherry	1 can (21 oz)	683	3	1	0	175	–	54
cherry	1/8 can (2.6 oz)	85	tr	tr	0	22	–	7
pumpkin pie mix	1 cup	282	3	tr	0	71	–	561

FOOD	PORTION	CALS	PROT	FAT	CHOL	CARB	FIBER	SOD
Comstock								
Blueberry	⅓ cup	100	0	0	0	24	1	10
Country Cherry	⅓ cup	90	0	0	0	23	1	25
Light Cherry	⅓ cup	60	0	0	0	15	1	15
Farmer's Market								
Organic Pumpkin Pie Mix	½ cup	100	0	0	0	25	2	0
PIEROGI								
potato	1 (1.3 oz)	70	3	2	22	11	1	95
Mrs. T's								
Potato & 4 Cheese Blend	3 (4.2 oz)	230	6	7	10	36	1	570
Potato & Cheddar	3 (4.2 oz)	180	6	3	5	34	1	530
PIGEON PEAS								
dried cooked	1 cup	204	11	1	0	39	–	9
dried cooked	½ cup	102	6	tr	0	20	–	5
PIGNOLIA (see PINE NUTS)								
PIG'S FEET								
cooked	1	201	19	14	93	0	0	204
pickled	1	177	12	14	70	tr	0	803
PIKE								
northern cooked	3 oz	96	21	1	43	0	0	42
northern cooked	½ fillet (5.4 oz)	176	38	1	78	0	0	76
northern raw	3 oz	75	16	1	33	0	0	33
roe raw	1 oz	37	7	tr	103	tr	–	–
walleye baked	3 oz	101	21	1	94	0	0	56
walleye fillet baked	4.4 oz	147	30	2	137	0	0	81
PILLNUTS								
canarytree dried	1 oz	204	3	23	0	1	–	1
PIMIENTOS								
canned	1 slice	0	tr	0	0	tr	–	0
canned	1 tbsp	3	tr	tr	0	1	–	2
PINE NUTS								
pignolia dried	1 tbsp	51	2	5	0	1	–	0
pignolia dried	1 oz	146	7	14	0	4	–	1
pinyon dried	1 oz	161	3	17	0	5	–	20

FOOD	PORTION	CALS	PROT	FAT	CHOL	CARB	FIBER	SOD
Frieda's								
Pine Nuts	¼ cup	150	7	15	0	4	1	0
Good Sense								
Pignolias	¼ cup	190	4	15	0	9	4	0
PINEAPPLE								
CANNED								
chunks in heavy syrup	1 cup	199	1	tr	0	52	–	3
chunks juice pack	1 cup	150	1	tr	0	39	–	4
crushed in heavy syrup	1 cup	199	1	tr	0	52	–	3
slices in heavy syrup	1 slice	45	tr	tr	0	12	–	1
slices in light syrup	1 slice	30	tr	tr	0	8	–	1
slices juice pack	1 slice	35	tr	tr	0	9	–	1
slices water pack	1 slice	19	tr	tr	0	5	–	1
tidbits in heavy syrup	1 cup	199	1	tr	0	52	–	3
tidbits in juice	1 cup	150	1	tr	0	19	–	4
tidbits in water	1 cup	79	1	tr	0	20	–	3
Del Monte								
Chunks In Heavy Syrup	½ cup	90	0	0	0	24	1	10
Chunks In Its Own Juice	½ cup	70	0	0	0	17	1	10
Crushed In Heavy Syrup	½ cup	90	0	0	0	24	1	10
Crushed In Its Own Juice	½ cup	70	0	0	0	17	1	10
Fruit Naturals Chunks	½ cup	70	tr	0	0	18	tr	5
Dole								
Chunks Juice Pack	½ cup	60	0	0	0	15	1	10
Liberty Gold								
Crushed No Sugar Added	½ cup	80	tr	0	0	21	2	10
Slices Natural Juice	½ cup	80	tr	0	0	21	1	10
DRIED								
Mrs. May's								
Fruit Chips	1 pkg	35	0	0	0	8	1	0
Sunsweet								
Pineapples	⅓ cup (1.4 oz)	130	0	0	0	34	1	25
FRESH								
diced	1 cup	77	1	tr	0	19	2	1
slice	1 slice	42	tr	tr	0	10	1	1
Cala Fruit								
Golden Sliced	1 serv (3.5 oz)	50	0	0	0	12	1	0

FOOD	PORTION	CALS	PROT	FAT	CHOL	CARB	FIBER	SOD
Frieda's								
Zululand Queen	1 cup (5 oz)	70	1	1	0	17	2	0
FROZEN								
chunks sweetened	½ cup	104	tr	tr	0	27	–	2
Europe's Best								
Aloha Gold	1 cup	70	1	0	0	20	2	0
Roast Works								
Flame Roasted	1 serv (3 oz)	80	1	0	0	22	1	15
PINEAPPLE JUICE								
canned	1 cup	139	1	tr	0	34	–	2
frzn as prep	1 cup	129	1	tr	0	32	–	3
frzn not prep	6 oz	387	3	tr	0	96	–	6
Adina								
Pineapple Ginger Gin-Jah	8 oz	80	0	0	0	19	–	11
Langers								
100% Juice	8 oz	130	0	0	0	33	–	15
Sundia								
Purely	½ cup	60	1	0	0	15	1	0
Walnut Acres								
Organic	8 oz	130	0	0	0	32	–	5
PINK BEANS								
dried cooked	1 cup	252	15	1	0	47	–	3
PINTO BEANS								
dried cooked	1 cup	245	15	1	0	45	15	2
Arrowhead Mills								
Organic Dried not prep	¼ cup	150	9	0	0	27	10	0
Eden								
Organic Spicy	½ cup	120	6	1	–	24	7	200
Organic Spicy Refried	½ cup	90	6	1	–	19	7	180
HamBeens								
Dried as prep	½ cup	120	7	1	0	22	6	63
TAKE-OUT								
stewed w/ viandas	1 cup	222	11	8	8	27	6	668
PISTACHIOS								
dry roasted w/ salt	49 nuts (1 oz)	161	6	13	0	8	3	115
dry roasted w/o salt	49 nuts (1 oz)	162	6	13	0	8	3	3

FOOD	PORTION	CALS	PROT	FAT	CHOL	CARB	FIBER	SOD
in shells	½ cup	165	6	13	0	8	3	89
Love'n Bake								
Pistachio Paste	2 tbsp	160	4	11	0	14	2	0

PITANGA

FOOD	PORTION	CALS	PROT	FAT	CHOL	CARB	FIBER	SOD
fresh	1	2	tr	tr	0	1	–	0
fresh	1 cup	57	1	1	0	13	–	5

PIZZA (see also PIZZA CRUST)

FOOD	PORTION	CALS	PROT	FAT	CHOL	CARB	FIBER	SOD
Alexia								
Pizza Snack Sweet Italian Sausage Roasted Peppers & Parmesan	6 pieces (3 oz)	210	7	10	10	23	1	210
Pizza Snacks Pesto Chicken w/ Fresh Mozzarella	6 pieces (3 oz)	220	9	11	10	23	1	310
Boca								
Supreme w/ Rising Crust Sausage & Pepperoni	⅓ pkg (4.3 oz)	280	13	8	10	38	3	810
Cedarlane								
Zone Cheese	1 (6.5 oz)	380	27	14	30	39	6	700
Celeste								
4 Cheese	1 (5.7 oz)	360	15	16	30	38	2	810
Ellio's								
All Cheesy	1 slice	160	7	5	10	23	1	330
Cheese	1 slice	150	7	4	10	23	1	250
Microwave Single Slice	1 slice	360	16	8	15	53	4	660
Pepperoni	1 slice	160	7	5	10	20	1	310
Farm Rich								
Slices Pepperoni	2 (3.5 oz)	280	14	14	30	22	1	720
Freschetta								
Pepperoni	½ pie (5.8 oz)	470	19	21	45	51	2	1350
Glutino								
Gluten Free Duo Cheese	1 (6.1 oz)	420	10	12	25	68	2	560
Gluten Free Spinach & Feta	1 (6.1 oz)	430	10	16	25	62	4	1000
Healthy Choice								
French Bread Cheese	1 pie	340	22	5	10	51	5	600
French Bread Pepperoni	1 pie	340	21	5	20	52	5	600
French Bread Supreme	1 pie	340	21	5	20	52	5	600
French Bread Vegetable	1 pie	320	17	5	10	51	6	600

FOOD	PORTION	CALS	PROT	FAT	CHOL	CARB	FIBER	SOD
Ian's								
Cheese	1 slice (1.5 oz)	100	4	3	10	14	1	200
Jiffy								
Crust Mix as prep	⅕ crust	180	4	4	0	33	2	220
Kid Cuisine								
Cheese Pizza Painter	1 meal	320	12	6	10	53	5	440
Dip & Dunk Cheese Pizza Strips	1 meal	510	19	14	20	74	9	980
Primo Pepperoni Pizza	1 meal	400	10	7	10	71	6	450
Lean Cuisine								
Casual Eating Deluxe	1 pkg (6 oz)	370	17	9	25	55	3	590
Casual Eating Four Cheese	1 pkg (6 oz)	400	20	9	15	59	3	610
Casual Eating French Bread Cheese	1 serv (6 oz)	320	18	7	20	47	3	520
Casual Eating French Bread Deluxe	1 pkg (6.1 oz)	310	16	9	20	44	3	700
Casual Eating French Bread Pepperoni	1 pkg (5.25 oz)	300	16	7	15	44	2	560
Casual Eating Margherita	1 pkg (6 oz)	320	14	9	5	48	4	340
Casual Eating Pepperoni	1 pkg (6 oz)	380	20	9	25	55	3	680
Casual Eating Roasted Vegetable	1 pkg (6 oz)	330	14	5	10	58	3	450
Casual Eating Spinach & Mushroom	1 pkg (6.1 oz)	310	17	7	15	46	4	420
Casual Eating Three Meat	1 pkg (6.4 oz)	350	21	9	25	48	4	670
Lean Pockets								
Pepperoni	1 (4.5 oz)	280	14	7	25	42	3	720
Sausage & Pepperoni	1 (4.5 oz)	280	13	7	45	41	3	630
Lunchables								
Maxed Deep Dish	1 pkg	510	24	13	15	77	2	850
Mini Pizza	1 pkg	480	17	14	30	72	4	610
Pepperoni Sausage	1 pkg	440	16	12	30	68	3	590
Mr. P's								
Cheese	1 pie (6.5 oz)	410	21	11	25	58	5	510
Red Baron								
Classic Crust 4 Cheese	1 pie (8.6 oz)	740	33	39	65	62	3	1480

FOOD	PORTION	CALS	PROT	FAT	CHOL	CARB	FIBER	SOD
Deep Dish Single Pepperoni	1 pizza	460	17	22	35	41	2	910
French Bread Supreme	1 pie (5.8 oz)	370	16	15	30	43	2	1010
South Beach								
Deluxe w/ Wheat Crust	1 pie	340	30	11	25	37	10	650
Four Cheese w/ Wheat Crust	1 pie	340	31	11	20	36	10	650
Grilled Chicken & Vegetable w/ Wheat Crust	1 pie	330	30	10	25	37	10	600
Pepperoni w/ Wheat Crust	1 pie	350	31	12	25	36	9	700
Stouffer's								
Corner Bistro Flatbread Chicken Bacon & Spinach	1 pkg (9.13 oz)	640	31	29	65	65	3	990
Corner Bistro Flatbread Margherita	1 pkg (9.13 oz)	540	22	22	40	65	4	800
Corner Bistro Flatbread Shrimp & Roasted Garlic	1 pkg (9.33 oz)	600	33	19	115	75	5	610
French Bread Grilled Vegetable	1 pkg (11.63 oz)	340	13	12	15	44	4	570
French Bread Sausage	1 pkg (4.2 oz)	420	15	21	25	43	4	730
French Bread Sausage & Pepperoni	1 pkg (4.2 oz)	460	17	24	30	42	4	880
French Bread White Pizza	1 pkg (10.13 oz)	470	22	23	40	44	4	900
Tony's								
Pizza For One Cheese	1 (6.5 oz)	500	18	22	20	58	3	830
TAKE-OUT								
cheese	1/8 of 16 in pie	423	19	18	37	46	3	823
cheese	16 in pie	3384	151	144	294	372	23	6584
cheese deep dish individual	1 (5.5 oz)	460	15	24	20	47	2	750
cheese & vegetables	1/8 of 16 in pie	428	17	16	19	55	3	967
ground beef	16 in pie	3753	151	172	299	392	20	8642
ham & pineapple	1/8 of 16 in pie	439	19	16	29	55	3	1110
no cheese	1/8 of 16 in pie	262	6	7	0	43	2	356

FOOD	PORTION	CALS	PROT	FAT	CHOL	CARB	FIBER	SOD
pepperoni	⅛ of 16 in pie	469	19	22	37	49	3	1080
white pizza	⅛ of 16 in pie	484	20	17	38	61	2	903

PIZZA CRUST
crust	1 slice (1.7 oz)	130	4	2	0	25	1	230
whole wheat	⅛ crust	140	5	1	0	27	1	150

Alvarado Street Bakery
Sprouted Wheat California Style	⅛ pie	190	4	3	0	35	1	225

PLANTAINS
cooked mashed	1 cup	232	2	tr	0	62	5	10
sliced cooked	1 cup	179	1	tr	0	48	4	8

Chester's
Chips	1 oz	150	tr	9	0	17	2	35

Grab Em Snacks
Chips Black Pepper	1 oz	150	tr	8	0	19	2	180

TAKE-OUT
mofongo	1 serv	320	9	3	7	71	5	1019
ripe fried	2.8 oz	214	1	7	–	38	4	–
sweet baked w/ ice cream	1 serv	285	2	8	0	57	3	65

PLUM JUICE
Sunsweet
PlumSmart Light	8 oz	60	0	0	0	15	3	20

PLUMS
canned in heavy syrup	1 cup	163	1	tr	0	42	3	35
canned purple juice pack	1 cup	146	1	tr	0	38	2	3
canned purple water pack	1 cup	102	1	tr	0	27	2	2
dried japanese	1	9	tr	tr	0	2	tr	96
fresh	1	30	tr	tr	0	8	1	0
pickled	1	34	tr	tr	0	9	tr	0

Eden
Umeboshi Plum Paste	1 tsp	5	0	0	0	0	0	340
Umeboshi Plums	1 (8 g)	5	0	0	0	1	0	690

POI
poi	1 cup	240	1	0	0	65	1	29

FOOD	PORTION	CALS	PROT	FAT	CHOL	CARB	FIBER	SOD
POKEBERRY SHOOTS								
cooked	½ cup	16	2	tr	0	3	–	–
fresh	½ cup	18	2	tr	0	3	–	–
POLENTA								
Bob's Red Mill								
Corn Grits Polenta not prep	¼ cup	130	3	1	0	27	2	0
Frieda's								
Organic	2 slices (3.5 oz)	70	2	0	0	15	1	310
POLLACK								
altantic fillet baked	5.3 oz	178	38	2	137	0	0	166
atlantic baked	3 oz	100	21	1	77	0	0	94
POMEGRANATE								
fresh	1 (5.4 oz)	105	1	tr	0	26	1	5
POMEGRANATE JUICE								
Apple & Eve								
Organic	8 oz	130	0	0	0	33	–	25
Frutzzo								
Organic 100% Juice	1 bottle (12 oz)	130	0	0	0	32	0	25
Izze								
Sparkling Pomegranate	8 oz	80	0	0	0	19	–	5
Langers								
100% Juice	8 oz	150	0	0	0	37	–	15
Naked Juice								
Pomegranate Passion	8 oz	150	1	0	0	38	0	10
Odwalla								
PomaGrand 100% Juice	8 oz	160	0	0	0	40	0	30
Old Orchard								
100% Pure	8 oz	140	0	0	0	34	–	15
POM								
100% Juice	8 oz	140	1	0	0	35	0	30
Pomegranate Blueberry	8 oz	140	1	0	0	34	0	45
Pomegranate Cherry	8 oz	140	1	0	0	33	0	35
Pomegranate Mango	8 oz	140	1	0	0	34	0	70
Pomegranate Tangerine	8 oz	150	1	0	0	37	0	75

FOOD	PORTION	CALS	PROT	FAT	CHOL	CARB	FIBER	SOD
POMPANO								
broiled	4 oz	192	18	13	49	1	0	464
smoked	2 oz	109	12	6	33	0	0	215
steamed	4 oz	232	26	13	71	0	0	83
TAKE-OUT								
battered & fried	4 oz	304	20	21	67	8	tr	132
breaded & fried	4 oz	361	24	22	94	14	1	653
POPCORN (see also POPCORN CAKES)								
air popped	1 cup (0.3 oz)	31	1	tr	0	6	2	0
caramel coated	1 cup (1.2 oz)	152	1	5	–	28	2	72
caramel coated w/ peanuts	⅔ cup (1 oz)	114	2	2	0	23	1	84
cheese	1 cup (0.4 oz)	58	1	4	1	6	1	98
oil popped	1 cup (0.4 oz)	55	1	3	0	6	1	97
Cape Cod								
White Cheddar	2⅓ cups	170	4	12	8	13	2	270
Chester's								
Microwave Butter	3 cups	170	2	12	0	16	3	330
Microwave Cheddar Cheese	3 cups	200	3	13	<5	17	2	340
Cracker Jack								
Butter Toffee	¾ cup	140	2	4	0	22	1	100
Original	½ cup	120	2	2	0	23	1	70
Dale & Thomas								
Caramel	½ cup	75	0	4	0	17	0	72
Hall Of Fame Kettlecorn	½ cup	34	0	1	0	6	1	22
North Country Cheddar	½ cup	73	1	5	1	7	1	68
Peanut Butter & White Chocolate Drizzlecorn	½ cup	115	1	6	0	15	1	83
Purepopped Natural	½ cup	26	1	2	0	3	1	20
Sweet Georgia Pecan	½ cup	96	1	3	3	18	1	123
Toffee Crunch Drizzlecorn	½ cup	107	3	5	1	15	1	88
Jay's								
Caramel	¾ cup	110	tr	0	0	26	1	80
Ok-Ke-Doke Cheese	1 oz	160	2	11	10	13	2	270

FOOD	PORTION	CALS	PROT	FAT	CHOL	CARB	FIBER	SOD
Jolly Time								
America's Best 94% Fat Free	5 cups	100	3	2	0	20	5	200
America's Best White	5 cups	100	4	1	0	24	6	0
America's Best Yellow	5 cups	90	3	2	0	23	9	210
Blast O Butter Light	4 cups	120	3	6	0	16	4	300
Butter Licious Light	5 cups	130	3	5	0	22	4	230
Crispy'n White Light	5 cups	125	3	5	0	20	7	320
Healthy Pop 94% Fat Free	5 cups	100	3	2	0	20	5	200
Healthy Pop Caramel Apple	5 cups	110	4	2	0	23	6	380
Healthy Pop Kettle	4 cups	100	3	2	0	24	4	200
Healthy Pop Minis	4 cups	90	3	2	0	23	8	280
Mallow Magic	2½ cups	180	2	13	0	15	3	200
The Big Cheez	3½ cups	140	2	9	0	17	6	340
White	5 cups	100	4	1	0	24	6	0
Yellow	5 cups	100	4	1	0	24	6	0
LesserEvil								
Black&White	1 cup	120	1	2	0	25	1	180
KettleCorn	1 cup	120	1	2	5	25	2	400
MaplePecan	1 cup	120	1	2	0	25	3	140
PeanutButter & Choco	1 cup	120	2	2	0	24	1	180
SinNamon	1 cup	120	1	2	5	24	2	340
Newman's Own								
Microwave 94% Fat Free	3½ cups	110	3	2	0	20	4	250
Microwave Butter	3½ cups	130	2	5	0	18	3	180
Microwave Butter Boom	3½ cups	130	2	5	0	18	3	290
Microwave Light Butter	3½ cups	120	3	4	0	19	4	170
Microwave Low Sodium Butter	3½ cups	130	2	5	0	18	3	100
Microwave Natural	3½ cups	130	2	5	0	18	3	200
Organic Pop's Corn Butter	3½ cups	160	3	9	0	17	1	190
Organic Pop's Corn No Butter No Salt 94% Fat Free	3½ cups	120	3	2	0	21	1	30
Oogie's								
Romano & Pesto	1 oz	138	3	6	0	16	3	102
Smoked Gouda	1 oz	132	3	7	0	14	3	198
Spicy Chipotle & Lime	1 oz	143	2	7	0	17	3	91
White Cheddar	1 oz	142	3	7	0	17	3	182

FOOD	PORTION	CALS	PROT	FAT	CHOL	CARB	FIBER	SOD
Orville Redenbacher's								
Hot Air	1 cup	15	1	0	0	3	1	0
Kernel Original	1 cup	15	1	0	0	3	1	0
Microwave Butter Light	1 cup	20	3	1	0	3	1	24
Microwave Kettle Korn Sweet	1 cup	35	tr	3	tr	3	1	24
Microwave Movie Theater Butter Light	1 cup	20	1	1	0	3	1	24
Microwave Movie Theater Extra Butter	1 cup	35	tr	3	0	3	1	48
Microwave Natural Light	1 cup	20	3	1	0	3	1	48
Microwave Pour Over Butter	1 cup	40	tr	3	0	3	1	24
Microwave Pour Over Cheddar	1 cup	50	tr	3	0	6	1	72
Microwave Regular Butter	1 cup	35	2	2	0	3	1	300
Microwave Regular Corn On The Cob	1 cup	35	tr	3	0	3	1	24
Microwave Regular Natural	1 cup	15	2	2	0	3	1	72
Microwave Regular Old Fashioned Butter	1 cup	35	tr	2	0	3	1	48
Microwave Regular Tender White	1 cup	40	1	3	0	3	1	72
Microwave Smart Pop Butter	1 cup	15	4	0	0	3	1	24
Microwave Smart Pop Kettle Korn	1 cup	20	1	0	0	3	1	24
Microwave Smart Pop Movie Theater Butter	1 cup	20	4	0	0	3	1	24
Microwave Sweet Cinnabon	1 cup	50	tr	3	0	6	tr	24
Microwave Sweet Honey Butter	1 cup	35	tr	3	0	3	1	24
Microwave Sweet 'N Buttery	1 cup	40	tr	3	tr	3	1	24
Microwave Ultimate Butter	1 cup	30	tr	3	0	3	1	48
Microwave Sweet Caramel	1 cup	90	1	5	0	15	4	24
White	1 cup	15	1	0	0	3	1	0
Poppycock								
The Original	½ cup	160	2	8	10	20	1	90

FOOD	PORTION	CALS	PROT	FAT	CHOL	CARB	FIBER	SOD
Smart Balance								
Light as prep	4 cups	120	3	5	0	18	4	320
Low Fat as prep	5 cups	120	4	2	0	24	5	80
Movie Style as prep	3½ cups	170	2	9	0	18	3	360
Smartfood								
Reduced Fat White Cheddar	3 cups	140	4	6	<5	19	3	280
White Cheddar	1 pkg	160	3	10	5	14	2	290
Snyder's Of Hanover								
Butter	0.6 oz	100	1	8	0	6	1	150
Utz								
Butter	2 cups	170	2	12	0	13	2	250
Cheese	2 cups	160	2	11	5	14	3	300
Puff'n Corn Original Hulless	2 cups	150	1	17	0	11	0	150
Wise								
Butter	1 pkg (0.5 oz)	80	1	5	0	7	1	140
Hot Cheese	1 oz	150	2	10	<5	14	2	280

POPCORN CAKES
Orville Redenbacher's

FOOD	PORTION	CALS	PROT	FAT	CHOL	CARB	FIBER	SOD
Butter	2	60	2	1	0	14	2	65
Caramel	1	40	tr	0	0	10	tr	15
Chocolate	1	45	tr	0	0	10	tr	20
Mini Butter	8	60	2	1	0	12	1	70
Mini Caramel	7	50	1	0	0	13	1	35
Mini Peanut Caramel Crunch	6	60	1	1	0	12	1	30
Mini Peanut Crunch	6	60	2	1	0	12	2	25
Mini Sour Cream & Onion	8	60	2	1	0	12	2	105
White Cheddar	2	60	2	1	0	13	2	65

POPOVER

FOOD	PORTION	CALS	PROT	FAT	CHOL	CARB	FIBER	SOD
home recipe as prep w/ 2% milk	1 (1.4 oz)	87	4	3	46	11	–	82
home recipe as prep w/ whole milk	1 (1.4 oz)	90	4	3	47	11	–	82
mix as prep	1 (1.2 oz)	67	3	2	–	10	–	143

FOOD	PORTION	CALS	PROT	FAT	CHOL	CARB	FIBER	SOD
POPPY SEEDS								
poppy seeds	1 tbsp	47	2	4	0	2	1	2
Bob's Red Mill								
Poppy Seeds	3 tbsp	170	6	14	0	6	3	0
Love'n Bake								
Poppy Seed Filling	2 tbsp	120	2	5	0	18	tr	15
PORGY								
fresh	3 oz	77	18	tr	–	0	0	52

PORK (see also HAM, MEAT STICKS, PORK DISHES)
FRESH

FOOD	PORTION	CALS	PROT	FAT	CHOL	CARB	FIBER	SOD
boneless loin lean & fat roasted	3.5 oz	195	26	9	80	0	0	46
center loin chop bone in broiled	1 (3 oz)	178	22	9	71	0	0	46
center rib chop lean & fat bone in broiled	1 (3 oz)	189	21	11	57	0	0	46
country style ribs bone in lean & fat braised	3.5 oz	288	28	19	110	0	0	61
dehydrated oriental style	1 cup (0.8 oz)	135	3	14	15	tr	0	151
fresh ham rump half lean & fat roasted	4 oz	278	32	16	106	0	0	69
fresh ham shank half lean & fat roasted	4 oz	319	28	22	102	0	0	65
fresh ham whole lean & fat roasted	4 oz	302	30	19	104	0	0	66
ground cooked	4 oz	328	28	23	104	0	0	81
ham hock cooked	1	167	14	12	56	0	0	128
shoulder chop bone in braised	1 (3 oz)	229	23	15	84	0	0	49
sirloin roast lean & fat bone in roasted	4 oz	231	27	13	89	0	0	57
spareribs bone in roasted	3 oz	304	18	26	89	0	0	77
tail simmered	3 oz	336	15	30	110	0	0	21
tenderloin roast boneless lean & fat roasted	4 oz	145	26	4	73	0	0	49
top loin chop boneless lean & fat broiled	1 (3.5 oz)	195	27	9	73	0	0	44

FOOD	PORTION	CALS	PROT	FAT	CHOL	CARB	FIBER	SOD
Boar's Head								
Smoked Shoulder Butt Roast	3 oz	170	13	13	55	tr	–	760
Organic Prairie								
Ground	4 oz	300	19	24	80	0	0	65
Smithfield								
Smoked Pork Chop	3 oz	100	14	3	30	2	0	1070
Tyson								
Baby Back Ribs Buffalo	4 oz	300	16	24	80	4	0	1080
Ground Reduced Fat	4 oz	260	18	20	65	0	0	320
Half Loin Boneless	4 oz	190	20	12	45	0	0	270
Loin Chops Bone-In Center Cut	4 oz	190	20	13	45	0	0	330
Spareribs	4 oz	290	16	24	80	0	0	330
Stew Meat	4 oz	130	21	5	65	0	0	300
READY-TO-EAT								
Sara Lee								
Oven Roasted	2 oz	70	9	3	40	1	0	440
TAKE-OUT								
chicharrones pork cracklings fried	1 cup	492	34	38	100	1	0	2102
chop breaded & fried	1 med (3.4 oz)	304	20	18	87	13	1	577
chop breaded & fried	1 lg (5 oz)	441	30	26	126	19	1	835
chop stewed	1 lg (4.6 oz)	315	36	18	106	0	0	63

PORK DISHES

FOOD	PORTION	CALS	PROT	FAT	CHOL	CARB	FIBER	SOD
A La Carte Gourmet								
Pork Loin w/ Cream Spinach Feta Stuffing	1 serv (5 oz)	200	20	9	85	8	tr	600
Hormel								
Extra Lean Apple Bourbon	1 serv (4 oz)	140	19	5	50	5	0	500
Pork Roast Au Jus	1 serv (5 oz)	180	29	7	85	0	0	570
Morton's Of Omaha								
Tender Pork Roast w/ Gravy & Vegetables	1 serv (5 oz)	210	21	10	70	10	1	460
Tyson								
Roast Pork w/ Vegetables	1 serv (4 oz)	190	21	4	60	18	2	190
Wellshire								
Baby Back Ribs w/ Sauce	2 ribs (5 oz)	260	21	18	81	5	0	410

FOOD	PORTION	CALS	PROT	FAT	CHOL	CARB	FIBER	SOD
Shredded Pork In BBQ Sauce	¼ cup	90	9	2	15	9	0	270
TAKE-OUT								
kalua pork	1 cup (7 oz)	497	43	34	157	1	0	3498
spareribs barbecued w/ sauce	2 med (2.8 oz)	248	17	18	70	3	tr	267
tourtiere	1 piece (4.9 oz)	451	15	34	–	21	–	–

PORK RINDS (see SNACKS)

POT PIE
Hot Pockets

FOOD	PORTION	CALS	PROT	FAT	CHOL	CARB	FIBER	SOD
Pot Pie Express Chicken	1 piece (4.5 oz)	350	8	17	15	41	3	860

Ian's

FOOD	PORTION	CALS	PROT	FAT	CHOL	CARB	FIBER	SOD
Chicken	1 pkg (9.4 oz)	510	26	23	65	50	2	600

Mon Cuisine

FOOD	PORTION	CALS	PROT	FAT	CHOL	CARB	FIBER	SOD
Vegan	1 pkg (9 oz)	650	21	39	0	60	8	850

Pepperidge Farm

FOOD	PORTION	CALS	PROT	FAT	CHOL	CARB	FIBER	SOD
Chili Beans & Cornbread	1 cup	360	11	17	20	40	3	890
Reduced Fat Roasted White Meat Chicken	1 cup	470	14	21	25	56	0	900
Roasted White Meat Chicken	1 cup	510	13	32	30	43	3	870

Stouffer's

FOOD	PORTION	CALS	PROT	FAT	CHOL	CARB	FIBER	SOD
Chicken White Meat	1 pkg (10 oz)	660	19	37	50	62	2	1060

TAKE-OUT

FOOD	PORTION	CALS	PROT	FAT	CHOL	CARB	FIBER	SOD
beef	8 in pie (14.6 oz)	938	34	57	67	72	5	1660
chicken	8 in pie (14.6 oz)	897	37	52	113	69	6	1080
ham	1 serv (11 oz)	752	28	45	38	58	4	1937
oyster	1 serv (11.5 oz)	817	19	53	89	67	3	1056
st. stephen's day pie	1 serv (16.7 oz)	549	35	29	198	38	6	474

FOOD	PORTION	CALS	PROT	FAT	CHOL	CARB	FIBER	SOD
POTATO (see also CHIPS, KNISH, PANCAKES)								
CANNED								
potatoes	½ cup	54	1	tr	0	12	–	–
Del Monte								
Savory Sides Au Gratin	½ cup	80	2	3	0	13	1	470
FRESH								
baked skin only	1 skin (2 oz)	115	2	tr	0	27	2	12
baked w/ skin	1 (6.5 oz)	220	5	tr	0	51	–	16
baked w/o skin	½ cup	57	1	tr	0	13	1	3
baked w/o skin	1 (5 oz)	145	3	tr	0	34	2	8
boiled	½ cup	68	1	tr	0	16	1	3
microwaved	1 (7 oz)	212	5	tr	0	49	–	16
microwaved w/o skin	½ cup	78	2	tr	0	18	–	5
raw w/o skin	1 (3.9 oz)	88	2	tr	0	20	–	7
Frieda's								
Fingerling	4 (5 oz)	100	4	0	0	25	3	0
Green Giant								
Red Potatoes	1 med (5 oz)	100	4	0	0	26	3	0
Lucinda's								
Red "C"	1 med (5.2 oz)	100	4	0	0	26	3	0
SunLite								
SunLite	1 (5 oz)	87	3	0	0	18	4	5
FROZEN								
french fries	10 strips	111	2	4	0	17	2	15
french fries thick cut	10 strips	109	2	4	0	17	–	23
hashed brown	½ cup	170	2	9	–	22	–	27
potato puffs	½ cup	138	2	7	0	19	–	462
potato puffs as prep	1	16	tr	1	0	2	–	52
Alexia								
Hashed Brown	1 serv (3 oz)	80	2	0	0	17	2	300
Mashed Red w/ Garlic & Parmesan	½ cup	150	3	6	0	20	2	115
Mashed Yukon Gold & Sea Salt	½ cup	150	3	6	20	20	2	80
Oven Crinkles Classic	1 serv (3 oz)	120	2	4	0	19	3	140
Oven Crinkles Salt & Pepper	1 serv (3 oz)	120	2	4	0	19	3	330
Oven Fries Garlic	12 pieces	140	2	6	0	20	2	330

FOOD	PORTION	CALS	PROT	FAT	CHOL	CARB	FIBER	SOD
Oven Reds	1 serv (3 oz)	120	3	4	0	19	2	270
Waffle Fries	8 pieces	150	2	5	0	24	3	330
Yukon Gold Fries w/ Sea Salt	1 serv (3 oz)	130	2	4	0	22	2	180
Cascadian Farm								
Organic Country Style	¾ cup	50	1	0	0	12	1	10
Organic Hash Browns	1 cup	60	2	0	0	14	1	10
Funster								
BBQ Lite	14 pieces (3 oz)	140	2	3	0	25	<2	500
Cheddar	14 pieces (3 oz)	135	2	3	0	25	<2	385
Original	14 pieces (3 oz)	135	2	3	0	25	2	230
Green Giant								
Roasted Potatoes w/ Garlic & Herb Sauce as prep	½ cup	90	2	2	0	15	1	420
Healthy Choice								
Cheddar Broccoli Potatoes	1 pkg	270	11	7	20	41	7	600
Ian's								
Alphatots	1 serv (3.5 oz)	156	2	7	0	23	1	160
Fries Sweet Potato	7 pieces (2.5 oz)	70	1	3	0	13	1	25
Inland Valley								
Crinkle Cuts	15 pieces (3 oz)	150	2	5	0	25	2	330
Crisscut Fries	13 pieces (3 oz)	160	2	7	0	22	2	300
Curly QQQ's	1⅓ cups (3 oz)	180	2	8	0	25	2	390
Fajita Fries	17 pieces (3 oz)	170	3	8	0	22	2	400
French Fries	15 pieces (3 oz)	130	2	4	0	21	2	310
Hash Browns	⅔ cup	70	2	0	0	16	2	15
Home Browns	1 patty (2.2 oz)	130	2	7	0	15	2	250
Mashed Homestyle	⅔ cup	160	3	6	5	22	3	500
Simply Shreds	1 cup	70	2	0	0	15	2	

FOOD	PORTION	CALS	PROT	FAT	CHOL	CARB	FIBER	SOD
Stix	5 pieces (3 oz)	170	2	10	0	19	2	360
Stuffed Spudz w/ Cheese	5 pieces	210	7	11	20	20	2	570
Tater Babies	8 pieces (3 oz)	130	2	5	0	19	2	360
Tater Puffs	10 pieces	160	2	7	0	20	2	380
Twice Baked	1 (5.2 oz)	230	8	12	30	23	2	310
Twice Baked Sour Cream Bacon & Chives	1 (5.2 oz)	240	5	8	10	36	3	330
Twice Baked Triple Cheese	1 (5.2 oz)	250	7	10	20	33	3	410
Larry's								
Mashed Broccoli & Cheddar Cheese	1 serv (5 oz)	180	3	8	0	22	2	390
Mashed Cheddar Cheese	1 serv (5 oz)	190	4	8	5	25	2	460
Mashed Old Fashioned Butter	1 serv (5 oz)	190	3	9	10	25	2	370
Mashed Sour Cream & Chives	1 serv (5 oz)	180	3	8	5	25	2	440
Mashed Sweet Potatoes	1 serv (4 oz)	140	2	4	10	27	2	530
Lean Cuisine								
One Dish Favorites Deluxe Cheddar	1 pkg (10.4 oz)	260	13	7	25	36	5	620
McCain								
French Fries Crinkle Cut	18 pieces (3 oz)	130	2	4	0	21	2	320
Mash-Bites	1 serv (3 oz)	50	2	7	0	24	1	430
Roasters All American	1 serv (3 oz)	120	2	3	0	21	tr	370
Roasters Grilled Garlic & Onion	1 serv (3 oz)	120	2	3	0	22	2	590
Seasoned Wedges Skin On	1 serv (3 oz)	120	2	5	0	17	2	390
Shoestring French Fries	45 pieces (3 oz)	140	2	5	0	21	2	290
Smiles	6 pieces (3 oz)	160	2	6	0	24	2	390
Steak Fries	8 pieces (3 oz)	120	2	3	0	21	2	330
Tasti Tater	1 serv (3 oz)	160	2	7	0	20	3	410
Oh Boy!								
Stuffed w/ Onion Sour Cream & Chives	1 (5 oz)	110	2	2	<5	22	2	260

FOOD	PORTION	CALS	PROT	FAT	CHOL	CARB	FIBER	SOD
Roast Works								
Roasted Seasoned Wedge	1 serv (3 oz)	100	3	2	0	18	1	410
Roasted Wedges Rosemary Redskin	1 serv (3 oz)	110	2	3	0	17	2	130
Roasted Wedges Yukon Gold	1 serv (3 oz)	110	2	3	0	18	1	210
MIX								
au gratin as prep	½ cup	160	6	9	29	14	–	528
instant mashed flakes as prep w/ whole milk & butter	½ cup	118	2	6	15	16	–	349
instant mashed flakes not prep	½ cup	78	2	tr	0	18	–	24
instant mashed granules as prep w/ whole milk & butter	½ cup	114	2	5	15	15	–	270
instant mashed granules not prep	½ cup	372	8	1	0	86	–	67
scalloped	½ cup	105	4	5	14	13	–	409
Betty Crocker								
Mashed Butter & Herb	½ cup	160	2	7	3	21	1	400
Hungry Jack								
Casserole Potatoes Au Gratin as prep	½ cup	100	2	1	–	21	2	570
Casserole Potatoes Creamy Scalloped as prep	½ cup	150	2	1	–	21	2	570
Casserole Potatoes Four Cheese as prep	½ cup	150	2	1	–	21	2	570
Easy Mash'd Cheesy Homestyle not prep	¼ cup	150	2	2	–	17	2	430
Easy Mash'd Creamy Butter not prep	¼ cup	150	2	2	–	17	2	430
Easy Mash'd Premium Homestyle not prep	¼ cup	150	2	2	–	17	2	430
Original Mashed not prep	⅓ cup	80	2	0	–	19	1	20
REFRIGERATED								
Country Crock								
Garlic Mashed	⅔ cup	160	2	7	10	22	2	430
Homestyle Mashed	⅔ cup	190	3	10	20	22	2	450

FOOD	PORTION	CALS	PROT	FAT	CHOL	CARB	FIBER	SOD
Diner's Choice								
Mashed	⅔ cup	110	2	5	10	15	3	500
Simply Potatoes								
Diced w/ Onion	⅔ cup	60	1	0	0	13	1	220
Homestyle Slices	⅔ cup	70	2	0	0	16	1	135
Mashed	⅔ cup	170	2	10	20	17	1	520
Mashed Sweet Potatoes	⅔ cup	160	3	3	0	33	2	105
Red Potato Wedges	½ cup	50	2	0	0	10	2	85
Shredded Hash Browns	½ cup	50	1	0	0	12	tr	105
SHELF-STABLE								
TastyBite								
Bombay Potatoes	½ pkg (5 oz)	105	5	4	0	13	3	412
TAKE-OUT								
au gratin w/ cheese	½ cup	178	7	10	18	17	–	548
baked topped w/ cheese sauce	1	475	15	29	19	47	–	381
baked topped w/ cheese sauce & bacon	1	451	18	26	30	44	–	973
baked topped w/ cheese sauce & broccoli	1	402	14	14	20	47	–	484
baked topped w/ cheese sauce & chili	1	481	23	22	31	56	–	701
baked topped w/ sour cream & chives	1	394	7	22	23	50	–	182
french fries	1 reg	235	3	12	0	29	–	124
hash brown	½ cup (2.5 oz)	151	2	9	9	16	–	290
indian yogurt potatoes	1 serv	315	7	9	18	52	0	216
mashed	½ cup	111	2	4	2	18	–	309
o'brien	1 cup	157	5	3	7	30	–	421
potato dumpling	3.5 oz	334	7	1	–	74	3	1
potato pancakes	1 (1.3 oz)	101	2	7	35	11	–	188
potato salad	½ cup	179	3	10	85	14	2	661
red new boiled	5 sm (5 oz)	120	3	0	0	27	2	5
scalloped	½ cup	127	4	5	7	18	–	435
twice baked w/ cheese	1 half (10 oz)	392	8	18	54	48	4	810

FOOD	PORTION	CALS	PROT	FAT	CHOL	CARB	FIBER	SOD
POTATO STARCH								
potato starch	1 oz	96	tr	tr	0	24	–	1
Bob's Red Mill								
Potato Starch	1 tbsp	40	0	0	0	10	0	0
POUT								
ocean baked	3 oz	86	18	1	57	0	0	66
ocean fillet baked	4.8 oz	139	29	2	91	0	0	107
PRETZELS								
chocolate covered	1 (0.4 oz)	47	1	1	1	8	tr	110
soft	1 lg (5 oz)	483	12	4	4	99	2	2008
twists salted	10 (2.1 oz)	229	6	2	0	48	2	1029
twists w/o salt	10 (2.1 oz)	229	5	2	0	48	2	173
whole wheat	2 sm (1 oz)	103	3	1	0	23	2	58
yogurt covered	1 cup (3 oz)	391	7	13	1	61	1	588
yogurt covered	1 (4 g)	19	tr	1	0	3	tr	29
Cape Cod								
Pretzels	25	130	3	1	0	27	tr	410
Combos								
Cheddar Cheese Cracker	1 pkg (1.7 oz)	240	3	11	0	31	1	490
Nacho Cheese	1 pkg (1.7 oz)	230	5	8	0	34	1	820
Pizzeria Pretzel	1 pkg (1.7 oz)	230	4	8	0	35	1	810
Glenny's								
Organic Original Salted	8 (1 oz)	110	3	0	0	23	1	480
Organic Sourdough	6 (1 oz)	110	3	0	0	23	1	480
Glutino								
Gluten Free All Shapes	44 (1.4 oz)	190	1	8	0	28	0	540
Goodniks								
Yogurt Pretzels	15	180	4	7	0	28	0	200
Handi-Snack								
Mister Salty Pretzels 'N Cheese	1 pkg	90	3	4	5	12	0	380
Healthy Handfuls								
Python Pretzels	1 box (1.5 oz)	170	5	1	0	36	1	360
New York Style								
Pretzel Flatz Original Salt	12	110	3	1	0	23	1	250

FOOD	PORTION	CALS	PROT	FAT	CHOL	CARB	FIBER	SOD
Newman's Own								
Organic Bavarian Sour Dough	1	90	2	0	0	19	1	400
Organic Hi Protein	22	120	5	1	0	22	4	430
Organic Salt & Pepper Rounds	8	100	2	1	0	24	1	400
Organic Salt & Pepper Thins	10	120	2	1	0	24	tr	400
Organic Salted Nuggets	20	120	3	2	0	25	2	330
Organic Salted Rods	4	120	3	2	0	25	2	330
Organic Salted Rounds	8	110	2	1	0	24	tr	400
Organic Salted Sticks	13	110	2	1	0	24	1	350
Organic Salted Thins	10	110	2	1	0	24	1	400
Organic Spelt	20	120	4	1	0	23	4	240
Organic Unsalted Rounds	8	110	2	1	0	24	tr	105
Quinlan								
Low Fat Mini	1 oz	110	2	1	0	23	tr	420
Rold Gold								
Braided Twists	8	110	2	1	0	22	1	410
Braided Twists Honey Wheat	8	110	2	1	0	22	1	410
Checkers	20	110	3	2	<5	22	1	300
Rods	3	110	3	1	0	22	1	610
Sourdough Hard	1	100	2	1	0	21	1	500
Sourdough Specials	5	110	3	1	0	23	1	470
Sticks	48	100	2	0	0	23	1	460
Thins	9 pieces	110	2	1	0	23	1	560
Tiny Twists	18 pieces	110	3	0	0	23	1	420
Tiny Twists Cheddar	20	110	3	1	0	22	1	370
Tiny Twists Honey Mustard	13	110	3	1	0	23	1	430
Snyder's Of Hanover								
100 Calorie Pack Snaps	1 pkg (0.9 oz)	100	3	1	0	22	tr	340
100 Calorie Pack Stick	1 pkg (0.9 oz)	100	2	1	0	20	tr	260
Dips Milk Chocolate	1 oz	140	2	6	<5	19	tr	100
Dips Special Dark Chocolate	1 oz	140	2	5	<5	22	2	130
Mini Unsalted	1 oz	110	3	0	0	25	tr	75
MultiGrain Sticks Lightly Salted	1 oz	120	3	2	0	23	3	160

FOOD	PORTION	CALS	PROT	FAT	CHOL	CARB	FIBER	SOD
MultiGrain Twists	1 oz	120	3	2	0	22	2	170
Nibblers Sourdough	1 oz	120	3	0	0	25	tr	200
Old Tyme	1 oz	120	3	1	0	24	1	120
Organic Honey Wheat	1 oz	130	3	2	0	24	1	210
Organic Oat Bran	1 oz	120	3	0	0	25	2	320
Pieces Garlic Bread	1 oz	140	3	7	0	18	1	160
Pieces Honey Mustard & Onions	1 oz	140	2	7	0	18	tr	240
Pieces Hot Buffalo Wing	1 oz	140	2	7	0	17	tr	380
Pretzel Sandwich Peanut Butter	1 oz	140	4	7	0	16	tr	140
Rods	1 oz	120	3	1	0	24	1	290
Snaps	1 oz	120	3	1	0	25	1	270
Sourdough Unsalted	1 oz	100	3	0	0	22	1	90
Sticks 12 MultiGrain	1 oz	130	3	2	0	22	3	180
Superpretzel								
Mozzarella	2 (1.8 oz)	130	6	4	5	20	1	420
Pretzelfils Pizza	2 (1.8 oz)	130	5	2	5	22	1	180
Soft	1 (2.25 oz)	160	5	1	0	34	1	130
Soft Bites	5 (1.9 oz)	150	31	1	0	32	1	912
Softstix	2 (1.8 oz)	130	4	3	10	22	1	260
Utz								
Braided Twists Baked Honey Wheat	1 oz	110	3	2	0	23	1	280
Chocolate Covered	6 (1.1 oz)	140	2	5	0	22	tr	220
Hard	1	90	2	0	0	18	tr	470
Special	1 oz	110	3	1	0	21	1	470
Special Multigrain	1 oz	110	3	1	0	21	2	340
Sticks Organic Whole Grain	1 oz	120	3	2	0	22	3	200
Wise								
Fat Free Sticks	1 oz	100	2	0	0	23	tr	490
Low Fat Honey Wheat Braided Twists	1 oz	110	2	1	0	24	1	200
PRUNE JUICE								
jarred	1 cup	182	2	tr	0	45	3	10
L&A								
100% Juice	8 oz	180	0	0	0	41	3	10
Lakewood								
Organic	8 oz	165	1	0	0	40	3	5

FOOD	PORTION	CALS	PROT	FAT	CHOL	CARB	FIBER	SOD
Langers								
Plus 100% Juice	8 oz	180	0	0	0	41	1	10
Old Orchard								
Healthy Balance	8 oz	70	0	0	0	12	5	35
Sunsweet								
100% Juice	8 oz	180	2	0	0	43	3	30
PlumSmart	8 oz	160	0	0	0	39	3	15
PRUNES								
cooked w/o sugar	½ cup	133	1	tr	0	35	4	1
dried	1	20	tr	tr	0	5	1	0
Earthbound Farm								
Organic Dried Plums	5	110	1	0	0	25	3	0
Love'n Bake								
Prune Lekvar	2 tbsp	90	0	0	0	21	1	120
Newman's Own								
Organic	½ cup	110	1	0	0	26	2	5
Sunsweet								
Pitted Dried	5	100	1	0	0	24	3	5
PUDDING								
MIX								
Uncle Ben's								
Rice Pudding Cinnamon & Raisins as prep	½ cup	160	2	1	0	37	1	180
Rice Pudding French Vanilla as prep	½ cup	120	2	0	0	28	1	90
READY-TO-EAT								
Hunt's								
Dessert Favorites Banana Cream Pie	1 serv (3.5 oz)	140	1	6	0	20	0	150
Dessert Favorites Chocolate Brownie	1 serv (3.5 oz)	190	2	7	0	28	0	135
Dessert Favorites Chocolate Mud Pie	1 serv (3.5 oz)	170	2	7	0	25	0	130
Dessert Favorites Chocolate Peanut Butter Pie	1 serv (3.5 oz)	190	3	8	0	27	0	170
Dessert Favorites Dulce De Leche Caramel Cream	1 serv (3.5 oz)	140	1	5	0	23	0	190
Dessert Favorites Lemon Meringue Pie	1 serv (3.5 oz)	130	0	3	0	26	0	48

FOOD	PORTION	CALS	PROT	FAT	CHOL	CARB	FIBER	SOD
Snack Pack Butterscotch	1 serv (3.5 oz)	130	2	5	0	20	0	170
Snack Pack Chocolate	1 serv (3.5 oz)	104	2	5	1	22	0	140
Snack Pack Chocolate Fudge	1 serv (3.5 oz)	150	2	5	1	23	0	160
Snack Pack Chocolate Marshmallow	1 serv (3.5 oz)	130	2	5	1	21	0	140
Snack Pack Fat Free Chocolate	1 serv (3.5 oz)	90	2	0	0	20	0	135
Snack Pack Fat Free Tapioca	1 serv (3.5 oz)	80	2	0	0	18	0	150
Snack Pack Fat Free Vanilla	1 serv (3.5 oz)	80	1	0	0	19	0	140
Snack Pack Lemon	1 serv (3.5 oz)	120	0	3	0	23	0	60
Snack Pack Swirl Chocolate Caramel	1 serv (3.5 oz)	140	2	5	0	22	0	150
Snack Pack Swirl S'mores	1 serv (3.5 oz)	140	2	5	0	21	0	100
Snack Pack Tapioca	1 serv (3.5 oz)	130	2	5	0	20	0	135
Snack Pack Vanilla	1 serv (3.5 oz)	130	1	5	1	21	0	140
Jell-O								
100 Calorie Pack Fat Free Chocolate Vanilla Swirl	1 pkg (4 oz)	100	2	0	0	23	tr	190
100 Calorie Pack Fat Free Tapioca	1 pkg (4 oz)	100	1	0	0	23	0	210
Sugar Free Dulce De Leche	1 pkg (3.7 oz)	60	1	1	0	13	0	178
Kozy Shack								
Black Forest	1 pkg (4 oz)	120	3	3	5	22	1	105
Chocolate	1 pkg (4 oz)	139	3	4	13	24	1	143
Chocolate No Sugar Added	1 pkg (4 oz)	93	4	3	9	14	1	130
Rice	1 pkg (4 oz)	135	4	3	20	23	0	135
Tapioca	1 pkg (4 oz)	130	3	3	15	23	0	140
Tapioca No Sugar Added	1 pkg	90	3	3	15	11	4	140
Vanilla	1 pkg (4 oz)	130	3	3	17	22	0	147
Vanilla No Sugar Added	1 pkg (4 oz)	90	4	2	9	14	0	130

FOOD	PORTION	CALS	PROT	FAT	CHOL	CARB	FIBER	SOD
Lifeway								
Organic Chocolate	½ cup	170	4	4	–	30	–	–
Organic Rice	½ cup	140	4	4	–	22	–	–
Organic Vanilla	½ cup	150	3	4	–	24	–	–
Swiss Miss								
Low Fat Tapioca	1 pkg (4 oz)	130	3	3	0	24	0	190
TAKE-OUT								
blancmange	1 serv (4.7 oz)	154	4	5	–	25	tr	–
bread w/ raisins	1 cup	306	11	9	124	47	2	472
coconut	1 cup	291	8	9	15	45	2	451
corn	1 cup	328	11	13	185	43	4	703
indian pudding	½ cup	156	5	4	40	25	1	220
noodle pudding kugel	1 cup	297	9	10	144	44	2	94
plum pudding	1 slice (1.5 oz)	125	2	5	22	20	1	83
queen of puddings	1 serv (4.4 oz)	266	6	10	–	41	tr	–
rice pudding	1 cup	302	8	4	14	60	1	133
sweet potato	1 cup	215	4	6	2	37	5	603
tapioca	1 cup	236	10	7	156	35	0	312
yorkshire	1 serv (3 oz)	177	6	8	57	22	tr	168
PUFFERFISH								
raw	3 oz	72	17	0	–	0	0	120
PUMMELO								
fresh	1	228	5	tr	0	59	–	7
sections	1 cup	71	1	tr	0	18	–	2
Sunkist								
Fresh	¼	90	1	1	0	20	4	0
PUMPKIN								
butter	1 tbsp	32	0	0	0	8	–	0
canned	½ cup	41	1	tr	0	10	–	6
cooked mashed	½ cup	24	1	tr	0	6	–	2
flowers cooked	½ cup	10	1	tr	0	2	–	4
flowers raw	1	0	tr	0	0	tr	–	0
leaves cooked	½ cup	7	1	tr	0	1	–	3
leaves raw	½ cup	4	1	tr	0	tr	–	2

FOOD	PORTION	CALS	PROT	FAT	CHOL	CARB	FIBER	SOD
raw cubed	½ cup	15	1	tr	0	4	–	1
Farmer's Market								
Organic Puree	½ cup	50	1	0	0	10	4	0

PUMPKIN SEEDS

FOOD	PORTION	CALS	PROT	FAT	CHOL	CARB	FIBER	SOD
dried	1 oz	154	7	13	0	5	–	5
roasted	¼ cup	296	19	24	0	8	–	10
salted & roasted	¼ cup	296	19	24	0	8	–	324
whole roasted	1 oz	127	5	6	0	15	–	5
whole roasted	¼ cup	71	3	3	0	9	–	3
whole salted roasted	¼ cup	71	3	3	0	9	–	67
David								
All Natural	¼ cup	160	8	13	0	3	1	940
Eden								
Dry Roasted & Salted	¼ cup	200	10	16	0	5	5	100
Good Sense								
Roasted & Salted	½ cup	160	8	13	0	3	1	10
Mrs. May's								
Pumpkin Crunch	1 oz	164	9	11	0	8	1	41

PURSLANE

FOOD	PORTION	CALS	PROT	FAT	CHOL	CARB	FIBER	SOD
cooked	1 cup	21	2	tr	0	4	–	51
fresh	1 cup	7	1	tr	0	1	–	20

QUAIL

FOOD	PORTION	CALS	PROT	FAT	CHOL	CARB	FIBER	SOD
cooked bone removed	1 (2.7 oz)	177	19	11	65	0	0	163

QUICHE
Mrs. Smith's

FOOD	PORTION	CALS	PROT	FAT	CHOL	CARB	FIBER	SOD
Pour-A-Quiche Bacon & Onion	1 serv (4.3 oz)	230	14	16	195	6	0	700
TAKE-OUT								
cheese	⅛ (9 in) pie	566	17	44	240	27	1	459
lorraine	⅛ (9 in) pie	568	17	44	242	27	1	695
mushroom	1 slice (3 oz)	256	9	18	–	17	1	–
spinach	⅛ (9 in) pie	342	11	26	157	17	1	326

FOOD	PORTION	CALS	PROT	FAT	CHOL	CARB	FIBER	SOD
QUINCE								
fresh	1	53	tr	tr	0	14	–	4
QUINOA								
quinoa not prep	1 cup (6 oz)	636	22	10	0	117	10	36
Alti Plano Gold								
Natural	1 pkg	170	6	3	0	30	5	120
Eden								
Quinoa not prep	¼ cup	180	7	4	0	29	11	10
Seeds Of Change								
French Herb Quinoa Blend as prep	1 cup	290	8	4	0	56	3	860
RABBIT								
domestic w/o bone roasted	3 oz	167	25	7	70	0	0	40
wild w/o bone stewed	3 oz	147	28	3	104	0	0	38
RACCOON								
roasted	3 oz	217	25	12	–	0	0	–
RADICCHIO								
raw shredded	½ cup	5	tr	tr	0	1	–	4
RADISHES								
chinese dried	½ cup	157	5	tr	0	37	–	161
chinese raw	1 (12 oz)	62	2	tr	0	14	–	71
chinese raw sliced	½ cup	8	tr	tr	0	2	–	9
chinese sliced cooked	½ cup	13	tr	tr	0	3	–	10
daikon dried	½ cup	157	5	tr	0	37	–	161
daikon raw	1 (12 oz)	62	2	tr	0	14	–	71
daikon raw sliced	½ cup	8	tr	tr	0	2	–	9
daikon sliced cooked	½ cup	13	tr	tr	0	3	–	10
red raw	10	7	tr	tr	0	2	–	11
red sliced	½ cup	10	tr	tr	0	2	–	14
white icicle raw	1 (0.5 oz)	2	tr	tr	0	tr	–	3
white icicle raw sliced	½ cup	7	1	tr	0	1	–	8
Eden								
Daikon Dried Shredded	2 tbsp	45	1	0	0	9	3	20
Daikon Pickled	2 slices (0.5 oz)	5	0	0	0	1	–	250

FOOD	PORTION	CALS	PROT	FAT	CHOL	CARB	FIBER	SOD
Frieda's								
Black	¾ cup	15	1	0	0	3	1	20
Chinese Lo Bok	⅔ cup	25	1	0	0	5	2	55
Daikon	½ cup	15	1	1	0	1	0	0
Korean Moo	⅔ cup	15	1	0	0	3	1	20
TAKE-OUT								
korean kimchee	½ cup	31	2	1	–	6	–	–
moo namul saengche korean salad	1 serv (3.7 oz)	34	1	tr	0	8	2	547
RAISINS								
cinnamon coated	¼ cup	108	1	tr	0	29	1	4
cooked	¼ cup	162	1	tr	0	42	1	5
golden seedless	¼ cup	109	1	tr	0	29	1	4
jumbo golden	¼ cup	130	1	0	0	31	2	10
milk chocolate coated	28 (1 oz)	109	1	4	1	19	1	10
milk chocolate coated	¼ cup	176	2	7	1	31	2	16
seedless	55 (1 oz)	86	1	tr	0	23	1	3
sultanas	1 oz	88	1	0	–	23	2	–
Amazin'								
Raisin All Flavors	1 oz	84	1	0	0	22	2	4
Bob's Red Mill								
Unsulfured	⅓ cup	130	1	0	0	31	3	5
Brach's								
California Chocolate Covered	35 pieces	170	1	6	10	28	1	10
Earthbound Farm								
Organic Jumbo Flame Seedless	¼ cup	120	1	0	0	32	2	0
Estee								
Chocolate Covered Fructose Sweetened	¼ cup	180	3	6	<5	27	1	45
Fool								
Cinnamon Raisin Spread	1 tbsp	20	0	0	0	5	1	0
Godiva								
Milk Chocolate Covered	1 pkg (1.2 oz)	150	2	7	<5	21	1	20
Goodniks								
Yogurt Raisins	3 tbsp	145	1	5	0	23	1	35

FOOD	PORTION	CALS	PROT	FAT	CHOL	CARB	FIBER	SOD
Newman's Own								
Organic	¼ cup	130	1	0	0	26	2	10
Sun-Maid								
California Golden	¼ cup	130	1	0	0	31	2	10
California Seedless	¼ cup	130	1	0	0	31	2	10
Sunsweet								
Red Flame	¼ cup	130	1	0	0	31	2	10

RASPBERRIES

FOOD	PORTION	CALS	PROT	FAT	CHOL	CARB	FIBER	SOD
canned in heavy syrup	½ cup	117	1	tr	0	30	–	4
fresh	1 pint	154	3	2	0	36	–	0
fresh	1 cup	61	1	1	0	14	–	0
frzn sweetened	1 cup	256	2	tr	0	65	–	1
frzn sweetened	1 pkg (10 oz)	291	2	tr	0	74	–	1
frzn unsweetened	¾ cup	130	2	0	0	29	2	0
C&W								
Ultimate Red	¾ cup	70	2	0	0	15	7	0
Cascadian Farm								
Organic frzn	1 ¼ cup	60	1	0	0	17	6	0
Europe's Best								
Raspberries frzn	¾ cup	60	1	0	0	13	2	0
Frieda's								
Dried	⅓ cup (1.4 oz)	145	0	1	0	36	6	0
Oregon								
In Heavy Syrup	½ cup	120	tr	0	0	30	5	10

RASPBERRY JUICE

FOOD	PORTION	CALS	PROT	FAT	CHOL	CARB	FIBER	SOD
Crystal Light								
Raspberry Ice Sugar Free	8 oz	5	0	0	0	0	0	15
Naked Juice								
Raspberry Ade	8 oz	90	0	0	0	22	0	15
Newman's Own								
Razz-Ma-Tazz Raspberry	8 oz	120	0	0	0	28	–	5
Old Orchard								
Organic 100% Juice	8 oz	120	0	0	0	29	–	25

RELISH

FOOD	PORTION	CALS	PROT	FAT	CHOL	CARB	FIBER	SOD
hamburger	½ cup	158	1	1	0	42	–	1338
hamburger	1 tbsp	19	tr	tr	0	5	–	164

FOOD	PORTION	CALS	PROT	FAT	CHOL	CARB	FIBER	SOD
hot dog	1 tbsp	14	tr	tr	0	4	–	164
hot dog	½ cup	111	2	1	0	28	–	1332
piccalilli	1.4 oz	13	tr	tr	–	2	1	–
sweet	½ cup	159	tr	1	0	43	–	990
sweet	1 tbsp	19	tr	tr	0	5	–	122
B&G								
India	1 tbsp	15	0	0	0	4	–	140
Piccalilli	1 tbsp	20	0	0	0	5	–	120
Sweet	1 tbsp	15	0	0	0	4	–	120
Del Monte								
Hamburger	1 tbsp	20	0	0	0	5	tr	125
Hot Dog	1 tbsp	15	0	0	0	4	tr	140
Sweet Pickle	1 tbsp	20	0	0	0	5	0	125
Frieda's								
Kim Chee	¼ cup	15	1	0	0	2	1	340
Matouk's								
Hot Chow	2 tbsp	20	0	0	0	5	0	200
Kuchela	1 tsp	9	0	1	0	tr	0	80
Patak's								
Brinjal Eggplant Sweet Spicy	1 tbsp	70	0	4	0	8	1	250
Garlic	1 tbsp	45	0	3	0	4	0	300
Lime Mild	1 tbsp	30	0	3	0	0	0	530
Mango Mild	1 tbsp	40	0	4	0	1	0	660
Peloponnese								
Sun Dried Tomato	1 tbsp	25	0	2	0	2	0	200
RENNIN								
tablet	1 (0.9 g)	1	0	0	–	tr	–	234
RHUBARB								
fresh	½ cup	13	1	tr	0	3	–	2
frozen	½ cup	60	tr	tr	0	3	–	1
frzn as prep w/ sugar	½ cup	139	tr	tr	0	37	–	2
RICE (see also RICE CAKES, WILD RICE)								
arborio	½ cup	100	2	0	0	22	–	5
brown long grain cooked	1 cup (6.8 oz)	216	5	2	0	45	4	10
brown medium grain cooked	1 cup (6.8 oz)	218	5	2	0	46	4	2

FOOD	PORTION	CALS	PROT	FAT	CHOL	CARB	FIBER	SOD
glutinous cooked	1 cup (6.1 oz)	169	4	tr	0	37	2	9
starch	1 oz	98	tr	0	0	24	–	17
white long grain cooked	1 cup (5.5 oz)	205	4	tr	0	45	1	2
white long grain instant cooked	1 cup (5.8 oz)	162	3	tr	0	35	1	5
white medium grain cooked	1 cup (6.5 oz)	242	4	tr	0	53	1	0
white short grain cooked	1 cup (6.5 oz)	242	4	tr	0	53	–	0
A Taste Of Thai								
Coconut Garlic Basil as prep	¾ cup	160	5	0	0	35	0	370
Coconut Ginger as prep	¾ cup	190	5	0	0	42	2	430
Jasmine not prep	¼ cup	160	3	0	0	36	0	0
Yellow Curry as prep	¾ cup	180	3	2	0	38	0	390
Arrowhead Mills								
Organic Brown Basmati not prep	¼ cup	140	3	2	0	31	2	0
Organic Long Grain Brown not prep	¼ cup	160	3	1	0	32	1	0
Buitoni								
Risotto Garden Vegetable	1 serv	210	4	1	0	47	0	930
Risotto Portobello Mushrooms	1 serv	210	5	0	0	48	0	930
Risotto Rosemary & Potatoes	1 serv	210	4	1	10	47	2	810
Risotto Tomato Basil	1 serv	210	4	1	0	46	0	870
Country Crock								
Chicken Rice w/ Herbs	1 cup	210	5	4	<5	42	1	930
Fantastic								
Arborio not prep	¼ cup	160	3	4	0	36	tr	0
Basmati not prep	¼ cup	160	3	0	0	36	tr	0
Jasmine not prep	¼ cup	160	3	0	0	36	tr	0
Green Giant								
Rice Pilaf	1 pkg (9.9 oz)	200	5	3	5	40	3	1080
White & Wild & Green Beans	1 pkg (9.9 oz)	260	6	5	0	48	3	1260

FOOD	PORTION	CALS	PROT	FAT	CHOL	CARB	FIBER	SOD
Knorr								
Asian Side Dish Chicken Fried Rice as prep	1 cup	240	7	1	0	48	1	864
Rice Sides Rice Medley as prep	1 cup	250	6	5	<5	45	1	780
Rice Sides Sesame Chicken w/ Whole Grains as prep	2/3 cup	300	7	9	0	51	3	864
Lundberg								
Eco-Farmed Black Japonica not prep	1/4 cup	170	5	2	0	38	3	0
Eco-Farmed California Brown Basmati not prep	1/4 cup	160	4	2	0	34	2	0
Eco-Farmed White California Arborio not prep	1/4 cup	10	6	0	0	43	1	3
Organic Brown Golden Rose not prep	1/4 cup	160	3	1	0	34	1	0
Organic Rise Sensations Ginger Miso not prep	1/2 cup	116	3	1	0	24	1	150
Organic Risotto Porcini Mushroom not prep	1/2 cup	143	4	1	0	35	1	535
Organic White Sushi Rice no prep	1/4 cup	150	4	0	0	36	1	0
Organic Wild Blend not prep	1/4 cup	150	4	2	0	35	3	0
RiceXpress Chicken Herb	1/2 pkg (4.4 oz)	250	4	5	0	47	6	670
RiceXpress Santa Fe Grill	1/2 pkg (4.4 oz)	260	5	5	0	50	3	472
Risotto Butternut Squash not prep	1/2 cup	143	4	1	0	31	1	496
Marrakesh Express								
Pilaf Tomato & Basil as prep	1 cup	190	6	0	0	41	0	570
Risotto Parmesan as prep	1 cup	200	5	1	0	42	1	870
Nueva Cocina								
Arroz A La Mexicana	1 cup	190	4	1	–	41	2	650
Arroz Con Pollo	1 cup	150	3	0	0	35	1	590
Gallo Pinto	1/3 pkg	220	6	0	0	47	3	750
Moros Y Cristianos	1/3 pkg	220	6	0	0	47	3	760
Paella	1/5 pkg	160	4	0	0	35	1	560

FOOD	PORTION	CALS	PROT	FAT	CHOL	CARB	FIBER	SOD
Pacific Foods								
Ready-To-Serve Lemon & Herb	½ pkg	240	5	3	0	48	1	570
Ready-To-Serve Roasted Chicken	½ pkg	240	4	6	0	45	1	570
Ready-To-Serve Spanish Style	½ pkg	230	4	3	0	45	1	600
Ready-To-Serve Wild Rice & Mushroom	½ pkg	230	4	3	0	46	1	600
Patak's								
Basmati	1 pkg	430	9	5	0	87	2	440
Coconut	1 pkg	500	10	12	0	87	4	880
Yellow	1 pkg	440	10	5	0	89	2	1140
Rice A Roni								
Beef as prep	1 cup	310	7	9	0	51	2	1110
Chicken as prep	1 cup	310	7	9	0	51	2	1160
Express Asian Fried	1 cup	280	6	6	0	51	2	710
Fried Rice as prep	1 cup	320	7	11	0	49	2	1490
Garden Vegetable as prep	1 cup	270	6	10	0	41	2	910
Long Grain & Wild as prep	1 cup	250	5	7	0	43	1	760
Lower Sodium Chicken as prep	1 cup	270	7	5	0	51	2	730
Parmesan Chicken as prep	1 cup	370	8	15	5	51	3	1360
Red Beans & Rice as prep	1 cup	290	8	7	0	51	5	1170
Savory Whole Grain Blends Spanish as prep	1 cup	250	5	8	0	42	3	760
Spanish as prep	1 cup	260	6	7	0	44	2	1340
Rice Select								
Jasmati	1 serv	150	3	0	0	34	–	0
Kasmati	1 serv	150	3	1	–	34	–	0
Risotto	1 serv	150	3	0	0	37	–	0
Royal Blend	1 serv	160	4	1	–	34	–	0
Royal Blend w/ Lentils	1 serv	130	3	1	0	28	1	5
Royal Blend w/ Red Beans	1 serv	130	4	1	0	27	2	10
Sushi Rice not prep	¼ cup	190	3	0	0	45	–	0
Teriyaki Fried Rice not prep	¼ cup	160	4	1	–	34	–	330
Texmati Brown	1 serv	170	4	1	–	35	2	0
Texmati Light Brown	1 serv	170	4	1	–	33	1	0
Texmati White	1 serv	150	3	1	–	34	–	0

FOOD	PORTION	CALS	PROT	FAT	CHOL	CARB	FIBER	SOD
Texmati Royal Blend Brown & Wild	1 serv	160	5	2	0	34	–	5
Seeds Of Change								
Moroccan Lentil Rice Pilaf as prep	1 cup	180	5	1	0	38	3	750
Tuscan Rice & Beans as prep	1 cup	180	4	1	0	40	2	670
Success								
Boil-In-Bag Brown as prep	1 cup	150	4	1	0	33	2	0
Boil-In-Bag Jasmine as prep	¾ cup	150	3	0	0	36	0	0
Boil-In-Bag White as prep	1 cup	190	4	0	0	43	1	0
Ready To Serve Brown	1 cup	170	3	5	0	28	2	5
Ready To Serve White	1 pkg	190	3	4	0	34	0	0
Ready To Serve Yellow Rice Mix	1 pkg	190	3	4	0	35	1	1030
Whole Grain Herb Roasted Chicken as prep	1 cup	290	7	10	5	43	3	620
Whole Grain Multigrain Pilaf as prep	1 cup	230	7	3	10	43	3	680
Whole Grain Portobello Mushroom as prep	1 cup	220	6	2	0	45	3	520
TastyBite								
Pilaf Multigrain	½ pkg (5 oz)	200	9	5	0	33	4	440
Pilaf Tandoori	½ pkg (5 oz)	183	3	3	0	37	1	458
Uncle Ben's								
Boil-In-Bag	1 cup	190	4	1	0	44	1	0
Brown Natural as prep	1 cup	170	5	1	0	35	–	0
Country Inn Chicken & Broccoli as prep	1 cup	190	5	1	0	42	1	910
Country Inn Chicken & Vegetables as prep	1 cup	200	5	2	0	41	1	720
Country Inn Mexican Fiesta as prep	1 cup	200	5	1	0	42	1	680
Country Inn Oriental Fried as prep	1 cup	200	6	1	0	42	1	580
Country Inn Three Cheese as prep	1 cup	200	6	2	5	40	1	800

FOOD	PORTION	CALS	PROT	FAT	CHOL	CARB	FIBER	SOD
Country Inn Wheat	1 cup	200	5	1	0	43	1	640
Fast & Natural	1 cup	190	4	2	0	42	2	20
Flavorful Four Cheese as prep	1 cup	190	5	1	5	43	1	550
Flavorful Garlic & Butter as prep	1 cup	200	5	1	0	44	tr	750
Flavorful Lemon & Herb as prep	1 cup	200	4	1	0	45	tr	740
Flavorful Spanish as prep	1 cup	200	4	1	0	45	tr	880
Instant	1 cup	190	3	1	0	43	1	15
Long Grain & Wild Butter Herb as prep	1 cup	190	5	1	0	40	1	810
Long Grain & Wild Fast Cook as prep	1 cup	200	6	1	0	43	1	690
Long Grain & Wild Original as prep	1 cup	200	6	0	0	42	1	670
Long Grain & Wild Roasted Garlic as prep	1 cup	200	5	1	0	42	1	750
Ready Rice Long Grain & Wild as prep	1 cup	240	5	4	0	44	1	500
Ready Rice Original as prep	1 cup	230	4	4	0	44	1	0
Ready Rice Roasted Chicken as prep	1 cup	230	5	4	0	44	1	960
Ready Rice Teriyaki as prep	1 cup	190	5	4	0	51	1	730
Ready Rice Whole Grain Brown	1 cup	220	5	4	0	41	1	5
White Original as prep	1 cup	170	4	0	0	38	0	0
TAKE-OUT								
coconut rice	1 serv	500	6	42	–	30	2	27
congee	½ cup (4.1 oz)	44	1	–	–	10	–	–
nasi goreng (fried rice)	1 serv	206	10	4	–	35	5	356
nasi goreng indonesian rice & vegetables	1 cup (4.9 oz)	130	4	0	0	28	1	530
pea palau rice & peas fried in ghee	1 serv	144	4	5	21	21	2	145
pilaf	½ cup	84	4	3	22	11	3	362
risotto	1 serv (6.6 oz)	426	6	18	–	65	3	–
spanish	¾ cup	363	11	27	35	19	–	1339

FOOD	PORTION	CALS	PROT	FAT	CHOL	CARB	FIBER	SOD
RICE CAKES (see also POPCORN CAKES)								
Lundberg								
Eco-Farmed Apple Cinnamon	1 (0.7 oz)	80	2	1	0	18	tr	0
Eco-Farmed Brown Rice Salt Free	1 (0.7 oz)	70	1	0	0	14	tr	0
Eco-Farmed Toasted Sesame	1 (0.7 oz)	70	2	0	0	15	1	65
Organic Caramel Corn	1 (0.7 oz)	80	1	1	0	18	1	40
Organic Green Tea w/ Lemon	1 (0.7 oz)	80	1	0	0	17	1	0
Organic Mochi Sweet	1 (0.7 oz)	70	1	0	0	15	tr	55
Mr. Krispers								
Baked Rice Krisps Barbecue	37	110	1	3	0	21	1	380
Baked Rice Krisps Nacho	37	120	2	3	0	21	1	360
Baked Rice Krisps Sea Salt & Pepper	37	110	1	4	0	20	1	220
Baked Rice Krisps Sour Cream & Onion	37	110	2	4	0	19	1	360
Quaker								
Mini Delights Chocolatey Drizzle	1 pkg (0.7 oz)	90	1	4	0	14	1	85
Riceworks								
Sweet Chili	10 (1 oz)	140	2	6	0	19	1	170
Wasabi	10 (1 oz)	140	2	6	0	19	1	140
ROCKFISH								
pacific cooked	1 fillet (5.2 oz)	180	36	3	66	0	0	114
pacific cooked	3 oz	103	20	2	38	0	0	65
pacific raw	3 oz	80	16	1	29	0	0	51
ROE (see also individual fish names)								
fresh baked	1 oz	58	8	2	136	1	0	33
ROLL								
FROZEN								
Alexia								
Ciabatta	1 (1.5 oz)	100	3	2	0	19	1	220
French	1 (1.5 oz)	100	4	0	0	20	1	230

FOOD	PORTION	CALS	PROT	FAT	CHOL	CARB	FIBER	SOD
Three Cheese Focaccia	1 (1.5 oz)	110	4	2	0	19	tr	230
Whole Grain	1 (1.5 oz)	90	4	1	0	19	3	220
Eggo								
Toaster Swirlz Cinnamon Roll Minis	4 (1.6 oz)	120	2	3	5	20	tr	200
Sara Lee								
Deluxe Cinnamon Rolls w/ Icing	1 (2.7 oz)	320	5	15	40	41	1	300
READY-TO-EAT								
bialy	1 (2.2 oz)	138	14	0	0	32	1	167
brioche sweet roll	1 (3.5 oz)	410	10	23	190	41	3	495
brown & serve	1 (1 oz)	85	2	2	0	14	–	148
cheese	1 (2.3 oz)	238	5	12	–	29	–	236
cinnamon raisin	1 (2¾ in)	223	4	10	40	31	1	229
dinner	1 (1 oz)	85	2	2	0	14	–	148
egg	1 (2½ in)	107	3	2	–	18	1	191
french	1 (1.3 oz)	105	3	2	0	19	–	232
hamburger	1 (1½ oz)	123	4	2	–	22	–	241
hamburger multi-grain	1 (1½ oz)	113	4	2	0	19	2	197
hamburger reduced calorie	1 (1½ oz)	84	4	1	0	18	3	190
hard	1 (3½ in)	167	6	2	0	30	–	310
hot cross bun	1	202	5	4	–	38	1	–
hotdog	1 (1½ oz)	123	4	2	–	22	–	241
hotdog reduced calorie	1 (1½ oz)	84	4	1	0	18	3	190
hotdog whole wheat	1 (1.5 oz)	110	5	2	0	19	2	220
kaiser	1 (3½ in)	167	6	2	0	30	–	310
oat bran	1 (1.2 oz)	78	3	2	0	13	1	136
rye	1 (1 oz)	81	3	1	0	15	–	253
submarine	1 (4.7 oz)	155	5	2	tr	30	–	313
wheat	1 (1 oz)	77	2	2	0	13	–	96
whole wheat	1 (1 oz)	75	3	1	0	15	–	135
Alvarado Street Bakery								
Sprouted Wheat Burger Bun	1 (2.2 oz)	140	7	2	0	27	3	290
Nature's Own								
100% Whole Grain Sugar Free	1 (1.9 oz)	110	6	2	0	23	4	240
Butter Buns	1 (1.7 oz)	120	5	2	5	23	1	115

FOOD	PORTION	CALS	PROT	FAT	CHOL	CARB	FIBER	SOD
Pepperidge Farm								
Hamburger 100% Whole Wheat	1	120	6	2	0	18	2	190
Hoagie Soft w/ Sesame Seeds	1	210	7	6	0	35	2	350
Hot & Crusty Sourdough	1	100	4	1	0	21	1	190
Hot Dog	1	140	5	3	0	26	tr	190
Hot Dog Whole Grain White	1	110	6	1	0	21	2	220
Parker House Dinner	1	80	3	2	0	14	tr	95
Premium Wheat	1	220	8	5	0	36	1	310
Rudi's Organic Bakery								
100% Whole Wheat	1 (2.3 oz)	160	7	2	0	29	5	240
Hot Dog Spelt	1 (2 oz)	140	5	2	0	28	2	260
Hot Dog Wheat	1 (2 oz)	150	5	2	0	28	2	260
Hot Dog White	1 (2 oz)	150	5	2	0	28	tr	280
Sara Lee								
Hamburger Bun Classic	1 (2.6 oz)	200	6	3	0	37	1	390
Hamburger Bun Classic Wheat	1 (2.6 oz)	200	7	4	0	38	3	390
Heart Healthy Hamburger Bun Wheat	1 (2.6 oz)	190	7	3	0	37	3	370
Hot Dog Gourmet	1 (1.5 oz)	120	4	2	0	23	tr	230
Stroehmann								
Hot Dog Wheat	1 (1.8 oz)	140	5	3	0	25	2	240
Super Bakery								
Daily Donut Reduced Fat	1 (2.2 oz)	200	7	6	15	35	1	290
Organic Sandwich Bun	1 (3.6 oz)	250	13	3	0	42	10	235
Sub Roll	1 (3.6 oz)	250	13	3	0	42	10	235
REFRIGERATED								
cinnamon w/ frosting	1	109	2	4	–	17	–	250
crescent	1 (1 oz)	98	2	4	0	14	–	341
Pillsbury								
Crescent	1 (1.7 oz)	170	2	10	0	20	tr	370
ROSE APPLE								
fresh	3.5 oz	32	1	tr	0	7	–	–
ROSE HIP								
fresh	1 oz	26	1	0	0	5	–	42

FOOD	PORTION	CALS	PROT	FAT	CHOL	CARB	FIBER	SOD
ROSELLE								
fresh	1 cup	28	1	tr	0	6	–	3
ROSEMARY								
dried	1 tsp	4	tr	tr	0	1	1	1
fresh	1 tbsp	1	tr	tr	0	tr	tr	0
ROUGHY								
orange baked	3 oz	75	16	1	22	0	0	69
RUBS (see HERBS/SPICES)								
RUTABAGA								
cooked mashed	½ cup	41	1	tr	0	9	–	22
raw cubed	½ cup	25	1	tr	0	6	–	14
Glory								
Cut Fresh	1 cup	50	2	0	0	11	4	30
SABLEFISH								
baked	3 oz	213	15	17	53	0	0	61
fillet baked	5.3 oz	378	26	30	95	0	0	108
smoked	1 oz	72	5	6	18	0	0	206
smoked	3 oz	218	15	17	55	0	0	626
SAFFLOWER								
seeds dried	1 oz	147	5	11	0	10	–	–
SAFFRON								
dried	1 tsp	2	tr	tr	0	tr	tr	1
SAGE								
ground	1 tsp	2	tr	tr	0	tr	tr	0
SALAD (see also SALAD TOPPINGS)								
Dole								
American Blend	1½ cups	15	1	0	0	3	1	10
Baby Spinach Salad	1½ cups (3 oz)	20	2	0	0	3	2	65
Butter & Red Leaf	1½ cups (3 oz)	10	1	0	0	3	1	10
Classic Iceberg	1½ cups (3 oz)	15	1	0	0	4	1	15
Classic Romaine	1½ cups (3 oz)	15	1	0	0	4	1	10

FOOD	PORTION	CALS	PROT	FAT	CHOL	CARB	FIBER	SOD
European Blend	1½ cups (3 oz)	15	1	0	0	3	1	15
Field Greens	1½ cups (3 oz)	15	1	0	0	4	2	30
French Blend	1½ cups (3 oz)	15	1	0	0	4	2	20
Greener Selection	1½ cups (3 oz)	15	1	0	0	3	1	10
Hearts Delight	1½ cups (3 oz)	15	1	0	0	3	1	10
Italian Blend	1½ cups (3 oz)	15	1	0	0	3	1	10
Kits Asian Crunch	1½ cups (3.5 oz)	120	2	6	0	12	2	230
Kits Bacon Lettuce Toss	1½ cups (3.5 oz)	130	3	9	10	8	1	300
Kits Caesar	1½ cups (3 oz)	170	3	15	10	8	2	440
Kits Caesar Light	1½ cups (3 oz)	100	3	7	0	8	1	370
Kits Fall Harvest	1½ cups (3.5 oz)	150	2	11	0	10	–	220
Kits Romano	1½ cups (3 oz)	150	3	12	0	9	2	570
Kits Spring Garden	1½ cups (3.5 oz)	140	2	11	0	11	2	390
Kits Sunflower Ranch	1½ cups (3 oz)	160	2	16	5	5	2	220
Mediterranean Blend	1½ cups	15	1	0	0	3	2	20
Very Veggie Blend	1½ cups (3 oz)	20	1	0	0	4	1	15
Earthbound Farm								
Organic Baby Arugula Salad	2 cups	20	2	0	0	3	1	25
Organic Baby Lettuce Salad	2 cups	15	1	0	0	3	1	60
Organic Baby Spinach Salad	2 cups	10	2	0	0	7	7	100
Organic Fresh Herb Salad	2 cups	15	2	0	0	4	2	70
Organic Mixed Baby Greens	2 cups	15	2	0	0	4	2	70

FOOD	PORTION	CALS	PROT	FAT	CHOL	CARB	FIBER	SOD
Mann's								
Rainbow	3 oz	25	2	0	0	5	2	25
River Ranch								
American Blend	1½ cups	15	tr	0	0	3	1	10
Caesar Kit	1½ cups	110	3	12	6	7	2	340
European Blend	1¾ cups	10	1	0	0	2	1	10
Garden	1½ cups	15	tr	0	0	3	1	10
Garden Supreme	1½ cups	15	1	0	0	3	1	10
Italian Blend	1¾ cups	15	1	0	0	2	1	10
Raspberry Vinaigrette Kit	1¾ cups	130	2	8	0	13	2	105
Riviera Blend	1½ cups	10	1	0	0	2	tr	5
TAKE-OUT								
7-layer salad	2 cups	557	11	51	119	15	3	612
caesar	4 cups	734	22	61	173	28	7	1119
chef salad w/o dressing	3 cups	535	52	32	280	9	–	1487
cobb w/ dressing	4 cups	645	32	49	294	23	11	1512
greek w/ dressing	4 cups	424	28	29	475	14	4	1638
mixed salad greens shredded	1 cup	9	1	tr	0	2	1	16
somen w/ lettuce egg fish pork	2 cups	550	40	17	429	57	4	1229
spinach no dressing	4 cups	429	20	19	308	45	6	909
tossed w/ avocado w/o dressing	2 cups	90	2	6	0	9	5	35
tossed w/ chicken w/o dressing	3 cups	194	33	4	86	5	2	108
tossed w/ egg w/o dressing	2 cups	93	7	5	183	6	2	92
tossed w/ seafood w/o dressing	3 cups	120	19	1	145	8	3	502
tossed w/ shrimp & egg w/o dressing	3 cups	185	30	5	430	5	2	1006
tossed w/o dressing	2 cups	22	1	tr	0	5	2	30
waldorf	1 cup	242	2	21	7	15	3	119
wilted lettuce w/ bacon dressing	1 cup	99	3	8	11	3	1	159

SALAD DRESSING (see also SALAD TOPPINGS)
MIX
A Taste Of Thai

Peanut Dressing as prep	2 tbsp	40	1	2	0	7	1	340

FOOD	PORTION	CALS	PROT	FAT	CHOL	CARB	FIBER	SOD
Good Seasons								
Italian as prep	2 tbsp	130	0	14	0	3	–	336
READY-TO-EAT								
blue cheese	1 tbsp	77	1	8	–	1	–	–
french	1 tbsp	67	tr	6	–	3	–	214
french reduced calorie	1 tbsp	22	0	1	1	4	–	128
italian	1 tbsp	69	tr	7	–	2	–	116
italian reduced calorie	1 tbsp	16	tr	2	1	1	–	118
russian	1 tbsp	76	tr	8	–	2	–	133
russian reduced calorie	1 tbsp	23	tr	1	1	5	–	141
sesame seed	1 tbsp	68	1	7	0	1	–	153
thousand island	1 tbsp	59	tr	6	–	2	–	109
thousand island reduced calorie	1 tbsp	24	tr	2	2	3	–	153
Annie's Naturals								
Cilantro & Lime	2 tbsp	100	0	10	–	2	–	90
French	2 tbsp	90	0	9	–	3	–	170
Goddess Dressing	2 tbsp	130	1	13	–	2	–	320
Low Fat Mustard Vinaigrette	2 tbsp	45	0	2	–	6	–	200
Organic Buttermilk	2 tbsp	70	tr	7	10	1	–	210
Organic Papaya Poppy Seed	2 tbsp	120	0	11	–	4	–	200
Organic Red Wine	2 tbsp	160	0	17	–	1	–	120
Organic No Fat Yogurt w/ Dill	2 tbsp	20	1	0	0	3	–	320
Sea Veggie & Sesame	2 tbsp	110	1	11	–	1	–	330
Tuscany Italian	2 tbsp	80	0	7	–	5	–	240
Bernstein's								
Chunky Blue Cheese	2 tbsp	120	1	13	5	2	0	180
Creamy Caesar	2 tbsp	120	0	13	15	1	0	200
Italian Restaurant Recipe	2 tbsp	120	1	12	5	1	0	360
Light Fantastic Roasted Garlic Balsamic	2 tbsp	45	0	4	0	3	0	320
Red Wine & Garlic Italian	2 tbsp	110	0	1	0	2	0	250
Cains								
Caesar Creamy	2 tbsp	170	0	19	5	1	0	170
Caesar Fat Free	2 tbsp	30	0	0	0	6	0	600
Caesar Light	2 tbsp	70	2	6	5	5	0	490
Chianti Vinaigrette	2 tbsp	130	0	12	0	5	0	220

FOOD	PORTION	CALS	PROT	FAT	CHOL	CARB	FIBER	SOD
Creamy Dill Cucumber Fat Free	2 tbsp	35	0	0	0	8	0	370
French	2 tbsp	120	0	11	0	6	0	170
French Light	2 tbsp	80	0	5	0	10	0	170
Greek	2 tbsp	160	0	17	5	2	0	190
Italian Fat Free	2 tbsp	15	0	0	0	4	0	490
Ranch	2 tbsp	180	0	19	5	1	0	270
Ranch Light	2 tbsp	80	0	6	5	6	0	310
Consorzio								
Balsamic Vinaigrette	2 tbsp	60	0	1	0	2	0	250
Caesar Parmesan & Romano	2 tbsp	120	0	7	20	1	–	290
Honey Mustard	2 tbsp	100	0	8	0	6	0	130
Italian	2 tbsp	60	0	7	0	1	0	250
Mango	1 tbsp	15	0	0	0	4	0	10
Raspberry & Balsamic	1 tbsp	15	0	0	0	4	0	0
Strawberry Balsamic	1 tbsp	10	0	0	0	2	0	0
David Burke								
Flavor Spray Ranch	2 sprays	0	0	0	0	0	0	10
Emeril's								
Bleu Cheese	2 tbsp	110	tr	12	–	tr	–	280
Honey Mustard	2 tbsp	100	0	9	–	3	–	250
House Herb Vinaigrette	2 tbsp	100	0	10	–	1	–	70
Kicked Up French	2 tbsp	80	0	5	–	8	–	200
Girard's								
White Balsamic Vinaigrette	2 tbsp	140	0	13	0	5	–	190
Ken's								
Bacon Ranch	2 tbsp	140	1	15	0	2	0	270
Caesar	2 tbsp	170	0	18	0	1	0	430
Country French w/ Vermont Honey	2 tbsp	150	0	12	0	10	0	220
Fat Free Italian	2 tbsp	25	0	0	0	5	0	380
Fat Free Raspberry Pecan	2 tbsp	50	0	0	0	12	0	280
Honey Mustard	2 tbsp	130	0	11	15	7	0	210
Italian w/ Aged Romano	2 tbsp	110	0	12	0	11	0	300
Lite Italian	2 tbsp	50	0	5	0	2	0	440
Lite Ranch	2 tbsp	80	0	6	10	6	0	310
Lite Red Wine Vinegar & Olive Oil	2 tbsp	50	0	5	0	2	0	280

FOOD	PORTION	CALS	PROT	FAT	CHOL	CARB	FIBER	SOD
Lite Vinaigrette Balsamic & Basil	2 tbsp	50	0	5	0	3	0	410
Lite Chunky Blue Cheese	2 tbsp	80	1	7	0	4	0	350
Red Wine Vinegar & Olive Oil	2 tbsp	120	0	12	0	2	0	360
Russian	2 tbsp	140	0	14	15	52	0	280
Thousand Island	2 tbsp	140	0	13	15	4	0	300
Kraft								
Free French	2 tbsp	50	0	0	0	11	0	350
Free Ranch	2 tbsp	50	0	0	0	11	1	350
Free Thousand Island	2 tbsp	45	0	0	0	10	0	260
LiteHouse								
Bleu Cheese Bacon	2 tbsp	150	1	16	15	1	0	240
Organic Vinaigrette Raspberry Lime	2 tbsp	40	0	2	0	5	0	55
Ranch Homestyle	2 tbsp	120	0	12	10	2	0	240
Ranch Lite	2 tbsp	70	0	6	5	2	0	220
Sesame Ginger	2 tbsp	35	0	0	0	8	0	230
Spinach Salad	2 tbsp	50	1	0	0	11	0	260
Vinaigrette Huckleberry	2 tbsp	20	0	0	0	4	0	90
Vinaigrette Lite Honey Dijon	2 tbsp	130	0	13	10	3	0	250
Marie's								
Blue Cheese Lite Chunky	2 tbsp	80	1	6	5	7	4	280
Blue Cheese Vinaigrette	2 tbsp	120	2	11	5	4	0	200
Caesar	2 tbsp	170	1	19	15	1	0	170
Coleslaw	2 tbsp	120	0	13	10	8	0	170
Creamy Ranch	2 tbsp	170	1	19	15	1	0	150
Red Wine Vinaigrette	2 tbsp	60	0	5	0	6	0	210
Sesame Ginger	2 tbsp	70	0	8	0	7	0	250
Milo's								
Gorgonzola Pear Riesling	2 tbsp	70	0	7	0	2	0	85
Pomegranate Port	2 tbsp	90	0	7	0	6	0	0
Nasoya								
Creamy Dill	1 tbsp	30	tr	3	0	1	0	140
Creamy Italian	2 tbsp	70	tr	7	0	1	0	140
Garden Herb	2 tbsp	60	tr	7	0	1	0	140
Sesame Garlic	2 tbsp	60	tr	7	0	1	0	130
Newman's Own								
Balsamic Vinaigrette	2 tbsp	90	0	9	0	3	0	350

FOOD	PORTION	CALS	PROT	FAT	CHOL	CARB	FIBER	SOD
Caesar	2 tbsp	150	1	16	0	1	0	420
Creamy Caesar	2 tbsp	150	1	16	<5	1	0	450
Family Recipe Italian	2 tbsp	120	1	13	0	1	0	400
Lighten Up Balsamic Vinaigrette	2 tbsp	45	0	4	0	2	0	470
Lighten Up Caesar	2 tbsp	70	2	6	5	3	0	520
Lighten Up Honey Mustard	2 tbsp	70	0	4	0	7	0	290
Lighten Up Italian	2 tbsp	60	0	6	0	0	0	260
Lighten Up Low Fat Sesame Ginger	2 tbsp	35	0	2	0	5	0	390
Lighten Up Raspberry & Walnut	2 tbsp	70	0	5	0	7	0	120
Lighten Up Red Wine Vinegar & Olive Oil	2 tbsp	110	0	10	0	3	–	430
Olive Oil & Vinegar	2 tbsp	150	0	16	0	1	0	150
Parmesan & Roasted Garlic	2 tbsp	110	0	11	0	2	0	250
Ranch	2 tbsp	140	0	15	10	2	0	250
Two Thousand Island	2 tbsp	140	0	14	10	4	0	260
San-J								
Tamari Mustard	2 tbsp	25	1	0	0	5	–	240
Tamari Peanut	2 tbsp	60	3	2	–	9	–	230
Tamari Sesame	2 tbsp	45	1	2	–	5	–	600
School House Kitchen								
Balsamic Vinaigrette Basico	2 tbsp	160	0	17	0	3	0	260
Seeds Of Change								
Vinaigrette Balsamic	2 tbsp	60	0	4	0	6	0	105
Vinaigrette Greek Feta	2 tbsp	60	1	5	0	5	0	270
Vinaigrette Roasted Garlic	2 tbsp	60	0	4	<5	6	0	125
Vinaigrette Sweet Basil	2 tbsp	60	0	5	0	6	0	160
Sonoma								
Creamy Tomato Bacon	2 tbsp	150	0	15	5	3	0	310
South Beach								
Balsamic Vinaigrette	2 tbsp	50	0	4	0	4	0	350
Italian	2 tbsp	60	0	4	0	3	0	300
Ranch	2 tbsp	70	1	7	0	2	0	300
Spectrum								
Provencal Garlic Lover's	2 tbsp	50	0	5	0	2	0	260
Vino De Milo								
Gorgonzola Pear Riesling	2 tbsp	80	0	7	0	2	0	75
Pomegranate Port	2 tbsp	90	0	7	0	5	0	0

FOOD	PORTION	CALS	PROT	FAT	CHOL	CARB	FIBER	SOD
Wishbone								
Blue Cheese w/ Gorgonzola	2 tbsp	140	0	15	<5	1	0	310
Caesar w/ Aged Romano	2 tbsp	80	0	8	0	3	0	530
Classic Ranch Extra Thick	2 tbsp	140	0	15	10	2	0	230
Creamy Caesar	2 tbsp	170	tr	18	10	1	0	300
Creamy Italian	2 tbsp	110	tr	10	0	4	0	240
Deluxe French	2 tbsp	50	0	2	0	8	tr	250
Fat Free Chunky Blue Cheese	2 tbsp	35	tr	0	0	7	tr	280
Fat Free Italian	2 tbsp	20	0	0	0	4	0	390
Fat Free Ranch	2 tbsp	30	0	0	0	7	tr	280
Fat Free Western	2 tbsp	45	0	0	0	12	–	260
Five Cheese Italian	2 tbsp	120	tr	10	0	6	0	410
Italian	2 tbsp	90	0	8	0	3	0	490
Just 2 Good Blue Cheese	2 tbsp	45	tr	2	0	6	0	310
Just 2 Good Creamy Caesar	2 tbsp	50	tr	2	10	7	0	300
Just 2 Good Deluxe French	2 tbsp	50	0	2	0	8	tr	250
Just 2 Good Italian	2 tbsp	35	0	2	0	4	0	490
Just 2 Good Ranch	2 tbsp	40	0	2	0	5	0	290
Just 2 Good Thousand Island	2 tbsp	50	0	2	5	9	0	290
Just 2 Good Western	2 tbsp	70	0	2	0	13	0	270
Light Vinaigrette Asian Sesame	2 tbsp	70	0	5	0	6	0	290
Light Vinaigrette Raspberry Walnut	2 tbsp	80	0	5	0	7	0	260
Light Ranch Extra Thick	2 tbsp	70	0	6	10	2	0	250
Ranch	2 tbsp	160	tr	17	10	1	0	200
Russian	2 tbsp	110	0	6	0	14	0	360
Salad Spritzers Balsamic Breeze	10 sprays	10	0	1	0	1	0	130
Salad Spritzers Italian	10 sprays	10	0	1	0	1	0	100
Salad Spritzers Red Wine Mist	10 sprays	10	0	1	0	1	0	95
Thousand Island	2 tbsp	130	0	12	10	6	0	330
Vinaigrette Berry	2 tbsp	50	0	5	0	2	0	135

FOOD	PORTION	CALS	PROT	FAT	CHOL	CARB	FIBER	SOD
Vinaigrette Lemon Garlic & Herb	2 tbsp	70	0	5	0	5	0	430
Vinaigrette Olive Oil	2 tbsp	60	0	5	0	4	0	250
Western	2 tbsp	160	0	12	0	12	0	230
TAKE-OUT								
vinegar & oil	1 tbsp	72	0	8	0	tr	–	tr

SALAD TOPPINGS
Fresh Gourmet

FOOD	PORTION	CALS	PROT	FAT	CHOL	CARB	FIBER	SOD
Crispy Onions Garlic Pepper	1½ tbsp	35	–	2	0	4	–	50
Tortilla Strips Lightly Salted	2 tbsp	35	–	2	0	5	0	25
Wonton Strips Wasabi Ranch	2 tbsp	35	1	2	0	4	0	45
Salad Pizazz!								
Asian Medley	1 tbsp	40	1	3	0	2	tr	50
Cherry Cranberry Pecano	1 tbsp	35	3	2	0	4	tr	10
Honey Toasted Delites	1 tbsp	40	1	3	0	2	1	20
Orange Cranberry Almondine	1 tbsp	35	1	2	0	4	tr	10
Raspberry Cranberry Walnut Frisco	1 tbsp	30	0	2	0	4	0	19
Tomato 'N Bacon Parmesano	1 tbsp	30	1	1	0	3	tr	35
Tomato Pinenut Tuscano	1 tbsp	130	1	2	0	2	tr	25

SALMON
CANNED

FOOD	PORTION	CALS	PROT	FAT	CHOL	CARB	FIBER	SOD
w/ bone	½ cup	106	15	5	39	0	0	410
Bumble Bee								
Blueback	¼ cup	110	13	7	40	0	0	270
Keta	¼ cup	90	13	4	40	0	0	270
Pink	¼ cup	90	12	5	40	0	0	270
Red	¼ cup	110	13	7	40	0	0	270
Skinless & Boneless	¼ cup	50	11	1	20	0	0	150
Smoked Fillets In Oil	⅓ cup	150	16	9	55	0	0	400
Chicken Of The Sea								
Pink	1 pkg (3 oz)	90	15	3	30	0	0	420
Red	¼ cup	110	13	7	40	0	0	270
Smoked Pacific	1 pkg (3 oz)	120	21	4	45	1	0	490

FOOD	PORTION	CALS	PROT	FAT	CHOL	CARB	FIBER	SOD
Libby's								
Red	¼ cup	110	13	7	40	0	0	270
FRESH								
atlantic farmed baked	4 oz	233	25	14	71	0	0	69
cloudberry native alaska	3.5 oz	51	2	1	–	9	–	–
coho wild poached	4 oz	209	31	9	65	0	0	30
pink baked	4 oz	169	29	5	76	0	0	97
roe raw	1 oz	59	7	3	–	tr	–	–
sockeye baked	4 oz	245	31	12	99	0	0	75
FROZEN								
Gorton's								
Fillets Classic Grilled	1 (3 oz)	100	15	3	35	2	–	270
Phillips Seafood								
Salmon Cakes	1 (3 oz)	180	13	13	40	3	–	270
SMOKED								
lox	1 oz	33	5	1	7	0	0	567
TAKE-OUT								
guisado salmon stew	1 serv (7.4 oz)	320	26	16	66	18	3	1130
roulette w/ spinach stuffing	1 serv (4 oz)	160	13	6	45	10	tr	400
salmon cake	1 (4.2 oz)	264	16	16	56	14	1	671
salmon loaf	1 slice (3.7 oz)	206	16	11	120	9	tr	819
SALSA								
black bean & corn	2 tbsp	15	1	0	0	3	tr	45
citrus	2 tbsp (1 oz)	10	0	0	0	2	0	7
peach	2 tbsp	15	0	0	0	4	0	90
tomatoless corn & chile	2 tbsp	45	1	0	0	10	tr	95
Bone Suckin'								
Fat Free Gluten Free	2 tbsp	40	0	0	0	10	0	110
Cape Cod								
Medium & Mild	2 tbsp	15	tr	0	0	3	1	210
Chi-Chi's								
Fiesta Mild	2 tbsp	10	0	0	0	2	0	150
Emeril's								
Original Recipe	2 tbsp	10	0	0	0	3	0	190
Muir Glen								
Organic Medium	2 tbsp	10	0	0	0	3	0	130

FOOD	PORTION	CALS	PROT	FAT	CHOL	CARB	FIBER	SOD
Newman's Own								
Bandito Pineapple	2 tbsp	15	0	0	0	3	1	90
Bandito Mild	2 tbsp	10	0	0	0	2	1	105
Bandito Peach	2 tbsp	25	0	0	0	6	tr	90
Bandito Roasted Garlic	2 tbsp	10	1	0	0	2	1	150
Bandito Tequila Lime	2 tbsp	15	0	0	0	3	–	170
Ortega								
Garden Style Mild	2 tbsp	10	tr	0	0	2	tr	220
Picante Mild	2 tbsp	10	0	0	0	2	–	220
Pace								
Black Bean & Corn	2 tbsp	25	1	0	0	5	1	150
Organic Picante	2 tbsp	10	0	0	0	2	tr	220
Thick & Chunky	2 tbsp	10	0	0	0	2	tr	230
Robert Rothchild Farm								
Tomatillo & Pepper	2 tbsp	20	0	0	0	5	tr	95
Seeds Of Change								
Black Bean & Tomato Mild	2 tbsp	15	1	0	0	3	tr	170
Garlic & Cilantro Mild	2 tbsp	15	0	0	0	2	tr	170
Snyder's Of Hanover								
Sweet	2 tbsp	20	0	0	0	5	0	95
Tostitos								
All Natural	2 tbsp	15	tr	0	0	3	1	260
Con Queso	2 tbsp	40	tr	3	<5	5	tr	280
Monterey Jack Queso	2 tbsp	40	1	3	<5	4	0	210
Restaurant Style	2 tbsp	15	0	<1	0	3	tr	210
Utz								
Sweet	2 tbsp	10	0	0	0	2	tr	160
Walnut Acres								
Organic Fiesta Cilantro	2 tbsp	10	0	0	0	2	0	135
Organic Sweet Southwestern Peach	2 tbsp	20	03	0	0	5	0	85
SALSIFY								
fresh sliced cooked	½ cup	46	2	tr	0	10	–	11
Frieda's								
Salsify	¾ cup	70	3	0	0	16	3	15
SALT SUBSTITUTES								
gomasio sesame salt	2 tsp	34	1	3	–	2	1	388
AlsoSalt								
Butter Flavored	¼ tsp	1	0	0	0	0	0	0

FOOD	PORTION	CALS	PROT	FAT	CHOL	CARB	FIBER	SOD
Garlic Flavored	¼ tsp	1	0	0	0	0	0	0
Salt Substitute	¼ tsp	tr	0	0	0	0	0	0
Chef Paul Prudhomme's								
Magic Salt Free Seasoning	¼ tsp	0	0	0	0	0	0	0
Eden								
Organic Seaweed Gomasio Sesame Salt	1 tsp	15	tr	2	0	tr	0	80
Organic Gomasio Sesame Salt	1 tsp	15	tr	2	0	tr	0	80
French's								
No Salt	¼ cup	0	0	0	0	0	0	0
SALT/SEASONED SALT								
salt	1 tbsp	0	0	0	0	0	0	6976
salt	1 tsp	0	0	0	0	0	0	2325
sea salt coarse	¼ tsp	0	0	0	0	0	0	330
sea salt fine	¼ tsp	0	0	0	0	0	0	440
BaconSalt								
Original	¼ tsp	0	0	0	0	0	0	150
Peppered	¼ tsp	0	0	0	0	0	0	135
Bob's Red Mill								
Garlic Salt Blend	¼ tsp	0	0	0	0	0	0	335
Sea Salt	¼ tsp	0	0	0	0	0	0	390
Eden								
French Celtic Salt	¼ tsp	0	0	0	0	0	0	390
Portuguese Coast Salt	¼ tsp	0	0	0	0	0	0	410
Maine Coast								
Sea Salt w/ Sea Veg	¼ tsp	0	0	0	0	0	0	396
Morton								
Iodized	¼ tsp	0	0	0	0	0	0	590
Kosher	1 tsp	0	–	0	0	–	–	–
Spice Hunter								
Celery Salt	¼ tsp	0	0	0	0	0	0	270
Garlic Salt	¼ tsp	0	0	0	0	0	0	290
SANDWICHES								
Aunt Jemima								
Biscuit Sausage Egg & Cheese	1 (4 oz)	340	12	21	110	27	1	830
Croissant Sausage Egg & Cheese	1 (4 oz)	350	13	23	145	22	1	680

FOOD	PORTION	CALS	PROT	FAT	CHOL	CARB	FIBER	SOD
Griddlecake Sausage Egg & Cheese	1 (4.4 oz)	350	13	20	150	30	tr	900
Aunt Trudy's								
Classic Samosa Fillo Pocket	1 (5 oz)	280	6	10	0	43	3	350
Fillo Pocket Cheese & Tomato	1 (5 oz)	320	11	15	20	36	2	490
Fillo Pocket Mediterranean Olive & Veggies	1 (5 oz)	270	6	10	0	41	2	550
Organic Fillo Pocket Roasted Sweet Potato	1 (5 oz)	310	5	12	0	45	4	270
Cedarlane								
Wrap Low Fat Couscous & Vegetable Veggie	1 (6 oz)	220	14	3	0	36	3	580
Fillo Factory								
Organic Fillo Pocket Asian Vegetable	1 (5 oz)	240	5	10	0	34	3	390
Gardenburger								
100% Meatless Margherita Pizza Wrap	1 (4.7 oz)	240	12	8	10	34	5	590
Wrap Black Bean Chipotle	1 (4.7 oz)	240	13	8	10	32	6	600
Guiltless Gourmet								
Wrap California Veggie	1 (5.7 oz)	270	9	5	0	47	4	290
Wrap Mediterranean Spinach	1 (5.7 oz)	270	10	5	<5	45	4	270
Ian's								
Mini Chicken Patty	2 (5.3 oz)	368	20	10	34	54	1	608
Lean Pockets								
Bacon Egg & Cheese	1 (4.5 oz)	150	7	5	40	21	2	280
Barbecue Sauce w/ Beef	1 (4.5 oz)	290	11	7	20	47	3	850
Chicken Cheddar & Broccoli	1 (4.5 oz)	260	11	7	20	39	3	590
Chicken Fajita	1 (4.5 oz)	260	11	7	25	38	3	730
Chicken Parmesan	1 (4.5 oz)	280	13	7	30	43	3	620
Ham & Cheese	1 (4.5 oz)	280	14	7	25	40	3	700
Meatballs & Mozzarella	1 (4.5 oz)	290	13	7	20	44	3	700
Philly Steak & Cheese	1 (4.5 oz)	280	13	7	25	40	3	590
Sausage Egg & Cheese	1 (4.5 oz)	140	7	5	45	19	2	310
Steak Fajita	1 (4.5 oz)	260	11	7	25	39	3	730
Three Cheese & Chicken Quesadilla	1 (4.5 oz)	280	14	7	25	41	3	630

FOOD	PORTION	CALS	PROT	FAT	CHOL	CARB	FIBER	SOD
Turkey & Ham w/ Cheddar	1 (4.5 oz)	280	13	7	30	43	3	710
Turkey Broccoli & Cheese	1 (4.5 oz)	270	13	7	25	39	3	530
Lunchables								
Chicken Dunks	1 pkg	310	12	6	30	52	0	550
Stackers Ham & American	1 pkg	430	15	17	50	56	tr	840
Stackers Turkey & American	1 pkg	420	13	17	45	55	tr	780
Madalena's Masterpiece								
Calzone Artichoke Parmesan	1 (10 oz)	570	27	29	45	51	2	1180
Calzone Grilled Chicken	1 (10 oz)	520	38	22	75	43	1	1190
Calzone Sausage Pepperoni	1 (10 oz)	640	34	36	90	48	tr	1770
Panini Garlic Chicken	1 (8 oz)	450	32	25	85	42	2	1310
Panini Honey Ham	1 (8 oz)	520	26	25	50	46	tr	1440
Panini Turkey Pesto	1 (8 oz)	500	25	26	55	43	0	1140
Panini Veggie	1 (8 oz)	480	20	26	40	43	1	1050
Quesabake Mexican Sausage	1 (7 oz)	510	21	26	45	48	2	820
Quesabake Roasted Veggie	1 (7 oz)	460	19	24	35	47	1	460
Oscar Mayer								
Deli Creations Honey Ham & Swiss	1 pkg (6.8 oz)	440	28	14	55	51	4	1490
Deli Creations Steakhouse Cheddar	1 pkg (7.1 oz)	450	29	15	60	50	3	1420
Deli Creations Turkey & Cheddar Dijon	1 pkg (6.7 oz)	430	26	15	50	48	5	1410
PBJammerz								
Peanut Butter & Jelly All Flavors	1 (2 oz)	220	8	13	0	22	3	150
Smucker's								
Uncrustables Grilled Cheese	1 (1.8 oz)	150	6	6	15	17	tr	500
Uncrustables Peanut Butter & Grape Jelly	1 (2 oz)	210	7	9	0	25	2	260
Uncrustables Peanut Butter & Strawberry Jam	1 (2 oz)	210	7	9	0	25	2	260
South Beach								
Breakfast Wraps All American	1 serv (4.6 oz)	200	19	9	15	26	15	620

FOOD	PORTION	CALS	PROT	FAT	CHOL	CARB	FIBER	SOD
Breakfast Wraps Denver	1 serv (4.6 oz)	180	16	7	15	27	15	620
Wrap Kit Deli Ham & Turkey	1 pkg	220	22	10	40	23	15	1110
Wrap Kit Grilled Chicken Caesar	1 pkg	230	24	10	50	23	14	1030
Wrap Kit Southwestern Style Chicken	1 pkg	250	26	10	55	26	15	1040
Wrap Kit Turkey & Bacon Club	1 pkg	250	24	13	40	24	15	1130
Stouffer's								
Corner Bistro Panini Southwestern Chicken	1 pkg (6 oz)	360	20	16	45	31	3	920
Corner Bistro Panini Philly Style Steak & Cheese	1 pkg (6 oz)	340	20	16	40	33	3	680
TAKE-OUT								
bacon & egg	1 (6.2 oz)	388	21	21	421	28	1	938
bacon lettuce & tomato w/ mayo	1 (5.8 oz)	344	12	17	21	35	3	945
beef barbecue w/ bun	1 (6.7 oz)	417	32	12	69	42	2	647
calzone beef & cheese	1 (14 oz)	1476	62	76	187	131	6	1726
calzone cheese	1 (15 oz)	1632	80	93	254	117	5	2519
chicken salad	1 (5 oz)	333	19	16	49	28	2	565
crab cake w/ bun	1	308	21	8	97	36	2	578
croque monsieur	1 (12.4 oz)	765	41	46	152	43	2	1018
egg salad	1 (5.6 oz)	485	14	35	329	28	1	706
french dip w/ roll	1 (6.8 oz)	357	26	13	54	34	1	562
fried egg	1 (3.4 oz)	226	10	9	206	26	1	439
grilled cheese	1 (2.9 oz)	290	9	16	22	28	1	764
gyro	1 (13.7 oz)	593	44	12	82	74	4	874
ham & egg	1 (4.4 oz)	272	15	11	222	27	2	802
ham w/ cheese w/ lettuce & mayo	1 (5.4 oz)	369	19	18	57	32	2	1525
hot turkey w/ gravy	1	389	40	10	88	32	2	1349
peanut butter & jelly	1 (3.3 oz)	327	10	14	0	42	3	483
reuben w/ sauerkraut & cheese	1 (6.4 oz)	463	21	29	81	30	4	1377
roast beef w/ gravy	1 (7.8 oz)	386	30	16	69	30	2	1083
sloppy joe pork on bun	1 (6.5 oz)	318	23	9	50	34	2	908

FOOD	PORTION	CALS	PROT	FAT	CHOL	CARB	FIBER	SOD
tuna melt	1 (5.3 oz)	350	20	16	34	30	1	832
tuna salad w/ lettuce	1 (5.9 oz)	289	19	7	22	37	2	785
turkey w/ mayo	1 (5 oz)	329	29	11	67	26	1	565

SAPODILLA

fresh	1	140	1	2	0	34	–	20
fresh cut up	1 cup	199	1	3	0	48	–	29

SAPOTES

fresh	1	301	5	1	0	76	–	21

SARDINES
CANNED

FOOD	PORTION	CALS	PROT	FAT	CHOL	CARB	FIBER	SOD
atlantic in oil w/ bone	2	50	6	3	34	0	0	121
atlantic in oil w/ bone	1 can (3.2 oz)	192	23	11	131	0	0	465
pacific in tomato sauce w/ bone	1 can (13 oz)	658	61	44	225	0	0	1532
pacific in tomato sauce w/ bone	1	68	6	5	23	0	0	157

Beach Cliff

FOOD	PORTION	CALS	PROT	FAT	CHOL	CARB	FIBER	SOD
In Louisiana Hot Sauce	1 can (3.7 oz)	150	18	8	110	2	0	420
In Mustard Sauce	1 can (3.7 oz)	150	20	8	110	2	0	460
In Olive Oil	1 can (3.7 oz)	200	20	14	105	0	0	270
In Tomato Sauce	1 can (3.7 oz)	140	17	6	90	2	0	520
In Water	1 can (3.7 oz)	150	19	8	115	0	0	240
Small In Soybean Oil	1 can (3.7 oz)	200	22	12	115	1	0	260
W/ Hot Green Chilies	1 can (3.7 oz)	180	19	12	100	1	0	250

Brunswick

FOOD	PORTION	CALS	PROT	FAT	CHOL	CARB	FIBER	SOD
In Louisiana Hot Sauce	1 can (3.7 oz)	150	18	8	110	2	0	420
In Mustard Sauce	1 can (3.7 oz)	150	20	8	110	2	0	460

FOOD	PORTION	CALS	PROT	FAT	CHOL	CARB	FIBER	SOD
In Soybean Oil	1 can (3.7 oz)	110	22	12	115	1	0	260
In Spring Water	1 can (3.7 oz)	150	19	8	115	0	0	240
In Tomato Sauce	1 can (3.7 oz)	150	16	8	100	3	0	520
W/ Hot Tabasco Peppers	1 can (3.7 oz)	110	21	12	110	0	0	280
Bumble Bee								
In Hot Sauce	¼ cup	90	8	6	30	0	0	250
In Mustard	¼ cup	70	8	4	20	1	1	260
In Oil	1 can (3.7 oz)	130	13	9	35	0	0	340
In Water	1 can (3.7 oz)	120	13	7	35	0	0	340
Chicken Of The Sea								
In Hot Sauce	1 can (3.75 oz)	130	17	6	60	2	2	490
In Mustard Sauce	1 can (3.75 oz)	150	17	8	60	2	2	490
In Oil	1 can (3.75 oz)	190	12	14	45	2	0	430
In Tomato Sauce	1 can (3.75 oz)	130	17	6	60	2	2	490
In Water	1 can (3.75 oz)	100	13	4	45	2	0	430
Goya								
In Tomato Sauce	2 pieces (2.2 oz)	50	8	1	45	20	2	15
King Oscar								
In Olive Oil	1 can (3.75 oz)	150	14	11	120	0	0	340
FRESH								
raw	3.5 oz	135	19	5	–	0	0	100

SAUCE (*see also* BARBECUE SAUCE, GRAVY, PIZZA SAUCE, SPAGHETTI SAUCE)

FOOD	PORTION	CALS	PROT	FAT	CHOL	CARB	FIBER	SOD
adobo fresco	2 tbsp	81	1	8	0	7	1	6175
bearnaise	1 oz	177	1	19	21	1	tr	257
cheese mix as prep w/ milk	1 cup	307	16	17	53	23	–	1566

FOOD	PORTION	CALS	PROT	FAT	CHOL	CARB	FIBER	SOD
curry mix as prep	1 cup	120	3	6	0	14	–	1142
curry mix as prep w/ milk	1 cup	270	11	15	35	26	–	1276
enchilada sauce green	¼ cup	46	1	4	11	3	1	113
enchilada sauce red	¼ cup	79	1	8	22	2	1	86
fish sauce chinese	1 tbsp	9	2	0	–	tr	0	1224
fish sauce vietnamese nuoc mam	1 tbsp	6	1	0	0	1	0	1390
hoisin	1 tbsp	35	1	1	0	7	tr	258
morroccan tagine	½ cup (4 oz)	70	2	3	0	10	1	1140
mushroom mix as prep w/ milk	1 cup	228	11	10	34	24	–	1533
oyster	1 tbsp	8	tr	0	0	2	0	437
plum sauce	0.5 oz	42	0	0	–	10	0	281
satay peanut sauce	1 oz	77	2	6	0	3	1	138
sour cream mix as prep w/ milk	1 cup	509	19	30	91	45	–	1007
stroganoff mix as prep	1 cup	271	12	11	38	34	–	1829
sweet & sour mix as prep	1 cup	294	1	tr	0	73	–	779
teriyaki	1 tbsp	15	1	0	0	3	–	690
teriyaki mix as prep	1 cup	131	4	1	0	28	–	4791
white sauce mix as prep w/ milk	1 cup	241	10	13	34	21	–	796
A Taste Of Thai								
Chili Sauce Garlic Pepper	1 tsp	10	2	0	0	2	0	230
Chili Sauce Sweet Red	1 tsp	10	0	0	0	2	0	40
Fish Sauce	1 tbsp	15	2	0	0	1	–	1730
Pad Thai Sauce Mix	2 tbsp	90	1	1	0	20	1	790
Peanut Satay	2 tbsp	80	1	5	0	9	1	180
Peanut Sauce Mix	¼ pkg	45	1	2	0	7	1	190
Annie Chun's								
Marinade & Dressing Lemongrass Herb	1 tbsp	25	0	2	0	4	0	105
Noodle Sauce & Dressing Sesame Cilantro	1 tbsp	60	0	4	0	4	0	400
Shiitake Mushroom	1 tbsp	15	1	0	0	3	0	190
Annie's Naturals								
Marinade Organic Spicy Ginger	2 tbsp	35	1	2	–	3	–	450

FOOD	PORTION	CALS	PROT	FAT	CHOL	CARB	FIBER	SOD
Marinade Organic Teriyaki	1 tbsp	30	0	1	–	6	–	340
Organic Worcestershire	1 tbsp	20	tr	0	0	5	–	460
Asian Creations								
Marvelous Mango	¼ cup	20	0	0	0	6	0	20
Pad Thai Pizzazz	2 oz	110	2	6	0	14	tr	310
Peanut Passion	¼ cup	130	4	9	0	12	1	420
Asian Gourmet								
Duck Sauce Peking Style	2 tbsp	40	0	0	0	13	–	65
Boar's Head								
Ham Glaze Sugar & Spice	2 tbsp	120	0	0	0	30	0	95
Bone Suckin'								
Hiccuppin' Hot	1 tsp	10	0	0	0	2	0	25
Yaki Stir Fry	1 tbsp	30	0	0	0	7	0	260
Cains								
Tartar	2 tbsp	160	0	16	15	2	0	160
Consorzio								
Marinade Baja Lime	1 tbsp	60	0	6	–	3	–	20
Marinade California Teriyaki	1 tbsp	40	1	2	–	5	–	420
Marinade Dijon Peppercorn	1 tbsp	15	0	0	0	3	–	150
Marinade Jamaican Jerk	1 tbsp	10	0	0	0	3	–	390
Marinade Lemon Pepper	1 tbsp	60	0	6	–	1	–	150
Marinade Roasted Garlic	1 tbsp	35	0	2	0	5	0	230
Marinade Sesame Ginger	1 tbsp	25	1	1	–	4	–	380
Marinade Southwestern Chipotle	1 tbsp	30	0	2	0	4	0	250
Marinade Tropical Grill	1 tbsp	40	0	3	0	3	0	50
Del Monte								
Seafood Cocktail	¼ cup	100	1	0	0	24	0	910
Sloppy Joe Original	¼ cup	50	1	0	0	11	0	620
D'Oni								
Happy Together Orange Chili Garlic	2 tbsp	50	0	0	0	12	–	80
Moondance Marinade	1 tbsp	10	–	0	0	0	–	150
Eden								
Ponzu Sauce	1 tbsp	5	0	0	0	1	–	340
Emeril's								
Marinade Hickory Maple Chipotle	1 tbsp	35	0	3	–	2	–	75

FOOD	PORTION	CALS	PROT	FAT	CHOL	CARB	FIBER	SOD
Marinade Lemon Rosemary Gaaahlic	1 tbsp	70	0	8	–	1	–	120
Marinade Orange Herb Poppyseed	1 tbsp	150	0	15	–	4	–	170
Steak Sauce	1 tbsp	20	0	0	0	4	–	200
Fage								
Tzatziki	2 tbsp	30	1	2	5	2	0	120
Frank's								
Buffalo Wing Sauce	1 tbsp	5	0	0	0	0	0	380
RedHot Chile & Lime Sauce	1 tsp	0	0	0	0	0	0	200
RedHot Original Cayenne Pepper Sauce	1 tsp	0	0	0	0	0	0	200
RedHot X-tra Hot	1 tsp	0	0	0	0	0	0	210
French's								
Worchestershire	1 tsp	0	0	0	0	1	0	50
Good Clean Food								
Simmer Sauce Balsamic Mushroom	⅜ cup (3 oz)	100	2	6	5	9	tr	250
Simmer Sauce Cacciatore	⅜ cup (3 oz)	70	2	4	–	7	2	350
Simmer Sauce Creole	⅜ cup (3 oz)	45	2	2	5	7	1	330
Simmer Sauce Dill	⅜ cup (3 oz)	60	2	4	5	5	–	250
Simmer Sauce French Tarragon	⅜ cup (3 oz)	90	2	6	5	8	tr	290
Simmer Sauce Mediterranean	⅜ cup (3 oz)	50	1	3	–	6	1	180
House Of Tsang								
General Tsao	1 tsp	45	0	1	0	10	0	230
Hoisin	1 tsp	15	0	0	0	4	0	120
Kobe Steak Grill	1 tbsp	50	0	4	0	2	0	560
Korean Teriyaki Stir Fry	1 tbsp	35	0	2	0	5	0	460
Peanut Sauce Bangkok Padang	1 tbsp	45	1	3	0	4	0	250
Spicy Brown Bean	1 tbsp	15	0	0	0	3	0	130
Sweet & Sour	1 tbsp	35	0	0	0	8	0	50
Sweet Ginger Sesame	1 tbsp	40	0	1	0	8	0	401
Thai Peanut	1 tbsp	50	1	3	0	4	0	280

FOOD	PORTION	CALS	PROT	FAT	CHOL	CARB	FIBER	SOD
Ken's								
Marinade Herb & Garlic	1 tbsp	20	0	1	0	3	0	370
Marinade Lemon & Pepper	1 tbsp	10	0	0	0	2	0	350
Marinade Teriyaki	1 tbsp	20	0	0	0	4	0	260
Knorr								
Alfredo Mix as prep	2 oz	60	2	3	5	5	–	390
Bearnaise Mix as prep	2 oz	35	2	1	5	5	–	190
Curry Indian Madras	1 oz	30	tr	2	5	2	–	140
Curry Thai	1 oz	35	tr	3	0	3	–	90
Demi-Glace Mix as prep	2 oz	30	1	1	0	4	–	500
Green Peppercorn Mix as prep	2 oz	35	1	1	5	5	–	390
Hollandaise Mix as prep	2 oz	35	2	1	5	5	–	170
Mango Habanero	1 oz	20	tr	0	0	6	–	95
Sweet Red Chili	1 oz	80	1	0	0	19	–	300
White Mix as prep	2 oz	20	tr	1	0	3	–	290
Las Palmas								
Enchilada Green	¼ cup	25	0	2	0	3	0	340
Enchilada Mild	¼ cup	20	0	1	0	2	1	310
Red Chili	¼ cup	20	0	1	0	2	1	310
Latino Chef								
Chimichurri Sun Dried Tomato	2 tbsp	120	2	10	0	8	2	210
Sofrito	2 tbsp	20	0	1	0	3	–	160
Lea & Perrins								
Worcestershire	1 tsp	5	0	0	0	1	–	65
Lee Kum Kee								
Plum Sauce	2 tbsp	100	0	0	0	26	–	520
Lollipop Tree								
Grilling & Glazing Chipotle	1 tbsp	50	0	0	0	14	0	120
Grilling & Glazing Mango Garlic	2 tbsp	60	0	0	0	14	0	10
Matouk's								
Calypso	1 tsp	0	0	0	0	0	0	115
Milo's								
Simmer Sauce Bombay Cabernet	3 oz	35	1	0	0	7	1	220
Mrs. Dash								
10 Minute Marinade Lemon Herb Peppercorn	1 tbsp	25	0	2	–	2	–	0

FOOD	PORTION	CALS	PROT	FAT	CHOL	CARB	FIBER	SOD
10 Minute Marinade Mesquite Grille	1 tbsp	25	0	2	–	2	–	0
10 Minute Marinade Southwestern Chipotle	1 tbsp	20	0	2	–	2	–	0
10 Minute Marinade Zesty Garlic Herb	1 tbsp	25	0	2	–	3	–	0
Nando's								
Curry Coconut	¼ cup	71	–	5	4	6	1	389
Fresh Lemon	¼ cup	61	–	5	3	5	0	185
Marinade Lime & Cilantro	1 tbsp	27	0	2	0	2	0	173
Marinade Sundried Tomato	1 tbsp	15	0	1	0	1	0	164
Peri-Peri Pepper Extra Hot	1 oz	17	1	1	0	2	–	1
Peri-Peri Pepper Garlic	1 oz	12	tr	1	0	1	–	tr
Peri-Peri Pepper Hot	1 oz	16	tr	1	0	2	–	1
Peri-Peri Pepper Wild Herb	1 oz	14	tr	1	0	2	–	tr
Roasted Red	¼ cup	70	–	5	0	7	1	777
Sweet Apricot	¼ cup	51	–	0	0	12	0	445
Newman's Own								
Fra Diavolo	½ cup	70	0	3	0	10	3	510
Steak Sauce	1 tbsp	20	0	1	0	4	0	85
Old El Paso								
Enchilada Mild	¼ cup	25	0	1	0	4	0	250
Ortega								
Enchilada	¼ cup	15	tr	1	0	4	tr	340
Taco	1 tbsp	10	0	0	0	1	–	60
Pace								
Taco Sauce Green	1 tbsp	5	0	0	0	1	0	100
Taco Sauce Red	2 tbsp	10	0	0	0	2	0	130
Patak's								
Dopiaza	½ cup	90	2	5	0	11	0	750
Jalfrezi Sweet Peppers & Coconut	½ cup	140	2	8	0	15	1	620
Korma Rich Creamy Coconut	½ cup	240	2	20	15	13	1	750
Rogan Josh Spicy Tomato & Cardamon	½ cup	90	2	4	0	12	2	750
Tikka Masala Tangy Lemon & Cilantro	½ cup	120	1	8	0	12	1	900

FOOD	PORTION	CALS	PROT	FAT	CHOL	CARB	FIBER	SOD
Road's End Organics								
Alfredo Style Dairy Free Gluten Free	⅓ pkg	35	3	0	0	5	1	240
Cheddar Style Dairy Free	⅓ pkg	35	2	0	0	6	1	260
Robert Rothchild Farm								
Anne Mae's Smoky Sweet Chipotle	2 tbsp	35	tr	0	0	9	0	80
San-J								
Japanese Steak	1 tbsp	13	2	0	0	2	–	930
Sweet & Tangy	1 tbsp	50	1	0	0	13	–	320
Szechuan	1 tsp	5	0	0	0	1	–	180
Teriyaki	1 tbsp	10	1	0	0	3	–	450
Thai Peanut	2 tbsp	70	3	3	–	7	–	710
South Beach								
Steak Sauce	1 tbsp	5	0	0	0	1	0	230
The Wizard's								
Organic Worcestershire Vegetarian Wheat Free	1 tsp	0	0	0	0	1	0	115
Ty Ling								
Duck	2 tbsp	70	0	0	0	19	1	260
WildWood								
Aioli	1 tbsp	80	0	9	0	0	0	80
Pesto Basil & Pine Nuts	¼ cup	230	5	23	8	2	1	360
Wingers								
Hotter Than Hot	1 tsp	0	0	0	0	0	0	120
TAKE-OUT								
cucumber yogurt sauce	1½ tbsp	20	2	0	2	3	0	20
SAUERKRAUT								
canned	½ cup	22	1	tr	0	5	–	780
Boar's Head								
Sauerkraut	2 tbsp (1 oz)	5	0	0	0	1	tr	180
Del Monte								
Bavarian Style	2 tbsp	15	0	0	0	4	0	180
Eden								
Organic	½ cup	25	2	0	0	4	3	580
Hebrew National								
Sauerkraut	2 tbsp	5	0	0	0	1	1	180

FOOD	PORTION	CALS	PROT	FAT	CHOL	CARB	FIBER	SOD
SAUSAGE								
beef & pork	1 link (2.3 oz)	196	8	17	51	1	0	560
beef & pork w/ cheddar cheese	1 link (2.7 oz)	228	10	20	49	2	0	653
bierschinken	3.5 oz	174	18	11	–	tr	–	753
bierwurst	3.5 oz	258	16	21	–	0	0	–
blutwurst uncooked	3.5 oz	424	13	39	–	0	0	680
bockwurst	3.5 oz	276	12	25	–	0	0	700
bratwurst pork cooked	1 link (2.5 oz)	226	10	19	44	2	0	778
brotwurst pork & beef	1 link (2.5 oz)	226	10	19	44	2	0	778
chipolata	3.5 oz	342	14	32	66	1	0	747
chorizo	1 link (2.1 oz)	273	14	23	53	1	0	741
fleischwurst	3.5 oz	305	12	29	–	0	0	829
free range chicken breakfast	2 links (2.7 oz)	110	14	6	45	1	0	570
gelbwurst uncooked	3.5 oz	363	12	33	–	0	0	640
italian pork cooked	1 (2.4 oz)	230	13	18	38	3	1	809
jagdwurst	3.5 oz	211	16	16	–	0	0	818
knockwurst pork & beef	1 (2.5 oz)	221	8	20	43	2	0	670
mettwurst uncooked	3.5 oz	483	13	45	–	0	0	1090
plockwurst uncooked	3.5 oz	312	19	45	–	0	0	–
polish kielbasa	2 oz	127	7	10	39	2	0	672
pork cooked	2 links (1.7 oz)	163	9	14	40	0	0	360
regensburger uncooked	3.5 oz	354	13	31	–	0	0	–
turkey italian smoked	1 (2 oz)	88	8	5	30	3	1	520
vienna canned	1 can (4 oz)	260	12	22	98	3	0	1095
vienna canned	1 link (0.5 oz)	37	2	3	14	tr	0	155
weisswurst uncooked	3.5 oz	305	11	27	–	0	0	620
zungenwurst (tongue)	3.5 oz	285	17	24	–	0	0	–
Al Fresco								
Apple Maple	1 (1.2 oz)	70	5	4	25	4	–	240
Buffalo Style	1 (3 oz)	160	19	8	50	4	–	630
Country Style	1 (1.2 oz)	60	6	4	35	1	–	230
Italian Sweet	1 (3 oz)	170	19	8	65	2	–	440

FOOD	PORTION	CALS	PROT	FAT	CHOL	CARB	FIBER	SOD
Roasted Garlic	1 (3 oz)	170	19	8	70	4	–	420
Spicy Jalapeno	1 (3 oz)	120	19	7	65	1	–	550
Sundried Tomato & Basil	1 (3 oz)	180	19	8	70	3	–	440
Sweet Apple	1 (3 oz)	160	19	8	65	9	–	580
Teriyaki Ginger	1 (3 oz)	180	19	8	70	7	–	660
Wild Blueberry	1 (1.2 oz)	90	5	4	25	4	–	200
Armour								
Brown'N Serve Lite Original	3	120	9	8	45	3	0	410
Brown'N Serve Turkey	3 links	120	10	8	35	2	0	370
Banquet								
Brown 'N Serve Lite Original	3 (2.1 oz)	120	9	9	25	2	0	430
Brown'N Serve Lite Maple	3 (2 oz)	130	9	9	35	4	0	450
Boar's Head								
Bratwurst	1 (4 oz)	300	19	25	75	0	0	650
Hot Smoked	1 (3.2 oz)	250	12	22	55	1	0	740
Kielbasa	2 oz	120	9	10	50	0	0	440
Knockwurst Beef	1 (4 oz)	310	15	27	70	1	0	950
Healthy Ones								
Smoked	2 oz	80	7	3	25	6	0	480
Hebrew National								
Knockwurst Beef	1 (3 oz)	260	10	24	55	1	0	670
Honeysuckle White								
Turkey Roll Mild Italian	2.5 oz	100	13	5	40	1	0	460
Jennie-O								
Turkey Italian Sweet	1 link (3.9 oz)	160	17	10	60	0	0	670
Johnsonville								
Bratwurst Original	1 (3 oz)	270	15	22	60	2	–	810
Breakfast Patty Original	2 (2 oz)	180	10	15	40	1	–	450
Grilling Chorizo	1 (3 oz)	280	16	22	55	3	–	840
Italian Mild	1 (3 oz)	270	15	22	60	3	–	710
Original Summer	1 (2 oz)	170	9	15	45	1	0	680
Polish	1 (2.7 oz)	240	9	21	60	2	–	640
Pork	2 oz	180	10	15	40	1	–	440
Smoked Turkey	1 (3 oz)	110	10	6	45	4	0	710
Jones								
Light 50% Less Fat	2 (1.6 oz)	110	6	8	25	3	–	270
Little Pork	3	190	8	17	45	1	–	420

FOOD	PORTION	CALS	PROT	FAT	CHOL	CARB	FIBER	SOD
Organic Prairie								
Bratwurst Pork	1 (3 oz)	210	13	19	50	1	0	720
Shady Brook								
Turkey Breakfast	1 (2.3 oz)	80	10	4	35	0	0	480
Turkey Sweet Italian	1 (2.5 oz)	110	13	7	50	1	–	570
Turkey Bratwurst	3 oz	160	18	9	75	1	–	690
Soy Lean								
Pork Breakfast Patty	1 (2 oz)	75	11	3	15	–	–	250
Wellshire								
Andouille	1 link (3 oz)	197	19	9	84	4	0	490
Andouille Turkey	2 oz	59	9	3	14	1	0	280
Chorizo	1 piece (2 oz)	130	17	6	50	2	0	350
Chorizo Dried	1 oz	100	8	8	30	1	0	530
Italian Turkey Mild	1 link (2 oz)	70	8	4	25	1	0	280
Kielbasa Polska	1 piece (2 oz)	130	17	6	50	2	0	350
Kielbasa Turkey	1 piece (2 oz)	59	9	3	14	1	0	280
Turkey Maple Breakfast	1 link (2 oz)	70	8	4	25	1	0	280
SAUSAGE DISHES								
TAKE-OUT								
italian sausage w/ peppers & onions	1 cup	210	17	11	70	14	–	1120
sausage roll	1 (2.3 oz)	311	5	24	–	22	1	–
SAUSAGE SUBSTITUTES								
meatless	1 patty (1.3 oz)	98	7	7	0	4	1	337
meatless	1 link (0.9 oz)	64	5	5	0	2	1	222
Boca								
Bratwurst	1 (2.5 oz)	140	14	7	0	6	1	760
Breakfast Patties	1 (1.3 oz)	60	7	3	0	5	2	280
Breakfast Links	2 (1.6 oz)	70	8	3	0	5	2	330
Italian	1 (2.5 oz)	130	13	6	0	6	1	650
Gardenburger								
Veggie Breakfast	1 (1.5 oz)	45	5	3	0	3	2	270
Veggie Breakfast	1 patty (1.5 oz)	45	5	3	0	3	2	270

FOOD	PORTION	CALS	PROT	FAT	CHOL	CARB	FIBER	SOD
Lightlife								
Gimme Lean	2 oz	50	8	0	0	4	2	330
Smart Brats	1 (2 oz)	120	13	5	0	5	1	580
Smart Links Breakfast	2 (2 oz)	100	10	4	0	8	4	580
Smart Links Italian	1 (2 oz)	120	10	5	0	7	3	650
Smart Menu Breakfast Patty	1	45	5	2	0	3	1	280
Morningstar Farms								
Breakfast Patties	1 (1.3 oz)	80	8	3	0	4	1	250
Quorn								
Links	2 (1.6 oz)	70	8	3	0	2	1	210
Tofurky								
Turkey Beerbrats	1 (3.5 oz)	280	24	16	0	8	5	650
Turkey Breakfast Links	1 (1.6 oz)	130	11	6	0	6	4	330
Turkey Italian Sweet	1 (3.5 oz)	280	29	13	0	12	8	620
Turkey Kielbasa	1 (3.5 oz)	240	26	12	0	12	8	650
Worthington								
Saucettes Breakfast Links	1 (1.3 oz)	90	6	6	0	1	1	200
Yves								
Veggie Brats Classic	1 (3.3 oz)	160	19	5	0	5	1	640
SAVORY								
ground	1 tsp	4	tr	tr	0	1	tr	0
SCALLOP								
raw	3 oz	75	14	1	28	2	–	137
Mrs. Paul's								
Fried	13 (3.7 oz)	260	12	11	25	28	tr	700
TAKE-OUT								
breaded & fried	2 lg	67	6	3	19	3	–	144
SCONE								
King Arthur								
English Cream Tea Scone not prep	⅓ cup	180	5	1	0	38	tr	130
TAKE-OUT								
apricot	1	232	5	7	34	39	–	201
blueberry	1 (3 oz)	270	7	9	10	41	2	600
cheese	1 (3.5 oz)	364	10	18	–	44	2	–
orange poppy	1 (3 oz)	260	6	6	30	47	2	400
plain	1 (3.5 oz)	362	8	14	–	54	2	–
raisin	1 (3 oz)	270	6	8	10	43	2	490

FOOD	PORTION	CALS	PROT	FAT	CHOL	CARB	FIBER	SOD
SCUP								
fresh baked	3 oz	115	21	3	–	0	0	46
SEA BASS (see BASS)								
SEA CUCUMBER								
dried	1 oz	74	14	1	17	1	0	1411
fresh	1 oz	20	5	tr	14	tr	0	143
SEA TROUT (see TROUT)								
SEA URCHIN								
canned	1 oz	39	4	1	–	3	0	–
fresh	1 oz	36	4	1	–	3	tr	32
roe paste	1 tbsp	19	2	tr	–	3	0	658
SEAWEED								
agar dried	1 oz	87	2	tr	0	23	–	29
agar fresh	1 oz	tr	tr	tr	0	2	–	3
hijiki dried	1 tbsp	9	1	0	0	2	1	–
irishmoss fresh	1 oz	14	tr	tr	0	4	–	19
kelp fresh	1 oz	12	tr	tr	0	3	–	66
kombu fresh	1 oz	12	tr	tr	0	3	–	66
laver fresh	1 oz	10	2	tr	0	1	–	14
nori fresh	1 oz	10	2	tr	0	1	–	14
nori sheet dried	1 (8 x 8 in)	5	1	0	0	1	1	18
seahair dried	1 tbsp	13	1	0	0	3	tr	–
spirulina dried	1 oz	83	16	2	0	7	–	309
spirulina fresh	1 oz	7	2	tr	0	1	–	28
tangle fresh	1 oz	12	tr	tr	0	3	–	66
wakame fresh	1 oz	13	1	tr	0	3	–	249
Eden								
Agar Agar Bars	1 bar (7 g)	25	0	0	0	5	5	0
Agar Agar Flakes	1 tbsp	0	0	0	0	1	1	10
Arame Wild	½ cup	30	1	0	0	7	7	120
Hiziki Wild	½ cup	30	0	0	0	6	6	160
Kombu Wild	½ piece (3.3 g)	5	0	0	0	1	1	90
Nori Sheets	1 (2.5 g)	10	1	0	0	0	0	5
Organic Dulse Flakes	1 tsp	3	0	0	0	0	0	15
Maine Coast								
Organic Alaria Whole Leaf	⅓ cup	18	1	tr	–	3	3	297

FOOD	PORTION	CALS	PROT	FAT	CHOL	CARB	FIBER	SOD
Organic Dulse Whole Leaf	½ cup	19	2	tr	–	3	2	122
Organic Kelp Whole Leaf	⅓ cup	17	1	tr	–	3	2	312
Organic Laver Whole Leaf	⅓ cup	22	2	tr	–	3	2	113
Organic Dulse Granules	1 tsp	6	0	0	0	2	–	22
Organic Kelp Granules	½ tsp	5	0	0	0	2	–	45

SEITAN (see WHEAT)

SEMOLINA

FOOD	PORTION	CALS	PROT	FAT	CHOL	CARB	FIBER	SOD
dry	1 cup (5.9 oz)	601	21	2	0	122	7	2

SESAME

FOOD	PORTION	CALS	PROT	FAT	CHOL	CARB	FIBER	SOD
seeds	1 tsp	16	1	2	0	tr	–	1
sesame butter	1 tbsp	95	3	8	0	4	1	2
sesame crunch candy	1 oz	146	3	9	0	14	–	–
sesame crunch candy	20 pieces (1.2 oz)	181	4	12	0	18	–	–
tahini from roasted & toasted kernels	1 tbsp	89	3	8	0	3	–	17
tahini from stone ground kernels	1 tbsp	86	3	7	0	4	–	11
tahini from unroasted kernels	1 tbsp	85	3	8	0	3	–	0
Arrowhead Mills								
Organic Tahini	2 tbsp	190	8	18	0	3	tr	10
Organic Seeds	¼ cup	210	9	19	0	3	1	15
Mrs. May's								
Black Sesame Crunch	1 oz	165	4	11	0	14	4	43
Peloponnese								
Tahini	1 tbsp	100	4	9	0	2	1	50
Sabra								
Tahini Sauce Taratore	1 oz	80	3	7	0	1	0	55

SESBANIA

FOOD	PORTION	CALS	PROT	FAT	CHOL	CARB	FIBER	SOD
flower	1	1	tr	0	0	tr	–	0
flowers	1 cup	5	tr	tr	0	1	–	3
flowers cooked	1 cup	23	1	tr	0	5	–	11

SHAD

FOOD	PORTION	CALS	PROT	FAT	CHOL	CARB	FIBER	SOD
american baked	3 oz	214	18	15	–	0	0	56
cooked	1 oz	55	7	3	121	1	0	149

FOOD	PORTION	CALS	PROT	FAT	CHOL	CARB	FIBER	SOD
roe baked w/ butter & lemon	1 oz	36	6	1	–	tr	–	21

SHALLOTS (see ONION)

SHARK
| fin dried | 1 oz | 32 | 7 | tr | – | – | – | 5 |
| raw | 3 oz | 111 | 18 | 4 | 43 | 0 | 0 | 67 |

TAKE-OUT
| batter-dipped & fried | 3 oz | 194 | 16 | 12 | 50 | 5 | – | 103 |

SHEEPSHEAD FISH
cooked	1 fillet (6.5 oz)	234	48	3	–	0	0	136
cooked	3 oz	107	22	1	–	0	0	62
raw	3 oz	92	17	2	–	0	0	61

SHELLFISH (see individual names, SHELLFISH SUBSTITUTES)

SHELLFISH SUBSTITUTES
crab imitation	1 cup (4.4 oz)	144	17	1	60	16	tr	1065
scallop imitation	3 oz	84	11	tr	18	9	–	676
shrimp imitation	3 oz	86	11	1	31	8	–	599
surimi	3 oz	84	13	1	25	6	–	122
surimi	1 oz	28	4	tr	8	2	–	40

Chicken Of The Sea
| Imitation Crab | 1 pkg (2.5 oz) | 40 | 3 | 0 | 9 | 6 | 1 | 360 |

Louis Kemp
Crab Delights	½ cup (3 oz)	80	8	0	10	11	0	470
Crab Delights Chunk Style	½ cup (3 oz)	80	8	0	10	11	0	470
Crab Delights Easy Shred	½ cup (3 oz)	80	7	0	10	13	0	620
Crab Delights Leg Style	½ cup (3 oz)	80	8	0	10	11	0	470

TAKE-OUT
| crab salad | 1 cup | 395 | 18 | 26 | 77 | 21 | 1 | 1739 |

SHELLIE BEANS
| canned | ½ cup | 37 | 2 | tr | 0 | 8 | – | 408 |

FOOD	PORTION	CALS	PROT	FAT	CHOL	CARB	FIBER	SOD
SHERBET								
orange	½ gal	2158	17	31	113	469	–	706
orange	½ cup (4 fl oz)	132	1	2	5	29	–	44
orange	1 bar (2.75 fl oz)	91	1	1	3	20	–	30
Blue Bunny								
Cool Tubes Orange Sherbet	1 (3 oz)	110	0	1	5	24	0	30
Lime	½ cup	110	0	0	0	25	0	30
Rainbow	½ cup	110	0	0	0	25	0	30
Raspberry	½ cup	110	0	0	0	26	0	30
Hola Fruta								
Margarita	½ cup	140	1	1	0	30	0	20
Peach	½ cup	130	8	1	0	30	0	35
Pomegranate	½ cup	140	1	1	0	32	0	20
Hood								
Orange Burst	½ cup	120	1	1	<5	27	0	40
SHRIMP								
CANNED								
canned	1 can (6 oz)	136	26	2	195	1	0	191
chinese shrimp paste	1 tbsp	46	1	0	9	10	tr	273
Bumble Bee								
Broken Shrimp	¼ cup	40	10	0	115	0	0	650
Medium Or Large Or Jumbo	¼ cup	40	10	0	115	0	0	650
Small	¼ cup	40	10	0	115	0	0	650
Tiny	¼ cup	40	10	0	115	0	0	430
Chicken Of The Sea								
Tiny, Small or Medium	½ can (2 oz)	45	10	1	145	1	0	400
DRIED								
dried	10	15	3	tr	22	tr	0	21
FRESH								
broiled	6 med	46	7	2	55	tr	0	154
steamed	6 med	41	8	1	59	tr	0	177
FROZEN								
Chicken Of The Sea								
Cooked Large Peeled Deveined Tail On	3 oz	80	18	1	165	0	0	190
Large Raw Cleaned Tail Off	4 oz	120	23	2	170	1	0	170

FOOD	PORTION	CALS	PROT	FAT	CHOL	CARB	FIBER	SOD
Contessa								
Orange Shrimp	11 to 13 (6 oz)	250	14	8	95	33	5	1150
Ragin' Cajun	8 to 10 (4 oz)	170	11	10	100	9	3	910
Shrimp Scampi	8 to 10 (4 oz)	290	9	27	85	4	2	810
Gorton's								
Popcorn Crunchy Golden	20 (3.2 oz)	240	8	12	55	24	0	630
Temptations Breaded Butterfly	5 (3.5 oz)	250	11	11	55	27	4	430
Temptations Scampi Sauced	1 serv (4 oz)	120	10	6	65	8	tr	630
Margaritaville								
Calypso Coconut + Sauce	5 pieces	350	12	17	70	39	0	690
Island Lime	6 pieces	130	16	7	155	2	0	720
Jammin' Jerk	7 pieces	140	16	7	145	4	0	1040
Paradise Cocktail + Sauce	5 pieces	85	12	0	130	6	tr	731
Sunset Scampi	1 serv (½ pkg)	270	12	20	130	10	0	460
Surfside Skewers + Sauce	2 skewers	105	14	1	185	11	0	875
Mrs. Paul's								
Butterfly	7 (4 oz)	250	12	11	65	27	1	540
Phillips Seafood								
Breaded Shrimp	5 pieces	230	12	13	50	20	–	620
Buffalo Shrimp	5 pieces	260	12	13	50	26	–	920
Coconut Shrimp	5 pieces	330	11	20	100	27	–	420
Crab Stuffed Shrimp	3 pieces	160	16	10	125	1	–	400
Van de Kamp's								
Battered	6 (4 oz)	200	14	6	90	22	1	750
Breaded Popcorn	20 (4 oz)	260	11	11	80	30	2	780
TAKE-OUT								
breaded & fried	6 med (2.3 oz)	162	14	8	121	8	tr	321
cocktail w/ sauce	4 shrimp	87	11	1	78	7	2	451
curried	1 cup	295	27	14	175	14	tr	621
gingered	4	80	–	tr	140	–	–	920
jambalaya	1 cup	309	27	9	180	28	1	330
scampi	1 cup	310	26	22	246	1	0	330
shrimp newburg	1 serv (6.4 oz)	456	22	37	313	8	tr	664

FOOD	PORTION	CALS	PROT	FAT	CHOL	CARB	FIBER	SOD
shrimp salad	¾ cup	212	20	12	152	4	1	292
shrimp w/ crab stuffing	5	158	16	8	126	5	tr	393

SMELT
rainbow cooked	3 oz	106	19	3	76	0	0	65
rainbow raw	3 oz	83	15	2	60	0	0	51

SMOOTHIES (see also FRUIT DRINKS, YOGURT DRINKS)
8th Continent
Refresher Orange Pineapple Banana	8 oz	150	6	0	0	30	0	90
Refresher Strawberry Banana	8 oz	150	6	0	0	30	0	90

Bolthouse Farms
Green Goodness	8 oz	140	2	0	0	33	1	25
Mango Lemonade	8 oz	120	tr	0	0	30	tr	0
Passion Fruit Apple Carrot Juice	8 oz	120	2	0	0	29	2	95
Strawberry Banana Fruit	8 oz	124	1	0	0	29	tr	10

C&W
Berry Blend	½ cup	90	2	2	10	15	2	65
Peach	½ cup	80	2	2	10	15	1	65

E4B
100% Fruit Puree Blueberry Raspberry	4 oz	70	0	0	0	18	3	10
100% Fruit Puree Kiwi	4 oz	70	0	0	0	16	1	15
100% Fruit Puree Mango	4 oz	70	0	0	0	18	1	10
100% Fruit Puree Pear Caramel	4 oz	70	0	0	0	18	1	15
100% Fruit Puree Strawberry Banana	4 oz	70	0	0	0	18	1	10

Horizon Organic
Tropical Punch	1 bottle (6.2 oz)	120	4	0	0	25	1	75

Jammin' Juice
Mambo Mango	6 oz	92	1	0	0	25	1	4

Jammin' Nectars
C-Beta Carrot	6 oz	96	0	0	0	23	1	5
Ginger Party	6 oz	6	0	0	0	19	1	3
Guanabana Limbo	6 oz	78	0	0	0	20	2	4
Pure Passion	6 oz	78	0	0	0	20	1	2
Razz-Ade	6 oz	89	1	0	0	21	1	4

FOOD	PORTION	CALS	PROT	FAT	CHOL	CARB	FIBER	SOD
Kidz Dream								
Orange Cream	1 box	120	4	2	0	21	tr	30
LightFull								
Satiety Smoothie Cafe Latte	1 (11 oz)	90	6	1	0	39	5	160
Satiety Smoothie Chocolate Fudge	1 (11 oz)	90	6	1	0	39	6	150
Satiety Smoothie Peaches & Cream	1 (11 oz)	100	6	0	0	41	6	95
Satiety Smoothie Strawberries & Cream	1 (11 oz)	90	6	0	0	40	6	240
Luna								
Berry Pomegranate	1 pkg	140	2	2	0	30	2	140
Orange Blossom	1 pkg	130	2	2	0	30	3	140
Vanilla Macaadamia	1 pkg	150	2	4	0	28	3	140
Naked Juice								
Chocolate Karma	8 oz	190	11	3	0	31	3	280
Vanilla Chai	8 oz	170	11	3	0	27	2	125
Nutiva								
Organic HempShake Amazon Acai not prep	4 tbsp	100	9	3	0	15	8	5
Organic HempShake Chocolate not prep	4 tbsp	80	7	2	0	19	12	5
Odwalla								
Bluberry B Monster	8 oz	140	0	0	0	33	0	10
Citrus C Monster	8 oz	150	2	0	0	36	0	15
Mango Tango	8 oz	150	1	1	0	34	0	10
Sambazon								
Acai Amazon Cherry	8 oz	156	5	0	0	16	1	5
Acai Mango Banana	8 oz	190	2	5	0	38	3	90
Acai Mango Uprising	8 oz	190	2	5	0	38	3	90
Acai Protein Warrior Chocolate	8 oz	215	8	6	0	33	3	75
Acai Protein Warrior Vanilla	8 oz	215	8	6	0	33	3	142
Acai Shaman's Immunity	8 oz	90	1	0	0	24	1	28
Acai Soy Energy	8 oz	210	6	6	0	25	4	142
Acai Strawberry Sensation	8 oz	210	1	4	0	42	2	10
Acai Supergreens Revolution	8 oz	200	2	4	0	40	3	12
Organic Acai	1 bottle	155	1	3	0	31	2	16

FOOD	PORTION	CALS	PROT	FAT	CHOL	CARB	FIBER	SOD
Smooze								
Mango + Coconut	1 box (8.5 oz)	250	2	10	0	33	0	–
Passion Fruit + Coconut	1 box (8.5 oz)	225	2	8	0	33	3	38
Pineapple + Coconut	1 box (8.5 oz)	200	2	8	0	33	0	25
Soy Blendz								
Mango Orange Dream	1 bottle (10 oz)	220	8	3	0	40	3	105
Mixed Berry Medley	1 bottle (10 oz)	210	8	3	0	38	3	120
Orange Citrus Splash	1 bottle (10 oz)	220	8	4	0	37	3	115
Strawberry Banana Blast	1 bottle (10 oz)	230	8	3	0	43	3	15
Soy Fusion								
Berry	1 box (8.45 oz)	120	2	1	–	24	–	20
Matcha Green Tea	1 box (8.45 oz)	110	3	2	–	19	–	120
Tropicana								
Fruit Smoothie Mixed Berry	1 bottle (11 oz)	220	1	0	0	54	2	30
Fruit Smoothie Tropical Fruit	1 bottle (11 oz)	220	1	0	0	53	1	15
V8								
Splash Tropical Colada	8 oz	100	3	0	0	21	1	50
WholeSoy & Co.								
Orgainic Soy Strawberry	8 oz	210	7	3	0	34	0	10
Organic Soy Peach	8 oz	210	7	3	0	34	0	20
Organic Soy Raspberry	8 oz	210	7	3	0	35	0	10
Yo On The Go								
All Flavors	1 box (8 oz)	180	6	3	0	31	0	80
Yoplait								
Go-Gurt All Fruit Flavors	1 bottle (5 oz)	120	4	1	5	23	0	100
Light All Flavors	1 bottle (8.3 oz)	90	6	0	5	16	3	120

FOOD	PORTION	CALS	PROT	FAT	CHOL	CARB	FIBER	SOD
Smoothie All Flavors	1 bottle (8.3 oz)	220	6	3	15	44	3	150

SNACKS

FOOD	PORTION	CALS	PROT	FAT	CHOL	CARB	FIBER	SOD
cheese puffs	1 oz	157	2	10	1	15	tr	298
corn puffs cheese	1 bag (8 oz)	1256	17	78	9	122	2	2383
corn twists cheese	1 oz	157	2	10	1	15	tr	298
corn twists cheese	1 bag (8 oz)	1256	17	78	9	122	2	2383
oriental mix	1 oz	155	6	12	0	9	–	235
pork skins	1 oz	154	17	9	27	0	0	521
pork skins barbecue	1 oz	152	16	9	33	1	–	756
Baken-ets								
Fried Pork Skins	9 pieces	80	7	5	20	0	0	310
Fried Pork Skins Hot'n Spicy	9 pieces	80	7	5	20	tr	tr	470
Fried Pork Skins Sweet & Tangy BBQ	9 pieces	80	7	5	20	1	0	400
Pork Cracklins	8 pieces	90	7	6	15	tr	tr	550
Pork Cracklins Hot'n Spicy	8 pieces	80	7	5	20	tr	tr	330
Barbara's Bakery								
Cheese Puffs Bakes Original	¾ cup	160	2	11	0	13	–	190
Cheese Puffs Original	¾ cup (1 oz)	150	2	10	0	16	–	130
Carole's								
Soycrunch Cinnamon & Raisins	½ cup	110	6	1	0	19	2	0
Soycrunch Original	½ cup	120	5	2	0	16	2	0
Soycrunch Toffee	½ cup	110	7	2	0	15	2	15
Cheetos								
Asteriods Go Snack	¾ cup (1 oz)	160	2	10	0	15	1	320
Baked Crunchy	34 pieces (1 oz)	130	2	5	0	19	0	240
Crunchy	1 pkg (1.25 oz)	200	2	13	5	19	1	370
Natural White Cheddar	32 pieces (1 oz)	150	2	8	<5	16	tr	290

FOOD	PORTION	CALS	PROT	FAT	CHOL	CARB	FIBER	SOD
Puffs	13 pieces (1 oz)	160	2	10	0	13	0	350
Twisted	7 pieces (1 oz)	160	2	10	0	13	0	350
Chester's								
Puffcorn Butter	3 cups	160	0	11	0	12	tr	300
Puffcorn Cheese	3 cups	160	2	11	0	12	0	310
Funyuns								
Mini Onion Rings Go Snacks	1 pkg	260	3	14	0	30	1	400
Onion Rings	13 pieces	140	2	7	0	18	tr	270
Garden Of Eatin'								
Organic Baked Cheese Puffs	32 pieces	150	2	10	<5	15	1	220
Organic Baked Chunchitos	35 pieces	140	2	7	<5	18	1	310
Good Sense								
Snack Mix Cajun Corn 'N Sesame	¼ cup	150	4	8	0	17	2	160
Kangaroo								
Pita Snackers Crispy Cinnamon	10 pieces (1 oz)	90	3	2	0	19	1	140
Pita Snackers Sea Salt	10 pieces (1 oz)	90	3	2	0	18	1	100
Munchies								
Snack Mix Flamin' Hot	1 oz	140	2	6	0	17	tr	190
Snack Mix Kids	1 oz	130	2	4	0	20	1	250
Sabritones								
Chile & Lime	23 pieces	150	2	10	0	13	1	690
Snyder's Of Hanover								
CheddAirs	1 oz	130	3	5	0	20	tr	140
MultiGrain Cheese Puffs	1 oz	130	2	6	0	19	2	200
Tumaro's								
Organic Krispy Crunchy Puffs Cheddar	22	120	2	3	0	21	1	130
Organic Krispy Crunchy Puffs Natural Corn	22	120	2	2	0	23	1	200
Organic Krispy Crunchy Puffs Ranch & Herb	22	130	3	4	0	20	tr	160
Organic Krispy Crunchy Puffs Tangy BBQ	22	120	2	4	0	21	tr	140

FOOD	PORTION	CALS	PROT	FAT	CHOL	CARB	FIBER	SOD
Utz								
Cheese Balls	50 (1 oz)	150	2	9	0	16	tr	260
Cheese Curls	18 (1 oz)	150	2	9	0	16	tr	260
Onion Rings	41 (1 oz)	130	1	5	0	20	0	500
Party Mix	1 oz	150	2	7	0	19	1	250
Pork Cracklins	0.5 oz	90	6	7	15	0	0	300
Pork Rinds Original	0.5 oz	80	9	5	15	0	0	210
Wise								
Cheez Doodles Crunchy	1 pkg (1 oz)	150	1	9	0	17	0	220
Cheez Doodles Crunchy Reduced Fat	1 oz	130	2	5	<5	20	tr	220
Cheez Doodles Puffed	1 pkg (0.7 oz)	110	1	6	0	13	0	240
Doodle O's	1 oz	160	2	11	<5	14	0	310
Onion Rings	1 oz	140	0	6	0	20	0	420
Pork Rinds Original	1 oz	90	9	6	25	0	0	330
SNAIL								
cooked	3 oz	233	41	1	110	13	–	350
raw	3 oz	117	20	tr	55	7	–	175
TAKE-OUT								
escargot cooked	5	25	4	0	15	1	0	25
SNAKE								
fresh	3 oz	78	17	tr	–	3	0	57
SNAPPER								
cooked	3 oz	109	22	1	40	0	0	48
cooked	1 fillet (6 oz)	217	45	3	80	0	0	96
raw	3 oz	85	17	1	31	0	0	54
SODA								
club	12 oz	0	0	0	0	0	0	75
cola	12 oz	151	tr	tr	0	39	–	14
cream	12 oz	191	0	0	0	49	–	43
diet cola	12 oz	2	tr	0	0	tr	–	21
diet cola w/ equal	12 oz	2	tr	0	0	tr	–	21
ginger ale	12 oz	124	tr	0	0	32	–	25
grape	12 oz	161	0	0	0	42	–	57
lemon lime	12 oz	149	0	0	0	38	–	41
orange	12 oz	177	0	0	0	46	–	49
pepper type	12 oz	151	0	tr	0	38	–	38

FOOD	PORTION	CALS	PROT	FAT	CHOL	CARB	FIBER	SOD
quinine	12 oz	125	0	0	0	32	–	15
root beer	12 oz	152	tr	0	0	39	–	49
shirley temple	1 serv	159	0	0	0	41	0	34
tonic water	12 oz	125	0	0	0	32	–	15
7 Up								
Diet	8 oz	0	0	0	0	0	0	45
Original	8 oz	100	0	0	0	26	–	50
Plus	12 oz	10	0	0	0	3	–	25
AJ Stephans								
Birch Beer	1 bottle	170	0	0	0	45	–	35
Black Cherry	1 bottle	180	0	0	0	46	–	35
Cream	1 bottle	170	0	0	0	45	–	35
Jamaican Style Ginger Beer	1 bottle	170	0	0	0	45	–	35
Lemon & Lime	1 bottle	190	0	0	0	46	–	35
Olde Style Root Beer	1 bottle	170	0	0	0	45	–	35
Barq's								
Diet French Vanilla Creme	8 oz	1	0	0	0	tr	0	44
Diet Red Creme	8 oz	4	0	0	0	0	0	43
Diet Root Beer	8 oz	1	0	0	0	tr	0	48
Floatz	8 oz	127	0	0	0	34	0	44
French Vanilla Creme	8 oz	112	0	0	0	30	0	44
Red Creme	8 oz	115	0	0	0	31	0	43
Root Beer	8 oz	111	0	0	0	30	0	48
Blumers								
Black Cherry	12 oz	138	0	0	0	34	–	31
Blueberry Cream	12 oz	190	0	0	0	47	–	21
Cream	12 oz	181	0	0	0	45	–	21
Orange Cream	12 oz	187	0	0	0	47	–	23
Root Beer	12 oz	190	0	0	0	46	–	15
Bubble Yum								
All Flavors	8 oz	110	0	0	0	31	–	35
Cape Cod Dry								
Cranberry	8 oz	120	0	0	0	29	–	0
Diet Cranberry	8 oz	10	0	0	0	2	–	0
Carver's								
Ginger Ale	8 oz	94	0	0	0	24	0	22
Chronic 187								
Orange	12 oz	300	0	0	0	77	–	53
Coca-Cola								
Blak	8 oz	46	0	0	0	12	0	32

FOOD	PORTION	CALS	PROT	FAT	CHOL	CARB	FIBER	SOD
C2	8 oz	45	0	0	0	12	–	30
Classic	8 oz	97	0	0	0	27	0	33
W/ Lime	8 oz	98	0	0	0	27	0	25
Coke								
Cherry	8 oz	104	0	0	0	28	0	28
Diet	8 oz	1	0	0	0	tr	0	28
Diet Cherry	8 oz	1	0	0	0	tr	0	28
Diet Plus	8 oz	0	0	0	0	0	0	30
Diet Vanilla	8 oz	1	0	0	0	tr	0	28
Diet w/ Lime	8 oz	2	0	0	0	tr	0	28
Vanilla	8 oz	100	0	0	0	28	0	25
Dr Pepper								
Original	12 oz	150	0	0	0	40	0	55
DRY								
Kumquat	12 oz	50	0	0	0	14	–	0
Lavender	12 oz	70	0	0	0	19	–	0
Lemongrass	12 oz	50	0	0	0	14	–	0
Rhubarb	12 oz	60	0	0	0	16	–	0
Fanta								
Apple	8 oz	121	0	0	0	33	0	39
Citrus	8 oz	91	0	0	0	25	0	16
Orange	8 oz	111	0	0	0	35	0	35
Fresca								
Soda	8 oz	2	0	0	0	tr	0	24
Frostie								
Diet Cherry Limeade	12 oz	0	0	0	0	0	0	105
Diet Root Beer	12 oz	0	0	0	0	0	0	30
Vanilla Root Beer	12 oz	180	0	0	0	46	–	50
Hansen's								
Natural Creamy Root Beer	12 oz	160	0	0	0	43	–	0
Hiball								
Club	10 oz	5	1	0	0	0	0	20
Tonic Water	10 oz	120	1	0	0	31	–	15
IBC								
Cream	12 oz	180	0	0	0	48	–	75
Inca Kola								
Diet	8 oz	1	0	0	0	tr	0	34
Soda	8 oz	96	0	0	0	26	0	31
Jolt								
Blue	8 oz	120	0	0	0	32	–	50

FOOD	PORTION	CALS	PROT	FAT	CHOL	CARB	FIBER	SOD
Cherry Bomb	8 oz	90	0	0	0	25	–	25
Cola	8 oz	100	0	0	0	27	–	10
Red	8 oz	120	0	0	0	33	–	40
Ultra	8 oz	0	0	0	0	0	0	30
Jones Soda								
Blue Bubble Gum	12 oz	190	0	0	0	48	0	25
Cream	12 oz	190	0	0	0	48	0	25
Crushed Melon	12 oz	190	0	0	0	48	0	25
FuFu Berry	12 oz	190	0	0	0	46	0	70
Green Apple	12 oz	180	0	0	0	46	0	25
Orange Cream	12 oz	180	0	0	0	46	0	25
Lucozade								
Soda	7 oz	136	0	0	0	36	0	–
Maine Root								
All Flavors	12 oz	165	0	0	0	49	–	35
Manzana Mia								
Soda	8 oz	99	0	0	0	27	0	47
Mello Yellow								
Diet	8 oz	3	0	0	0	tr	0	25
Soda	8 oz	118	0	0	0	32	0	33
Mr. Pibb								
Diet	8 oz	1	0	0	0	tr	0	26
Nesbitt's								
Orange	12 oz	190	0	0	0	48	–	90
Northern Neck								
Diet Ginger Ale	8 oz	4	0	0	0	0	0	24
Ginger Ale	8 oz	94	0	0	0	24	0	22
Nuky								
Rose Soda	8 oz	120	0	0	0	32	–	0
Olde Brooklyn								
Coney Island Cream	8 oz	130	0	0	0	33	–	25
Williamsburg Root Beer	8 oz	120	0	0	0	32	–	25
Pibb								
Zero	8 oz	2	0	0	0	tr	0	31
Polar								
Birch Beer	8 oz	110	0	0	0	28	–	0
Bitter Lemon Mixer	8 oz	120	0	0	0	29	–	0
Collins Mixer	8 oz	90	0	0	0	22	–	0
Cream	8 oz	120	0	0	0	30	–	0
Diet Pomegranate Dry	8 oz	10	0	0	0	2	–	0

FOOD	PORTION	CALS	PROT	FAT	CHOL	CARB	FIBER	SOD
Orange	8 oz	130	0	0	0	32	–	0
Pomegranate Dry	8 oz	120	0	0	0	30	–	0
Seltzer All Flavors	8 oz	0	0	0	0	0	0	0
Strawberry	8 oz	120	0	0	0	30	–	0
Tonic Water	8 oz	90	0	0	0	23	–	0
Vichy Water	8 oz	0	0	0	0	0	0	300
Red Flash								
Soda	8 oz	105	0	0	0	28	0	21
Santa Cruz								
Organic Cherry	1 can	140	0	0	0	34	–	220
Schweppes								
Ginger Ale	8 oz	120	0	0	0	34	0	60
Sex Kola								
Diet All Flavors	12 oz	0	0	0	0	0	0	0
Sierra Mist								
Lemon Lime	12 oz	140	0	0	0	39	0	35
Snow								
Sparkling Mint	8 oz	75	0	0	0	18	–	0
Souix City								
Cream	12 oz	180	0	0	0	45	–	30
Orange Cream	12 oz	200	0	0	0	50	–	45
Root Beer	12 oz	170	0	0	0	42	–	45
Sprite								
Diet Zero	8 oz	2	0	0	0	0	0	24
ReMix Aruba Jam	8 oz	97	0	0	0	26	–	44
Soda	8 oz	96	0	0	0	26	0	47
Steaz								
Organic Green Tea Soda Cola	8 oz	90	0	0	0	23	–	35
Organic Green Tea Soda Diet Black Cherry	8 oz	20	0	0	0	5	–	20
Organic Green Tea Soda Ginger Ale	8 oz	90	0	0	0	23	–	35
Organic Green Tea Soda Lemon	8 oz	90	0	0	0	23	–	35
Stirrings								
Club	1 bottle (6.3 oz)	0	0	0	0	0	0	15
Ginger Ale	1 bottle (6.3 oz)	100	0	0	0	24	0	0

FOOD	PORTION	CALS	PROT	FAT	CHOL	CARB	FIBER	SOD
Tonic Water	1 bottle (6.3 oz)	85	0	0	0	20	0	20
Sunkist								
Diet Orange	8 oz	0	0	0	0	0	0	65
Orange	8 oz	130	0	0	0	35	0	30
Tab								
Soda	8 oz	1	0	0	0	tr	–	28
Tava								
Sparkling Brazilian Samba	8 oz	0	0	0	0	0	0	35
Sparkling Mediterranean Fiesta	8 oz	0	0	0	0	0	0	40
Tommyknocker								
Almond Creme	12 oz	150	0	0	0	40	–	19
Key Lime Creme	12 oz	180	0	0	0	45	–	29
Orange Creme	12 oz	180	0	0	0	45	–	29
Root Beer	12 oz	150	0	0	0	40	–	19
Root Beer Float	12 oz	110	0	0	0	29	–	20
Strawberry Creme	12 oz	150	0	0	0	40	–	19
Uno Mas								
All Flavors	12 oz	130	0	0	0	31	0	200
Vignette								
Wine Country Soda Chardonnay	12 oz	130	0	0	0	33	–	20
Wine Country Soda Pinot Noit	12 oz	130	0	0	0	31	–	15
White Rock								
Organics Raspberry Creme	1 can (12.4 oz)	120	0	0	0	30	–	0
Organics Red Peach	1 can (12.4 oz)	120	0	0	0	30	–	0
Windy City								
Root Beer	12 oz	170	0	0	0	43	0	45
SOLE								
cooked	3 oz	99	21	1	58	0	0	89
cooked	1 fillet (4.5 oz)	148	31	2	86	0	0	133
lemon raw	3.5 oz	85	17	1	–	0	0	80
TAKE-OUT								
breaded & fried	3.2 oz	211	13	11	31	15	–	484

FOOD	PORTION	CALS	PROT	FAT	CHOL	CARB	FIBER	SOD
SORGHUM								
sorghum	1 cup (6.7 oz)	651	22	6	0	143	–	12
SOUFFLE								
TAKE-OUT								
cheese	1 cup	194	9	15	134	6	tr	307
corn	1 cup	257	10	11	152	34	3	666
lime chilled	1 cup	388	11	18	306	48	2	102
seafood	1 cup	245	17	15	231	9	tr	668
spinach	1 cup	124	6	8	97	7	1	170
SOUP								
CANNED								
Butterball								
Chicken Broth 99% Fat Free	1 cup	10	tr	0	0	2	0	840
Campbell's								
25% Less Sodium Chicken Noodle as prep	1 cup	60	3	2	15	8	1	660
25% Less Sodium Cream of Mushroom as prep	1 cup	110	2	8	5	8	2	650
98% Fat Free Cream Of Broccoli as prep	1 cup	70	2	2	<5	10	2	700
98% Fat Free Cream Of Celery as prep	1 cup	60	1	3	5	8	1	580
98% Fat Free Cream Of Chicken as prep	1 cup	70	2	3	10	10	1	590
Cheddar Cheese as prep	1 cup	110	2	5	5	12	1	890
Chunky Beef and Country Vegetables	1 cup	150	10	3	15	21	4	890
Chunky Chicken Mushroom Chowder	1 cup	210	7	12	10	19	3	910
Chunky Classic Chicken Noodle	1 cup	120	9	3	20	16	2	860
Chunky Grilled Chicken w/ Vegetables & Pasta	1 cup	100	8	2	15	15	2	880
Chunky Hearty Vegetable w/ Pasta	1 cup	120	4	2	5	23	4	870
Chunky New England Clam Chowder	1 cup	210	7	9	10	25	5	890

FOOD	PORTION	CALS	PROT	FAT	CHOL	CARB	FIBER	SOD
Chunky Old Fashioned Vegetable Beef	1 cup	130	9	3	15	18	4	890
Chunky Roadhouse Beef & Bean Chili	1 cup	230	15	8	30	25	8	870
Chunky Sirloin Burger w/ Country Vegetables	1 cup	180	10	7	15	20	4	900
Healthy Request Chicken Noodle as prep	1 cup	60	3	2	10	8	1	480
Healthy Request Chicken Rice as prep	1 cup	70	2	2	5	13	1	480
Healthy Request Cream Of Chicken as prep	1 cup	80	2	3	5	12	1	460
Healthy Request Italian Style Wedding	1 cup	120	7	3	10	15	2	480
Healthy Request Minestrone as prep	1 cup	80	3	1	0	15	3	460
Healthy Request Tomato as prep	1 cup	90	2	2	0	10	1	470
Low Sodium Chicken Broth	1 can	25	4	1	5	1	0	140
Microwavable Bowl Chicken Noodle	1 cup	70	4	2	15	10	tr	870
Microwavable Bowl Vegetable	1 cup	110	4	1	<5	22	3	800
Select Beef w/ Roasted Barley	1 cup	130	9	1	10	22	2	920
Select Blended Red Pepper Black Bean	1 cup	110	3	2	<5	21	4	820
Select Chicken With Egg Noodles	1 cup	90	9	2	20	12	2	960
Select Harvest Tomato w/ Basil	1 cup	80	1	0	0	18	1	750
Select Honey Roasted Chicken w/ Golden Potatoes	1 cup	110	7	1	15	19	3	860
Select Italian Sausage w/ Pasta & Pepperoni	1 cup	150	7	6	15	18	2	800
Select Italian Style Wedding	1 cup	110	7	3	15	15	2	790
Select Mexican Chicken Tortilla	1 cup	130	8	3	10	19	3	850

FOOD	PORTION	CALS	PROT	FAT	CHOL	CARB	FIBER	SOD
Select Potato Broccoli Cheese	1 cup	120	3	4	<5	18	4	890
Select Savory Chicken & Long Grain Rice	1 cup	90	7	1	10	15	1	970
Select Split Pea w/ Roasted Ham	1 cup	160	10	1	5	29	5	830
Soup At Hand 25% Less Sodium Chicken w/ Mini Noodles	1 pkg (10.75 oz)	80	4	2	10	11	2	730
Soup At Hand Chicken & Stars	1 pkg	70	3	2	5	11	2	960
Soup At Hand Creamy Chicken	1 pkg (10.75 oz)	130	4	8	5	13	4	890
Soup At Hand Italian Style Wedding	1 pkg	90	3	5	10	10	2	860
Soup At Hand Vegetable Medley	1 pkg (10.75 oz)	100	3	2	<5	19	4	890
Soup At Hand Velvety Potato	1 pkg (10.75 oz)	160	2	7	<5	21	4	870
College Inn								
Beef Broth Fat Free Lower Sodium	1 cup	15	3	0	0	0	0	450
Chicken Broth Light & Fat Free	1 cup	5	1	0	0	0	0	450
Gold's								
Borscht Low Calorie	1 cup	20	1	0	0	5	1	920
Borscht Unsalted	1 cup	70	1	0	0	13	tr	30
Hungarian Cabbage	6 oz	70	1	0	0	18	2	210
Schav	1 cup	15	1	1	15	1	1	880
Health Valley								
Organic Split Pea No Salt Added	1 cup	110	10	0	0	23	8	45
Healthy Choice								
Bean & Ham	1 cup	180	11	2	<5	29	10	480
Beef & Potato	1 cup	110	8	1	10	19	2	480
Chicken & Dumplings	1 cup	140	9	3	20	21	3	480
Chicken & Pasta	1 cup	110	6	2	5	18	2	480
Chicken Corn Chowder	1 cup	140	7	2	5	26	3	480
Chicken Fiesta	1 cup	100	6	2	5	17	3	480
Chicken w/ Roasted Garlic	1 cup	120	8	2	10	19	2	480

FOOD	PORTION	CALS	PROT	FAT	CHOL	CARB	FIBER	SOD
Chicken w/ Rice	1 cup	90	6	2	15	14	2	480
Chili Beef	1 cup	170	13	2	15	31	6	480
Clam Chowder	1 cup	110	4	2	15	21	4	480
Country Vegetable	1 cup	110	5	1	<5	19	4	480
Creamy Tomato	1 cup	100	3	2	0	22	2	480
Garden Vegetable	1 cup	120	6	1	0	25	4	480
Hearty Chicken	1 cup	120	8	2	20	20	3	480
Italian Bean & Pasta	1 cup	100	6	2	0	18	3	480
Old Fashioned Chicken Noodle	1 cup	100	9	2	15	13	2	480
Roasted Italian Style Chicken	1 cup	120	9	2	15	18	4	480
Split Pea w/ Ham	1 cup	170	11	3	5	30	4	480
Turkey w/ Rice	1 cup	90	6	2	10	16	3	480
Vegetable Beef	1 cup	130	9	1	15	22	4	480
Vegetable Clam Chowder	1 cup	230	4	1	0	16	3	480
Zesty Gumbo	1 cup	100	6	2	20	16	4	480
Imagine								
Lobster Bisque	1 cup	130	5	5	15	15	–	690
Organic Creamy Butternut Squash	1 cup	90	0	2	0	18	2	480
Organic Creamy Chicken	1 cup	70	3	2	0	12	1	680
Organic Creamy Sweet Corn	1 cup	120	4	3	0	20	3	450
Organic Sweet Potato	1 cup	110	2	2	0	23	1	400
Organic Bistro Cuban Black Bean Bisque	1 cup	170	8	4	0	30	6	480
Organic Broth Beef	1 cup	20	2	1	5	1	0	700
Organic Broth Free Range Chicken	1 cup	10	1	0	0	1	0	570
Organic Broth Vegetable	8 oz	20	2	0	0	2	0	550
Manischewitz								
Clear Chicken Condensed	½ cup	15	tr	1	0	2	2	740
Muir Glen								
Organic Garden Vegetable	1 cup	80	3	1	0	16	3	560
Organic Southwest Black Bean	1 cup	140	7	1	0	27	8	670
Pacific Foods								
Beef Broth	1 cup	20	4	0	0	1	0	570
Creamy Roasted Carrot	1 cup	100	3	1	0	18	2	780

FOOD	PORTION	CALS	PROT	FAT	CHOL	CARB	FIBER	SOD
Creamy Roasted Red Pepper & Tomato	1 cup	100	5	2	10	16	1	720
Hearty Beef Barley	1 cup	110	6	2	10	16	2	790
Hearty Chicken Noodle	1 cup	80	7	1	20	12	1	680
Hearty Chicken Tortilla	1 cup	130	8	2	5	22	5	670
Hearty Roasted Red Pepper & Corn Chowder	1 cup	210	3	12	45	21	3	–
Organic Creamy Tomato	1 cup	100	5	2	10	16	1	750
Organic Free Range Chicken Broth	1 cup	10	1	0	0	1	–	570
Organic French Onion	1 cup	35	1	0	0	6	tr	600
Organic Low Sodium Chicken Broth	1 cup	10	1	0	0	1	–	100
Organic Mushroom Broth	1 cup	5	0	0	0	1	–	530
Organic Vegetarian Broth	1 cup	15	0	0	0	3	tr	530
Progresso								
50% Less Sodium Chicken Gumbo	1 cup	110	7	2	15	18	2	450
50% Less Sodium Chicken Noodle	1 cup	90	7	2	20	12	1	470
50% Less Sodium Garden Vegetable	1 cup	100	3	0	0	22	3	450
50% Less Sodium Minestrone	1 cup	120	5	2	0	24	4	470
99% Fat Free Beef Barley	1 cup	120	7	2	10	20	4	720
Carb Monitor Chicken Vegetable	1 cup	70	7	2	15	7	1	860
Rich & Hearty Chicken & Homestyle Noodles	1 cup	110	8	2	25	14	1	920
Rich & Hearty Chicken Pot Pie	1 cup	170	8	6	15	21	2	940
Rich & Hearty Sirloin Steak & Vegetables	1 cup	130	8	2	15	21	2	870
Traditional Beef & Vegetable	1 cup	100	7	1	15	17	2	850
Traditional Beef Barley	1 cup	140	9	4	15	18	2	650
Traditional Chickarina	1 cup	120	8	5	20	12	2	950
Traditional Chicken & Herb Dumplings	1 cup	100	5	3	30	14	tr	790

FOOD	PORTION	CALS	PROT	FAT	CHOL	CARB	FIBER	SOD
Traditional Chicken & Wild Rice	1 cup	100	6	2	15	15	1	870
Traditional Chicken Noodle	1 cup	100	8	2	25	13	1	950
Traditional Hearty Chicken & Rotini	1 cup	100	7	2	15	14	1	970
Traditional Homestyle Chicken	1 cup	100	6	2	10	14	1	830
Traditional Italian Style Wedding	1 cup	100	6	4	10	12	1	840
Traditional New England Clam Chowder	1 cup	190	5	10	30	20	2	900
Traditional Split Pea w/ Ham	1 cup	140	9	1	5	26	4	790
Vegetable Classics 99% Fat Free Minestrone	1 cup	100	4	1	0	19	4	630
Vegetable Classics Creamy Mushroom	1 cup	130	2	3	10	9	1	820
Vegetable Classics French Onion	1 cup	50	1	2	<5	8	1	850
Vegetable Classics Green Split Pea w/ Bacon	1 cup	170	9	1	<5	28	5	910
Vegetable Classics Hearty Tomato	1 cup	110	2	1	0	23	3	980
Vegetable Classics Lentil	1 cup	150	9	2	0	28	4	870
Vegetable Classics Macaroni & Bean	1 cup	160	7	4	<5	25	6	890
Vegetable Classics Vegetable	1 cup	80	3	1	0	16	2	950
Rienzi								
Chicken & Rice	1 cup	110	6	3	5	17	2	930
Italian Wedding Bell	1 cup	130	5	7	15	12	tr	860
Swanson								
100% Fat Free Lower Sodium Beef Broth	1 cup	15	3	0	0	1	0	440
99% Fat Free Chicken Broth	1 cup	10	1	1	5	1	–	960
Organic Beef Broth	1 cup	15	2	1	0	1	0	550
Organic Chicken Broth	1 cup	15	1	1	0	1	0	550
Organic Vegetable Broth	1 cup	15	0	0	0	3	0	550
Valley Fresh								
Chicken Broth	1 cup	30	2	2	<5	1	–	1000

FOOD	PORTION	CALS	PROT	FAT	CHOL	CARB	FIBER	SOD
Chicken Broth 40% Less Sodium	1 cup	15	2	0	<5	1	–	600
Wolfgang Puck								
Chicken Parmesan w/ Pasta	1 cup	300	9	12	0	15	1	890
Hearty Lentil & Vegetable	1 cup	170	10	3	<5	29	6	580
FROZEN								
Kettle Cuisine								
Gluten Free Angus Beef Steak Chili w/ Beans	1 pkg (10 oz)	250	19	12	55	17	4	760
Gluten Free Chicken w/ Rice Noodles	1 pkg (10 oz)	140	15	3	45	12	1	560
Gluten Free New England Clam Chowder	1 pkg (10 oz)	330	15	18	80	26	1	800
Phillips Seafood								
Cream Of Crab	1 cup	310	9	25	130	12	–	750
Shrimp Bisque	1 cup	280	11	18	195	18	–	1340
Tabatchnick								
Barley Mushroom	1 serv (7.5 oz)	80	3	1	0	17	3	420
Chicken w/ Dumplings	1 serv (7.5 oz)	150	5	6	65	19	tr	740
Cream Of Broccoli	1 serv (7.5 oz)	130	4	5	20	18	2	440
Macaroni & Cheese	1 serv (7.5 oz)	250	9	8	20	34	tr	770
No Salt Pea	1 serv (7.5 oz)	140	13	0	0	34	14	50
Old Fashioned Potato	1 serv (7.5 oz)	100	3	2	0	21	2	330
Southwest Bean	1 serv (7.5 oz)	220	11	5	0	35	9	440
Vegetable	1 serv (7.5 oz)	90	3	2	0	17	4	350
Vegetarian Chili	1 serv (7.5 oz)	180	12	4	0	28	8	360
Wild Rice	1 serv (7.5 oz)	80	3	1	0	16	1	220
MIX								
beef broth cube	1 cube	6	1	tr	tr	1	–	864
chicken broth cube	1 cube (4.8 g)	9	1	tr	1	1	–	1152

FOOD	PORTION	CALS	PROT	FAT	CHOL	CARB	FIBER	SOD
A Taste Of Thai								
Coconut Ginger	2 tsp	15	0	1	0	2	0	620
Annie Chun's								
Noodle Bowl Chicken Noodle	1 pkg	260	8	2	0	52	2	990
Noodle Bowl Hot & Sour	1 pkg	280	8	3	0	55	2	910
Noodle Bowl Korean Kimchi	½ pkg	140	6	2	0	28	1	720
Noodle Bowl Miso	1 pkg	230	6	3	0	45	2	890
Noodle Bowl Thai Tom Yum	½ pkg	150	5	2	0	30	1	730
Noodle Bowl Udon	1 pkg	220	6	2	0	45	1	920
Azumaya								
Asian Style Thin Noodle	1 cup	120	5	0	0	24	tr	820
Asian Style Wide Noodle	1 cup	120	5	0	0	24	tr	800
Edward & Sons								
Bouillon Cubes Not-Beef	½ cube	20	1	2	0	1	0	920
Bouillon Cubes Not-Chicken	½ cube	15	1	2	0	1	0	800
Veggie Low Sodium	½ cup	20	1	2	0	1	0	135
Fantastic								
Noodle Bowl Hot & Sour as prep	2 cups	138	4	2	0	22	1	710
Noodle Bowl Miso w/ Tofu as prep	1 cup	100	4	1	0	19	tr	580
Noodle Bowl Sesame Miso as prep	2 cups	90	3	1	0	17	tr	550
Noodle Bowls Spring Vegetable as prep	2 cups	90	4	0	0	19	tr	590
Noodle Soup Spicy Thai as prep	2 cups	110	3	1	0	22	1	460
Noodle Soup Cup Vegetarian Chicken as prep	1 cup	90	4	1	0	19	1	590
Soup Cup Italian Tomato as prep	2 cups	130	5	1	0	26	2	480
Soup Cup Mandarin Broccoli as prep	2 cups	110	5	0	0	20	2	630
HamBeens								
15 Bean as prep	½ cup	120	8	1	0	20	9	70

FOOD	PORTION	CALS	PROT	FAT	CHOL	CARB	FIBER	SOD
15 Bean Beef as prep	½ cup	120	8	1	0	20	9	310
15 Bean Chicken as prep	½ cup	120	8	1	0	20	9	250
15 Bean Soup Cajun as prep	½ cup	120	8	1	0	20	9	100
Spanish American Black Bean as prep	½ cup	120	7	1	0	22	8	280
Leahey Gardens								
No Beef Noodle	1½ cups	89	7	1	0	16	6	415
No Chicken Noodle	1½ cups	94	7	1	0	16	6	495
Miso-Cup								
Golden Vegetable as prep	1 cup	30	2	1	0	3	tr	780
Japanese Restaurant Style as prep	1 cup	60	4	2	0	7	tr	1170
Organic Traditional w/ Tofu as prep	1 cup	35	2	1	0	4	tr	480
Reduced Sodium as prep	1 cup	25	2	1	0	3	tr	270
Savory Seaweed as prep	1 cup	30	3	1	0	3	tr	690
Nissin								
Chicken Vegetable as prep	1 pkg	290	6	13	<5	38	2	1430
White Cheddar as prep	1 pkg	290	6	13	0	38	2	1120
Nueva Cocina								
Frijoles Negros Con Chipotle Chile	1 cup	140	9	1	0	27	9	680
Sopa De Calabaza	1 cup	180	2	8	15	25	1	730
Sopa De Frijoles Colorados	1 cup	140	9	1	0	27	7	790
Sopa De Frijoles Negros	1 cup	140	9	0	0	27	9	790
Sopa De Maiz	1 cup	150	3	7	5	28	2	940
Sopa De Tortilla	1 cup	140	3	4	0	34	2	980
San-J								
Miso Dark	1 pkg	40	3	2	–	3	1	1200
Miso Mild	1 pkg	45	3	2	–	5	1	1340
Simply Asia								
Soy Noodle Bowl	1 pkg	70	7	0	0	10	3	100
Uncle Ben's								
Black Bean & Rice as prep	1 cup	150	7	2	0	28	7	720
Broccoli Cheese & Rice as prep	1 cup	110	3	2	5	19	1	680
REFRIGERATED								
Organic Classics								
French Onion w/ Croutons	1 cup	140	3	6	0	17	2	790
Seafood Chowder	1 cup	160	11	6	50	17	1	800

FOOD	PORTION	CALS	PROT	FAT	CHOL	CARB	FIBER	SOD
TAKE-OUT								
ban mien fish head	1 serv (10 oz)	277	20	10	59	27	4	851
beef stew soup	1 cup (8.8 oz)	221	23	5	60	20	–	461
black bean turtle soup	1 cup	241	15	1	0	45	10	6
broccoli cheese	1 cup	165	6	9	14	15	2	875
brunswick stew soup	1 cup (8.5 oz)	232	27	6	71	17	–	438
caldo de res beef soup	1 cup	143	12	5	22	12	2	784
chinese velvet corn	1¼ cups	135	–	0	1	–	–	708
corn & cheese chowder	¾ cup	215	9	12	66	21	3	386
egg drop	1 cup	73	8	4	102	1	0	730
gazpacho	1 cup	46	1	tr	0	5	–	63
greek lemon	¾ cup	63	4	2	83	7	2	386
hot & sour	1 serv (14 oz)	173	15	8	87	8	1	475
matzo ball soup	1 cup	118	7	5	63	10	1	757
minestrone	1 cup	233	9	13	9	22	4	700
miso w/ tofu	1 cup	84	6	3	0	8	2	989
onion soup gratinee	1 serv	492	25	27	77	38	4	1325
oxtail	1 cup	68	3	2	2	9	1	1166
pasta e fagioli	1 cup (8.8 oz)	194	9	5	3	30	–	790
ratatouille	1 cup (7.5 oz)	266	2	25	0	12	–	329
shark fin	1 bowl (10 oz)	164	15	9	84	9	00	1164
shrimp bisque	1 cup	263	22	14	129	13	tr	263
sopa de albondigas	1 cup	171	10	11	50	9	1	187
thai lemon grass	1 bowl	100	10	4	65	5	–	553
vietnamese pho beef noodle	1 serv (7.8 oz)	480	15	12	46	78	1	43
wonton soup	1 cup	183	14	7	53	14	1	769
zupa koprowa polish dill soup	1 bowl	54	11	2	55	6	–	524
SOUR CREAM								
sour cream	1 cup (8 oz)	493	7	48	102	10	–	123

FOOD	PORTION	CALS	PROT	FAT	CHOL	CARB	FIBER	SOD
sour cream	1 tbsp (0.4 oz)	26	tr	3	5	1	–	6
Cabot								
Light	2 tbsp	35	1	3	10	2	0	25
Sour Cream	2 tbsp	50	1	5	15	1	0	35
Daisy								
No Fat	2 tbsp	20	2	0	0	1	0	15
Sour Cream	2 tbsp	60	1	5	0	1	0	15
Hood								
Fat Free	2 tbsp	20	1	0	0	4	0	25
Low Fat	2 tbsp	35	1	2	5	3	0	20
Sour Cream	2 tbsp	60	1	5	20	2	0	15
Horizon Organic								
Lowfat	2 tbsp	35	1	2	10	3	0	25
Sour Cream	2 tbsp	60	1	5	20	1	0	15
Organic Valley								
Lowfat	2 tbsp	40	1	2	10	1	0	15

SOUR CREAM SUBSTITUTES

FOOD	PORTION	CALS	PROT	FAT	CHOL	CARB	FIBER	SOD
nondairy	1 oz	59	1	6	0	2	–	29
nondairy	1 cup	479	6	45	0	15	–	235

SOURSOP

FOOD	PORTION	CALS	PROT	FAT	CHOL	CARB	FIBER	SOD
fresh	1	416	6	2	0	105	–	87
fresh cut up	1 cup	150	2	1	0	38	–	31

SOY (*see also* CHEESE SUBSTITUTES, ICE CREAM AND FROZEN DESSERTS, MILK SUBSTITUTES, MISO, SMOOTHIES, SOY SAUCE, SOYBEANS, TEMPEH, TOFU, YOGURT FROZEN)

FOOD	PORTION	CALS	PROT	FAT	CHOL	CARB	FIBER	SOD
lecithin	1 tbsp	104	0	14	0	0	0	–
soya cheese	1.4 oz	128	7	11	–	tr	0	–
Bob's Red Mill								
Lecithin Granules	1 tbsp	60	0	4	0	1	0	0
Protein Powder	1 tbsp	20	5	0	0	0	0	60
Good Sense								
Soynuts Honey Roasted	1/3 cup	140	10	6	0	11	4	65
Soynuts Roasted & Salted	1/3 cup	140	10	7	0	10	5	90
Soynuts Roasted w/o Salt	1/3 cup	140	10	7	0	10	5	0
South Beach								
Soy Nuts Dark Chocolate	1 pkg (0.7 oz)	100	3	6	0	9	2	0

SOY DRINKS (*see* MILK SUBSTITUTES, SMOOTHIES)

FOOD	PORTION	CALS	PROT	FAT	CHOL	CARB	FIBER	SOD
SOY SAUCE								
shoyu	1 tbsp	9	1	tr	0	2	–	1029
soy sauce	1 tbsp	7	tr	tr	0	1	–	1024
tamari	1 tbsp	11	2	tr	0	1	–	1005
Eden								
Organic Shoyu	1 tbsp	15	2	0	0	2	0	1040
Organic Shoyu Reduced Sodium	1 tbsp	10	2	0	0	2	0	500
Organic Tamari	1 tbsp	15	2	0	0	2	0	860
House Of Tsang								
Ginger Soy Sauce	1 tbsp	20	0	0	0	4	0	760
Less Sodium	1 tbsp	5	0	0	0	0	0	300
San-J								
Shoyu Organic	1 tbsp	15	2	0	0	1	–	960
Tamari	1 tbsp	15	2	0	0	1	–	960
Tamari Reduced Sodium	1 tbsp	20	2	0	0	1	–	700
Tamari Organic Wheat Free	1 tbsp	15	2	0	0	1	–	940
Tamari Organic Wheat Free Reduced Sodium	1 tbsp	20	2	0	0	2	–	700
SOYBEANS								
dried cooked	1 cup	298	29	15	0	17	–	1
dry roasted	½ cup	387	34	19	0	28	–	2
green cooked	½ cup	127	11	6	0	10	4	13
roasted	½ cup	405	30	22	0	29	–	140
roasted & toasted	1 cup	490	40	26	0	33	–	4
roasted & toasted salted	1 cup	490	40	26	0	33	–	176
sprouts raw	½ cup	43	5	2	0	3	–	5
sprouts steamed	½ cup	38	4	2	0	3	–	5
sprouts stir fried	1 cup	125	13	7	0	9	–	14
Arrowhead Mills								
Organic Dried not prep	¼ cup	160	14	8	0	11	4	0
C&W								
In the Pod	½ cup	110	9	4	0	12	9	0
Eden								
Organic Blacksoy	½ cup	120	11	6	0	8	7	30
Frieda's								
Edamame	½ cup (2.6 oz)	100	8	3	0	10	3	10

FOOD	PORTION	CALS	PROT	FAT	CHOL	CARB	FIBER	SOD
Soyafarm								
Edamame Yuba Sticks	7 pieces (2.5 oz)	123	10	6	–	9	4	440

SPAGHETTI (see PASTA, PASTA DINNERS, PASTA SALAD, SPAGHETTI SAUCE)

SPAGHETTI SAUCE
JARRED

FOOD	PORTION	CALS	PROT	FAT	CHOL	CARB	FIBER	SOD
marinara sauce	1 cup	171	4	8	0	25	–	1572
spaghetti sauce	1 cup	272	12	12	0	40	–	1236
Barilla								
Arrabbiata Tomato & Spicy Pepper	½ cup	90	2	3	0	11	3	560
Basilico Tomato & Basil	½ cup	70	2	2	0	12	3	560
Boscaiola Mushrooms & Garlic	½ cup	90	2	3	0	11	3	560
Campagnola Roasted Garlic & Onion	½ cup	60	2	2	0	11	3	560
Garden Vegetable	½ cup	70	2	2	0	11	2	460
Rustica Sweet Peppers & Garlic	½ cup	70	2	3	0	11	3	620
Catelli								
Garden Select Country Mushroom	½ cup	80	3	2	0	13	3	320
Garden Select Diced Tomatoes & Basil	½ cup	80	2	2	0	13	3	330
Garden Select Fine Herbs	½ cup	80	3	2	0	13	3	340
Garden Select Garlic & Onion	½ cup	80	3	2	0	13	3	340
Garden Select Parmesan & Romano	½ cup	80	3	3	0	12	4	360
Garden Select Zucchini Primavera	½ cup	80	3	2	0	15	4	320
Classico								
Tomato & Basil	½ cup	60	2	1	0	11	2	310
Del Monte								
Chunky Garlic & Herb	½ cup	60	2	2	0	11	tr	490
Garlic & Onion	½ cup	80	2	1	0	16	2	490
W/ Four Cheese	½ cup	70	2	2	0	15	3	680
W/ Green Peppers & Mushrooms	½ cup	80	2	1	0	16	3	490

FOOD	PORTION	CALS	PROT	FAT	CHOL	CARB	FIBER	SOD
W/ Meat	½ cup	60	3	1	2	14	3	720
W/ Mushrooms	½ cup	60	2	1	0	14	2	630
Eden								
Organic	½ cup	80	3	3	0	12	3	320
Organic No Salt	½ cup	80	3	3	0	12	3	10
Organic Pizza Pasta Sauce	½ cup	65	2	3	0	9	5	300
Emeril's								
Homestyle Marinara	½ cup	90	2	4	0	11	3	700
Roasted Gaaahlic	½ cup	70	2	3	–	9	2	480
Sicilian Gravy	½ cup	90	1	5	0	10	1	520
Vodka	½ cup	130	2	8	10	13	2	490
Francesco Rinaldi								
Chunky Garden Tomato Garlic & Onion	½ cup	70	2	3	0	12	tr	640
Hearty Mushroom Pepper & Onion	½ cup	70	2	3	0	11	tr	650
Three Cheese	½ cup	80	3	2	0	15	tr	470
Traditional No Salt Added	½ cup	70	2	3	0	10	tr	25
Hunt's								
Basil Garlic & Oregano	¼ cup	15	tr	0	0	3	tr	350
Cheese & Garlic	½ cup	50	3	1	0	9	2	600
Chunky Vegetable	½ cup	50	2	1	0	11	3	560
Family Favorites Lasagna	¼ cup	30	1	0	0	6	1	330
Family Favorites Pizza Sauce	¼ cup	25	1	0	0	5	1	270
Four Cheese	½ cup	50	3	1	0	10	3	600
Italian Sausage	½ cup	60	3	2	0	10	3	590
Light	½ cup	45	2	0	0	9	3	430
Meat	½ cup	60	3	1	0	11	3	610
No Added Sugar	½ cup	45	2	1	0	9	3	580
Roasted Garlic & Onion	½ cup	50	2	1	0	10	3	540
Traditional	½ cup	50	2	1	0	10	2	580
With Mushrooms	½ cup	45	2	1	0	10	3	290
Joey Pots & Pans								
Arrabbiata	½ cup	100	1	9	0	7	1	740
Marinara	½ cup	50	1	4	0	6	1	430
Vodka Sauce	½ cup	110	1	9	30	6	1	530
Knorr								
W/ Meat	4 oz	110	6	5	20	9	–	820

FOOD	PORTION	CALS	PROT	FAT	CHOL	CARB	FIBER	SOD
Milo's								
Portobello Shiraz	4 oz	40	2	5	0	8	2	320
Muir Glen								
Organic Chunky Tomato	¼ cup	15	tr	0	0	4	tr	230
Organic Garlic Roasted Garlic	½ cup	60	2	1	0	12	2	380
Organic Pizza Sauce	¼ cup	40	1	2	0	6	1	290
Organic Tomato Sauce No Salt Added	¼ cup	25	1	0	0	5	1	10
Newman's Own								
Bambolina	½ cup	90	2	5	0	13	tr	620
Cabernet Marinara	½ cup	70	2	3	0	10	2	590
Five Cheese	½ cup	80	3	3	5	10	tr	610
Italian Sausage & Peppers	½ cup	90	4	4	10	11	tr	630
Marinara	½ cup	70	2	2	0	12	tr	510
Marinara w/ Mushrooms	½ cup	70	2	2	0	12	tr	520
Pesto & Tomato Sauce	½ cup	80	2	4	0	10	tr	640
Roasted Garlic & Green Peppers	½ cup	70	2	3	0	11	4	460
Sockarooni	½ cup	70	2	2	0	12	tr	520
Tomato & Roasted Garlic	½ cup	70	2	3	0	11	tr	580
Vodka Sauce	½ cup	110	5	5	5	11	0	440
Pomi								
Marinara	½ cup	80	1	4	0	5	3	650
Prego								
100% Natural Roasted Garlic Parmesan	½ cup	100	3	1	5	20	3	550
Heart Smart Traditional Italian	½ cup	100	2	3	0	15	3	430
Italian	½ cup	70	2	2	0	13	3	470
Italian Roasted Red Pepper & Garlic	½ cup	90	2	4	0	13	3	530
Italian Three Cheese	½ cup	80	3	2	0	14	3	430
Italian Tomato Basil & Garlic	½ cup	80	2	3	0	12	3	420
Italian Marinara	½ cup	100	2	5	0	11	4	550
Italian Meat	½ cup	130	2	4	5	19	3	570
Organic Mushroom	½ cup	90	2	3	0	13	4	540

FOOD	PORTION	CALS	PROT	FAT	CHOL	CARB	FIBER	SOD
Ragu								
Chunky Garden Style Tomato Garlic & Onion	½ cup (4.5 oz)	110	2	3	0	18	2	520
Fresh Italian	4 oz	110	2	3	0	19	–	590
Marinara	4 oz	100	1	3	0	16	–	610
Pizza Quick Fresh Italian	2 oz	35	1	1	0	5	–	270
Robert Rothchild Farm								
Artichoke	½ cup	80	2	5	0	8	0	90
Seeds Of Change								
Balsamic Olive & Onion	½ cup	80	3	2	0	14	2	650
Garden Vegetable	½ cup	70	2	1	0	14	2	550
Mushroom & Onion	½ cup	70	2	2	0	12	2	550
Three Cheese Marinara	½ cup	70	2	2	5	12	2	590
Traditional Herb	½ cup	70	2	0	0	16	2	550
Tuttorosso								
Pasta Sauce Meat	½ cup	90	3	3	0	15	3	620
Vino De Milo								
Mediterranean Pinot Grigio	½ cup	90	2	4	0	12	2	320
Portobella Shiraz	½ cup	40	1	1	0	9	2	340
Tuscan Merlot	½ cup	80	–	3	0	2	2	470
Walnut Acres								
Organic Garlic Garlic	½ cup	125	2	1	0	10	1	280
Organic Marinara & Zinfandel	½ cup	125	2	1	0	9	1	330
Organic Roasted Garlic	½ cup	125	2	1	0	11	1	280
Organic Tomato & Basil	½ cup	125	2	1	0	9	1	330
REFRIGERATED								
Buitoni								
Alfredo	¼ cup	140	4	12	35	5	0	430
Alfredo Portabello Mushroom	¼ cup	100	2	8	20	5	0	340
Alfredo Light	¼ cup	80	4	5	20	5	0	370
Marinara	½ cup	80	2	3	0	11	2	580
Marinara Roasted Garlic	½ cup	60	2	2	0	9	1	580
Pesto	¼ cup	330	10	27	20	11	6	560
Pesto w/ Basil	¼ cup	300	7	26	20	9	2	560
Pesto w/ Basil Reduced Fat	¼ cup	230	7	18	15	9	2	560
Pesto w/ Sun Dried Tomatoes	¼ cup	210	4	18	5	9	2	400
Tomato Herb Parmesan	½ cup	120	0	8	10	9	2	790

FOOD	PORTION	CALS	PROT	FAT	CHOL	CARB	FIBER	SOD
TAKE-OUT								
bolognese	5 oz	195	11	15	–	4	tr	–

SPANISH FOOD
FROZEN
Cedarlane

FOOD	PORTION	CALS	PROT	FAT	CHOL	CARB	FIBER	SOD
Organic Burrito Low Fat Rice & Cheese	1 (6 oz)	260	13	1	0	48	7	490
Organic Enchilada Low Fat Black Bean & Tofu	1 (9 oz)	220	10	3	0	42	6	390
Roasted Chile Relleno	1 pkg (10 oz)	400	23	20	55	37	5	770
Zone Burrito Beans & Cheese	1 (6 oz)	350	27	13	15	37	8	380
Contessa								
Fajitas Shrimp	2 (8 oz)	230	11	4	45	37	5	940
Paella w/ Chicken & Seafood	1½ cups	200	17	3	50	28	2	780
Seafood Veracruz not prep	1¾ cups	180	15	2	35	27	6	920
El Monterey								
Quesadillas Chicken Breast & Cheese	1 (5 oz)	280	20	13	60	21	tr	820
Healthy Choice								
Chicken Enchiladas	1 pkg	360	13	7	30	59	8	580
Enchilada Chicken	1 pkg	300	13	7	40	46	6	600
Helen's Kitchen								
Cheese Enchiladas w/ Toful Steaks In Spicy Red Sauce	½ pkg (5 oz)	150	5	9	10	20	5	300
Jose Ole								
Burrito Beef & Cheese	1 (5 oz)	300	13	10	25	39	2	510
Burrito Chicken	1 (5 oz)	270	9	7	20	41	2	630
Chimichanga Chicken & Cheese	1 (5 oz)	330	11	12	20	44	2	550
Chimichanga Shredded Beef	1 (5 oz)	350	13	15	25	39	2	510
Mini Burrito Chicken & Cheese	3	200	6	8	10	25	1	440
Mini Chimichanga Beef & Cheddar	3	240	8	12	10	25	1	520

FOOD	PORTION	CALS	PROT	FAT	CHOL	CARB	FIBER	SOD
Mini Quesadilla Grilled Chicken	3	220	9	8	20	28	1	600
Mini Tacos Beef & Cheese	4	200	7	11	20	19	3	390
Mini Taquitos Beef & Cheese	4	180	7	8	5	21	2	390
Soft Taco Beef & Cheese	1 (5 oz)	280	14	11	25	31	1	850
Taquitos Beef & Cheese Flour Tortilla	2	220	8	10	10	24	1	430
Taquitos Buffalo Chicken Flour Tortilla	2	200	7	10	15	23	tr	480
Taquitos Chicken Flour Tortilla	3	180	6	8	10	23	2	430
Taquitos Chicken & Cheese Flour Tortilla	2	220	8	10	15	25	1	430
Taquitos Pepperoni Pizza Flour Tortilla	2	240	7	14	15	23	1	490
Taquitos Shredded Beef Corn Tortilla	3	180	7	7	<5	21	2	440
Lean Cuisine								
One Dish Favorites Chicken Enchilada	1 pkg (9 oz)	280	10	5	20	49	3	540
Patio								
Burrito Bean & Cheese	1 (5 oz)	280	8	8	5	44	5	630
Burrito Beef & Bean Medium	1 (5 oz)	300	10	10	<5	44	5	740
Burrito Chicken	1 (5 oz)	280	9	8	15	42	2	740
Stouffer's								
Chicken Enchilada w/ Cheese Sauce & Rice	1 pkg (7.13 oz)	280	12	12	40	30	3	720
Tyson								
Meal Kit Chicken Fajita	1 (3.8 oz)	130	8	4	15	17	2	350
Meal Kit Quesadilla Chicken	1 (4 oz)	250	15	10	35	26	3	430
READY-TO-EAT								
taco shell corn	1 (6.5 inch)	98	2	5	0	13	2	77
taco shell flour	1 (7 inch)	173	3	9	0	19	1	168
Ortega								
Tostada Shells	2 (1 oz)	140	2	6	0	19	1	180

FOOD	PORTION	CALS	PROT	FAT	CHOL	CARB	FIBER	SOD
SHELF-STABLE								
Fantastic								
Spanish Paella	1 pkg (8 oz)	280	6	5	0	55	4	650
TAKE-OUT								
arroz con coco	1 cup	532	7	38	4	46	4	108
burrito w/ beans	1 med (5 oz)	295	10	8	6	45	7	501
burrito w/ beans & rice	1 (3.5 oz)	221	7	5	2	37	4	397
burrito w/ beef	1 sm (3.4 oz)	297	18	13	49	25	1	460
burrito w/ beef & beans	1 med (5 oz)	331	17	13	34	36	6	524
burrito w/ beef beans & cheese	1 med (5 oz)	379	21	19	57	30	5	596
burrito w/ chicken & beans	1 med (5 oz)	295	18	9	37	34	5	498
burrito w/ pork & beans	1 med (5 oz)	320	18	12	34	35	6	494
chiles rellenos meat & cheese filled	1 (5 oz)	213	10	16	109	9	2	430
chimichanga w/ bean cheese lettuce & tomato	1 (4.1 oz)	271	8	18	17	22	3	301
chimichanga w/ beef & rice	1 (10 oz)	634	19	36	35	58	5	573
chimichanga w/ beef beans lettuce & tomato	1 (4.1 oz)	254	9	15	15	22	3	225
chimichanga w/ beef cheese lettuce & tomato	1 (4.1 oz)	337	13	24	37	19	1	348
chimichanga w/ chicken sour cream lettuce & tomato	1 (4 oz)	277	9	20	30	17	1	153
enchilada w/ beans	1 (4.1 oz)	179	6	6	4	27	6	297
enchilada w/ beans & cheese	1 (4.6 oz)	233	9	11	21	25	5	381
enchilada w/ beef	1 (4 oz)	214	11	10	30	21	3	179
enchilada w/ beef & beans	1 (4 oz)	195	8	8	15	25	4	303
frijoles	1 cup	278	18	2	0	49	9	606
frijoles w/ cheese	1 cup	225	11	8	37	29	–	882
nachos w/ beans & cheese	1 serv (9.4 oz)	616	25	33	56	57	13	990

FOOD	PORTION	CALS	PROT	FAT	CHOL	CARB	FIBER	SOD
nachos w/ beef beans cheese & sour cream	1 serv (19 oz)	1620	59	97	171	133	19	1846
paella	1 serv (7 oz)	308	23	16	92	17	3	580
pupusa meat filled	1 (3.6 oz)	187	8	6	20	26	3	88
quesadilla w/ cheese	1 (5 oz)	498	20	28	60	40	3	1234
quesadilla w/ meat & cheese	1 (6.5 oz)	605	32	35	98	40	2	1268
taco de jueye w/ crab meat	1 (4.2 oz)	266	16	14	79	18	2	800
taco w/ beans lettuce tomato & salsa	1 (2.8 oz)	117	4	5	2	16	4	214
taco w/ chicken lettuce tomato & salsa	1 (2.5 oz)	114	8	5	22	10	1	134
taco w/ fish lettuce tomato & salsa	1 (2.7 oz)	101	8	4	39	10	1	190
tostada w/ beef lettuce tomato & salsa	1 (2.7 oz)	143	8	8	21	11	2	152

SPICES (see individual names, HERBS/SPICES)

SPINACH
CANNED

FOOD	PORTION	CALS	PROT	FAT	CHOL	CARB	FIBER	SOD
drained	1 cup	49	6	1	0	7	5	58
Popeye								
Spinach	½ cup	45	5	1	0	5	3	200
FRESH								
baby raw	2 cups	20	1	0	0	5	3	80
cooked	1 cup	41	5	tr	0	7	4	126
malabar cooked	1 cup	10	1	tr	0	1	1	24
mustard cooked	1 cup	29	3	tr	0	5	4	25
new zealand cooked	1 cup	22	2	tr	0	4	–	193
raw	1 cup	7	1	tr	0	1	1	24
Fresh Express								
Spicy Spinach	3 cups (3 oz)	10	2	0	0	6	6	80
FROZEN								
chopped cooked	1 cup	30	4	tr	0	5	4	92
Birds Eye								
Chopped	⅓ cup	20	2	0	0	2	2	115
C&W								
Baby Chopped	1 cup	30	2	0	0	3	1	120
Creamed	½ cup	100	4	7	20	6	.4	410

FOOD	PORTION	CALS	PROT	FAT	CHOL	CARB	FIBER	SOD
Cascadian Farm								
Organic Cut	⅓ cup	25	2	0	0	3	1	160
Cedarlane								
Organic Spanakopita Spinach & Feta Pie	½ pkg (5 oz)	260	12	8	20	38	2	650
Fillo Factory								
Spanakopita Spinach & Cheese Fillo Appetizers	3 (3 oz)	190	6	9	20	20	1	280
Green Giant								
No Sauce	½ cup	25	2	0	0	3	1	200
Stouffer's								
Creamed	½ pkg (4.5 oz)	200	5	16	25	8	2	490
Taverna								
Spinach Pie	1 piece (4.8 oz)	190	11	6	55	24	5	508
TAKE-OUT								
indian saag	1 serv	28	2	2	0	2	1	44
spanakopita spinach pie	1 serv (3 oz)	148	5	11	60	8	1	289
SPINACH JUICE								
juice	7 oz	14	2	0	0	2	–	146
SPORTS DRINKS (see ENERGY DRINKS)								
SPOT								
baked	3 oz	134	20	5	–	0	0	32
SPROUTS								
kidney bean	½ cup	27	4	tr	0	4	–	–
lentil sprouts	½ cup	40	3	tr	0	8	–	4
mung bean	½ cup	16	2	tr	0	3	–	3
mung bean canned	½ cup	8	1	tr	0	1	–	–
mung bean cooked	½ cup	13	1	tr	0	3	–	6
pea	½ cup	77	5	tr	0	17	–	12
radish	½ cup	8	1	tr	0	1	–	1
Brassica								
Broccoli Sprouts	½ cup (1 oz)	16	.1	0	0	2	1	3
TAKE-OUT								
mung bean stir fried	½ cup	31	3	tr	0	7	–	–

FOOD	PORTION	CALS	PROT	FAT	CHOL	CARB	FIBER	SOD
SQUAB								
boneless baked	1 (4 oz)	242	26	14	129	0	0	243
SQUASH (see also SQUASH SEEDS, ZUCCHINI)								
CANNED								
crookneck sliced	½ cup	14	1	tr	0	3	–	5
Farmer's Market								
Organic Butternut	½ cup	50	1	tr	0	12	2	5
FRESH								
acorn cooked mashed	½ cup	41	1	tr	0	11	3	3
acorn cubed baked	½ cup	57	1	tr	0	15	2	4
butternut baked	½ cup	41	1	tr	0	11	2	4
crookneck sliced cooked	½ cup	18	1	tr	0	4	1	1
hubbard baked	½ cup	51	3	tr	0	11	3	8
hubbard cooked mashed	½ cup	35	2	tr	0	8	3	6
scallop sliced cooked	½ cup	14	1	tr	0	3	1	1
spaghetti cooked	½ cup	23	1	tr	0	5	2	14
Frieda's								
Acorn	¾ cup (3 oz)	35	1	0	0	9	2	0
Baby Crookneck	⅔ cup (3 oz)	15	1	0	0	3	1	0
Baby Scallop	⅔ cup (3 oz)	15	1	0	0	3	1	0
Eight Ball	2 (4.4 oz)	18	2	0	0	4	1	4
Hubbard	¾ cup (3 oz)	35	2	0	0	7	2	5
Mini Pumpkin	¾ cup (3 oz)	20	1	0	0	6	2	0
Spaghetti	¾ cup (3 oz)	30	1	0	0	6	1	15
Star Spangled	⅔ cup (3 oz)	20	2	0	0	3	1	0
Turban	¾ cup (3 oz)	30	1	0	0	7	1	0
Glory								
Yellow Sliced	¾ cup	20	1	0	0	3	1	20
FROZEN								
butternut cooked mashed	½ cup	47	1	tr	0	12	3	2
crookneck sliced cooked	½ cup	24	1	tr	0	5	–	6

FOOD	PORTION	CALS	PROT	FAT	CHOL	CARB	FIBER	SOD
C&W								
Butternut	½ cup	45	1	0	0	10	1	2
McKenzie's								
Southland Butternut	½ cup	70	1	3	0	10	1	270
TAKE-OUT								
fritter	1 (0.8 oz)	81	2	5	15	8	1	79
SQUASH SEEDS								
roasted	1 oz	148	9	12	0	4	–	5
salted & roasted	1 oz	148	9	12	0	4	–	5
seeds dried	1 oz	154	7	13	0	5	–	5
seeds whole roasted	1 oz	127	5	6	0	15	–	5
SQUID								
baked	1 cup	192	26	6	393	5	0	540
canned in its own ink	1 can (4 oz)	122	21	2	308	4	0	360
dried	1 sm (1.5 oz)	147	25	2	371	5	0	255
pickled	1 oz	26	4	tr	63	1	0	431
steamed	1 cup	147	25	2	374	5	0	587
Contessa								
Calamari + Sauce	13 pieces + 2 tbsp sauce	160	5	6	55	21	1	370
Margaritaville								
Captain's Calamari Strips + Sauce	⅓ pkg	330	9	20	85	28	0	730
Van de Kamp's								
Fried Calamari	15 pieces (4 oz)	270	10	13	105	26	1	650
TAKE-OUT								
arroz con calamares	1 cup	400	14	17	150	47	1	906
calamari breaded & fried	1 cup	296	26	12	378	17	1	584
SQUIRREL								
roasted	3 oz	147	26	4	103	0	0	102
STARFRUIT								
fresh	1	42	1	tr	0	10	–	2
Frieda's								
Dried	⅓ cup (1.4 oz)	120	2	0	0	29	1	5

FOOD	PORTION	CALS	PROT	FAT	CHOL	CARB	FIBER	SOD
STRAWBERRIES								
canned in heavy syrup	½ cup	117	1	tr	0	30	2	5
fresh halves	1 cup	49	1	tr	0	12	3	2
fresh whole	1 cup	46	1	tr	0	11	3	1
fresh whole	1 pint	114	2	1	0	27	7	4
frzn sweetened sliced	½ cup	122	1	tr	0	33	2	4
frzn whole unsweetened	1 cup	77	1	tr	0	20	5	4
organic fresh whole	8 med	45	1	0	0	12	4	0
whole sweetened frzn	1 cup	199	1	tr	0	54	5	3
C&W								
Ultimate Sliced frzn	⅔ cup	50	0	0	0	12	1	5
Europe's Best								
Sliced frzn	¾ cup	40	1	1	0	10	3	0
Frieda's								
Dried	½ cup (1.4 oz)	150	1	0	0	34	3	0
LiteHouse								
Glaze Sugar Free	3 tbsp	35	0	0	0	8	0	55
Marie's								
Glaze	2 tbsp	40	0	0	0	10	0	40
STRAWBERRY JUICE								
Adina								
California Kiss Hibiscus Strawberry	8 oz	80	0	0	0	21	–	15
STUFFING/DRESSING								
Fresh Gourmet								
All Natural Multi-Grain w/ Cranberries not prep	⅓ cup (1 oz)	110	3	3	0	19	1	360
Organic Seasoned not prep	⅓ cup (1 oz)	110	3	3	0	19	1	350
Kellogg's								
Stuffing Mix as prep	1 cup	240	5	13	0	26	1	800
Pepperidge Farm								
Corn Bread	¾ cup	170	4	2	0	33	2	480
Cube	¾ cup	140	4	1	0	28	2	530
Herb Seasoned	¾ cup	170	5	2	0	33	3	600
One Step Turkey	½ cup	170	4	7	0	23	1	540
Tofurky								
Wild Rice & Mushroom	½ cup	110	3	2	0	21	1	421

FOOD	PORTION	CALS	PROT	FAT	CHOL	CARB	FIBER	SOD
TAKE-OUT								
bread	1 cup	352	6	17	0	44	2	1028
cornbread	½ cup	179	3	9	0	22	3	455
oyster	1 cup	304	7	18	23	29	2	953
sausage	½ cup	292	8	11	12	40	1	258
STURGEON								
broiled	3 oz	115	18	4	65	0	0	59
roe raw	1 oz	59	7	3	–	tr	–	–
smoked	1 oz	49	9	1	23	0	0	210
TAKE-OUT								
breaded & fried	4 oz	252	19	15	85	9	1	416
SUCKER								
white baked	3 oz	101	18	3	45	0	0	44
SUGAR								
brown packed	1 cup (7.7 oz)	828	0	0	0	214	–	86
brown unpacked	1 cup (5.1 oz)	547	0	0	0	141	0	57
brown organic	1 tsp	17	0	0	0	4	0	0
cinnamon sugar	1 tsp	16	tr	tr	0	4	tr	0
maple	1 piece (1 oz)	99	tr	tr	0	25	0	3
powdered	1 tbsp (0.3 oz)	31	0	0	0	8	–	0
powdered unsifted	1 cup (4.2 oz)	467	tr	tr	0	119	–	2
raw	1 pkg (5 g)	19	0	0	0	5	0	2
sugarcane stem	3 oz	54	1	0	0	14	3	–
white	1 packet (3 g)	12	0	0	0	3	0	0
white	1 cup (7 oz)	773	0	0	0	200		3
white	1 tsp (4 g)	15	0	0	0	4	–	0
Bob's Red Mill								
Date Sugar	1 tsp	11	0	0	0	3	0	0
Turbinado	1 tsp	10	0	0	0	3	0	0
Domino								
Dark Brown	1 tsp	15	0	0	0	4	–	0
Organic Cane Sugar	1 tsp	15	0	0	0	4	–	0
White	1 tsp	15	0	0	0	4	–	0

FOOD	PORTION	CALS	PROT	FAT	CHOL	CARB	FIBER	SOD
Equinox								
Organic Maple Flakes	2 tsp	15	0	0	0	4	–	0
Gluco Burst								
Arctic Cherry	1 pkg (1.3 oz)	70	0	0	0	16	–	30

SUGAR SUBSTITUTES

FOOD	PORTION	CALS	PROT	FAT	CHOL	CARB	FIBER	SOD
Equal								
Flavor Sticks	1 pkg	0	0	0	0	tr	–	0
Packet	1 pkg	0	0	0	0	tr	–	0
Spoonful	1 tsp	0	0	0	0	tr	–	0
Sugar Lite	1 tsp	8	0	0	0	2	0	0
Nature's Family								
Sun Crystals	1 pkg (4.5 g)	4	0	0	0	1	–	0
Neway								
Sweet Sensation	¼ tsp	0	0	0	0	tr	0	0
Splenda								
Flavor Blends All Flavors	1 pkg	0	0	0	0	tr	0	0
No Calorie Granules	1 tsp	0	0	0	0	tr	0	0
Sugar Blend For Baking	½ tsp	10	0	0	0	2	–	0
Sweetener	1 pkg	0	0	0	0	tr	0	0
Sun Crystals								
Natural Sweetener	1 pkg (5 g)	4	0	0	0	5	–	–
Sweet Fiber								
All Natural	1 pkg	0	0	0	0	tr	tr	0
Sweet Simplicity								
Sweetener	1 pkg	0	0	0	0	6	–	0
Sweete								
Sugar Free	1 pkg	0	0	0	0	tr	0	10
SweetLeaf								
SteviaPlus	1 pkg	0	0	0	0	0	1	–
Whey Low								
Gold	1 tsp	4	0	0	0	4	0	0
Granular	1 tsp	4	0	0	0	4	0	0
Maple Buzz	¼ cup	57	0	0	0	57	0	0
Powder	1 tsp	4	0	0	0	4	0	0
Zsweet								
All Natural	1 pkg (1 g)	0	0	0	0	tr	0	0

SUGAR-APPLE

FOOD	PORTION	CALS	PROT	FAT	CHOL	CARB	FIBER	SOD
fresh	1	146	3	tr	0	37	–	15
fresh cut up	1 cup	236	5	1	0	59	–	24

FOOD	PORTION	CALS	PROT	FAT	CHOL	CARB	FIBER	SOD
SUNCHOKE								
fresh raw sliced	½ cup	57	2	tr	0	13	–	–
Frieda's								
Sunchoke	½ cup (3 oz)	70	2	0	0	14	1	0
SUNFISH								
pumpkinseed baked	3 oz	97	21	1	73	0	0	87
SUNFLOWER								
seeds dry roasted w/ salt	¼ cup	186	6	16	0	8	3	131
seeds dry roasted w/o salt	¼ cup	186	6	16	0	8	4	1
seeds w/ hulls dried	¼ cup	66	3	6	0	2	1	0
Arrowhead Mills								
Organic Seeds	¼ cup	170	7	15	0	6	3	0
Bob's Red Mill								
Seeds Roasted & Salted	3 tbsp	186	6	15	0	6	5	104
David								
Kernals Original	¼ cup	200	6	17	0	5	2	140
Seeds BBQ	¼ cup	190	7	15	0	5	2	160
Seeds BBQ Sizzlin	¼ cup	190	6	16	0	6	2	260
Seeds Jalapeno	¼ cup	190	7	15	0	5	2	160
Seeds Nacho Cheese	¼ cup	180	7	15	0	6	2	180
Seeds Original	¼ cup	190	7	15	0	5	2	130
Seeds Ranch	¼ cup	190	7	15	0	6	2	180
Seeds Reduced Sodium	¼ cup	190	7	15	0	5	2	85
Frito Lay								
Seeds	3 tbsp	180	7	15	0	5	2	150
Good Sense								
Nuts Honey Roasted	¼ cup	190	6	15	0	7	2	120
Nuts Raw	¼ cup	170	7	15	0	6	4	0
Nuts Roasted & Salted	¼ cup	190	8	15	0	5	2	120
Seeds In Shell Roasted & Salted	½ cup	150	5	9	0	13	13	1290
Sunflower Nuts Roasted w/o Salt	¼ cup	190	8	16	0	5	2	5
SunButter								
Creamy	2 tbsp	200	7	16	0	7	4	120
Organic	2 tbsp	203	8	16	0	7	3	100
SunGold								
Seeds Roasted Salted	1 oz	172	7	15	0	4	2	168

FOOD	PORTION	CALS	PROT	FAT	CHOL	CARB	FIBER	SOD

SUSHI
TAKE-OUT

FOOD	PORTION	CALS	PROT	FAT	CHOL	CARB	FIBER	SOD
california roll	1 piece (0.8 oz)	28	1	1	1	4	–	37
fresh salmon rolls	4 pieces	250	11	7	20	37	3	590
inari	1 sm	46	1	1	0	9	0	79
sashimi	1 serv (6 oz)	198	24	7	63	4	–	718
tuna roll	1 piece (0.7 oz)	23	2	tr	3	3	–	33
vegetable roll	1 piece (1.2 oz)	27	1	1	0	5	–	47
vinegared ginger	⅓ cup (1.6 oz)	48	1	tr	0	12	–	6
wasabi	2 tsp (0.3 oz)	5	tr	tr	0	1	–	124
yellowtail roll	1 piece (0.6 oz)	25	1	1	0	3	–	32

SWAMP CABBAGE

FOOD	PORTION	CALS	PROT	FAT	CHOL	CARB	FIBER	SOD
chopped cooked w/o salt	1 cup	20	2	tr	0	4	2	120

SWEET POTATO (see also YAM)

FOOD	PORTION	CALS	PROT	FAT	CHOL	CARB	FIBER	SOD
baked w/ skin	1 (3.5 oz)	118	2	tr	0	28	3	12
canned in syrup	½ cup	106	1	tr	0	25	–	38
canned pieces	1 cup	183	3	tr	0	42	–	107
frzn cooked	½ cup	88	2	tr	0	21	–	7
leaves cooked	½ cup	11	1	tr	0	2	–	4
mashed	½ cup	172	3	tr	0	40	3	21
Diner's Choice								
Mashed	⅔ cup	160	3	3	0	33	2	105
Framer's Market								
Organic Puree	½ cup	96	2	0	0	22	2	6
Glory								
Casserole	½ cup	180	2	0	0	43	2	250
Cut Fresh	1 serv (5 oz)	140	2	0	0	36	4	50
Sweet Potatoes	⅔ cup	160	3	0	0	37	2	35
Green Giant								
Candied	¾ cup	240	2	7	0	41	3	430
Mann's								
Fresh Cubes	1 serv (3 oz)	60	1	0	0	15	3	10
Mrs. Paul's								
Candied	1 serv (5 oz)	300	1	1	0	73	3	130

FOOD	PORTION	CALS	PROT	FAT	CHOL	CARB	FIBER	SOD
Princella								
In Light Syrup	⅔ cup	160	0	0	0	39	3	35
Sugary Sam								
In Syrup	⅔ cup	160	3	0	0	37	2	35
TAKE-OUT								
candied	3.5 oz	144	1	3	0	29	–	73
SWEETBREAD (PANCREAS)								
beef braised	3 oz	230	23	15	223	0	0	51
lamb braised	3 oz	199	19	13	340	0	0	44
pork braised	3 oz	186	24	9	268	0	0	36
testicals cooked	1 pair (6.8 oz)	241	44	6	673	0	0	739
veal braised	3 oz	218	25	12	–	0	0	58
SWISS CHARD								
cooked	½ cup	18	2	tr	0	4	–	158
raw chopped	½ cup	3	tr	tr	0	1	–	38
Frieda's								
Bright Lights	1 cup (3 oz)	15	2	0	0	3	1	180
SWORDFISH								
cooked	3 oz	132	22	4	43	0	0	98
raw	3 oz	103	17	3	33	0	0	76
SYRUP								
corn dark & light	¼ cup	240	0	tr	0	65	0	99
date syrup	1 tbsp	63	tr	tr	–	15	0	–
maple	1 tbsp	52	0	0	0	13	–	2
maple	1 cup (11.1 oz)	824	tr	1	0	212	–	27
raspberry	1 oz	76	tr	0	0	19	–	1
rose hip	1 oz	9	0	0	–	2	0	–
sorghum	1 tbsp (0.7 oz)	61	0	0	0	16	–	2
sorghum	1 cup (11.6 oz)	957	0	0	0	247	–	28
sugar syrup	¼ cup	76	0	0	0	20	0	1
Cary's								
Maple	¼ cup	210	0	0	0	53	–	5
Eden								
Organic Barley Malt	1 tbsp	60	1	0	0	14	0	0

FOOD	PORTION	CALS	PROT	FAT	CHOL	CARB	FIBER	SOD
Estee								
Blueberry	¼ cup	30	tr	0	0	8	–	–
Karo								
Corn Syrup Dark	2 tbsp	120	0	0	0	30	–	45
Corn Syrup Light	2 tbsp	120	0	0	0	31	–	35
Lundberg								
Organic Sweet Dreams Brown Rice	2 tbsp	110	1	0	0	31	0	30
Navitas Naturals								
Yacon	2 tbsp	90	0	0	0	22	0	25
Nesquik								
Strawberry Calcium Fortified	2 tbsp	100	0	0	0	27	1	55
Neway								
Sweet Sensation Luo Han Guo Syrup	1 tsp	8	0	0	0	2	0	0
Pacifica Culinaria								
Pomegranate	1 tbsp	60	0	0	0	16	–	0
Watermelon	1 tbsp	60	0	0	0	16	–	0
Smucker's								
Blackberry	¼ cup	210	0	0	0	52	–	0
Blueberry	¼ cup	210	0	0	0	52	–	0
Boysenberry	¼ cup	210	0	0	0	52	–	0
Red Raspberry	¼ cup	210	0	0	0	52	–	0
Strawberry	¼ cup	210	0	0	0	52	–	0
Sundae Syrup 3 Musketeers	2 tbsp	110	1	2	0	23	–	60
Sundae Syrup Butterscotch	2 tbsp	100	1	0	0	25	–	110
Sundae Syrup Caramel	2 tbsp	100	1	0	0	25	–	110
Sundae Syrup Strawberry	2 tbsp	110	0	0	0	26	–	5

TAHINI (see SESAME)

TAMARILLOS
Frieda's

FOOD	PORTION	CALS	PROT	FAT	CHOL	CARB	FIBER	SOD
Gold Or Red	2 (4.2 oz)	40	2	0	0	9	4	0

TAMARIND

FOOD	PORTION	CALS	PROT	FAT	CHOL	CARB	FIBER	SOD
dried sweetened pulpitas	½ cup	279	3	1	0	73	5	28
dried sweetened pulpitas	1 piece (0.8 oz)	56	1	tr	0	15	1	6

FOOD	PORTION	CALS	PROT	FAT	CHOL	CARB	FIBER	SOD
fresh	1 (2 g)	5	tr	tr	0	1	tr	1
fresh cut up	1 cup	143	2	tr	0	38	3	17

TAMARIND JUICE

nectar	1 cup	143	tr	tr	0	37	1	18

TANGERINE
CANNED

in light syrup	1 cup	154	1	tr	0	41	2	15
juice pack	1 cup	92	2	tr	0	24	2	12

FRESH

fresh	1 sm (2.7 oz)	40	1	tr	0	10	1	2
fresh	1 med (3.1 oz)	47	1	tr	0	12	2	2
fresh	1 lg (4.2 oz)	64	1	tr	0	16	2	2
sections	1 cup	103	2	1	0	26	4	4
River Pride								
Sweet	1 (3.8 oz)	50	1	1	0	15	3	0
Sunkist								
Fresh	1 (3.8 oz)	50	1	1	0	15	3	0

TANGERINE JUICE

canned sweetened	1 cup	124	1	1	0	30	1	2
fresh	1 cup	106	1	tr	0	25	1	2
Italian Volcano								
Organic	1 serv (6.75 oz)	94	2	1	0	20	tr	0
Naked Juice								
Tangerine Scream	8 oz	110	1	0	0	25	0	0
Odwalla								
100% Juice	8 oz	110	1	0	0	25	0	0
SSips								
Drink	1 box (7 oz)	120	0	0	0	31	–	10

TAPIOCA

pearl dry	¼ cup (1.3 oz)	136	tr	tr	0	34	tr	0
starch	1 oz	98	17	tr	–	24	–	1
Let's Do Organic								
Granulated	1 tbsp	35	0	0	0	9	0	0
Starch	1 tbsp	0	0	0	0	9	0	0

FOOD	PORTION	CALS	PROT	FAT	CHOL	CARB	FIBER	SOD
TARO								
chips	10 (0.8 oz)	115	1	6	0	16	–	79
leaves cooked	½ cup	18	2	tr	0	3	–	2
raw sliced	½ cup	56	1	tr	0	14	–	6
shoots sliced cooked	½ cup	10	1	tr	0	2	–	1
sliced cooked	½ cup (2.3 oz)	94	tr	tr	0	23	–	10
tahitian sliced cooked	½ cup	30	3	tr	0	5	–	37
Frieda's								
Taro Root	⅔ cup (3 oz)	90	0	0	0	22	3	10
TARPON								
fresh	3 oz	87	17	2	–	0	0	70
TARRAGON								
dried crumbled	1 tsp	2	tr	tr	0	tr	0	0
ground	1 tsp	5	tr	tr	0	1	tr	1
TEA/HERBAL TEA *(see also* ICED TEA*)*								
HERBAL								
chamomile brewed	1 cup	2	0	tr	0	tr	0	2
Celestial Seasonings								
Chamomile	1 cup	0	0	0	0	0	0	0
Dessert Tea English Toffee	1 cup	0	0	0	0	0	0	0
Moroccan Pomegranate Red	1 cup	0	0	0	0	0	0	0
Peppermint	1 cup	0	0	0	0	0	0	0
Red Safari Spice	1 cup	0	0	0	0	0	0	0
Roastaroma Herb	1 cup	0	0	0	0	0	0	0
Wellness Tea Ginseng Energy	1 tea bag	0	0	0	0	0	0	0
Zinger Acai Mango	1 cup	0	0	0	0	tr	0	0
Zinger Lemon	1 cup	0	0	0	0	0	0	0
Eden								
Organic Genmaicha Tea	1 tea bag	0	0	0	0	0	0	0
Organic Kukicha Tea	1 tea bag	0	0	0	0	0	0	0
Lipton								
Cinnamon Apple	1 tea bag	0	0	0	0	tr	–	0
Ginger Twist	1 tea bag	0	0	0	0	0	0	0
Honey Lemon	1 tea bag	0	0	0	0	1	–	0

FOOD	PORTION	CALS	PROT	FAT	CHOL	CARB	FIBER	SOD
Lemon	1 tea bag	0	0	0	0	1	–	0
Mango	1 tea bag	0	0	0	0	0	0	0
Orange	1 tea bag	0	0	0	0	1	–	0
Peach	1 tea bag	0	0	0	0	tr	–	0
Peppermint	1 tea bag	0	0	0	0	0	0	0
Quietly Chamomile	1 tea bag	0	0	0	0	tr	–	0
Raspberry	1 tea bag	0	0	0	0	tr	–	0
Tetley								
Chamomile	1 cup	0	0	0	0	0	0	0
Orange & Peach	1 cup	0	0	0	0	0	0	10
Peppermint	1 cup	0	0	0	0	tr	0	10
REGULAR								
brewed tea	6 oz	2	0	0	0	1	0	5
Celestial Seasonings								
Black Fast Lane	1 cup	0	0	0	0	0	0	0
Black Decafe Victorian Earl Grey	1 cup	0	0	0	0	tr	–	0
Chai White Honey Vanilla	1 tea bag	0	0	0	0	0	0	0
Green Antioxidant	1 cup	0	0	0	0	0	0	0
Green Tropical Acai	1 cup	0	0	0	0	0	0	0
Green Tea	1 cup	0	0	0	0	0	0	0
Morning Thunder	1 cup	0	0	0	0	0	0	0
TeaHouse Chai Cinnamon Spice as prep	1 serv	110	2	0	0	25	–	80
White Tea Antioxidant Plum	1 tea bag	0	0	0	0	0	0	0
Daily Detox								
Original	1 teabag	0	0	0	0	0	0	0
Eden								
Organic Bancha Green Tea	1 tea bag	0	0	0	0	0	0	0
Organic Hojicha Tea	1 tea bag	0	0	0	0	0	0	0
General Foods								
International Tea Chai Latte	1 serv	70	0	2	0	12	–	60
Lipton								
Black Tea as prep	1 teabag	0	0	0	0	0	0	0
Black Tea French Vanilla	1 tea bag	0	0	0	0	0	0	0
Black Tea Honey & Lemon	1 tea bag	0	0	0	0	1	–	0
Black Tea Mint	1 tea bag	0	0	0	0	0	0	0
Black Tea Orange & Spice	1 tea bag	0	0	0	0	0	0	0
Black Tea Spiced Chai	1 tea bag	0	0	0	0	1	–	0

FOOD	PORTION	CALS	PROT	FAT	CHOL	CARB	FIBER	SOD
Decaffeinated Black Tea as prep	1 serv	0	0	0	0	0	0	0
Earl Grey	1 tea bag	0	0	0	0	0	0	0
English Breakfast	1 tea bag	0	0	0	0	0	0	0
English Estate	1 tea bag	0	0	0	0	0	0	0
Green Tea as prep	1 tea bag	0	0	0	0	0	0	0
Green Tea Citrus Blossom	1 tea bag	5	0	0	0	2	–	0
Green Tea Decaffeinated	1 tea bag	0	0	0	0	0	0	0
Green Tea Lemon Ginseng	1 tea bag	0	0	0	0	0	0	0
Green Tea Mint	1 tea bag	0	0	0	0	0	0	0
Raspberry Truffle	1 tea bag	0	0	0	0	tr	–	0
Vanilla Hazelnut	1 tea bag	0	0	0	0	tr	–	0
Oregon Chai								
Chai Tea Latte Original Caffeine Free Concentrate	½ cup	78	0	0	0	18	–	8
Chai Tea Latte Original Concentrate	½ cup	78	0	0	0	19	–	8
Chai Tea Latte Spiced Original Mix	1 pkg	100	2	1	5	20	–	135
Chai Tea Latte Vanilla Mix	1 pkg	120	2	2	5	25	–	130
Organic Chai Cider Concentrate	½ cup	110	0	0	0	26	–	10
Organic Chai Nog Concentrate	½ cup	90	0	0	0	15	–	15
Red Rose								
Black Tea Teabag	1	0	0	0	0	0	0	0
Decaffeinated	1 cup	0	0	0	0	0	0	0
English Breakfast Teabag	1 cup	0	0	0	0	0	0	0
Salada								
Original Blend Black Tea	1 tea bag	0	0	0	0	0	0	0
Tea Tech								
Instant Green Tea All Flavors	1 tube	0	0	0	0	tr	–	0
XtraGreen Tea Mix All Flavors	1 tube	0	0	0	0	tr	–	0
Tetley								
Chai Black Tea	1 cup	0	0	0	0	tr	0	10
Earl Grey	1 cup	0	0	0	0	0	0	15
English Breakfast	1 cup	0	0	0	0	tr	0	0
Honey Lemon Green Tea	1 cup	0	0	0	0	0	0	10

FOOD	PORTION	CALS	PROT	FAT	CHOL	CARB	FIBER	SOD
TEMPEH								
tempeh	½ cup	165	16	6	0	14	–	5
Lightlife								
Garden Veggie	1 serv (4 oz)	230	21	10	0	14	10	190
Organic Flax	1 serv (4 oz)	230	21	10	0	14	11	30
Organic Grilles Lemon	1 patty (2.7 oz)	140	11	6	0	11	0	280
Organic Grilles Tamari	1 patty (2.7 oz)	130	11	5	0	9	0	260
Organic Soy	1 serv (4 oz)	210	19	9	0	14	10	0
Organic Three Grain	1 serv (4 oz)	240	18	9	0	21	8	0
Organic Wild Rice	1 serv (4 oz)	280	19	11	0	14	10	10
Tofurky								
Edamame Veggie	3 oz	145	13	4	0	20	7	25
Five Grain	3 oz	190	11	6	0	20	6	10
Soy	3 oz	160	13	4	0	20	7	10
WildWood								
Organic Nori Seaweed	3 oz	170	13	7	0	16	4	0
TESTICLES (see SWEETBREAD)								
THYME								
dried crumbled	1 tsp	3	tr	tr	0	1	tr	1
fresh	1 tsp	1	tr	tr	0	tr	tr	0
ground	1 tsp	4	tr	tr	0	1	1	1
TILAPIA								
Beacon Light								
Farm Raised Fillets	3 oz	85	15	1	50	1	0	35
Gorton's								
Fillets Crunchy Breaded frzn	1 (3 oz)	80	14	3	50	tr	–	150
Van de Kamp's								
Lightly Breaded Fillets	1 (4 oz)	240	16	11	35	17	1	280
TAKE-OUT								
battered & fried	1 filet (4 oz)	206	21	9	109	8	tr	133
breaded & fried	1 filet (4 oz)	300	26	14	142	16	1	708
broiled w/o fat	1 filet (3.5 oz)	128	26	3	57	0	0	56

FOOD	PORTION	CALS	PROT	FAT	CHOL	CARB	FIBER	SOD
TILEFISH								
cooked	½ fillet (5.3 oz)	220	37	7	–	0	0	88
cooked	3 oz	125	21	4	–	0	0	50
raw	3 oz	81	15	2	–	0	0	45
TOFU								
firm	¼ block (3 oz)	118	13	7	0	3	1	11
firm	½ cup	183	20	11	0	5	2	17
fresh fried	1 piece (0.5 oz)	35	2	3	0	1	tr	2
fuyu salted & fermented	1 block (0.33 oz)	13	1	1	0	1	tr	316
koyadofu dried frozen	1 piece (0.5 oz)	82	8	5	0	2	tr	1
okara	½ cup	47	2	1	0	8	1	6
regular	¼ block (4 oz)	88	9	6	0	2	1	8
regular	½ cup	94	6	6	0	2	1	9
Azumaya								
Extra Firm	1 serv (2.8 oz)	70	7	4	0	2	1	0
Firm	1 serv (2.8 oz)	70	7	4	0	2	tr	0
Lite Silken	1 serv (3.2 oz)	40	5	1	0	3	0	45
Lite Extra Firm	1 serv (2.8 oz)	60	7	2	0	3	1	30
Seasoned Oriental Spice	1 serv (3 oz)	90	8	5	0	3	1	220
Seasoned Zesty Garlic & Onion	1 serv (3 oz)	90	8	5	0	3	1	250
Silken	1 serv (3.2 oz)	40	4	2	0	1	tr	0
Eden								
Dried	1 piece (0.4 oz)	50	5	3	0	0	2	0
Nasoya								
Chinese Spice	¼ pkg (3 oz)	90	8	5	0	3	1	220

FOOD	PORTION	CALS	PROT	FAT	CHOL	CARB	FIBER	SOD
Extra Firm	⅕ pkg (2.8 oz)	80	8	4	0	2	1	0
Firm	⅕ pkg (2.8 oz)	70	7	3	0	2	tr	0
Garlic & Onion	¼ pkg (3 oz)	90	8	5	0	3	1	250
Lite Firm	⅕ pkg (2.8 oz)	40	7	2	0	0	tr	25
Lite Silken	⅕ pkg (3.2 oz)	30	6	1	0	0	tr	65
Seasoned Ginger Sesame	½ pkg (5.5 oz)	210	9	6	0	27	2	630
Seasoned Sweet & Sour	½ pkg (5.5 oz)	190	8	4	0	26	1	690
Seasoned Teriyaki	½ pkg (5.5 oz)	190	10	4	0	24	2	1150
Seasoned Thai Peanut	½ pkg (5.5 oz)	240	12	9	0	24	2	770
Silken	⅕ pkg (3.2 oz)	45	4	3	0	2	0	5
Soft	⅕ pkg (2.8 oz)	60	6	3	0	1	tr	0
TofuMate Breakfast Scramble	¼ pkg	15	1	0	0	3	–	330
TofuMate Eggless Salad	¼ pkg	15	0	0	0	4	–	310
TofuMate Mandarin Stirfry	¼ pkg	25	1	0	0	6	–	310
TofuMate Mediterranean Herb	¼ pkg	15	1	0	0	3	–	330
TofuMate Szechwan StirFry	¼ pkg	25	1	0	0	4	–	280
TofuMate Texas Taco	¼ pkg	15	1	0	0	3	0	360
Soyafarm								
Baked Tofu	10 pieces (3.5 oz)	147	8	10	–	6	1	15
Nuggets	4 pieces (3.5 oz)	162	9	8	–	14	1	270
Tofu & Yuba Patties	1 (3.5 oz)	243	16	14	–	12	1	450
WildWood								
Organic Baked Aloha	1 piece (3.5 oz)	180	20	5	0	15	3	239

FOOD	PORTION	CALS	PROT	FAT	CHOL	CARB	FIBER	SOD
Organic Calcium Rich Medium	3 oz	70	7	4	0	2	1	5
Organic Golden Pineapple Teriyaki	3 oz	160	13	12	0	5	1	230
Organic High Protein Super Firm	3 oz	100	14	4	0	5	1	45
Organic Smoked Mild Szechuan	3 oz	150	14	6	0	11	2	368
TAKE-OUT								
breaded deep fried w/ soy sauce japanese style	1 piece (0.4 oz)	15	0	1	1	1	tr	16
soy sauce marinated & grilled	1 serv (4 oz)	181	19	11	0	6	1	294

TOMATILLO

FOOD	PORTION	CALS	PROT	FAT	CHOL	CARB	FIBER	SOD
fresh	1 (1.2 oz)	11	tr	tr	0	2	–	0
fresh chopped	½ cup	21	1	1	0	4	–	1
Las Palmas								
Tomatillos Crushed	½ cup	45	1	2	0	7	2	0

TOMATO

CANNED

FOOD	PORTION	CALS	PROT	FAT	CHOL	CARB	FIBER	SOD
paste	½ cup	110	5	1	0	25	6	86
puree	1 cup	102	4	tr	0	25	6	532
puree w/o salt	1 cup	102	4	tr	0	25	6	49
red whole	½ cup	24	1	tr	0	5	–	195
sauce	½ cup	37	2	tr	0	9	2	738
sauce spanish style	½ cup	40	2	tr	0	9	2	–
sauce w/ mushrooms	½ cup	42	2	tr	0	10	–	552
sauce w/ onion	½ cup	52	1	tr	0	12	–	672
stewed	½ cup	34	1	tr	0	8	–	325
w/ green chiles	½ cup	18	1	tr	0	4	–	481
wedges in tomato juice	½ cup	34	1	tr	0	8	–	285
Cento								
Crushed	¼ cup	35	2	0	0	7	2	20
Paste	2 tbsp	30	2	0	0	6	1	20
Puree	¼ cup	25	1	0	0	5	1	15
Contadina								
Crushed w/ Italian Herbs	¼ cup	20	tr	0	0	3	tr	150
Paste Italian Herbs	2 tbsp	35	1	1	0	7	1	290
Petite Cut Diced	½ cup	25	1	0	0	6	2	250

FOOD	PORTION	CALS	PROT	FAT	CHOL	CARB	FIBER	SOD
Del Monte								
Chunky Pasta Style	½ cup	45	1	0	0	11	2	560
Diced No Salt Added	½ cup	25	1	0	0	6	2	50
Diced w/ Garlic & Onion	½ cup	40	2	1	0	8	tr	610
Diced w/ Green Pepper& Onion	½ cup	40	1	0	0	9	2	480
Diced Zesty Chili Style	½ cup	30	1	0	0	8	2	600
Diced Zesty w/ Mild Green Chilies	½ cup	30	1	0	0	6	1	550
Garden Select Petite Diced	½ cup	15	1	0	0	3	tr	230
Organic Diced	½ cup	25	1	0	0	6	2	250
Organic Tomato Paste	2 tbsp	30	2	0	0	6	1	20
Organic Diced w/ Basil Garlic & Oregano	½ cup	50	2	0	0	11	tr	650
Petite Cut	½ cup	25	1	0	0	6	2	250
Petite Cut Garlic & Olive Oil	½ cup	45	1	1	0	10	1	620
Sauce	¼ cup	20	1	0	0	4	tr	340
Stewed Italian Recipe	½ cup	30	1	0	0	8	2	420
Stewed Mexican Recipe	½ cup	35	1	0	0	9	2	400
Eden								
Organic Crushed	¼ cup	20	1	0	0	3	1	0
Organic Diced	½ cup	30	1	0	0	6	2	5
Organic Whole Roma	½ cup	30	1	0	0	4	1	10
Hunt's								
Crushed	½ cup	30	2	0	0	7	2	350
Diced In Tomato Sauce	½ cup	30	tr	0	0	7	1	430
Diced Original	½ cup	20	1	0	0	5	tr	380
Diced w/ Basil Garlic & Oregano	½ cup	25	1	0	0	6	1	230
Diced w/ Green Pepper Celery & Onions	½ cup	45	1	0	0	10	1	340
Diced w/ Mild Green Chilies	½ cup	30	2	0	0	6	2	360
Diced w/ Roasted Garlic	½ cup	30	1	0	0	6	1	480
Diced w/ Sweet Onion	½ cup	45	1	0	0	10	tr	460
Family Favorites Meatloaf	¼ cup	30	1	0	0	7	2	390
Paste	2 tbsp	25	1	0	0	6	2	90
Paste No Salt Added	2 tbsp	30	1	0	0	6	2	15
Paste w/ Basil Garlic & Oregano	2 tbsp	25	1	0	0	6	2	260

FOOD	PORTION	CALS	PROT	FAT	CHOL	CARB	FIBER	SOD
Petite Diced	½ cup	20	1	0	0	5	1	330
Petite Diced w/ Mushrooms	½ cup	40	1	1	0	6	tr	380
Puree	½ cup	30	1	0	0	7	2	450
Sauce	¼ cup	15	tr	0	0	3	tr	360
Sauce Garlic & Herb	½ cup	40	2	1	0	8	3	610
Sauce No Salt Added	2 tbsp	30	1	0	0	6	2	15
Sauce Roasted Garlic	¼ cup	15	tr	0	0	3	tr	380
Stewed	½ cup	35	1	0	0	8	1	390
Stewed No Salt Added	½ cup	40	2	0	0	9	1	30
Whole No Salt Added	¼ cup	20	tr	0	0	4	1	15
Muir Glen								
Organic Chunky Tomato & Herb	½ cup	60	2	1	0	11	2	350
Organic Diced Fire Roasted	½ cup	30	1	0	0	6	1	290
Organic Diced w/ Basil & Garlic	½ cup	30	1	0	0	6	1	290
Pomi								
Chopped	½ cup	20	1	0	0	4	3	10
Redpack								
Crushed In Puree	¼ cup	20	0	0	0	4	1	120
Diced In Juice	½ cup	25	1	0	0	5	1	220
Paste	2 tbsp	0	2	0	0	6	1	20
Petite Diced Onion Celery & Green Pepper	½ cup	45	1	0	0	10	1	370
Rienzi								
Paste	2 tbsp	25	1	0	0	5	1	60
Ro-Tel								
Diced In Sauce	½ cup	40	1	0	0	8	tr	490
Mexican Festival	½ cup	30	tr	0	0	6	1	540
Original	½ cup	20	tr	0	0	4	1	520
Tillen Farms								
Sunnyside Tomatoes	3 pieces (1 oz)	40	1	3	0	4	1	5
Tuttorosso								
Puree	¼ cup	20	1	0	0	4	1	15
DRIED								
sun dried	1 piece	5	tr	tr	0	1	–	42
sun dried	1 cup	140	8	2	0	30	–	1131
sun dried in oil	1 piece (3 g)	6	tr	tr	0	1	–	8
sun dried in oil	1 cup (4 oz)	235	6	15	0	26	–	293

FOOD	PORTION	CALS	PROT	FAT	CHOL	CARB	FIBER	SOD
Frieda's								
Red Chopped	⅓ cup (1.1 oz)	100	2	1	0	19	2	10
FRESH								
bruschetta	¼ cup	50	2	3	0	6	tr	360
cooked	½ cup	32	1	1	0	7	–	13
grape tomatoes	20	30	1	0	0	6	1	0
green	1	30	1	tr	0	6	–	16
red	1 (4.5 oz)	26	1	tr	0	6	2	11
red chopped	1 cup	35	2	tr	0	8	2	16
Earthbound Farm								
Organic Roma	1 med (5.2 oz)	35	1	1	0	7	1	5
Eurofresh								
Tomatoes On The Vine	1 med (5.2 oz)	35	1	1	0	7	1	5
Foxy								
Roma	1 med (5 oz)	35	1	1	0	7	1	5
Frieda's								
Baby Roma	⅔ cup (3 oz)	120	1	0	0	4	1	10
Tear Drop	⅔ cup (3 oz)	20	1	0	0	4	1	10
TAKE-OUT								
bruschetta on toasted italian bread	1 slice	106	4	3	0	18	tr	355
stewed	1 cup	80	2	3	0	13	–	460
TOMATO JUICE								
beef broth & tomato	1 can (5.5 oz)	62	1	tr	0	14	tr	220
clam & tomato	1 can (5.5 oz)	77	1	tr	–	18	–	664
tomato juice	½ cup	21	1	tr	0	5	–	441
tomato juice	6 oz	32	1	tr	0	8	–	658
Campbell's								
Healthy Request	8 oz	50	2	0	0	10	2	480
Low Sodium	8 oz	50	2	0	0	10	2	140
Organic	8 oz	50	2	0	0	10	2	680

FOOD	PORTION	CALS	PROT	FAT	CHOL	CARB	FIBER	SOD
Del Monte								
Juice	8 oz	50	2	0	0	10	1	760
Kagome								
Sweet Summer	8 oz	50	2	0	0	11	1	100
Lakewood								
Organic	8 oz	35	1	0	0	7	1	140
Luvli Juices								
Smashing Tomato	1 bottle (10 oz)	125	3	1	0	28	4	140
Spicy Tomato	1 bottle (10 oz)	125	3	1	0	28	4	140

TONGUE

FOOD	PORTION	CALS	PROT	FAT	CHOL	CARB	FIBER	SOD
beef simmered	3 oz	241	16	19	112	0	0	55
lamb braised	3 oz	234	18	17	161	0	0	57
pork braised	3 oz	230	20	16	124	0	0	93
veal braised	3 oz	172	22	9	202	0	0	54

TORTILLA

FOOD	PORTION	CALS	PROT	FAT	CHOL	CARB	FIBER	SOD
corn	1 (6 in diam)	56	1	1	0	12	1	40
corn w/o salt	1 (6 in diam)	56	1	1	0	12	1	3
flour w/o salt	1 (8 in diam)	114	3	3	0	20	1	167
Alvarado Street Bakery								
Sprouted Wheat Burrito Size	1 (2.2 oz)	170	5	4	0	30	1	480
Food For Life								
Sprouted Corn	2 (1.7 oz)	120	2	1	0	25	4	0
French Meadow Bakery								
Organic Fat Flush	1 (1 oz)	100	5	1	0	18	3	105
La Tortilla Factory								
Carb Cutting Original	1 (1.3 oz)	60	5	2	0	11	7	150
Organic Yellow Corn	2 (2.4 oz)	120	3	2	0	25	2	0
Smart & Delicious Low Fat Low Sodium	1 (2.5 oz)	150	5	2	0	32	6	170
Manny's								
Burrito Tortilla	1 (2.1 oz)	180	5	5	0	30	4	520
Fajita Tortilla	1 (2 oz)	170	5	5	0	28	4	490
Fat Free	1 (1 oz)	65	2	0	0	14	1	210
Low Carb	1 (1.7 oz)	140	6	7	0	13	6	490
Soft Taco Tortilla	1 (1 oz)	80	2	2	0	14	tr	240
Tortilla Wrap Tomato Basil	1 (1.4 oz)	100	2	2	tr	19	2	150

FOOD	PORTION	CALS	PROT	FAT	CHOL	CARB	FIBER	SOD
White Corn Gluten Free	1 (2 oz)	60	1	1	0	11	tr	0
Whole Wheat	1 (2 oz)	170	5	4	0	27	3	460
Rudi's Organic Bakery								
Spelt	1 (2 oz)	140	5	3	0	27	1	200
Super Bakery								
Organic	1 (2.5 oz)	210	10	5	0	35	13	320
Tumaro's								
Honey Wheat	1 (8 in)	110	3	2	0	23	2	135
Low In Carbs Garden Vegetable	1 (8 in)	100	7	3	0	12	8	115
Low In Carbs Green Onion	1 (8 in)	100	7	3	0	13	7	115
Low In Carbs Multi Grain	1 (8 in)	100	7	3	0	13	8	115
Low In Carbs Salsa	1 (8 in)	100	7	3	0	13	8	115
Pesto & Garlic	1 (8 in)	110	3	1	0	23	1	135
Premium White	1 (8 in)	120	3	2	0	23	tr	130
Soy-full Heart 8 Grain 'N Soy	1 (1.4 oz)	100	6	0	0	14	4	60
Soy-full Heart Apple 'N Cinnamon	1 (1.4 oz)	90	6	3	0	13	4	65
Soy-full Heart Wheat Soy & Flax	1 (1.4 oz)	90	6	3	0	10	4	65
Spinach & Vegetables	1 (8 in)	110	3	2	0	23	1	140

TORTILLA CHIPS (see CHIPS)

TRAIL MIX
Enjoy Life

FOOD	PORTION	CALS	PROT	FAT	CHOL	CARB	FIBER	SOD
Gluten Free Not Nuts! Beach Bash	1 oz	130	4	7	0	13	2	45
Gluten Free Not Nuts! Mountain Mambo	1 oz	140	5	8	0	12	2	45
Good Sense								
Dietary Snack Mix	¼ cup	130	4	6	0	14	2	10
Organic Tropical	⅓ cup	160	2	10	0	16	2	20
Mrs. May's								
Coconut Almond Crunch	1 oz	183	4	15	0	10	2	40
Navitas Naturals								
3 Berry Cacao Nibs & Cashews	1 oz	110	3	5	0	16	4	45
Goji Cacao Nibs & Cashews	1 oz	120	4	6	0	13	3	70

FOOD	PORTION	CALS	PROT	FAT	CHOL	CARB	FIBER	SOD
Goji Golden Berry & Mulberry	1 oz	90	3	0	0	19	2	65
Organic Trails								
Summit Blend	¼ cup	150	3	8	0	19	2	40
Planters								
Berry Nut & Chocolate	3 tbsp (1 oz)	120	2	5	0	18	1	20
SunRise								
Honey Coated	3 tbsp (1 oz)	137	5	6	1	14	4	67
W/ Fruit	3 tbsp (1 oz)	130	4	6	0	16	2	50

TREE FERN

FOOD	PORTION	CALS	PROT	FAT	CHOL	CARB	FIBER	SOD
chopped cooked	½ cup	28	tr	tr	0	8	–	3

TRIPE

FOOD	PORTION	CALS	PROT	FAT	CHOL	CARB	FIBER	SOD
beef simmered	3 oz	80	10	3	133	2	0	58
TAKE-OUT								
mondongo w/ potatoes	1 cup	300	24	11	148	26	6	1565

TRITICALE

FOOD	PORTION	CALS	PROT	FAT	CHOL	CARB	FIBER	SOD
dry	½ cup (3.4 oz)	323	13	2	0	69	–	5

TROUT

FOOD	PORTION	CALS	PROT	FAT	CHOL	CARB	FIBER	SOD
baked	3 oz	162	23	7	63	0	0	57
rainbow cooked	3 oz	129	22	4	62	0	0	29
sea trout baked	3 oz	113	18	4	90	0	0	63

TRUFFLES

FOOD	PORTION	CALS	PROT	FAT	CHOL	CARB	FIBER	SOD
fresh	0.5 oz	4	2	tr	0	9	2	39

TUNA (*see also* TUNA DISHES)
CANNED

FOOD	PORTION	CALS	PROT	FAT	CHOL	CARB	FIBER	SOD
light in oil	3 oz	169	25	7	15	0	0	301
light in oil	1 can (6 oz)	399	50	14	30	0	0	606
light in water	1 can (5.8 oz)	192	42	1	49	0	0	558
light in water	3 oz	99	22	1	25	0	0	287
white in oil	3 oz	158	23	7	26	0	0	336
white in oil	1 can (6.2 oz)	331	47	14	55	0	0	704
white in water	1 can (6 oz)	234	46	4	72	0	0	673
white in water	3 oz	116	23	2	35	0	0	333

FOOD	PORTION	CALS	PROT	FAT	CHOL	CARB	FIBER	SOD
Bumble Bee								
Chunk Light In Water	2 oz	60	13	1	30	0	0	250
Chunk Light Touch Of Lemon In Water	¼ cup	60	13	1	30	0	0	250
Chunk Light In Oil	¼ cup	110	13	6	20	0	0	250
Chunk White In Water	¼ cup	60	13	1	25	0	0	250
Chunk White In Oil	¼ cup	100	13	5	25	0	0	250
Chunk White In Water Very Low Sodium	¼ cup	70	15	1	25	0	0	35
Light In Oil	¼ cup	110	13	6	30	0	0	290
Sensations Lemon & Pepper w/ Crackers	1 pkg (3.6 oz)	200	19	8	25	13	0	460
Solid White In Oil	¼ cup	90	14	3	25	0	0	250
Solid White In Water	2 oz	70	15	1	25	0	0	250
Tonno In Olive Oil	¼ cup	120	15	6	0	0	0	330
Chicken Of The Sea								
Albacore Solid In Water	2 oz	70	15	1	25	0	0	250
Chunk Light In Oil	2 oz	110	13	6	30	0	0	250
Chunk White Low Sodium In Spring Water	1 can (3 oz)	80	18	1	35	0	0	50
Chunk White In Spring Water	½ can	60	13	1	25	0	0	250
Premium Albacore Pouch	2 oz	60	13	1	25	0	0	250
Coral								
Light In Water	¼ cup	60	13	1	30	0	0	290
StarKist								
Solid White Albacore In Water	¼ cup	70	15	1	25	0	0	250
FRESH								
bluefin cooked	3 oz	157	25	5	42	0	0	43
bluefin raw	3 oz	122	20	4	32	0	0	33
skipjack baked	3 oz	112	24	1	51	0	0	40
yellowfin baked	3 oz	118	25	1	49	0	0	40
MIX								
Chicken Of The Sea								
Salad Kit	1 serv (3.5 oz)	380	22	24	22	18	1	640
Tuna Salad Kit Single Mayo & Onion	1 pkg	380	22	24	55	18	1	640

FOOD	PORTION	CALS	PROT	FAT	CHOL	CARB	FIBER	SOD
SHELF-STABLE								
Bumble Bee								
Steak Entrees Ginger & Soy	1 pkg (4 oz)	170	34	3	40	3	0	1030
Steak Entrees Lemon & Cracked Pepper	1 pkg (4 oz)	160	36	1	50	0	0	370
Steak Entrees Mesquite Grilled	1 pkg (4 oz)	150	35	2	40	0	0	370
TAKE-OUT								
tuna salad	1 cup	383	33	19	27	19	–	824
TURBOT								
european baked	3 oz	104	17	3	–	0	0	163
TURKEY (*see also* MEAT STICKS, TURKEY DISHES, TURKEY SUBSTITUTES)								
CANNED								
w/ broth	1 cup	220	32	9	89	0	0	630
Valley Fresh								
Chunk White	2 oz	80	16	2	55	0	0	150
FRESH								
breast pre-basted w/ skin roasted	3.5 oz	126	22	3	42	0	0	397
breast roasted w/ skin	4 oz	212	32	8	83	0	0	71
breast w/ skin roasted	4 oz	212	32	8	83	0	0	70
dark meat w/o skin roasted	1 cup (5 oz)	262	40	10	119	0	0	110
dark meat w/o skin roasted	3 oz	170	26	7	78	0	0	72
ground cooked	3 oz	193	22	11	84	0	0	88
leg w/ skin roasted	1 (19 oz)	1136	152	54	464	0	0	420
light meat w/ skin roasted half turkey	2.3 lbs	2069	87	87	794	0	0	658
light meat w/o skin roasted	4 oz	183	35	4	81	0	0	75
neck simmered	1 (5.3 oz)	274	41	11	186	0	0	84
skin roasted	1 oz	141	13	13	36	0	0	17
skin roasted from half turkey	8.7 oz	1096	49	98	281	0	0	132
tail cooked	1 (2 oz)	197	13	16	53	0	0	223
w/ skin roasted	8.4 oz	498	67	23	196	0	0	164
w/ skin roasted	½ turkey (4 lbs)	3857	522	181	1514	0	0	1269
w/o skin roasted	7.3 oz	354	61	10	159	0	0	147
w/o skin roasted	1 cup (5 oz)	238	41	7	107	0	0	99

FOOD	PORTION	CALS	PROT	FAT	CHOL	CARB	FIBER	SOD
wing w/ skin roasted	1 (6.5 oz)	426	51	23	151	0	0	114
wing w/o skin roasted	1	237	45	5	147	0	0	584
Honeysuckle White								
85% Lean Ground	4 oz	240	20	17	85	0	0	70
93% Lean Patties	1 (4 oz)	160	22	8	80	0	0	200
97% Lean Ground White	4 oz	130	26	2	65	0	0	70
99% Fat Free Breast Tenderloin	4 oz	120	28	1	70	0	0	55
99% Fat Free Breast Cutlets	4 oz	120	28	1	70	0	0	55
Drumettes	4 oz	180	24	8	75	0	0	75
Marinated Strips Asian Grill	4 oz	160	17	7	55	8	0	490
Necks	4 oz	150	23	6	90	0	0	105
Tenderloins Creamy Dijon Mustard	4 oz	140	21	4	50	0	0	500
Tenderloins Homestyle	4 oz	130	21	4	55	0	0	440
Tenderloins Teriyaki	4 oz	140	21	4	50	5	0	530
Thighs	4 oz	190	21	11	75	0	0	75
Whole Honey Roasted	4 oz	180	20	9	70	5	0	250
Wings	4 oz	220	23	14	80	0	0	60
Shady Brook								
Breast Tenderloin	4 oz	130	28	1	70	0	0	55
Breast Tenderloin Creamy Dijon Mustard	4 oz	140	21	4	50	4	0	500
Breast Tenderloin Teriyaki	4 oz	140	21	4	50	5	0	530
Breast Cutlets	4 oz	110	25	1	60	0	0	240
Ground 85% Lean	4 oz	220	21	17	75	1	–	75
Ground 93% Lean	4 oz	160	22	8	80	0	0	85
Ground 99% Lean	4 oz	120	28	1	70	0	0	55
Marinated Strips Asian Grill	4 oz	160	17	7	55	8	0	490
Marinated Strips Mild Herb	4 oz	130	18	4	60	6	0	450
Necks	4 oz	150	23	6	90	0	0	105
Tenderloins Turkey Breast Homestyle	4 oz	130	21	1	55	1	0	530
Thigh	4 oz	145	20	7	75	0	0	0
Whole Turkey	4 oz	180	23	9	85	–	–	75
Wing	4 oz	210	24	12	110	0	0	70
FROZEN								
roast boneless seasoned light & dark meat roasted	3.5 oz	155	21	6	53	3	0	680
sticks breaded fried	1 (2.2 oz)	179	9	11	41	11	–	536

FOOD	PORTION	CALS	PROT	FAT	CHOL	CARB	FIBER	SOD
Honeysuckle White								
Breast Boneless Roast	4 oz	170	21	7	60	0	0	700
Jennie-O								
Burger	1 (4 oz)	160	19	9	100	0	0	90
Organic Prairie								
Whole Young	4 oz	190	23	10	70	0	0	70
READY-TO-EAT								
bologna	1 slice (1 oz)	59	3	4	21	1	tr	351
breast	1 slice (0.7 oz)	22	4	tr	9	1	tr	213
ham	1 slice (1 oz)	35	5	1	20	1	tr	312
pastrami	2 oz	70	9	2	39	2	tr	559
salami	1 slice (1 oz)	48	5	3	21	tr	0	281
Boar's Head								
Breast 50% Lower Sodium Skin On	2 oz	60	12	2	25	0	0	320
Breast Cracked Pepper Smoked	2 oz	60	13	1	30	1	0	460
Breast Hickory Smoked Black Forest	2 oz	60	13	1	25	0	0	360
Breast Maple Glazed Honey Coat	2 oz	70	14	1	30	2	0	440
Breast Ovengold	2 oz	60	12	2	35	1	0	360
Breast Ovengold Skinless	2 oz	60	13	1	20	0	0	350
Breast Roasted Mesquite Smoked Skinless	2 oz	60	13	1	25	1	0	440
Breast Roasted Salsalito	2 oz	60	13	1	25	1	0	480
Carl Buddig								
Honey Roasted Sliced	2 oz	90	9	5	–	2	–	–
Turkey Sliced	2 oz	90	9	5	–	tr	–	–
Healthy Choice								
Smoked Breast	4 slices (1.8 oz)	60	9	2	25	2	0	450
Healthy Ones								
Oven Roasted 97% Fat Free	7 slices (2 oz)	60	9	2	20	2	–	460
Hebrew National								
98% Fat Free Oven Roasted	5 slices (2 oz)	50	11	1	20	1	–	430

FOOD	PORTION	CALS	PROT	FAT	CHOL	CARB	FIBER	SOD
98% Fat Free Smoked Breast	5 slices (2 oz)	60	12	1	25	0	0	380
Honeysuckle White								
Simply Done Whole Breast	4 oz	160	21	7	60	2	0	500
Organic Prairie								
Roasted Breast Slices	2 oz	60	14	1	30	0	0	330
Oscar Mayer								
Breast Smoked Shaved	2 oz	50	8	1	20	2	0	570
Sara Lee								
Breast Hardwood Smoked	4 slices (1.8 oz)	50	11	1	20	1	0	490
Breast Cracked Pepper	4 slices (1.8 oz)	50	9	1	25	1	0	480
Shady Brook								
Breast Bone-In Oven Roasted	3 oz	160	20	7	60	1	–	610
Hickory Smoked Breast Fat Free	2 oz	50	11	0	25	1	–	470
Turkey Ham Smoked	2 oz	60	9	2	30	0	0	590
Whole Oven Roasted	3 oz	160	19	8	65	1	–	620
Tyson								
Breast Oven Roasted	2 slices (1.6 oz)	40	8	1	15	1	0	560

TURKEY DISHES
FROZEN

FOOD	PORTION	CALS	PROT	FAT	CHOL	CARB	FIBER	SOD
gravy & turkey	1 cup (8.4 oz)	160	14	6	–	11	–	1328

READY-TO-EAT
Perdue

FOOD	PORTION	CALS	PROT	FAT	CHOL	CARB	FIBER	SOD
Meal Time Starters Turkey Breast Roast W/ Homestyle Gravy	½ cup (4.6 oz)	144	16	5	45	7	0	710

TAKE-OUT

FOOD	PORTION	CALS	PROT	FAT	CHOL	CARB	FIBER	SOD
boneless breast w/ cranberry apple stuffing	1 serv (5 oz)	260	32	9	80	10	1	250
fricassee	1 cup	322	29	18	85	8	tr	693
salad	1 cup	417	29	32	100	3	1	288
tetrazzini	1 cup	369	19	18	49	29	2	657
turkey creole w/o rice	1 cup	189	29	4	69	9	2	585

FOOD	PORTION	CALS	PROT	FAT	CHOL	CARB	FIBER	SOD
turkey croquette	1 (2 oz)	158	10	9	28	8	tr	226
turkey divan	1 cup	321	40	14	135	9	3	387
turkey meatloaf	1 lg slice (5 oz)	243	29	9	122	11	1	658

TURKEY SUBSTITUTES
Lightlife
Smart Deli Roast Turkey	4 slices (2 oz)	80	15	0	0	4	1	560

Tofurky
Deli Slices Cranberry	3 slices (1.8 oz)	98	11	3	0	8	3	368
Deli Slices Hickory Smoked	3 slices (1.8 oz)	100	13	3	0	6	3	250
Deli Slices Italian	3 slices (1.8 oz)	103	11	4	0	7	4	359
Deli Slices Original	3 slices (1.8 oz)	103	13	3	0	6	3	300
Deli Slices Peppered	3 slices (1.8 oz)	103	13	3	0	6	3	300
Deli Slices Philly Steak	3 slices (1.8 oz)	110	12	3	0	7	3	368
Roast	1 serv (4 oz)	190	26	5	0	10	2	396

Worthington
Turkee Slices	3 slices (3.3 oz)	180	14	12	0	5	0	530

Yves
Meatless Ground Turkey	1/3 cup	60	12	1	0	8	2	330
Meatless Deli Turkey Slices	4 slices	100	16	2	0	5	0	340

TURMERIC
ground	1 tsp	8	tr	tr	0	1	tr	1

TURNIPS
canned greens	1/2 cup	17	2	tr	0	3	–	325
cooked mashed	1/2 cup (4.2 oz)	47	2	tr	0	10	–	25
cubed cooked	1/2 cup (3 oz)	33	1	tr	0	7	–	17
frzn greens cooked	1/2 cup	24	3	tr	0	4	2	12
greens chopped cooked	1/2 cup	15	1	tr	0	3	2	21

FOOD	PORTION	CALS	PROT	FAT	CHOL	CARB	FIBER	SOD
greens raw chopped	½ cup	7	tr	tr	0	2	1	11
raw cubed	½ cup (2.4 oz)	25	1	tr	0	6	–	14
Allens								
Green	½ cup	30	2	0	0	5	2	650
Seasoned Southern Style								
Glory								
Greens Fresh	2 cups	20	1	0	0	5	3	30
Greens Seasoned canned	½ cup	35	1	0	0	4	2	490
Root Cut Fresh	½ cup	20	1	0	0	4	1	45
Sensibly Seasoned Greens	½ cup	20	1	0	0	4	2	240
TURTLE								
raw	3.5 oz	85	18	1	–	0	0	–
TUSK FISH								
raw	3.5 oz	79	17	tr	–	0	0	113
VANILLA								
vanilla extract	1 tsp	12	0	0	0	1	0	0
Bob's Red Mill								
Organic Extract	1 tsp	0	0	0	0	0	0	0
Virginia Dare								
Extract	1 tsp	10	–	0	0	–	–	–
VEAL (*see also* VEAL DISHES)								
breast braised	3 oz	226	23	14	96	0	0	55
chop cooked	1 med (6.5 oz)	230	26	13	109	0	0	444
chop breaded fried	1 med (6.5 oz)	290	35	12	142	13	tr	577
cubed braised	3 oz	160	30	4	123	0	0	79
cutlet cooked	3 oz	141	26	4	83	0	0	311
ground broiled	3 oz	146	21	6	88	0	0	71
leg roasted	3 oz	136	24	4	88	0	0	58
loin roasted	3 oz	184	21	10	88	0	0	79
patty breaded fried	1 (2.8 oz)	211	16	13	80	7	tr	329
shank braised	3 oz	162	27	5	105	0	0	79
VEAL DISHES								
TAKE-OUT								
cordon bleu	1 serv (8 oz)	490	33	35	172	4	1	552

FOOD	PORTION	CALS	PROT	FAT	CHOL	CARB	FIBER	SOD
parmigiana	1 serv (6.4 oz)	362	27	21	146	15	2	790
scallopini	1 slice + sauce (3.4 oz)	238	18	17	64	2	tr	304
stew	1 serv (8.8 oz)	192	15	6	50	18	3	605
veal marengo	1 serv (8.8 oz)	274	33	9	118	7	1	607
veal marsala	1 slice + sauce (3.4 oz)	268	12	19	69	6	tr	191
veal paprikash	1 serv (8.6 oz)	280	36	12	138	5	1	829
veal picatta	1 piece + sauce (3.5 oz)	154	16	9	72	2	tr	546

VEGETABLE JUICE

FOOD	PORTION	CALS	PROT	FAT	CHOL	CARB	FIBER	SOD
low sodium tomato & vegetable juice	1 cup	53	1	tr	0	11	2	169
vegetable juice cocktail	8 oz	46	2	tr	0	11	2	653
Bolthouse Farms								
Vedge Tomato Carrot Celery	8 oz	60	3	0	0	11	2	440
Lakewood								
Super Veggie	6 oz	40	2	0	0	9	4	135
V8								
100% Vegetable Essential Antioxidants	8 oz	50	2	0	0	11	2	480
Calcium Enriched	8 oz	50	2	0	0	11	2	460
High Fiber	8 oz	60	2	0	0	13	5	480
Low Sodium	8 oz	50	2	0	0	10	2	140
Organic	8 oz	50	2	0	0	10	2	480
V-Fusion Acai Mixed Berry	8 oz	110	0	0	0	27	0	70
Walnut Acres								
Organic Incredible Vegetable	8 oz	50	2	0	0	12	1	580

FOOD	PORTION	CALS	PROT	FAT	CHOL	CARB	FIBER	SOD
VEGETABLES MIXED								
CANNED								
mixed vegetables	½ cup	39	2	tr	0	8	–	122
peas & carrots	½ cup	48	3	tr	0	11	–	332
peas & onions	½ cup	30	2	tr	0	5	–	265
succotash	½ cup	102	4	1	0	23	–	325
Del Monte								
Mixed	½ cup	40	2	0	0	8	2	360
Mixed Vegetables w/ Potatoes	½ cup	45	2	0	0	10	2	360
Peas And Carrots	½ cup	60	2	0	0	11	2	360
Savory Sides Homestyle Vegetable Medley	½ cup	70	1	3	0	11	2	380
Savory Sides Rio Grande Vegetables	½ cup	70	2	0	0	14	2	470
Veg-All								
Original Mixed	½ cup	40	1	0	0	8	2	290
FRESH								
Mann's								
Broccoli & Cauliflower	1 serv (3 oz)	25	2	0	0	4	2	25
California Stir Fry	1 serv (3 oz)	30	2	0	0	6	2	30
Medley	1 serv (3 oz)	25	2	0	0	5	2	25
Veggies On The Go w/ Dip	1 cup + 1 tbsp dip	100	1	8	5	7	2	180
River Ranch								
Broccoli & Carrots	1 cup	25	2	0	0	5	2	25
Broccoli & Cauliflower	1 cup	25	2	0	0	4	2	25
Stir Fry Blend	1 cup	30	2	0	0	5	2	22
Vegetable Medley	1 cup	25	2	0	0	6	2	25
FROZEN								
mixed vegetables cooked	½ cup	54	3	tr	0	12	2	32
peas & carrots cooked	½ cup	38	3	tr	0	8	–	55
peas & onions cooked	½ cup	40	2	tr	0	8	–	–
succotash cooked	½ cup	79	4	1	0	17	–	38
Birds Eye								
Broccoli & Cauliflower	1 cup	30	1	0	0	4	2	25
Italian Herb Harvest Vegetables	1¼ cups	90	2	6	15	6	2	150
Spring Vegetables In Citrus Sauce	1¼ cups	70	2	4	10	8	2	280

FOOD	PORTION	CALS	PROT	FAT	CHOL	CARB	FIBER	SOD
Steamfresh Asian Medley	1 cup	50	2	2	0	6	2	310
Steamfresh Broccoli Cauliflower & Carrots	¾ cup	30	1	0	0	5	2	30
Steamfresh Broccoli Carrots Sugar Snap Peas & Water Chestnuts	¾ cup	35	1	0	0	6	2	25
Steamfresh Mixed Vegetables	⅔ cup	40	2	0	0	12	2	20
C&W								
Early Harvest Peas & Baby Carrots	⅔ cup	60	3	0	0	10	3	150
Petite Peas & Pearl Onions	⅔ cup	60	4	0	0	11	3	160
Cascadian Farm								
Organic Peas & Carrots	⅔ cup	50	2	0	0	10	3	75
Organic Mixed Vegetables	⅔ cup	60	2	0	0	12	2	20
Europe's Best								
Zen Garden	¾ cup	60	2	1	0	12	3	15
Green Giant								
Broccoli & Carrots w/ Garlic & Herbs as prep	½ cup	40	2	1	0	7	2	200
Garden Vegetable Medley as prep	½ cup	70	2	1	0	14	2	220
Mixed Vegetables as prep	½ cup	50	2	0	0	11	2	20
Southwestern Style as prep	½ cup	90	4	1	0	18	4	190
Szechuan Vegetables as prep	½ cup	50	2	1	0	9	2	410
Lean Cuisine								
Cafe Classics Roasted Potatoes w/ Broccoli & Cheddar Cheese Sauce	1 pkg (10.25 oz)	230	11	5	15	35	5	660
McKenzie's								
Gumbo Mixture	1 serv (2.9 oz)	35	1	0	0	8	2	30
Okra Tomatoes w/ Onions	1 serv (2.8 oz)	20	1	0	0	4	2	30
Melrose Made Gourmet								
Vegetable Souffle Fat Free	1 serv (4 oz)	70	12	0	0	5	3	530
Pictsweet								
Peas & Carrots	⅔ cup	50	2	0	0	9	3	125

FOOD	PORTION	CALS	PROT	FAT	CHOL	CARB	FIBER	SOD
Roast Works								
Flame Roasted Redskins & Vegetables	1 serv (3 oz)	90	2	3	0	14	3	190
TAKE-OUT								
buddha's delight	1 serv (16 oz)	174	17	5	35	17	3	1368
pakoras	1 (2 oz)	108	5	5	–	12	3	–
ratatouille	1 serv (3.5 oz)	96	2	7	0	7	4	812
samosa	1 (2.4 oz)	206	4	11	12	22	2	311
succotash	½ cup	111	5	1	0	23	–	16
tapenade grilled vegetables	¼ cup	40	0	3	0	4	tr	150
VENISON (*see also* MEAT STICKS)								
roasted	4 oz	215	41	4	127	0	0	20
VINEGAR								
balsamic	1 tbsp	14	tr	0	0	3	–	4
cider	1 tbsp	3	0	0	0	tr	0	1
red wine	1 tbsp	3	tr	0	0	tr	0	1
vinegar	1 tbsp	3	0	0	0	tr	0	0
Carapelli								
Balsamic	1 tbsp	15	0	0	0	4	0	0
Red Wine	1 tbsp	5	0	0	0	0	0	0
White Wine	1 tbsp	5	0	0	0	0	0	0
Eden								
Organic Apple Cider	1 tbsp	0	0	0	0	0	0	0
Organic Brown Rice	1 tbsp	2	0	0	0	0	0	0
Red Wine	1 tbsp	0	0	0	0	0	0	0
Ume Plum	1 tsp	0	0	0	0	0	0	1050
Latino Chef								
Lulo	1 tbsp	35	1	3	0	1	–	0
Passion Fruit	1 tbsp	40	0	3	–	2	tr	0
Newman's Own								
Organic Balsamic	1 tbsp	20	0	0	0	5	0	0
Pacifica Culinaria								
Balsamic Dark Sweet Cherry	1 tbsp	15	0	0	0	4	–	0
Pear Pomegranate	1 tbsp	10	0	0	0	2	–	0
Regina								
Red Wine	1 tbsp	0	0	0	0	tr	–	0

FOOD	PORTION	CALS	PROT	FAT	CHOL	CARB	FIBER	SOD
Spectrum								
Apple Cider Organic	1 tbsp	7	0	0	0	2	0	0
Balsamic Organic	1 tbsp	6	0	0	0	2	0	5

WAFFLES
FROZEN
Aunt Jemima

FOOD	PORTION	CALS	PROT	FAT	CHOL	CARB	FIBER	SOD
Blueberry	2 (2.5 oz)	190	4	5	5	32	1	450
Low Fat	2 (2.5 oz)	160	4	3	0	30	1	420
Eggo								
Buttermilk	2	180	5	6	15	26	1	420
Homestyle	2	190	5	6	20	29	1	440
Homestyle Minis	12	250	7	9	30	38	1	600
Nutri-Grain Low Fat Whole Wheat	2	140	5	3	0	28	3	430
Special K	3	190	8	1	0	37	1	400
Waf-Fulls Strawberry	1	150	3	5	10	25	tr	300
EnviroKidz								
Organic Gorilla Banana	2 (2.7 oz)	230	4	8	0	34	2	410
Kashi								
Heart To Heart Honey Oat	2 (3 oz)	160	6	3	0	31	3	370
Lifestream								
Organic Fig + Flax	2 (2.8 oz)	210	5	0	0	29	6	410
Organic Pomegran Plus	2 (2.8 oz)	190	5	5	0	31	5	370
Van's								
Belgian 7 Grain	2	230	7	4	0	42	7	290
Belgian Blueberry	2	184	5	4	0	33	2	196
Belgian Original	2	172	5	4	0	30	2	196
Carb Manager Flax	2	200	12	13	0	21	6	310
Carb Manager Homestyle	2	200	12	12	65	21	6	330
Gourmet 97% Fat Free	2	230	4	8	0	37	4	410
Gourmet Blueberry	2	190	5	6	0	30	5	306
Gourmet Buckwheat	2	145	5	4	0	24	2	152
Gourmet Flax	2	157	5	4	0	24	2	162
Gourmet Multi Grain	2	260	6	11	0	34	6	340
Gourmet Original	2	180	5	2	0	30	5	306
Hearty Oat Berry Boost	2	200	4	8	0	31	4	280
Hearty Oat Maple Fusion	2	210	4	9	0	31	4	280
Hearty Oat Oats 'N Honey	2	200	4	8	0	30	4	290
Mini Blueberry	4	110	3	5	0	21	2	114
Mini Chocolate Chip	4	119	3	4	0	16	2	114

FOOD	PORTION	CALS	PROT	FAT	CHOL	CARB	FIBER	SOD
Mini Homestyle	4	116	3	4	0	18	2	114
Organic Blueberry	2	240	5	10	0	29	4	320
Organic Original	2	190	6	5	0	30	6	230
Organic Soy Flax	2	230	6	11	0	26	6	290
Wheat Free Blueberry	2	201	4	5	0	35	5	390
Wheat Free Cinnamon Apple	2	189	4	5	0	32	5	390
Wheat Free Flax	2	230	3	6	0	42	5	390
Wheat Free Mini	4	160	1	5	0	30	tr	290
Wheat Free Original	2	189	4	5	0	32	5	390
MIX								
plain as prep 7 in diam	1 (2.6 oz)	218	6	11	52	25	–	383
READY-TO-EAT								
Kashi								
GoLean Blueberry	2 (3 oz)	170	8	3	0	33	6	300
GoLean Original	2 (3 oz)	170	8	3	0	33	6	330
TAKE-OUT								
belgian	1 (4.7 oz)	412	10	13	19	65	3	958
blueberry 9 in sq	1 (7 oz)	556	13	16	24	90	5	1232
round 10 in diam	1 (6.8 oz)	598	14	18	27	94	5	1390
square 9 in	1 (7 oz)	620	15	19	28	98	5	1440
whole wheat 9 in sq	1 (7 oz)	534	18	22	188	67	5	990

WALNUTS

FOOD	PORTION	CALS	PROT	FAT	CHOL	CARB	FIBER	SOD
black chopped	¼ cup	193	8	18	0	3	2	1
english chopped	¼ cup	191	4	19	0	4	2	1
english ground	¼ cup	131	3	13	0	3	1	0
english halves	14 (1 oz)	185	4	18	0	4	2	1
english in shell	7 (1 oz)	183	4	18	0	4	2	1
honey roasted	¼ cup	172	4	16	0	7	2	5
Diamond								
Chopped	¼ cup	200	5	20	0	4	2	0
Emerald								
Glazed	¼ cup	140	2	10	0	12	1	125
Good Sense								
Organic Raw Walnuts	¼ cup	210	5	20	0	3	3	0

WASABI (see HORSERADISH)

WATER

FOOD	PORTION	CALS	PROT	FAT	CHOL	CARB	FIBER	SOD
ice cubes	3	0	0	0	0	0	0	2
tap water	8 oz	0	0	0	0	0	0	7

FOOD	PORTION	CALS	PROT	FAT	CHOL	CARB	FIBER	SOD
Aloe Breeze								
Organic All Flavors	8 oz	0	0	0	0	0	0	10
Aloe Splash								
All Flavors	8 oz	0	0	0	0	0	0	0
Apple & Eve								
Water Fruits All Flavors	10 oz	90	0	0	0	21	–	10
Aquafina								
Alive Wellness Berry Pomegranate	8 oz	10	0	0	0	2	0	65
Sparkling Citrus Twist	8 oz	0	0	0	0	0	0	45
Aroma Water								
All Flavors	8 oz	0	0	0	0	0	0	0
Ayala's								
Herbal All Flavors	1 bottle	0	0	0	0	0	0	0
Base Energy + Water								
All Flavors	8 oz	28	0	0	0	7	–	45
Bot								
Fortified All Flavors	12 oz	40	0	0	0	10	0	0
Carpe Diem								
Botanic Water All Flavors	8 oz	35	0	0	0	9	–	0
Clearly Canadian								
Sparkling Blackberry	8 oz	90	0	0	0	22	–	10
Sparkling Cherry	8 oz	85	0	0	0	23	–	10
Sparkling Raspberry	8 oz	75	0	0	0	20	–	10
Sparkling Strawberry	8 oz	85	0	0	0	20	–	10
Zero Sparkling All Flavors	8 oz	0	0	0	0	0	0	10
Crystal Geyser								
Spring Water	8 oz	0	0	0	0	0	0	0
Dasani								
Purified Water	8 oz	0	0	0	0	0	0	0
w/ Lemon	8 oz	2	0	0	0	0	0	5
w/ Raspberry	8 oz	1	0	0	0	0	0	35
Eden								
Springs Artesian	8 oz	0	0	0	0	0	0	0
Fiji								
Natural Artesian	1 bottle (16.9 oz)	0	0	0	0	0	0	–
FlavH20								
All Flavors	1 can (12.3 oz)	80	0	0	0	21	–	0

FOOD	PORTION	CALS	PROT	FAT	CHOL	CARB	FIBER	SOD
Fruit 2 0								
Grape	8 oz	0	0	0	0	0	0	5
Natural Berry	8 oz	0	0	0	0	0	0	10
Watermelon Kiwi	8 oz	0	0	0	0	0	0	10
Fruit Refreshers								
Lemonade	8 oz	0	0	0	0	0	0	35
Gerolsteiner								
Sparkling Mineral	8 oz	0	0	0	0	0	0	30
Glaceau Vitamin Water								
Balance Cran Grapefruit	8 oz	50	0	0	0	13	–	0
Energy Tropical Citrus	8 oz	40	0	0	0	9	–	0
Essential Orange Orange	8 oz	40	0	0	0	9	–	0
Focus Kiwi Strawberry	8 oz	40	0	0	0	9	–	0
Formula 50	8 oz	50	0	0	0	13	–	0
Perform Lemon Lime	8 oz	50	0	0	0	13	–	0
Power-C Dragonfruit	8 oz	40	0	0	0	9	–	0
Rescue Green Tea	8 oz	40	0	0	0	9	–	0
Revive Fruit Punch	8 oz	50	0	0	0	13	–	0
Stress-B Lemon Lime	8 oz	40	0	0	0	9	–	0
H2Odwalla								
Enhanced Tropical Orange	20 oz	120	0	0	0	33	2	15
Organic Enhanced Blueberry Tea	20 oz	120	0	0	0	29	–	20
Organic Enhanced Jasmine Lime	20 oz	120	0	0	0	30	–	20
Hint								
All Flavors	15 oz	0	0	0	0	0	0	0
IQ								
H2O Orange Mango	8 oz	40	0	0	0	10	–	0
Jones Soda								
24C Multi Vitamin Enhanced All Flavors	1 bottle	100	0	0	0	24	–	30
Klear Splash								
Mini Sip	1 pkg (4 oz)	0	0	0	0	0	0	0
Liquid Salvation								
Ultra Hydrating	1 bottle	0	0	0	0	0	0	0
Nestle								
Pure Life Splash All Flavors	8 oz	0	0	0	0	0	0	10

FOOD	PORTION	CALS	PROT	FAT	CHOL	CARB	FIBER	SOD
Nui								
All Natural Kid Water	10 oz	90	0	0	0	21	3	10
O Water								
Hydrate Black Raspberry	8 oz	25	0	0	0	7	0	0
Replenish Lemon Lime	8 oz	25	0	0	0	7	0	0
Vitalize Peach Mango	8 oz	25	0	0	0	7	0	0
Pellegrino								
Mineral Water	8 oz	0	0	0	0	0	0	10
Pink2O								
Fortified	20 oz	0	0	0	0	0	0	88
Propel								
Fitness Water All Flavors	1 bottle (23.7 oz)	30	0	0	0	7	–	15
Rapid								
Hydra-Cell Water	1 bottle (16.9 oz)	0	0	0	0	0	0	0
SoBe								
All Flavors	8 oz	50	0	0	0	13	–	25
SoNu								
Water All Flavors	8 oz	45	0	0	0	13	0	5
Special K2O								
Protein Water All Flavors	1 bottle (16.6 oz)	50	5	0	0	8	–	30
Splash								
All Flavors	8 oz	0	0	0	0	0	0	0
Stacker 2								
Protein Water All Flavors	1 bottle (19.44 oz)	80	20	0	0	1	0	40
Sulinka								
Sparkling Mineral	8 oz	0	0	0	0	0	0	202
TalkingRain								
Ice All Flavors	8 oz	5	0	0	0	1	0	0
Tao Tea								
Lychee Water	8 oz	67	0	0	0	21	–	23
Thorpedo								
Ultra Low GI Energy Water	8 oz	45	0	0	0	11	0	60
Tipperary								
Mineral Water	1 liter	0	0	0	0	0	0	25
Trinity								
Energize	8 oz	50	0	0	0	12	–	150

FOOD	PORTION	CALS	PROT	FAT	CHOL	CARB	FIBER	SOD
Multi-Essential	8 oz	50	0	·0	0	12	–	15
Revive	8 oz	50	0	0	0	12	–	15
Strength	8 oz	50	0	0	0	12	–	15
Think	8 oz	50	0	0	0	12	–	15
Twist								
Organics All Flavors	8 oz	10	0	0	0	2	0	0
Vasa								
Natural Spring	8 oz	0	0	0	0	0	0	0
Volvic								
Mineral Water	1 liter	0	0	0	0	0	0	12
Natural Lemon	8 oz	0	0	0	0	1	0	0
Natural Orange	8 oz	30	0	0	0	7	0	0
W20 For Women								
All Flavors	8 oz	40	0	0	0	10	0	10
Wateroos								
All Flavors	1 box (8 oz)	0	0	0	0	0	0	0
WaterPlus								
Antioxidants Acai Berry	8 oz	50	0	0	0	13	–	0
Electrolytes Fruit Punch	8 oz	50	0	0	0	13	–	0
Extra-C Orange Tangerine	8 oz	50	0	0	0	13	0	0
Vitamins Dragonfruit Kiwi	8 oz	50	0	0	0	13	–	0
Wild Waters								
All Flavors	8 oz	50	0	0	0	15	–	0
WATER CHESTNUTS								
chinese sliced canned	½ cup	35	1	tr	0	9	–	6
fresh sliced	½ cup	66	1	tr	0	15	–	9
WATERCRESS								
cooked w/o fat	1 cup	15	3	tr	0	2	1	427
raw chopped	1 cup	4	1	tr	0	tr	tr	14
Frieda's								
Watercress	1 cup	10	2	0	0	1	2	35
WATERMELON								
cut up	1 cup	46	1	tr	0	12	1	2
seeds dried	¼ cup	150	8	13	0	4	–	27
wedge	1 sm (2.5 oz)	21	tr	tr	0	5	tr	1
wedge	1 med (10 oz)	86	2	tr	0	22	1	3
wedge	1 lg (20 oz)	172	3	1	0	43	2	6

FOOD	PORTION	CALS	PROT	FAT	CHOL	CARB	FIBER	SOD
whole melon	1 (9 lb)	1227	25	6	0	309	16	41
Dulcinea								
Fresh Mini Seedless	2 cups	88	1	0	0	27	2	–
Frieda's								
Yellow Seedless	½ cup (3 oz)	25	0	0	0	6	0	0
Sundia								
Fresh	2 cups	80	1	0	0	27	2	10

WATERMELON JUICE

FOOD	PORTION	CALS	PROT	FAT	CHOL	CARB	FIBER	SOD
juice	8 oz	71	1	tr	0	18	1	2
Sundia								
100% Natural	8 oz	110	1	1	0	27	1	15
Tang								
Watermelon Wallop	1 box (7 oz)	90	0	0	0	24	0	30

WHALE

FOOD	PORTION	CALS	PROT	FAT	CHOL	CARB	FIBER	SOD
alaskan	3.5 oz	97	12	5	–	1	–	–
beluga dried	1 oz	92	20	2	34	0	0	62

WHEAT

FOOD	PORTION	CALS	PROT	FAT	CHOL	CARB	FIBER	SOD
sprouted	1 cup (3.8 oz)	214	8	1	0	46	1	17
starch	3.5 oz	348	tr	tr	–	86	–	2
Arrowhead Mills								
Whole Grain Wheat	¼ cup (1.6 oz)	150	7	1	0	31	5	0
Bob's Red Mill								
Vital Wheat Gluten	¼ cup	120	23	1	0	6	0	9
Hodgson Mill								
Vital Wheat Gluten	4 tsp	40	8	0	0	3	1	0

WHEAT GERM

FOOD	PORTION	CALS	PROT	FAT	CHOL	CARB	FIBER	SOD
plain	¼ cup	108	8	3	0	14	4	1
Bob's Red Mill								
Wheat Germ	2 tbsp	59	4	2	0	7	2	2
Hodgson Mill								
Untoasted	2 tbsp	55	4	1	0	7	4	0
Kretschmer								
Original Toasted	2 tbsp	50	4	1	0	6	2	0

FOOD	PORTION	CALS	PROT	FAT	CHOL	CARB	FIBER	SOD
WHEY								
acid dry	1 tbsp	10	tr	tr	0	2	0	28
sweet dry	1 tbsp	26	1	tr	0	6	0	81
sweet fluid	½ cup	33	1	tr	2	6	0	66
whey cheese	1 oz	126	4	8	–	9	0	146
Bob's Red Mill								
Protein Concentrate	¼ cup	80	16	1	30	1	0	40
Sweet Dairy	1 tbsp	30	1	0	1	6	0	70
Wellements								
Whey Protein Chocolate	1 scoop (1 oz)	120	22	2	42	4	0	55
Whey Protein Vanilla	1 scoop (1 oz)	120	22	2	39	4	0	55
WHIPPED TOPPINGS								
cream pressurized	1 cup (2.1 oz)	154	2	13	46	7	–	78
cream pressurized	1 tbsp (3 g)	8	tr	tr	2	tr	–	4
nondairy frzn	1 tbsp	13	tr	1	0	1	–	1
nondairy powdered as prep w/ whole milk	1 cup	151	3	10	8	13	–	53
nondairy pressurized	1 cup	184	1	16	0	11	–	43
nondairy pressurized	1 tbsp (4 g)	11	tr	1	0	1	–	2
Cabot								
Whipped Cream	2 tbsp	15	0	2	<5	1	0	0
Estee								
Whipped Topping as prep	1 serv	10	0	1	0	1	0	5
Hood								
Light Sugar Free Whipped Cream	2 tbsp	10	0	1	<5	tr	0	5
Whipped Light Cream	2 tbsp	20	0	2	5	tr	0	0
Reddiwip								
Chocolate	2 tbsp	15	0	1	<5	1	0	0
Extra Creamy	2 tbsp	15	0	2	5	tr	0	0
Fat Free	2 tbsp	5	0	0	0	1	0	0
Original	2 tbsp	15	0	1	<5	tr	0	0
Soyatoo								
Soy Whip	2 tbsp	10	0	1	0	1	0	0
WHITE BEANS								
canned	1 cup	306	19	1	0	58	–	13

FOOD	PORTION	CALS	PROT	FAT	CHOL	CARB	FIBER	SOD
dried regular cooked	1 cup	249	17	1	0	45	–	11
dried small cooked	1 cup	253	16	1	0	46	–	4

WHITEFISH

FOOD	PORTION	CALS	PROT	FAT	CHOL	CARB	FIBER	SOD
baked	3 oz	146	21	6	65	0	0	56
smoked	1 oz	39	7	tr	9	0	0	285
smoked	3 oz	92	20	1	28	0	0	866

WHITING

FOOD	PORTION	CALS	PROT	FAT	CHOL	CARB	FIBER	SOD
cooked	3 oz	98	20	1	71	0	0	113
hake raw	3.5 oz	84	17	1	–	0	0	101
raw	3 oz	77	16	1	57	0	0	61

WILD RICE

FOOD	PORTION	CALS	PROT	FAT	CHOL	CARB	FIBER	SOD
cooked	1 cup (5.7 oz)	166	7	1	0	35	3	5
Lundberg								
Organic Quick not prep	¼ cup	150	6	1	0	33	2	0

WINE

FOOD	PORTION	CALS	PROT	FAT	CHOL	CARB	FIBER	SOD
chinese cooking	1 bottle (15 oz)	559	0	0	0	3	0	43
cooking	1 oz	15	tr	0	0	2	0	182
dessert dry	1 glass (4 oz)	179	tr	0	0	14	0	11
haiku	1 serv	93	tr	0	0	3	0	2
japanese plum	3 oz	139	tr	tr	0	16	0	–
japanese sake	1 oz	33	tr	0	0	2	0	1
kir	1 serv	78	tr	0	0	3	0	4
madeira	3.5 oz	169	0	0	–	10	0	–
port	3.5 oz	156	tr	0	–	11	0	4
red	1 glass (4 oz)	85	tr	0	0	2	0	6
rosé	1 glass (4 oz)	84	tr	0	0	2	0	6
sake screwdriver	1 serv	175	2	tr	0	23	tr	3
sangria	1 serv	88	tr	tr	0	6	tr	4
sangria blanco	1 serv	155	1	tr	0	24	3	13
sherry	2 oz	84	tr	0	0	5	–	–
sweet dessert	1 glass (4 oz)	189	tr	0	0	16	0	11
vermouth dry	3.5 oz	105	–	0	0	1	–	–

FOOD	PORTION	CALS	PROT	FAT	CHOL	CARB	FIBER	SOD
vermouth sweet	3.5 oz	167	–	0	0	12	–	–
wassail wine	1 serv	142	1	tr	0	22	2	6
white	1 glass (4 oz)	80	tr	0	0	1	0	6
wine cooler	1 (7 oz)	118	tr	tr	0	14	0	15
Eden								
Mirin Rice Cooking Wine	1 tbsp	25	0	0	0	7	–	130

WINGED BEANS
dried cooked	1 cup	252	18	10	0	26	–	22

WRAPS (see BREAD, SANDWICHES)

YACON
Navitas Naturals
Slices Dried	1 oz	90	1	0	0	22	1	10

YAM (see also SWEET POTATO)
CANNED
Bruce's
In Syrup	⅔ cup	150	tr	1	0	36	3	45
Glory								
Candied	½ cup	210	1	0	0	52	1	240
FRESH								
mountain yam hawaii cooked w/o salt	1 cup	119	3	tr	0	29	–	17
yam cooked w/o salt	1 cup	158	2	tr	0	38	5	11
Earthbound Farm								
Organic	1 med (4.6 oz)	130	2	0	0	33	4	45
Frieda's								
Name	¾ cup	100	1	0	0	24	3	10

YARDLONG BEANS
sliced cooked w/o salt	1 cup	49	3	tr	0	10	–	4

YAUTIA (see MALANGA)

YEAST
baker's compressed	1 cake (0.6 oz)	18	1	tr	0	3	1	5
baker's dry	1 pkg (7 g)	21	3	tr	0	3	2	4
baker's dry	1 tbsp	35	5	1	0	5	3	6
brewer's dry	1 tbsp	35	5	1	0	5	3	6

FOOD	PORTION	CALS	PROT	FAT	CHOL	CARB	FIBER	SOD
Bob's Red Mill								
Active Dry	1 tbsp	25	0	1	0	5	2	0
Hodgson Mill								
Active Dry	1 tsp	30	4	0	0	3	1	0
Fast Rise	1 tsp (9 g)	25	3	0	0	4	1	0
YELLOW BEANS								
fresh cooked w/o salt	1 cup	44	2	tr	0	10	4	4
fresh raw	1 cup	34	2	tr	0	8	4	7
YELLOWTAIL								
baked	4 oz	199	32	7	75	0	0	53
YOGURT (see also YOGURT DRINKS, YOGURT FROZEN)								
plain low fat	8 oz	143	12	4	14	16	0	159
plain nonfat	8 oz	127	13	tr	5	17	0	175
plain whole milk	8 oz	138	8	7	30	11	0	104
tofu yogurt	1 cup	246	9	5	0	42	1	92
Breyers								
Creme Savers Orange & Creme	1 pkg (8 oz)	240	7	4	25	45	0	230
Creme Savers Raspberries & Creme	1 pkg (8 oz)	240	7	4	25	45	0	240
Light! Probiotic Plus Apple Cinnamon	1 pkg (8 oz)	100	8	2	15	15	0	105
Light! Probiotic Plus Blueberies 'N Cream	1 pkg (8 oz)	110	8	2	15	15	0	105
Light! Probiotic Plus Lemon Chiffon	1 pkg (8 oz)	100	8	2	15	14	0	105
Light! Probiotic Plus Peaches 'N Cream	1 pkg (8 oz)	100	8	2	15	15	0	105
Light! Probiotic Plus Strawberry Banana	1 pkg (8 oz)	110	8	2	15	16	0	105
Light! Probiotic Plus Strawberry Cheesecake	1 pkg (8 oz)	110	8	2	15	16	0	105
Smart! w/ DHA Mixed Berry	1 pkg (6 oz)	170	6	2	0	34	1	95
Smart! w/ DHA Strawberry	1 pkg (6 oz)	170	6	2	0	34	1	95
Smart! w/ DHA Strawberry Banana	1 pkg (6 oz)	170	6	2	10	34	1	95
Smart! w/DHA Black Cherry	1 pkg (6 oz)	170	6	2	10	35	1	95
Smart! w/DHA Peach	6 oz	170	6	2	10	34	1	95

FOOD	PORTION	CALS	PROT	FAT	CHOL	CARB	FIBER	SOD
Smart! w/DHA Pineapple	1 pkg (6 oz)	170	6	2	0	34	tr	95
Smooth & Creamy Peaches 'N Cream	1 pkg (8 oz)	240	7	2	20	48	0	105
Smooth & Creamy Strawberry	1 pkg (8 oz)	230	7	2	20	46	0	105
Smooth & Creamy Vanilla Cream	1 pkg (8 oz)	240	7	2	20	47	0	105
Cabot								
Non Fat French Vanilla	8 oz	130	8	0	10	24	0	115
Non Fat Plain	8 oz	100	10	0	0	19	0	135
Non Fat Raspberry	8 oz	130	8	0	5	24	0	115
Dannon								
Activia Blueberry	1 pkg (4 oz)	110	5	2	5	19	0	65
Activia Mixed Berry	1 pkg (4 oz)	110	5	2	5	19	0	75
Activia Peach	1 pkg (4 oz)	110	5	2	10	19	0	70
Activia Prune	1 pkg (4 oz)	110	5	2	10	19	0	75
Activia Strawberry	1 pkg (4 oz)	110	5	2	5	19	0	75
Activia Vanilla	1 pkg (4 oz)	110	5	2	10	19	0	70
Activia Vanilla Light Fat Free	4 oz	70	5	0	0	13	3	75
All Natural Blended Mini Blueberry	1 (3.3 oz)	110	5	1	5	20	0	65
All Natural Blended Mini Strawberry	1 (3.3 oz)	110	5	1	5	20	0	65
Creamy Fruit Blends Raspberry	6 oz	170	7	2	10	32	tr	125
Fruit On The Bottom Apple Cinnamon	6 oz	150	6	2	5	28	tr	130
Fruit On The Bottom Peach	6 oz	150	6	2	5	28	0	95
Fruit On The Bottom Pineapple	6 oz	150	6	2	5	28	0	125
Fruit On The Bottom Raspberry	6 oz	150	6	2	5	28	tr	115
La Creme Vanilla	4 oz	140	5	5	15	19	0	65
La Creme Mousse French Vanilla	1 (2.6 oz)	110	3	5	10	14	0	45
Light & Fit Carb & Sugar Control Blueberries & Cream	4 oz	60	5	3	10	3	0	25

FOOD	PORTION	CALS	PROT	FAT	CHOL	CARB	FIBER	SOD
Light & Fit Carb & Sugar Control Vanilla	4 oz	60	5	3	10	3	0	25
Light & Fit Nonfat Cherry Vanilla	6 oz	60	5	0	<5	11	0	85
Light & Fit Nonfat Lemon Chiffon	6 oz	60	5	0	<5	10	0	90
Light & Fit Nonfat Raspberry	6 oz	60	5	0	<5	11	0	95
Light & Fit Nonfat White Chocolate Raspberry	6 oz	90	5	0	0	10	0	80
Fage								
Sheep & Goat's Milk	1 pkg (7 oz)	190	10	12	35	10	0	100
Horizon Organic								
Fat Free Peach	1 pkg (6 oz)	140	7	0	<5	27	1	105
Fat Free Vanilla	1 cup	180	9	0	5	33	0	140
Kids Strawberry	1 pkg (4 oz)	110	4	1	5	20	1	75
Lowfat Blended Blueberry	1 pkg (6 oz)	160	7	2	10	30	2	110
Tube Lowfat Blueberry	1 (2 oz)	70	2	1	5	12	0	40
Whole Milk Plain	1 cup	160	10	7	30	14	0	150
La Yogurt								
Lowfat Blueberries 'N' Cream	1 pkg (6 oz)	200	7	2	10	39	0	90
Lowfat Fruit On The Bottom Cherry	1 pkg (8 oz)	230	6	3	10	47	tr	85
Lowfat Fruit On The Bottom Probiotic Peach	1 pkg (6 oz)	160	6	2	5	31	0	100
Lowfat Fruit On The Bottom Strawberry	1 pkg (8 oz)	220	9	2	10	43	tr	140
Lowfat Peaches 'N' Cream	1 pkg (6 oz)	200	7	2	10	39	0	90
Lowfat Pina Colada	1 pkg (6 oz)	160	5	2	5	30	0	90
Lowfat Probiotic Pina Colada	1 pkg (6 oz)	160	5	2	5	30	0	90
Lowfat Probiotic Plain	1 pkg (6 oz)	100	9	2	10	12	0	130
Lowfat Probiotic Vanilla	1 pkg (6 oz)	150	8	2	10	26	0	120
Lowfat Probiotic Vanilla	1 pkg (6 oz)	170	5	2	5	32	0	110
Lowfat Vanilla 'N' Cream	1 pkg (6 oz)	200	7	2	10	39	0	90
Nonfat Banana Cream	1 pkg (6 oz)	100	6	0	0	18	0	90
Nonfat Probiotic Cherry	1 pkg (6 oz)	100	6	0	0	17	0	90
Nonfat Probiotic Peach	1 pkg (6 oz)	90	6	0	0	16	0	85
Nonfat Probiotic Raspberry	1 pkg (6 oz)	90	6	0	0	15	0	85

FOOD	PORTION	CALS	PROT	FAT	CHOL	CARB	FIBER	SOD
Nonfat Probiotic Vanilla	1 pkg (6 oz)	90	6	0	0	15	0	85
Sabor Latino Lowfat Dulce De Leche	1 pkg (6 oz)	190	7	2	10	36	0	105
Sabor Latino Lowfat Guava	1 pkg (6 oz)	190	7	2	10	37	0	110
Sabor Latino Lowfat Horchata	1 pkg (6 oz)	210	7	2	10	41	0	105
Sabor Latino Lowfat Papaya	1 pkg (6 oz)	190	7	2	10	37	0	105
Rachel's								
Essence Berry Jasmine w/ Zinc	1 pkg (6 oz)	160	8	3	10	28	2	115
Essence Plum Honey Lavander	1 pkg (6 oz)	160	8	3	10	28	2	115
Essence Pomegranate Acai	1 pkg (6 oz)	170	8	3	10	29	2	125
Exotic Kiwi Passion Fruit Lime	1 pkg (6 oz)	160	8	3	10	28	2	135
Exotic Orange Strawberry Mango	1 pkg (6 oz)	160	8	3	10	28	2	120
Exotic Pomegranate Blueberry	1 pkg (6 oz)	170	8	3	10	29	2	135
Redwood Hill Farm								
Goat Milk Apricot Mango	1 cup	180	6	5	15	31	2	130
Goat Milk Cranberry Orange	1 cup	180	6	5	15	31	2	130
Goat Milk Plain	1 cup	130	8	6	20	14	1	65
Goat Milk Strawberry	1 cup	180	6	5	15	31	2	130
Goat Milk Vanilla	1 cup	190	7	5	25	31	2	110
Stonyfield Farm								
Kids' Lowfat BaNilla	1 pkg (4 oz)	110	4	1	5	21	2	65
Light Black Cherry	1 pkg (6 oz)	100	6	0	0	28	3	105
Light Blueberry	1 pkg (4 oz)	100	6	0	0	28	3	105
Light Peach	1 pkg (6 oz)	100	6	0	0	28	3	110
Light Strawberry	1 pkg (4 oz)	100	6	0	0	28	3	110
Nonfat French Vanilla	1 pkg	90	5	0	0	18	2	70
Nonfat Strawberry	1 pkg	140	6	0	0	26	2	130
O'Soy Chocolate	1 pkg (6 oz)	160	7	3	0	28	4	30
O'Soy Peach	1 pkg (4 oz)	100	5	2	0	16	3	20
Squeezers Lowfat Strawberry	1 tube (2 oz)	60	2	1	5	11	tr	30
Whole Milk French Vanilla	1 pkg (6 oz)	190	6	6	25	27	3	95

FOOD	PORTION	CALS	PROT	FAT	CHOL	CARB	FIBER	SOD
Total								
Greek Yogurt 0% Fat	1 pkg (5.3 oz)	80	13	0	0	6	0	55
Greek Yogurt 2% Fat	1 pkg (7 oz)	130	17	4	10	8	0	65
Greek Yogurt Classic	1 pkg (7 oz)	180	14	20	35	6	0	60
Greek Yogurt Light	1 pkg (5.3 oz)	130	11	8	20	5	0	70
Honey	1 pkg (3.5 oz)	250	8	12	20	28	0	35
Wallaby								
Organic Banana Vanilla	1 pkg (6 oz)	150	6	3	15	25	0	75
Organic Lemon	1 pkg (6 oz)	150	6	3	15	25	0	75
Organic Maple	1 pkg (6 oz)	150	6	3	15	26	0	80
Organic Plain	1 cup	150	11	5	25	18	0	120
Organic Raspberry	1 pkg (6 oz)	150	7	3	15	25	0	75
Organic Vanilla	1 pkg (6 oz)	150	6	3	15	25	0	75
Organic Nonfat Mango Lime	1 pkg (6 oz)	140	7	0	0	28	0	90
Organic Nonfat Plain	1 cup	130	12	0	15	19	0	150
Organic Nonfat Vanilla Bean	1 pkg (6 oz)	140	7	0	0	28	0	90
WholeSoy & Co.								
Organic Soy Apricot Mango	1 pkg (6 oz)	160	6	3	0	30	2	35
Organic Soy Lemon	1 pkg (6 oz)	160	6	3	0	29	2	15
Organic Soy Plain	1 pkg (6 oz)	150	6	3	0	27	2	25
Organic Soy Raspberry	1 pkg (6 oz)	170	5	3	0	32	2	25
Organic Soy Vanilla	1 pkg (6 oz)	150	6	3	0	28	2	25
WildWood								
Organic Soyogurt Low Fat Peach	1 pkg (6 oz)	160	5	3	0	29	5	40
Organic Soyogurt Low Fat Vanilla	1 pkg (6 oz)	160	5	3	0	30	5	40
Organic Soyogurt Plain Unsweetened	1 pkg (6 oz)	110	6	4	0	14	4	45
Yoplait								
Go-Gurt All Fruit Flavors	1 pkg (2.25 oz)	80	2	2	5	13	0	40
Grande 99% Fat Free All Flavors	1 cup	250	9	3	15	48	0	130
Grande Fat Free Plain	1 cup	90	15	0	5	19	0	220

FOOD	PORTION	CALS	PROT	FAT	CHOL	CARB	FIBER	SOD
Kids Banana Vanilla	1 pkg (4 oz)	100	5	2	10	17	1	75
Kids Strawberry Vanilla	1 pkg (4 oz)	100	5	2	5	17	1	75
Light All Fruit Flavors	1 pkg (6 oz)	180	10	0	<5	19	0	85
Light Indulgent All Flavors	1 pkg (6 oz)	110	8	0	<5	20	0	90
Light Thick & Creamy All Fruit Flavors	1 pkg (6 oz)	100	5	0	50	20	–	90
Original All Fruit Flavors	1 pkg (6 oz)	170	5	2	10	33	0	80
Original Coconut Cream	1 pkg (6 oz)	190	5	3	10	34	0	86
Original Lemon Burst	1 pkg (6 oz)	180	5	2	10	36	0	80
Original Pina Colada	1 pkg (6 oz)	170	5	2	10	33	0	95
Trix All Fruit Flavors	1 pkg (4 oz)	120	4	2	5	23	0	55
Yo Plus All Flavors	1 pkg (4 oz)	110	4	2	10	21	3	70

YOGURT DRINKS (see also SMOOTHIES)

FOOD	PORTION	CALS	PROT	FAT	CHOL	CARB	FIBER	SOD
lassi	7 oz	78	0	5	19	8	0	–
Dannon								
DanActive Plain	1 bottle (3.3 oz)	90	3	2	5	15	0	40
DanActive Vanilla	1 bottle (3.3 oz)	90	3	2	5	17	0	40
Danimals Rockin' Raspberry	1 bottle (3.1 oz)	70	2	1	<5	15	0	35
Danimals Strawberry Explosion	1 bottle (3.1 oz)	70	2	1	<5	15	0	35
Danimals Strikin' Strawberry Kiwi	1 bottle (3.1 oz)	70	2	1	<5	15	0	30
Frusion Cherry Berry Blend	1 bottle (10 oz)	260	8	4	15	50	tr	190
Frusion Pina Colada	1 bottle (10 oz)	260	8	4	15	50	0	135
Frusion Strawberry Blend	1 bottle (10 oz)	260	7	4	15	50	0	125
Light & Fit Carb & Sugar Control Berries & Cream	1 bottle (7 oz)	60	6	3	15	4	0	35
Light & Fit Smoothie Peach Passion	1 bottle (7 oz)	70	5	0	<5	13	0	70
Light & Fit Smoothie Strawberry Banana	1 bottle (7 oz)	70	5	0	<5	13	0	65
Lifeway								
Lassi Lowfat All Flavors	8 oz	174	14	2	10	25	3	125

FOOD	PORTION	CALS	PROT	FAT	CHOL	CARB	FIBER	SOD
Promise								
Activ All Flavors	1 bottle (3.5 oz)	75	1	4	0	8	tr	20
Stonyfield Farm								
Kids' Juice Smoothie Orange Strawberry Banana Wave	1 bottle (6 oz)	160	6	2	5	29	2	90
Smoothie Light Strawberry	1 bottle (10 oz)	130	9	0	5	40	3	105
Smoothie Lowfat Strawberry	1 bottle (10 oz)	250	10	3	10	46	4	160
Yoplait								
Nouriche All Fruit Flavors	1 bottle (11 oz)	260	10	0	10	55	5	270
YOGURT FROZEN								
chocolate soft serve	1 cup	230	6	9	7	36	3	141
vanilla soft serve	1 cup	236	6	8	3	35	0	125
Edy's								
Black Cherry Vanilla Swirl	½ cup	90	3	0	0	19	–	45
Caramel Praline Crunch	½ cup	100	3	0	0	23	–	60
Chocolate	½ cup	90	3	0	0	19	–	40
Strawberry	½ cup	100	3	0	0	22	–	40
Vanilla	½ cup	90	3	0	0	19	–	45
Vanilla Chocolate Swirl	½ cup	90	3	0	0	19	–	45
Hood								
Fat Free Old Fashioned Vanilla	½ cup	110	3	0	0	24	tr	75
Fat Free Strawberry	½ cup	100	2	0	0	23	tr	70
Vanilla Swiss Almond	½ cup	150	3	5	10	25	tr	85
WholeSoy & Co.								
Organic All Flavors	½ cup	120	2	1	0	25	1	85
ZUCCHINI								
baby raw	1 (0.5 oz)	3	tr	tr	0	1	tr	0
canned italian style	1 cup	66	2	tr	0	16	–	849
fresh	1 sm (4.1 oz)	19	1	tr	0	4	1	12
pickled	¼ cup	16	tr	tr	0	4	1	71
raw sliced	1 cup	19	1	tr	0	4	1	11
sliced cooked w/o salt	1 cup	29	1	tr	0	7	3	5

FOOD	PORTION	CALS	PROT	FAT	CHOL	CARB	FIBER	SOD
C&W								
Yellow & Green	⅔ cup	20	1	0	0	3	tr	5
Frieda's								
Baby	⅔ cup (3 oz)	20	2	0	0	3	0	0
TAKE-OUT								
breaded & fried	6 slices (3 oz)	141	2	11	2	10	1	105
indian pakora	1 serv	46	2	2	1	7	2	141
sticks breaded & fried	6 (2 oz)	90	1	7	2	6	1	67

PART TWO

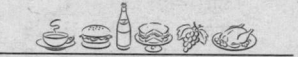

Restaurant Chains

FOOD	PORTION	CALS	PROT	FAT	CHOL	CARB	FIBER	SOD
A&W								
BEVERAGES								
Coke	1 sm (11 oz)	145	0	0	0	37	0	23
Diet Coke	1 sm (11 oz)	0	0	0	0	0	0	25
Diet Root Beer	1 sm (15 oz)	0	0	0	0	0	0	40
Float Diet Root Beer	1 sm (14 oz)	170	2	5	40	30	0	100
Float Root Beer	1 sm (14 oz)	330	2	5	40	70	0	100
Milkshake Chocolate	1 med	700	11	29	125	100	2	200
Milkshake Strawberry	1 med	670	11	29	115	90	0	180
Milkshake Vanilla	1 med	720	12	31	135	97	0	210
Root Beer	1 sm (15 oz)	220	0	0	0	57	0	40
DESSERTS								
Cone Vanilla	1 med	260	1	7	25	41	1	145
Freeze A&W Root Beef	1 med	480	25	10	40	89	0	230
Polar Swirl M&M	1 med	710	15	25	55	107	2	290
Polar Swirl Oreo	1 med	690	14	24	50	107	3	570
Polar Swirl Reese's	1 med	740	18	31	55	97	3	380
Sundae Caramel	1 med	340	8	9	35	57	0	250
Sundae Chocolate	1 med	320	8	8	30	53	0	180
Sundae Hot Fudge	1 med	350	8	11	30	54	4	140
Sundae Strawberry	1 med	300	7	8	30	47	0	140
Sundae Vanilla	1 med	310	7	8	30	52	0	140
MAIN MENU SELECTIONS								
Cheese Curds	1 serv	570	27	40	105	27	2	1220
Cheese Dog	1	320	11	20	40	25	1	910
Cheeseburger Original Bacon Double	1	800	45	48	165	47	2	1600
Cheeseburger Original Double	1	720	41	42	150	46	2	1370
Cheeseburger Original Bacon	1	570	27	33	90	41	2	1200
Chicken Strips	3	500	28	29	55	32	7	1050
Chili Bowl	1 serv	190	12	6	20	22	5	640
Coney Chili Dog	1	310	13	18	40	24	2	870
Coney Chili Dog Cheese	1	350	13	21	45	27	2	1070
Fries	1 lg	430	5	18	0	61	6	640
Fries Cheese	1 serv	380	4	19	5	50	4	870
Fries Chili	1 serv	370	8	16	10	49	5	780
Fries Chili & Cheese	1 serv	400	8	19	10	51	5	990
Hot Dog Plain	1	280	11	17	35	22	1	710

FOOD	PORTION	CALS	PROT	FAT	CHOL	CARB	FIBER	SOD
Onion Rings	1 serv	350	5	18	0	45	2	710
Papa Burger	1	720	41	42	145	46	2	1390
Sandwich Crispy Chicken	1	590	31	29	65	54	3	1170
Sandwich Grilled Chicken	1	440	31	19	90	54	2	860
SAUCES								
Dipping Sauce BBQ	1 serv (1 oz)	40	0	0	0	10	0	230
Dipping Sauce Honey Mustard	1 serv (1 oz)	100	0	6	0	12	0	170
Dipping Sauce Ranch	1 serv (1 oz)	160	0	17	15	2	0	240
Dipping Sauce Sweet & Sour	1 serv (1 oz)	45	0	0	0	12	0	120

ARBY'S
BEVERAGES

FOOD	PORTION	CALS	PROT	FAT	CHOL	CARB	FIBER	SOD
Dr Pepper	1 (16 oz)	180	0	0	0	52	0	60
Jamocha Shake	1 reg	498	13	13	34	81	0	393
Pepsi	1 (16 oz)	130	0	0	0	34	0	30
Shake Chocolate	1 reg	507	13	13	34	83	0	257
Shake Orange Cream	1 (17 oz)	637	15	17	41	105	0	423
Shake Strawberry	1 reg	498	13	13	34	81	0	363
Shake Strawberry Banana Swirl	1 (17 oz)	567	15	16	39	87	0	425
Sierra Mist	1 (16 oz)	100	0	0	0	27	0	25
Vanilla Shake	1 reg	437	13	13	34	66	0	350

BREAKFAST SELECTIONS

FOOD	PORTION	CALS	PROT	FAT	CHOL	CARB	FIBER	SOD
Biscuit	1	273	5	15	1	28	1	786
Biscuit Bacon Egg & Cheese	1	461	17	28	169	30	1	1446
Biscuit Chicken	1	417	15	23	17	39	1	1240
Biscuit Ham Egg & Cheese	1	437	20	23	169	31	1	1658
Biscuit Sausage Egg & Cheese	1	557	18	38	187	30	1	1579
Biscuit Suasage Gravy	1	961	7	68	12	107	1	3755
Biscuit w/ Bacon	1	340	9	21	13	29	1	1028
Biscuit w/ Ham	1	316	13	17	13	29	1	1240
Biscuit w/ Sausage	1	436	10	31	32	26	1	1160
Breakfast Syrup	1 serv (1 oz)	78	0	0	0	20	0	25
Cinnamon Roll Original Gourmet	1	507	10	10	7	73	4	373
Croissant	1	190	3	10	30	21	1	190
Croissant Bacon & Egg	1	337	11	22	187	23	1	651

FOOD	PORTION	CALS	PROT	FAT	CHOL	CARB	FIBER	SOD
Croissant Bacon Egg & Cheese	1	378	14	22	198	23	1	850
Croissant Ham & Cheese	1	274	13	12	53	22	1	842
Croissant Ham Egg & Cheese	1	434	22	24	343	26	1	1282
Croissant Sausage & Egg	1	433	12	32	206	23	1	784
Croissant Sausage Egg & Cheese	1	475	15	32	216	23	1	982
French Toastix	1 serv	312	6	13	0	44	1	492
Muffin Blueberry	1	320	4	12	20	49	1	490
Pecan Sticky Bun	1	688	12	22	7	91	5	420
Sourdough Bacon Egg & Cheese	1	437	20	16	174	40	2	1220
Sourdough Egg & Cheese	1	392	17	12	166	40	2	1058
Sourdough Ham Egg & Cheese	1	679	34	35	354	42	2	2104
Sourdough Sausage Egg & Cheese	1	514	19	27	186	40	2	1232
Twist Chocolate	1	250	4	12	5	34	2	110
Twist Cinnamon	1	260	3	14	5	33	1	190
Wrap Bacon Egg & Cheese	1	515	16	29	165	50	2	1367
Wrap Ham Egg & Cheese	1	568	24	31	183	51	2	1929
Wrap Sausage Egg & Cheese	1	689	21	45	202	50	2	1849
CHILDREN'S MENU SELECTIONS								
Kids Meal Chicken Tenders	1 serv	289	19	14	32	21	1	907
Kids Meal Junior Roast Beef Sandwich	1	272	16	10	29	34	2	740
Market Fresh Mini Ham & Cheese Sandwich	1	228	14	5	23	28	2	916
Market Fresh Mini Turkey & Cheese Sandwich	1	235	17	4	33	28	2	798
DESSERTS								
Cookie Chocolate Chip	1 (1.6 oz)	202	2	10	15	26	1	213
Turnover Apple	1	377	4	16	0	65	2	201
Turnover Cherry	1	377	4	15	0	65	2	201
SALAD DRESSINGS AND SAUCES								
Arby's Sauce	1 serv (0.5 oz)	15	0	0	0	4	0	177
Dipping Sauce BBQ	1 pkg (1 oz)	40	0	0	0	11	0	343

FOOD	PORTION	CALS	PROT	FAT	CHOL	CARB	FIBER	SOD
Dipping Sauce Bronco Berry	1 serv (2 oz)	122	0	0	0	30	0	36
Dipping Sauce Buffalo	1 serv (1 oz)	10	0	1	0	2	0	790
Dipping Sauce Cool Ranch Sour Cream	1 serv (1.5 oz)	158	1	16	0	2	0	277
Dipping Sauce Honey Mustard	1 serv (1 oz)	129	0	12	9	6	0	151
Dressing Buttermilk Ranch	1 serv (2.2 oz)	325	1	34	28	4	0	657
Dressing Buttermilk Ranch Light	1 serv (2 oz)	112	1	6	1	13	1	472
Dressing Sante Fe Ranch	1 pkg (2.2 oz)	296	1	31	21	4	0	692
Horsey Sauce	1 pkg (0.5 oz)	62	0	5	5	3	0	173
Ketchup	1 pkg	13	0	0	0	3	0	158
Sauce Cheddar Cheese	1 serv (0.7 oz)	30	0	2	1	2	0	181
Sauce Spicy Three Pepper	1 serv (0.5 oz)	22	0	1	0	3	0	140
Sauce Tangy Southwest	1 serv (2 oz)	333	1	35	29	5	0	371
SALADS								
Chicken Club	1 serv	487	32	25	178	31	4	1220
Martha's Vineyard	1 serv	277	26	8	72	24	4	451
Santa Fe	1 serv	477	29	21	53	42	6	1131
SANDWICHES								
Arby's Melt	1	302	16	12	30	36	2	921
Beef 'N Cheddar	1	445	22	21	51	44	2	1274
Chicken Bacon & Swiss Crispy	1	624	36	29	68	52	2	1320
Chicken Bacon & Swiss Grilled	1	462	38	17	25	38	2	1333
Chicken Cordon Bleu Crispy	1	650	40	31	74	49	2	1548
Chicken Cordon Bleu Grilled	1	488	42	19	32	35	2	1561
Chicken Fillet Crispy	1	576	30	30	52	50	3	901
Chicken Fillet Grilled	1	414	32	17	9	36	3	913
Chicken Salad w/ Pecans	1	769	30	39	74	79	9	1240

FOOD	PORTION	CALS	PROT	FAT	CHOL	CARB	FIBER	SOD
Corned Beef Reuben	1	606	34	33	83	55	3	1849
Fish	1	543	21	25	55	61	3	956
French Dip	1	391	26	16	58	37	3	1282
French Dip & Swiss	1	473	32	18	79	28	3	1679
Ham & Swiss Melt	1	275	18	6	27	35	1	1118
Roast Beef Regular	1	320	21	14	44	34	2	953
Roast Beef Super	1	398	21	19	44	40	2	1060
Roast Beef & Swiss	1	777	37	41	89	73	5	1743
Roast Beef 'N Cheddar	1	521	27	27	64	45	2	1573
Roast Ham & Swiss	1	705	36	31	63	75	5	2103
Roast Turkey Ranch & Bacon	1	834	49	38	109	75	5	2258
Roast Turkey Rueben	1	611	44	30	94	56	3	1429
Roast Turkey & Swiss	1	725	45	30	91	75	5	1788
Sourdough Melt Beef	1	355	18	14	30	40	2	1047
Sourdough Melt Ham	1	380	19	13	31	39	2	1280
Spicy Cajun Fish	1	603	21	32	68	61	3	883
Sub Toasted Classic Italian	1	828	37	46	89	69	3	2496
Sub Toasted French Dip & Swiss	1	622	37	20	79	68	3	3397
Sub Toasted Philly Beef	1	739	32	37	85	64	3	1881
Sub Toasted Turkey Bacon Club	1	619	42	18	82	65	3	2052
Swiss Melt	1	303	16	12	29	37	2	919
Ultimate BLT	1	779	23	45	51	75	6	1571
Wrap Chicken Salad w/ Pecans	1	638	30	38	74	48	8	1199
Wrap Corned Beef Reuben	1	577	38	29	83	42	1	1721
Wrap Roast Turkey Ranch & Bacon	1	700	49	37	109	44	4	2215
Wrap Roast Turkey Reuben	1	581	48	27	94	43	1	1301
Wrap Southwest Chicken	1	567	36	29	88	42	4	1451
Wrap Ultimate BLT	1	648	23	44	51	45	5	1530
SIDES								
Bites Jalapeno	5	305	5	21	28	29	2	526
Bites Loaded Potato	5	353	11	22	13	27	2	800
Cheddar Fries	1 med	465	6	28	2	51	5	1311
Chicken Tenders	3 pieces	379	25	18	42	28	2	1188
Croutons Cheese & Garlic	1 pkg	77	2	5	1	7	0	116
Curly Fries	1 sm	338	4	20	0	39	4	791

FOOD	PORTION	CALS	PROT	FAT	CHOL	CARB	FIBER	SOD
Curly Fries	1 lg	631	8	37	0	73	7	1476
Fruit Cup	1 serv	35	0	0	0	9	1	0
Homestyle Fries	1 sm	302	3	20	0	44	3	549
Homestyle Fries	1 lg	566	6	37	0	82	6	1029
Mozzarella Sticks	8 pieces	849	36	56	90	75	4	2730
Onion Petals	1 reg	331	4	23	1	35	2	332
Popcorn Chicken	1 reg	365	24	18	40	27	2	1145
Potato Cakes	2	246	2	18	0	26	2	391
Seasoned Tortilla Strips	1 serv	71	1	3	0	9	1	25

AU BON PAIN
BAKED SELECTIONS

FOOD	PORTION	CALS	PROT	FAT	CHOL	CARB	FIBER	SOD
Bagel Asiago Cheese	1	360	15	4	10	64	3	590
Bagel Cinnamon Raisin	1	320	11	1	0	67	3	440
Bagel Everything	1	350	13	5	0	64	3	990
Bagel Honey 9 Grain	1	330	13	2	0	68	6	540
Bagel Jalapeno Double Cheddar	1	350	17	10	30	55	2	650
Bagel Onion Dill	1	350	13	1	0	72	4	530
Bagel Plain	1	290	11	1	0	59	2	440
Bagel Poppy Seed	1	290	11	1	0	59	2	440
Bagel Sesame Seed	1	330	12	5	0	61	3	440
Baguette Artisan Salad Size	1 (3.5 oz)	210	7	1	0	44	2	460
Baguette Artisan Sandwich Size	1 (4.7 oz)	290	10	1	0	59	2	610
Baguette Artisan Honey Multigrain Salad Size	1 (3.5 oz)	240	8	3	0	47	4	460
Baguette Artisan Honey Multigrain Sandwich Size	1 (4.7 oz	310	10	3	0	62	6	610
Blondie	1	330	7	19	35	61	3	350
Bread Artisan Multigrain	1 serv (4 oz)	260	9	3	0	51	4	610
Bread Artisan Sundried Tomato	1 serv (4 oz)	240	8	1	0	49	2	570
Bread Cheese	1 serv (4.8 oz)	290	14	8	2	55	3	730
Bread Country White	1 serv (4 oz)	240	6	1	0	50	2	590
Bread Bowl	1 (9.24 oz)	640	28	3	0	127	6	1830

FOOD	PORTION	CALS	PROT	FAT	CHOL	CARB	FIBER	SOD
Bread Stick Rosemary Garlic	1 (2.3 oz)	200	6	5	0	33	2	1430
Brownie Chocolate Chip	1	380	5	17	75	62	1	390
Brownie Hazelnut Mocha	1	430	6	21	65	58	3	360
Brownie Rocky Road	1	410	6	17	70	62	2	430
Ciabatta	1 sm	180	7	1	0	37	2	380
Cinnamon Roll	1	350	7	12	40	53	2	240
Cookie Chocolate Chip	1 (2 oz)	260	2	12	25	37	1	220
Cookie Confetti	1 (2.4 oz)	310	3	14	25	42	1	290
Cookie Gingerbread	1 (2.7 oz)	300	4	9	10	50	1	140
Cookie Hazelnut Fudge	1 (2.25 oz)	290	4	16	40	34	3	150
Cookie Oatmeal Raisin	1 (2 oz)	230	3	8	35	36	2	190
Cookie Shortbread	1 (2.3 oz)	310	3	9	25	34	1	270
Cookie English Toffee	1 (2 oz)	210	2	11	20	26	1	240
Creme De Fleur	1 serv	550	12	26	110	71	1	540
Croissant Almond	1	560	12	36	110	52	4	270
Croissant Apple	1	230	4	10	25	31	2	230
Croissant Chocolate	1	330	6	17	30	42	3	180
Croissant Plain	1 (2.8 oz)	260	5	15	55	28	1	190
Croissant Raspberry Cheese	1	330	7	16	60	41	1	280
Croissant Sweet Cheese	1	320	4	16	60	39	1	280
Danish Cherry	1	370	7	19	85	44	1	290
Danish Sweet Cheese	1	380	7	20	90	44	1	300
Focaccia	1 piece (4.4 oz)	310	11	4	0	57	3	640
Lahvash	1 (4 oz)	320	15	1	0	62	2	190
Macaroon Chocolate Dipped Cranberry Almond	1	320	4	16	0	42	3	190
Mini Loaf Bacon & Cheese	1 (4.8 oz)	540	13	31	95	50	1	790
Muffin Blueberry	1	510	9	19	20	76	5	550
Muffin Carrot Walnut	1	520	8	25	55	66	4	800
Muffin Corn	1	460	9	16	60	69	2	550
Muffin Cranberry Walnut	1	500	10	24	20	61	5	460
Muffin Double Chocolate Chunk	1	590	10	20	25	83	5	480
Muffin Pumpkin	1	490	9	17	65	75	2	520
Muffin Raisin Bran	1	410	10	9	30	74	9	590
Muffin Low Fat Triple Berry	1	290	5	2	25	61	2	310

FOOD	PORTION	CALS	PROT	FAT	CHOL	CARB	FIBER	SOD
Pastry Hazelnut Creme	1	540	10	34	85	50	3	380
Poundcake Cappuccino	1 slice (5.2 oz)	530	3	26	85	68	1	490
Poundcake Chocolate	1 slice (4.7 oz)	500	7	29	100	58	3	580
Poundcake Lemon	1 slice (4.9 oz)	520	5	27	85	64	0	460
Poundcake Marble	1 slice (4.7 oz)	490	6	27	90	59	1	520
Roll Soft	1 (4.7 oz)	410	11	11	20	65	3	700
Roll Pecan	1	630	10	32	30	80	3	330
Scone Cinnamon	1	430	9	24	130	48	1	360
Scone Orange	1	410	9	20	130	51	2	370
Shortbread Chocolate Dipped	1	350	3	20	25	38	1	280
Toasts Basil Pesto Cheese	3 pieces (2 oz)	140	5	2	0	26	1	330
Tulip Blueberry	1	370	4	20	65	44	1	300
Tulip Chocolate Raspberry	1	430	5	21	70	55	1	410
Tulip Key Lime	1	440	5	22	70	55	1	360
BEVERAGES								
Blast Caramel	1 med (16 oz)	540	6	17	60	104	0	105
Blast Coffee	1 med (16 oz)	440	8	21	75	71	0	115
Blast Mocha	1 med (16 oz)	440	7	17	60	80	2	95
Blast Vanilla	1 med (12 oz)	540	6	17	60	104	0	100
Caffe Americano	1 sm (12 oz)	5	0	0	0	1	0	15
Caffe Latte	1 sm (12 oz)	200	11	11	45	17	0	170
Cappuccino	1 sm (12 oz)	120	6	7	20	10	0	85
Caramel Macchiato	1 sm (12 oz)	350	10	10	30	53	0	160
Chai Latte	1 sm (12 oz)	290	11	11	30	38	0	130
Chocolate Milk	1 (12 oz)	320	10	9	25	54	3	100
Hot Chocolate	1 sm (12 oz)	350	12	11	30	58	3	125
Iced Caffe Latte	1 sm (12 oz)	110	6	6	20	19	0	80
Iced Caramel Macchiato	1 sm (12 oz)	290	7	7	25	49	0	125
Iced Chai Latte	1 sm (12 oz)	190	5	5	15	31	0	65
Iced Mocha Latte	1 sm (12 oz)	210	6	11	35	27	1	70

FOOD	PORTION	CALS	PROT	FAT	CHOL	CARB	FIBER	SOD
Iced Tea Peach	1 med (22 oz)	120	0	0	0	30	0	35
Iced Vanilla Latte	1 sm (12 oz)	240	5	5	15	44	0	65
Iced White Chocolate Latte	1 sm (12 oz)	250	5	11	35	35	0	135
Lemonade	1 med (22 oz)	300	0	0	0	72	0	0
Mocha Latte	1 sm (12 oz)	300	11	16	60	35	1	160
Orange Juice	1 (8 oz)	110	2	0	0	26	1	0
Smoothie Peach	1 med (16 oz)	310	4	1	10	69	4	115
Smoothie Strawberry	1 med (16 oz)	310	4	1	10	66	3	110
Vanilla Latte	1 sm (12 oz)	320	9	9	30	50	0	120
White Chocolate Latte	1 sm (12 oz)	310	9	14	45	41	0	180
MAIN MENU SELECTIONS								
Fruit Cup	1 sm (6 oz)	70	1	0	0	16	1	10
Harvest Rice Bowl Cajun Shrimp	1 (20 oz)	520	16	17	145	69	2	1660
Harvest Rice Bowl Cajun Shrimp w/ Brown Rice	1 (20 oz)	56	14	20	145	73	5	1660
Harvest Rice Bowl Mayan Chicken	1 (19.25 oz)	490	25	14	70	67	4	1430
Harvest Rice Bowl Mayan Chicken w/ Brown Rice	1 (19.25 oz)	540	23	16	70	71	7	1430
Harvest Rice Bowl Steak Teriyaki	1 (19.25 oz)	530	30	15	60	72	2	1520
Harvest Rice Bowl Steak Teriyaki w/ Brown Rice	1 (19.25 oz)	570	28	18	60	76	5	1520
Macaroni & Cheese	1 med (12 oz)	440	19	26	95	31	2	1280
Stew Beef	1 med (12 oz)	300	18	16	55	25	3	1070
Stew Chicken Vegetable	1 med (12 oz)	290	11	17	40	26	3	930
SALAD DRESSINGS AND SPREADS								
Artichoke Aioli	1 serv (1 oz)	130	1	14	10	1	0	180
Basil Pesto	1 serv (1 oz)	140	2	15	5	1	0	160
Chili Dijon	1 serv (1 oz)	120	1	12	10	3	1	130
Cream Cheese Honey Pecan	1 serv (2 oz)	120	4	10	35	5	0	340

FOOD	PORTION	CALS	PROT	FAT	CHOL	CARB	FIBER	SOD
Cream Cheese Honey Walnut	1 serv (2 oz)	140	3	9	30	12	0	150
Cream Cheese Lite	1 serv (2 oz)	120	4	9	30	5	0	280
Cream Cheese Plain	1 serv (2 oz)	170	3	16	50	4	0	290
Cream Cheese Strawberry	1 serv (2 oz)	180	3	15	45	9	0	250
Cream Cheese Sundried Tomato	1 serv (2 oz)	120	4	10	35	5	.0	340
Cream Cheese Vegetable	1 serv (2 oz)	170	3	16	45	3	0	270
Dressing Balsamic Vinaigrette	1 serv (2.25 oz)	190	9	16	0	11	0	430
Dressing Blue Cheese	1 serv (1.75 oz)	230	2	24	20	2	0	550
Dressing Caesar	1 serv (2 oz)	280	2	28	20	4	0	400
Dressing Fat Free Raspberry Vinaigrette	1 serv (2.25 oz)	70	0	0	0	17	0	150
Dressing Light Honey Mustard	1 serv (2.25 oz)	180	1	11	10	21	1	590
Dressing Light Olive Oil Vinaigrette	1 serv (2.25 oz)	130	0	10	0	9	0	630
Dressing Light Ranch	1 serv (2.25 oz)	150	2	15	15	3	0	470
Dressing Thai Peanut	1 serv (2.25 oz)	230	5	13	0	24	1	840
Guacomole	1 serv (1 oz)	60	1	6	0	2	2	125
Honey Mustard	1 serv (2.5 oz)	210	1	13	15	23	1	650
Hummus Roasted Red Pepper	1 serv (2 oz)	80	2	5	0	6	2	250
Mayonnaise	1 serv (1 oz)	200	0	22	20	0	0	150
Mayonnaise Herb	1 serv (1 oz)	210	0	23	20	1	0	210
Mayonnaise Jalapeno	1 serv (1 oz)	140	2	15	15	0	0	260
Mayonnaise Tarragon Sauce	1 serv (2 oz)	420	0	45	40	2	0	420
Mustard	1 tsp	0	0	0	0	0	0	70
Spread Herb Bagel	1 serv (2 oz)	130	4	11	35	5	0	470
Spread Sundried Tomato	1 serv (0.53 oz)	70	1	6	0	4	0	85
SALADS								
Caesar Asiago	1 serv	210	11	12	25	18	3	470

FOOD	PORTION	CALS	PROT	FAT	CHOL	CARB	FIBER	SOD
Caesar Asiago Grilled Chicken	1 (8.5 oz)	340	29	13	65	19	3	680
Caesar Asiago Side	1 (3.2 oz)	120	6	6	15	12	2	260
Chef's	1 serv	230	22	14	60	7	3	1090
Garden	1 (7 oz)	80	4	2	0	14	4	210
Garden Side	1 (3.6 oz)	50	2	1	0	10	3	70
Mediterranean Chicken	1 (9.75 oz)	330	24	16	60	12	2	1170
Riviera	1 (9.5 oz)	260	7	7	15	46	5	250
Thai Peanut Chicken	1 (11 oz)	250	22	8	40	22	4	290
Tuna Garden	1 (10.5 oz)	350	21	25	55	14	4	470
Turkey Medallion Cobb	1 (11 oz)	340	27	19	260	15	3	980
Turkey Spinach Sonoma	1 (12.3 oz)	310	29	13	65	22	5	1310
SANDWICHES								
Arizona Chicken	1 (12 oz)	750	49	29	120	61	4	1480
Baguette Turkey & Swiss	1 (12.3 oz)	770	41	38	95	65	3	2120
Baja Turkey	1 (13 oz)	700	41	32	90	61	4	1970
Breakfast Asiago Bagel Prosciutto & Egg	1 (9.6 oz)	660	40	25	185	67	3	1580
Breakfast Asiago Bagel Sausage Egg & Cheddar	1 (10.2 oz)	770	36	45	215	55	0	1450
Breakfast Bagel & Bacon	1 (4.2 oz)	340	15	6	15	56	0	630
Breakfast Egg On A Bagel	1 (6.8 oz)	370	21	4	115	62	2	790
Breakfast Egg On A Bagel w/ Bacon	1 (7.2 oz)	410	25	8	130	58	0	980
Breakfast Egg On A Bagel w/ Bacon Cheese	1 (7.9 oz)	500	30	15	150	59	0	1120
Breakfast Egg On A Bagel w/ Cheese	1 (7.6 oz)	450	26	10	135	62	2	920
Breakfast Onion Dill Bagel Smoked Salmon & Wasabi	1 (7.1 oz)	490	18	11	45	77	3	1250
Caprese	1 (11.8 oz)	700	28	35	65	65	4	1120
Chicken Mozzarella	1 (14.5 oz)	800	50	27	105	71	2	1360
Chicken Pesto	1 (12.5 oz)	700	44	23	80	62	2	1340
Chicken Tarragon	1 (11 oz)	720	40	29	85	61	1	1190
Ciabatta Bacon & Egg Melt	1 (7 oz)	400	26	15	155	40	2	1160
Ciabatta Ham & Cheddar	1 (12 oz)	650	40	20	95	80	4	2330
Club Smoked Turkey	1 (11.6 oz)	780	43	43	115	56	2	2330
Croissant Ham & Cheese	1 (4.2 oz)	350	14	18	60	34	1	550
Croissant Spinach & Cheese	1	250	8	14	35	25	2	280

FOOD	PORTION	CALS	PROT	FAT	CHOL	CARB	FIBER	SOD
Hot BBQ Chicken On Farmhouse Roll	1 (14.3 oz)	970	50	44	130	78	4	1630
Hot Eggplant & Mozzarella	1 (12.4 oz)	710	26	37	60	68	6	1440
Hot Steakhouse On Ciabatta	1 (13 oz)	800	43	41	100	70	4	1850
Melt Tuna	1 (12.5 oz)	760	40	41	100	60	4	1240
Melt Turkey	1 (12.2 oz)	890	45	47	120	70	3	2360
Portobello & Goat Cheese	1 (10 oz)	610	18	33	35	61	6	1290
Portobello Egg & Cheddar	1 (8.5 oz)	590	22	37	200	42	3	1050
Prosciutto Mozzarella	1 (12.7 oz)	880	40	49	110	71	4	2270
Spicy Tuna	1 (10.3 oz)	640	28	34	65	57	6	1100
The Montana	1 (12.5 oz)	560	40	23	105	62	4	1370
Turkey & Cranberry Chutney	1 (10.9 oz)	680	30	24	60	63	3	1970
Wrap Chicken Caesar Asiago	1	700	42	25	75	69	3	930
Wrap Chopped Turkey Club	1 (12 oz)	660	35	27	165	70	4	1200
Wrap Mediterranean	1 (12.8 oz)	670	24	28	20	80	7	1240
Wrap Southwest Tuna	1 (14 oz)	900	46	51	110	72	5	980
Wrap Thai Peanut Chicken	1 (14.5 oz)	660	38	19	40	84	4	770
Wrap Turkey Spinach Sonoma	1 (12 oz)	630	35	19	45	80	5	1070
Wrap Hot Cajun Shrimp	1 (14.9 oz)	700	20	24	90	95	4	1680
Wrap Hot Mayan Chicken	1 (13.5 oz)	630	24	19	40	92	5	1400
Wrap Hot Steak Teriyaki	1 (13.5 oz)	660	28	19	40	93	5	1780
SOUPS								
Baked Stuffed Potato	1 med (12 oz)	350	9	21	60	30	2	990
Broccoli Cheddar	1 med (12 oz)	310	11	21	50	20	2	1000
Carrot Ginger	1 med (12 oz)	130	7	5	0	21	3	920
Chicken Florentine	1 med (12 oz)	240	8	13	35	25	1	1030
Chicken & Dumplings	1 med (12 oz)	210	11	7	50	28	2	1280
Chicken Noodle	1 med (12 oz)	130	9	3	15	20	2	1000
Clam Chowder	1 med (12 oz)	320	9	18	55	27	1	1020

FOOD	PORTION	CALS	PROT	FAT	CHOL	CARB	FIBER	SOD
Corn & Green Chili Bisque	1 med (12 oz)	250	5	14	35	29	3	1540
Corn Chowder	1 med (12 oz)	350	9	18	50	40	3	1120
Curried Rice & Lentil	1 med (12 oz)	150	9	2	0	30	8	1260
French Moroccan Tomato Lentil	1 med (12 oz)	180	10	2	0	32	8	1050
French Onion	1 med (12 oz)	130	4	5	10	19	2	1310
Garden Vegetable	1 med (12 oz)	80	3	2	0	14	3	1010
Harvest Pumpkin	1 med (12 oz)	190	8	10	25	26	2	1110
Hearty Cabbage	1 med (12 oz)	110	4	5	10	14	3	910
Italian Wedding	1 med (12 oz)	170	8	7	15	10	2	1300
Jamaican Black Bean	1 med (12 oz)	180	16	1	0	45	25	460
Mediterranean Pepper	1 med (12 oz)	100	5	3	0	18	5	580
Old Fashioned Tomato Rice	1 med (12 oz)	120	4	1	0	24	3	340
Pasta E Fagioli	1 med (12 oz)	240	11	8	5	36	9	930
Portuguese Kale	1 med (12 oz)	120	5	5	5	15	3	1130
Potato Cheese	1 med (12 oz)	250	7	14	50	25	2	1340
Potato Leek	1 med (12 oz)	300	5	20	60	28	2	1000
Red Beans Italian Sausage & Rice	1 med (12 oz)	200	15	5	10	28	16	1140
Southern Black Eyed Pea	1 med (12 oz)	180	12	2	5	31	12	950
Southwest Tortilla	1 med (12 oz)	200	4	11	10	24	4	1290
Southwest Vegetable	1 med (12 oz)	160	4	3	0	17	3	370

FOOD	PORTION	CALS	PROT	FAT	CHOL	CARB	FIBER	SOD
Split Pea	1 med (12 oz)	210	18	2	5	42	15	1190
Thai Coconut Curry	1 med (12 oz)	150	3	7	0	20	2	1150
Tomato Florentine	1 med (12 oz)	120	5	3	5	19	2	1390
Tomato Basil Bisque	1 med (12 oz)	210	6	8	25	29	5	490
Tomato Cheddar	1 med (12 oz)	240	12	15	25	17	2	1040
Tuscan Vegetable	1 med (12 oz)	170	7	5	10	24	3	1170
Vegetable Beef Barley	1 med (12 oz)	140	9	3	20	21	4	1000
Vegetarian Lentil	1 med (12 oz)	140	10	2	0	32	11	1260
Vegetarian Minestrone	1 med (12 oz)	120	5	2	0	21	4	1120
Vegetarian Chili	1 med (12 oz)	230	12	3	0	40	11	1000
Wild Mushroom Bisque	1 med (12 oz)	190	5	9	10	23	2	1010
YOGURT								
Blueberry w/ Fruit	1 sm (7.5 oz)	220	6	2	10	44	0	120
Blueberry w/ Granola & Fruit	1 sm (8.5 oz)	310	10	6	10	56	2	130
Strawberry w/ Blueberries	1 sm (7.5 oz)	220	6	2	10	44	0	120
Strawberry w/ Granola & Blueberries	1 sm (8.5 oz)	310	10	6	10	56	2	130
Vanilla w/ Blueberries	1 sm (7.5 oz)	190	10	2	10	32	0	160
Vanilla w/ Granola & Blueberries	1 sm (8.5 oz)	310	10	6	10	56	2	130

AUNTIE ANNE'S
BEVERAGES

FOOD	PORTION	CALS	PROT	FAT	CHOL	CARB	FIBER	SOD
Dutch Ice Blue Raspberry	1 (14 oz)	165	0	0	0	38	0	20
Dutch Ice Grape	1 (14 oz)	180	0	0	0	43	0	20

FOOD	PORTION	CALS	PROT	FAT	CHOL	CARB	FIBER	SOD
Dutch Ice Kiwi Banana	1 (14 oz)	190	0	0	0	44	0	30
Dutch Ice Lemonade	1 (14 oz)	315	0	0	0	77	0	0
Dutch Ice Lemonade Strawberry	1 (14 oz)	330	0	0	0	81	0	0
Dutch Ice Mocha	1 (14 oz)	400	0	10	0	74	0	100
Dutch Ice Orange Creme	1 (14 oz)	280	0	0	0	64	0	35
Dutch Ice Pina Colada	1 (14 oz)	220	0	0	0	53	0	15
Dutch Ice Strawberry	1 (14 oz)	220	0	0	0	50	0	40
Dutch Ice Watermelon	1 (14 oz)	200	0	0	0	50	0	35
Dutch Ice Wild Cherry	1 (14 oz)	210	0	0	0	48	0	25
Dutch Latte Caramel	1 (14 oz)	350	4	15	55	49	0	55
Dutch Latte Coffee	1 (14 oz)	290	4	14	50	38	0	135
Dutch Latte Mocha	1 (14 oz)	160	5	17	55	47	0	135
Dutch Shake Chocolate	1 (14 oz)	580	10	27	105	75	0	380
Dutch Shake Coffee	1 (14 oz)	590	10	27	105	77	0	304
Dutch Shake Strawberry	1 (14 oz)	610	10	27	105	78	0	304
Dutch Shake Vanilla	1 (14 oz)	510	10	27	105	58	0	300
Dutch Smoothie Blue Raspberry	1 (14 oz)	230	3	8	30	34	0	100
Dutch Smoothie Grape	1 (14 oz)	230	3	8	30	36	0	100
Dutch Smoothie Kiwi Banana	1 (14 oz)	240	3	8	30	38	0	100
Dutch Smoothie Lemonade	1 (14 oz)	300	3	8	30	53	0	80
Dutch Smoothie Mocha	1 (14 oz)	330	3	13	30	50	0	130
Dutch Smoothie Orange Creme	1 (14 oz)	280	3	8	30	46	0	100
Dutch Smoothie Pina Colada	1 (14 oz)	260	3	8	30	44	0	90
Dutch Smoothie Strawberry	1 (14 oz)	250	3	8	30	40	0	100
Dutch Smoothie Wild Cherry	1 (14 oz)	250	3	8	30	41	0	90
Lemonade	1 (22 oz)	180	0	0	0	43	0	0
Lemonade Strawberry	1 (22 oz)	190	0	0	0	48	0	0
DIPPING SAUCES								
Caramel Dip	1 serv (1.5 oz)	135	1	3	5	27	0	110
Cheese Sauce	1 serv (1.25 oz)	100	3	8	10	4	0	510

FOOD	PORTION	CALS	PROT	FAT	CHOL	CARB	FIBER	SOD
Cream Cheese Light	1 serv (1.25 oz)	70	3	6	25	1	0	140
Hot Salsa Cheese	1 serv (1.25 oz)	100	2	8	10	4	0	550
Marinara Sauce	1 serv (1.25 oz)	10	0	0	0	4	0	180
Sweet	1 serv (1.4 oz)	40	0	0	0	10	0	0
Sweet Mustard	1 serv (1.25 oz)	60	tr	2	40	8	0	120
PRETZELS								
Almond	1	400	9	8	20	72	2	400
Almond w/o Butter	1	350	9	2	0	72	2	390
Cinnamon Raisin w/o Butter	1	350	9	2	0	74	2	410
Cinnamon Sugar	1	450	8	9	25	83	3	430
Garlic	1	350	9	5	10	68	2	850
Garlic w/o Butter	1	320	9	1	0	66	2	830
Glazin' Raisin	1	510	11	4	10	107	4	480
Glazin' Raisin w/o Butter	1	470	11	1	0	104	3	460
Jalapeno	1	310	8	5	10	59	2	940
Jalapeno w/o Butter	1	270	8	1	0	58	2	780
Original	1	370	10	4	10	72	3	930
Original w/o Butter	1	340	10	1	0	72	3	900
Pretzel Dog	1	290	10	16	40	25	1	600
Sesame	1	410	12	12	15	64	7	860
Sesame w/o Butter	1	350	11	6	0	63	3	840
Sour Cream & Onion	1	340	9	5	10	66	2	930
Sour Cream & Onion w/o Butter	1	310	9	1	0	66	2	920
Stix	6	370	10	4	10	72	3	930
Stix w/o Butter	6	340	10	1	0	72	3	900
Whole Wheat	1	370	11	5	10	72	7	1120
Whole Wheat w/o Butter	1	350	11	2	0	72	7	1100

BABS DELI
BAGELS

FOOD	PORTION	CALS	PROT	FAT	CHOL	CARB	FIBER	SOD
Apple Cinnamon	1	332	12	2	0	70	4	472
Banana Nut	1	340	12	2	0	68	4	460
Blueberry	1	330	12	2	0	68	4	482

FOOD	PORTION	CALS	PROT	FAT	CHOL	CARB	FIBER	SOD
Blueberry Cobbler	1	392	10	8	12	70	2	440
Cheddar Herb	1	352	14	6	16	60	2	604
Cheddar Nacho	1	352	14	6	16	60	4	702
Chocolate Chip	1	348	12	2	0	68	4	472
Cinnamon Apple Pie	1	386	10	8	12	68	2	420
Cinnamon Bun	1	400	10	8	12	70	2	440
Cinnamon Danish	1	396	10	8	12	72	4	428
Cinnamon Raisin	1	336	12	2	0	70	4	464
Cinnamon Sugar	1	350	12	2	0	74	2	482
Cranberry Walnut	1	352	12	2	0	72	4	470
Egg	1	328	12	2	4	66	2	492
Everything	1	336	12	2	0	68	4	778
French Toast	1	372	12	4	0	74	2	464
Garlic	1	330	12	2	0	68	4	492
Honey Oat	1	320	12	2	0	68	2	446
Jalapeno	1	350	14	6	16	30	2	688
Onion	1	336	12	2	0	70	4	492
Plain	1	334	12	2	0	68	4	502
Poppy	1	344	12	2	0	68	4	490
Pumpernickel	1	332	12	2	0	68	4	492
Quiche Lorraine	1	354	16	8	20	54	2	125
Salt	1	324	12	2	0	66	2	1936
Sesame	1	358	14	4	0	66	4	476
Spinach	1	356	14	2	0	72	4	274
Strawberry	1	342	12	2	0	72	4	470
Strawberry White Chocolate	1	364	12	4	0	72	4	478
Swiss Melt	1	368	18	8	20	58	2	470
Tomato Basil	1	322	12	2	0	66	4	560
Vegetable	1	318	12	2	0	66	4	482
Wheat	1	330	12	2	0	78	4	476
White Chocolate Swirl	1	396	10	8	12	70	2	448
BEVERAGES								
Americano	1 (16 oz)	12	0	0	0	2	0	28
Cafe Caramello	1 (16 oz)	212	2	8	26	31	0	40
Cappuccino 2% Milk	1 (16 oz)	195	13	7	26	20	0	212
Cappuccino Fat Free Milk	1 (16 oz)	133	12	1	7	18	0	193
Coffee Black Forest	1 (16 oz)	198	1	5	16	37	1	35
Icepresso Caramel Decadence	1 (16 oz)	300	6	12	0	42	2	300

FOOD	PORTION	CALS	PROT	FAT	CHOL	CARB	FIBER	SOD
Icepresso Classic	1 (16 oz)	300	8	5	0	52	0	240
Icepresso Java Chip	1 (16 oz)	360	6	18	0	48	2	190
Icepresso Latte	1 (16 oz)	300	6	12	0	42	2	300
Icepresso Mocha	1 (16 oz)	300	6	12	0	42	2	300
Icepresso Strawberry	1 (16 oz)	340	2	12	0	56	0	120
Italiano 2% Milk	1 (16 oz)	131	9	5	18	13	0	139
Italiano Fat Free Milk	1 (16 oz)	89	8	1	5	12	0	126
Jittery Monkey 2% Milk	1 (16 oz)	482	13	11	39	82	1	230
Jittery Monkey Fat Free Milk	1 (16 oz)	429	12	6	22	80	1	214
Latte 2% Milk	1 (16 oz)	212	14	7	28	22	0	229
Latte Cinnamon Toast 2% Milk	1 (16 oz)	299	13	7	25	45	0	205
Latte Cinnamon Toast Fat Free Milk	1 (16 oz)	240	11	1	6	44	0	187
Latte Creme Caramel 2% Milk	1 (16 oz)	303	13	7	25	47	0	205
Latte Creme Caramel Fat Free Milk	1 (16 oz)	244	11	1	6	45	0	187
Latte Fat Free Milk	1 (16 oz)	145	13	1	7	20	0	209
Latte Oregon Chai Tea 2% Milk	1 (16 oz)	274	9	5	18	48	0	150
Latte Oregon Chai Tea Fat Free Milk	1 (16 oz)	231	8	1	5	47	0	137
Latte Raspberry Cheesecake 2% Milk	1 (16 oz)	319	13	7	25	51	0	209
Latte Raspberry Cheesecake Fat Free Milk	1 (16 oz)	259	11	1	6	50	0	191
Latte Vanilla Creme 2% Milk	1 (16 oz)	275	13	7	26	39	0	210
Mocha Whipped Cream 2% Milk	1 (16 oz)	454	15	12	42	71	2	272
Mocha Whipped Cream Fat Free Milk	1 (16 oz)	392	14	6	23	70	2	253
Turtle Mocha Fat Free Milk	1 (16 oz)	522	12	12	45	90	1	225
MUFFINS								
My Favorite Banana Nut	2 mini	195	4	11	21	21	1	121
My Favorite Blueberry	2 mini	168	2	8	24	22	0	136
My Favorite Blueberry Cheesecake	2 mini	199	3	12	38	20	0	145

FOOD	PORTION	CALS	PROT	FAT	CHOL	CARB	FIBER	SOD
My Favorite Boston Cream Pie	2 mini	176	2	7	22	26	0	144
My Favorite Cherry Cheesecake	2 mini	170	2	10	30	19	0	124
My Favorite Chocolate Cheesecake	2 mini	202	2	12	20	22	0	133
My Favorite Chocolate Chip	2 mini	211	3	11	25	27	1	142
My Favorite Cinnamon Crumb Cake	2 mini	212	3	13	37	21	0	135
My Favorite Cinnamon Swirl Cheesecake	2 mini	214	2	11	25	28	0	142
My Favorite Deep Dish Apple	2 mini	177	2	8	19	25	0	113
My Favorite Double Chocolate	2 mini	210	2	9	0	28	1	139
My Favorite Fat Free Blueberry	2 mini	108	2	0	0	26	1	192
My Favorite Fat Free Cherry Pie	2 mini	109	2	0	0	26	0	188
My Favorite Fat Free Chocolate Marble	2 mini	125	2	0	0	29	1	256
My Favorite Fat Free Cinnamon Bun	2 mini	168	1	0	0	42	0	176
My Favorite Fat Free Raspberry Amaretto	2 mini	127	2	0	0	31	1	186
My Favorite Golden Corn Bread	2 mini	197	3	9	24	26	1	135
My Favorite Lemon Poppyseed	2 mini	201	3	10	28	25	0	161
My Favorite Pumpkin Spice	2 mini	181	2	8	23	26	0	128
SALADS								
Calypso Chicken	1 (13.6 oz)	637	20	49	50	34	3	1229
Calypso Chicken w/ Lite Italian	1 (13.6 oz)	317	20	17	50	22	3	1823
Chicken Caesar	1 (11.5 oz)	524	23	41	83	15	3	1583
Chicken Caesar w/ Lite Italian	1 (11.5 oz)	268	20	12	56	17	3	1996
Classic Caesar	1 (8.4 oz)	414	9	36	33	12	3	1053
Classic Caesar Cafe	1 (4.3 oz)	225	5	19	16	9	2	573

FOOD	PORTION	CALS	PROT	FAT	CHOL	CARB	FIBER	SOD
Classic Caesar w/ Lite Italian	1 (8.4 oz)	158	6	8	6	14	3	1466
Garden Mix	1 (12.4 oz)	197	9	9	211	18	4	1352
Garden Mix Cafe	1 (6.5 oz)	100	5	5	105	9	2	684
Grilled Chicken Club	1 (17.9 oz)	820	35	69	104	16	3	2216
Grilled Chicken Club w/ Lite Italian	1 (17.9 oz)	500	35	31	104	18	3	2589
Low Carb Tuna Salad Plate	1 serv (8.9 oz)	356	28	25	58	3	1	652
Mediterranean Bread	1 (18.8 oz)	973	30	73	75	52	5	2371
Mediterranean Bread w/ Lite Italian ·	1 (18.8 oz)	626	30	32	75	55	5	2775
SANDWICHES								
Breakfast BLT	1	704	22	31 ·	91	83	4	1371
Breakfast Lox & Cream Cheese	1	602	29	21	58	78	4	1456
Breakfast Morning Classic	1	486	23	11	256	73	3	861
Breakfast Northern Omelette	1	699	31	31	296	73	3	1192
Breakfast So. Tradition w/ Ham	1	547	29	15	283	73	3	1362
Breakfast So. Tradition w/ Bacon	1	566	27	18	271	73	3	1151
Breakfast So. Tradition w/ Sausage	1	696	31	31.	296	73	3	1191
Build Your Own Ham	1	495	27	9	53	77	4	1734
Build Your Own Roast Beef	1	480	29	6	46	77	4	1689
Build Your Own Tuna	1	547	27	14	29	77	4	1039
Build Your Own Turkey	1	465	32	3	61	77	4	1567
Enchilada Bagellata	1	522	22	11	30	84	4	895
Gourmet Classic Turkey	1	552	32	14	66	74	4	1450
Gourmet Holey Guacamole	1	476	33	5	61	76	4	1449
Gourmet Kick-N Roast Beef	1	579	29	15	74	79	4	1802
Gourmet Mediterranean Veg-Out	1	506	20	9	0	90	8	818
Overstuffed Classic Reuben	1	962	60	43	156	57	4	3017
Overstuffed Corned Beef	1	661	43	19	97	77	3	2770
Overstuffed Ham & Cheese	1	889	60	36	147	79	4	2893
Overstuffed Manhattan Club	1	1122	69	40	178	120	6	2992

FOOD	PORTION	CALS	PROT	FAT	CHOL	CARB	FIBER	SOD
Overstuffed Pastrami	1	661	43	19	97	77	3	2770
Overstuffed TD Classic California	1	759	49	12	80	113	8	2089
Overstuffed TD Classic Club	1	1110	61	43	158	122	5	3062
Overstuffed TD Clubhouse	1	1079	69	37	171	117	5	2957
Pizzaah Bruschetta	1 piece	162	7	12	38	7	3	175
Pizzaah Cheese	1 piece	189	10	7	22	23	3	268
Pizzaah Grilled Chicken Bruschetta	1 piece	343	17	21	78	24	3	625
Pizzaah Sausage	1 piece	211	11	17	42	6	2	306
Pizzaah Veggie	1 piece	238	12	10	22	32	7	272
Specialty All American Duo	1	752	46	28	107	78	4	1767
Specialty Big Apple Club	1	797	41	37	110	75	4	2438
Specialty Chicken Caesar	1	611	31	19	64	78	4	1459
Specialty Roma Italian	1	764	40	34	109	76	4	2393
Specialty Turkey Club	1	782	43	34	113	75	4	2355
Toasted Cafe Chicken Melt	1	815	51	32	133	80	4	1767
Toasted Deli Style Turkey	1	732	48	25	115	76	4	1602
Toasted Roast Beef Parmesan Grinder	1	583	36	15	66	76	4	1896
Toasted Spicy Italian Sub	1	770	40	34	109	77	4	2505
Toasted Tuna Melt	1	641	32	23	54	75	4	1310
SOUPS								
Beef Barley Mushroom	1 serv (8 oz)	100	6	3	–	12	–	1040
Boston Clam Chowder	1 serv (8 oz)	210	2	13	–	20	–	900
Chicken & Wild Rice	1 serv (8 oz)	190	5	9	–	22	–	960
Chicken Gumbo	1 serv (8 oz)	130	8	3	–	19	–	920
Cream Of Potato	1 serv (8 oz)	240	4	14	–	24	–	1080
Hearty Vegetable Beef	1 serv (8 oz)	100	5	1	–	16	–	880
New England Clam Chowder	1 serv (8 oz)	220	6	13	–	21	–	1100
Split Pea w/ Ham	1 serv (8 oz)	90	5	2	–	15	–	950
Wisconsin Cheese	1 serv (8 oz)	210	8	11	–	20	–	1050
TOPPINGS								
Cream Cheese	2 tbsp	90	1	9	25	2	0	200
Cream Cheese Cheddar Jalapeno	2 tbsp	90	1	8	25	2	0	150
Cream Cheese Garden Vegetable	2 tbsp	90	1	9	25	2	0	140
Cream Cheese Lite	2 tbsp	60	2	5	15	3	0	170

FOOD	PORTION	CALS	PROT	FAT	CHOL	CARB	FIBER	SOD
Cream Cheese Onion Chive	2 tbsp	80	1	8	25	2	0	110
Cream Cheese Strawberry	2 tbsp	90	1	5	20	5	0	65
Cream Cheese Whipped	2 tbsp	70	1	7	20	1	0	65
Cream Cheese Whipped Brown Sugar Cinnamon	2 tbsp	70	tr	5	15	5	0	80
Cream Cheese Whipped Reduced Fat Spring Veggie	2 tbsp	60	1	5	15	2	0	100

BAJA FRESH
CHILDREN'S MENU SELECTIONS

FOOD	PORTION	CALS	PROT	FAT	CHOL	CARB	FIBER	SOD
Kid's Mini Burrito Bean & Cheese	1 serv	540	18	14	25	84	11	1050
Kid's Mini Burrito Bean & Cheese w/ Chicken	1 serv	590	28	15	50	84	12	1200
Kid's Mini Quesadilla Cheese	1 serv	610	19	26	50	72	5	940
Kid's Mini Quesadilla Cheese w/ Chicken	1 serv	650	28	27	75	72	5	1090
Kid's Taquitos Chicken	1 serv	630	18	33	70	60	4	990

MAIN MENU SELECTIONS

FOOD	PORTION	CALS	PROT	FAT	CHOL	CARB	FIBER	SOD
Baja Burrito Chicken	1 serv	790	52	38	120	65	8	2140
Baja Burrito Steak	1 serv	850	49	46	125	67	7	2260
Black Beans	1 serv	360	23	3	5	61	26	1120
Burrito Baja Breaded Fish	1 serv	850	40	44	80	78	7	1900
Burrito Baja Carnitas	1 serv	830	45	45	115	67	8	2280
Burrito Baja Mahi Mahi	1 serv	780	51	38	115	66	7	1840
Burrito Baja Shrimp	1 serv	760	47	37	295	66	7	2230
Burrito Bare Carnitas	1 serv	600	37	14	70	99	20	2480
Burrito Bare Chicken	1 serv	640	45	7	75	97	20	2330
Burrito Bare Steak	1 serv	700	41	15	80	99	19	2450
Burrito Bare Veggie & Cheese	1 serv	580	19	10	15	101	20	1950
Burrito Bean & Cheese Breaded Fish	1 serv	1030	54	41	95	108	20	1990
Burrito Bean & Cheese Carnitas	1 serv	1010	59	42	130	98	21	2370
Burrito Bean & Cheese Chicken	1 serv	970	67	35	135	96	21	2230

FOOD	PORTION	CALS	PROT	FAT	CHOL	CARB	FIBER	SOD
Burrito Bean & Cheese Mahi Mahi	1 serv	960	65	35	130	96	20	1930
Burrito Bean & Cheese No Meat	1 serv	840	39	33	65	96	20	1790
Burrito Bean & Cheese Shrimp	1 serv	950	61	34	310	96	20	2320
Burrito Bean & Cheese Steak	1 serv	1030	64	43	140	97	20	2350
Burrito Dos Manos Breaded Fish	1 serv	890	39	33	70	107	13	2025
Burrito Dos Manos Carnitas	1 serv	780	34	30	73	95	14	2115
Burrito Dos Manos Chicken	½ serv	760	38	26	75	94	14	2040
Burrito Dos Manos Mahi Mahi	1 serv	780	42	26	83	95	13	1915
Burrito Dos Manos Shrimp	1 serv	780	41	26	223	95	13	2220
Burrito Dos Manos Steak	½ serv	795	36	30	78	95	13	2105
Burrito Grilled Veggie	1 serv	506	32	33	65	94	16	1880
Burrito Mexicano Breaded Fish	1 serv	850	37	19	30	129	18	2040
Burrito Mexicano Carnitas	1 serv	830	42	20	70	119	19	2420
Burrito Mexicano Chicken	1 serv	790	50	13	75	117	20	2270
Burrito Mexicano Mahi Mahi	1 serv	790	49	13	70	117	18	1970
Burrito Mexicano Shrimp	1 serv	770	44	13	245	117	18	2370
Burrito Mexicano Steak	1 serv	860	47	21	118	118	18	2400
Burrito Ultimo Breaded Fish	1 serv	940	41	42	95	96	8	1950
Burrito Ultimo Carnitas	1 serv	920	46	44	130	86	9	2330
Burrito Ultimo Chicken	1 serv	880	54	36	140	84	9	2190
Burrito Ultimo Mahi Mahi	1 serv	880	52	36	130	84	8	1890
Burrito Ultimo Shrimp	1 serv	860	48	36	310	85	8	2280
Burrito Ultimo Steak	1 serv	950	50	44	140	85	8	2310
Chips & Guacamole	1 serv	1340	21	83	0	141	20	950
Chips & Salsa Baja	1 serv	810	13	37	0	98	14	1140
Fajitas Corn Tortillas Breaded Fish	1 serv	1060	51	37	85	130	22	2180
Fajitas Corn Tortillas Carnitas	1 serv	920	50	34	120	108	23	2610
Fajitas Corn Tortillas Chicken	1 serv	860	61	24	130	105	24	2400

FOOD	PORTION	CALS	PROT	FAT	CHOL	CARB	FIBER	SOD
Fajitas Corn Tortillas Mahi Mahi	1 serv	840	57	23	110	105	22	1960
Fajitas Corn Tortillas Shrimp	1 serv	840	55	23	390	106	22	2570
Fajitas Corn Tortillas Steak	1 serv	960	58	36	135	107	22	2600
Fajitas Flour Tortillas Breaded Fish	1 serv	1340	59	46	85	172	25	3020
Fajitas Flour Tortillas Carnitas	1 serv	1190	58	43	120	150	26	3450
Fajitas Flour Tortillas Chicken	1 serv	1140	69	33	130	147	27	3240
Fajitas Flour Tortillas Mahi Mahi	1 serv	1120	64	32	110	147	25	2800
Fajitas Flour Tortillas Shrimp	1 serv	1120	62	32	390	148	25	3410
Fajitas Flour Tortillas Steak	1 serv	960	58	36	135	170	22	2600
Guacamole Side	1 (3 oz)	110	2	13	0	5	2	270
Nachos Breaded Frish	1 serv	2090	78	116	185	176	31	2740
Nachos Carnitas	1 serv	2060	83	117	220	166	32	3120
Nachos Cheese	1 serv	1890	63	108	155	163	31	2530
Nachos Chicken	1 serv	2020	91	110	230	164	32	2980
Nachos Mahi Mahi	1 serv	2020	90	110	220	164	31	2600
Nachos Shrimp	1 serv	2000	85	110	395	164	31	3060
Nachos Steak	1 serv	2120	96	118	163	163	31	2990
Pico De Gallo Side	1 serv (8 oz)	50	2	1	0	12	3	890
Pinto Beans	1 serv	320	19	1	5	56	21	840
Pronto Guacamole Side	1 serv (6 oz)	560	9	34	0	60	8	370
Quesadilla Breaded Frish	1 serv	1400	62	86	170	96	8	2350
Quesadilla Carnitas	1 serv	1370	67	87	205	86	9	2730
Quesadilla Cheese	1 serv	1200	47	78	140	84	8	2140
Quesadilla Chicken	1 serv	1330	75	80	215	84	9	2590
Quesadilla Mahi Mahi	1 serv	1330	73	79	205	84	8	2290
Quesadilla Shrimp	1 serv	1310	69	79	385	84	8	2680
Quesadilla Steak	1 serv	1430	80	87	240	84	8	2600
Quesadilla Veggie	1 serv	1260	48	78	145	96	11	2310
Rice	1 serv	280	5	4	0	55	4	980
Rice & Beans Plate	1 serv	420	18	5	10	72	18	1320
Salsa Baja Side	1 serv (8 oz)	70	2	3	0	7	4	970
Salsa Roja Side	1 serv (8 oz)	70	3	1	0	13	4	1080

FOOD	PORTION	CALS	PROT	FAT	CHOL	CARB	FIBER	SOD
Salsa Verde Side	1 serv (8 oz)	50	2	0	0	11	3	1170
Soup Tortilla w/ Chicken	1 serv (13.6 oz)	320	17	14	40	29	4	2760
Soup Tortilla w/o Chicken	1 serv (12.4 oz)	270	8	14	45	29	4	2600
Taco Grilled Mahi Mahi	1 serv	230	12	9	20	26	4	300
Taco Baja Breaded Fish	1 serv	250	8	13	15	27	2	420
Taco Baja Chicken	1 serv	210	12	5	25	28	2	230
Taco Baja Shrimp	1 serv	200	11	5	90	28	2	280
Taco Baja Steak	1 serv	230	11	8	25	28	2	260
Taco Soft Breaded Fish	1 serv	240	10	11	20	23	2	490
Taco Soft Carnitas	1 serv	250	13	12	35	21	2	640
Taco Soft Chicken	1 serv	230	16	10	35	20	2	590
Taco Soft Mahi Mahi	1 serv	240	17	10	40	20	2	490
Taco Soft Shrimp	1 serv	230	15	10	105	21	2	640
Taco Soft Steak	1 serv	260	15	13	40	21	2	640
Taquitos Chicken w/ Beans	3	780	39	40	85	68	17	1810
Taquitos Chicken w/ Rice	3	740	30	40	85	66	8	1770
Veggie Mix	1 serv	110	3	0	0	24	6	330
SALAD DRESSINGS								
Chipotle Vinaigrette	1 serv (2.5 oz)	110	0	9	0	0	0	490
Fat Free Salsa Verde	1 serv (2.5 oz)	15	0	0	0	3	1	370
Olive Oil Vinaigrette	1 serv (2.5 oz)	290	0	31	0	2	0	290
Ranch	1 serv (2.5 oz)	260	2	26	50	4	0	470
SALADS								
Baja Ensalada Chicken	1 serv	310	46	7	18	18	7	1210
Baja Ensalada Chicken	1 serv	370	35	18	100	20	7	1410
Baja Ensalada Shrimp	1 serv	230	28	6	250	18	6	1110
Baja Ensalada Steak	1 serv	450	54	18	150	18	6	1240
Chipotle w/ Carnitas	1 serv	640	38	30	95	56	10	1280
Chipotle w/ Chicken	1 serv	590	47	22	105	54	11	1110
Chipotle w/ Steak	1 serv	700	54	31	135	54	9	1140
Side By Side Carnitas	1 serv	570	46	40	140	16	8	1560
Side By Side Chicken	1 serv	500	60	27	150	12	9	1310
Side By Side Steak	1 serv	620	55	42	160	14	6	1550
Side Salad	1 (6.5 oz)	130	5	6	5	16	4	430

FOOD	PORTION	CALS	PROT	FAT	CHOL	CARB	FIBER	SOD
Tostada Breaded Fish	1 serv	1200	47	61	71	111	25	2140
Tostada Carnitas	1 serv	1180	52	62	100	100	26	2520
Tostada Chicken	1 serv	1140	60	55	115	98	27	2370
Tostada Mahi Mahi	1 serv	1130	59	55	105	99	25	2070
Tostada No Meat	1 serv	1010	32	53	40	98	25	1930
Tostada Shrimp	1 serv	1120	55	55	285	99	25	2460
Tostada Steak	1 serv	1230	65	63	140	98	25	2380

BEAR ROCK CAFE
SANDWICHES

FOOD	PORTION	CALS	PROT	FAT	CHOL	CARB	FIBER	SOD
Colorado Turkey Club	1	855	38	37	126	95	5	2310
Coop's Chicken Salad Croissant	1	439	24	31	44	46	5	375
Garden Grill Ciabatta	1	406	12	25	33	55	4	907
Giant Panda Wrap	1	556	31	23	58	68	23	2045
Hoot Owl	1	641	34	42	92	32	2	1618
Rising Sunflower	1	596	35	35	86	35	2	1694
Roast Turkey & Bacon	1	522	32	30	71	31	2	1656
Rockslide Focaccia	1	958	43	62	129	57	3	2546
The Moose	1	976	54	54	142	64	7	2565

BEN & JERRY'S
FROZEN YOGURT

FOOD	PORTION	CALS	PROT	FAT	CHOL	CARB	FIBER	SOD
Low Fat Cherry Garcia	½ cup	170	4	3	20	32	tr	65
Low Fat Chocolate Fudge Brownie	½ cup	190	5	3	15	35	1	100
Low Fat Half Baked	½ cup	190	5	3	20	35	tr	100
Phish Food	½ cup	220	4	5	15	41	1	95

ICE CREAM

FOOD	PORTION	CALS	PROT	FAT	CHOL	CARB	FIBER	SOD
Bar Cherry Garcia	1	270	4	19	35	29	1	45
Bar Half Baked	1	340	5	16	40	46	2	125
Bar Vanilla	1	300	4	20	45	26	1	60
Bar Vanilla Almond	1	340	5	23	65	30	2	135
Black & Tan	½ cup	230	4	13	50	24	1	55
Brownie Batter	½ cup	310	5	18	70	32	1	115
Butter Pecan	½ cup	280	4	21	65	20	1	105
Cherry Garcia	½ cup	250	4	14	60	26	tr	50
Chocolate	½ cup	260	4	16	50	25	2	50
Chocolate Chip Cookie Dough	½ cup	270	4	15	65	32	0	85
Chocolate Fudge Brownie	½ cup	260	5	13	35	32	2	80

FOOD	PORTION	CALS	PROT	FAT	CHOL	CARB	FIBER	SOD
Chubby Hubby	½ cup	330	7	20	55	31	1	150
Chunky Monkey	½ cup	300	5	18	55	30	1	45
Coffee	½ cup	240	4	15	75	21	0	60
Coffee Heath Bar Crunch	½ cup	290	4	18	65	29	0	–
Dave Matthews Band Magic Brownies	½ cup	250	4	13	60	29	0	75
Dublin Mudslide	½ cup	270	4	16	65	28	tr	80
Everything But The	½ cup	310	5	19	50	30	1	85
Fossil Fuel	½ cup	280	4	17	60	30	1	60
Fudge Central	½ cup	300	4	18	55	31	1	60
Half Baked	½ cup	280	5	14	50	34	tr	90
In A Crunch	½ cup	350	6	23	55	30	1	150
Karamel Sutra	½ cup	280	4	15	50	32	1	75
Marsha Marsha Marshmallow	½ cup	300	4	17	30	33	1	60
Mint Chocolate Cookie	½ cup	260	4	16	65	26	0	100
Neapolitan Dynamite	½ cup	250	4	13	45	29	1	70
New York Super Fudge Chunk	½ cup	310	5	20	40	29	2	55
Oatmeal Cookie Chunk	½ cup	270	4	15	55	31	tr	120
Organic Chocolate Fudge Brownie	½ cup	270	4	13	35	30	2	55
Organic Strawberry	½ cup	210	3	12	55	21	0	40
Organic Sweet Cream & Cookies	½ cup	250	4	15	60	24	0	95
Organic Vanilla	½ cup	220	3	14	65	18	0	50
Peanut Butter Cup	½ cup	360	7	26	60	27	1	125
Phish Food	½ cup	280	4	13	30	37	1	85
Pistachio Pistachio	½ cup	260	5	17	65	21	tr	55
Sandwich Wich Ice Cream Cookie	1	350	4	18	55	45	1	220
Strawberry	½ cup	230	4	13	65	26	0	50
The Godfather	½ cup	270	4	14	30	32	2	50
Turtle Soup	½ cup	280	4	15	60	30	1	100
Uncanny Cashew	½ cup	290	4	19	70	27	0	130
Vanilla Caramel Fudge	½ cup	280	4	15	70	31	0	105
Vanilla Heath Bar Crunch	½ cup	290	4	18	65	29	0	120
Vermonty Python	½ cup	310	4	19	60	30	1	90
SORBETS								
Berried Treasure	½ cup	110	0	0	0	29	1	5

FOOD	PORTION	CALS	PROT	FAT	CHOL	CARB	FIBER	SOD
Jamaican Me Crazy	½ cup	130	0	0	0	33	4	10
Strawberry Kiwi Swirl	½ cup	110	0	0	0	28	1	10

BILLY'S BURGER HUT
BEVERAGES

FOOD	PORTION	CALS	PROT	FAT	CHOL	CARB	FIBER	SOD
Shake Chocolate	1 (20 oz)	420	9	10	30	63	0	260
Shake Vanilla	1 (20 oz)	320	8	10	25	49	0	157

MAIN MENU SELECTIONS

FOOD	PORTION	CALS	PROT	FAT	CHOL	CARB	FIBER	SOD
Big Billy's Roast Beef Sub	1	843	51	54	151	62	3	2860
Billyburger	1	426	20	22	63	35	3	1076
Billyburger w/ Cheese	1	498	23	35	57	35	4	1276
Billy's Best Red Potato Salad	1 serv	190	2	9	80	12	3	650
Billy's Biggest Burger ½ Pounder w/ Everything	1	852	70	58	140	61	4	2229
Billy's Famous 7 Layer Salad	1 serv	558	10	49	119	18	2	680
Billy's Seafood Sandwich	1	399	21	18	42	43	3	890
Caesar Side Salad	1 serv	360	11	28	70	12	4	610
Chili w/ Cheese & Onion	1 serv	380	33	12	64	35	7	1004
Cowboy Cobb Salad	1 serv	735	29	45	239	25	9	1450
Cowboy Coleslaw	1 serv	180	1	9	10	11	3	250
French Fries	1 reg	230	5	12	0	25	1	253
Onion Rings	1 serv	250	2	10	0	37	1	955
Super Billy Burger w/ Bacon	1	663	35	41	98	39	4	1869

BOB EVANS
BREAKFAST SELECTIONS

FOOD	PORTION	CALS	PROT	FAT	CHOL	CARB	FIBER	SOD
Bacon	1 piece	36	1	4	5	0	0	54
Benedict Ham & Cheese	1 serv	826	44	52	564	44	0	3137
Country Benedict Sausage	1 serv	936	44	66	536	40	0	2098
Country Benedict Spinach Bacon & Tomato	1 serv	729	30	48	494	42	1	1885
Country Biscuit Breakfast	1 serv	659	24	45	269	40	1	1703
Egg Hardcooked	1	60	6	4	190	1	0	55
Egg Over Easy	1	101	7	8	229	1	0	68
Egg Beaters	1 serv	173	28	12	5	3	0	581
Eggs Scrambled	1 serv	255	20	17	723	2	0	213
French Toast	1 slice	131	3	2	25	13	1	175
French Toast Stuffed Plain	1 serv	599	11	20	99	53	3	689

FOOD	PORTION	CALS	PROT	FAT	CHOL	CARB	FIBER	SOD
Fruit & Yogurt Plate	1 serv	403	9	2	5	93	9	109
Grits	1 serv	178	3	7	9	28	2	172
Ham Smoked	1 slice	87	14	2	52	2	0	1131
Hotcake Blueberry	1	328	6	9	0	55	2	749
Hotcake Buttermilk	1	318	6	9	0	53	2	746
Hotcake Cinnamon	1	417	6	15	0	66	2	749
Hotcake Multigrain	1	322	7	10	0	52	3	773
Mush	1 serv	79	1	3	0	11	2	466
Oatmeal	1 serv	172	6	3	0	32	4	394
Omelette Bacon & Cheese	1 serv	825	40	66	826	6	1	1603
Omelette Border Scramble	1	756	42	58	846	15	3	1059
Omelette Egg Beaters Bacon & Cheese	1 serv	615	57	47	108	7	1	1972
Omelette Egg Beaters Border Scramble	1 serv	517	48	37	72	16	3	1411
Omelette Egg Beaters Farmer's Market	1 serv	569	49	41	92	14	2	2108
Omelette Egg Beaters Garden Harvest	1 serv	444	40	31	64	14	2	1610
Omelette Egg Beaters Ham & Cheddar	1 serv	426	51	29	80	5	1	1789
Omelette Egg Beaters Sausage & Cheddar	1 serv	502	49	40	73	4	1	1295
Omelette Egg Beaters Three Cheese	1 serv	435	43	34	78	5	1	1394
Omelette Farmer's Market	1	778	42	60	810	13	2	1739
Omelette Garden Harvest	1 serv	654	33	50	782	13	2	1241
Omelette Ham & Cheddar	1 serv	634	44	48	798	3	1	1419
Omelette Sausage & Cheddar	1 serv	741	42	61	847	3	1	942
Omelette Three Cheese	1 serv	645	35	52	796	4	1	1025
Omelette Western	1 serv	654	44	48	798	8	2	1420
Pot Roast Hash	1 serv	652	38	39	533	34	4	1084
Sausage Gravy Bowl	1 serv	268	7	17	17	21	0	1238
Sausage Link	1	125	5	11	14	0	0	184
Skillet Sunshine	1 serv	842	37	60	819	36	4	1474
Waffles Sweet Cream	1 serv	598	15	12	149	100	3	1288
CHILDREN'S MENU SELECTIONS								
Fruit & Yogurt Dippers	1 serv	275	7	2	5	61	5	95

FOOD	PORTION	CALS	PROT	FAT	CHOL	CARB	FIBER	SOD
Hotcakes	1 serv	501	9	17	0	79	2	1071
Kid's Macaroni & Cheese	1 serv	320	11	11	23	45	2	778
Kids Pasta	1 serv	113	3	5	12	15	1	857
Mini Cheeseburgers	1 serv	306	12	19	40	21	1	525
Smiley Face Potatoes	1 serv	524	5	31	2	57	3	646
Sundae Fudge Blast	1 serv	244	3	11	25	33	0	81
Sundae Reese's I'm Smiling	1 serv	330	5	17	26	41	1	130
MAIN MENU SELECTIONS								
Seniors Chicken Parmesan	1 serv	522	38	26	127	33	3	2404
Seniors Garden Vegetable Alfredo Chicken	1 serv	452	26	26	74	29	5	1678
Seniors Garen Vegetable Alfredo	1 serv	363	11	23	36	29	5	1322
Seniors Steak Tips & Noodles	1 serv	422	33	22	101	23	2	2251
Seniors Stir-Fry Chicken	1 serv	368	21	13	37	44	5	1385
SOUPS								
Bean	1 cup	144	10	3	8	19	3	778
Cheddar Baked Potato	1 cup	294	10	20	34	19	1	1168
Sausage Chili	1 cup	268	16	17	42	18	7	687
Vegetable Beef	1 cup	135	6	5	14	17	3	370

BOJANGLES

FOOD	PORTION	CALS	PROT	FAT	CHOL	CARB	FIBER	SOD
Biscuit	1	243	4	12	2	29	2	663
Biscuit Sandwich Bacon	1	290	8	17	10	26	1	810
Biscuit Sandwich Bacon Egg Cheese	1	550	17	42	160	27	1	1250
Biscuit Sandwich Cajun Filet	1	454	20	21	41	46	1	949
Biscuit Sandwich Country Ham	1	270	9	15	20	26	1	1010
Biscuit Sandwich Egg	1	400	8	30	120	26	1	630
Biscuit Sandwich Sausage	1	350	9	23	20	26	1	810
Biscuit Sandwich Smoked Sausage	1	380	10	26	20	27	1	940
Biscuit Sandwich Steak	1	649	14	49	34	37	1	1126
Botato Rounds	1 serv	235	3	11	13	31	3	328
Buffalo Bites	1 serv	180	27	5	105	5	0	720
Cajun Pintos	1 serv	110	6	0	0	18	6	480
Cajun Spiced Breast	1 serv	278	18	17	75	12	tr	565

FOOD	PORTION	CALS	PROT	FAT	CHOL	CARB	FIBER	SOD
Cajun Spiced Leg	1 serv	264	19	16	96	11	tr	530
Cajun Spiced Thigh	1 serv	310	15	23	67	11	tr	465
Cajun Spiced Wing	1 serv	355	21	25	94	11	tr	630
Chicken Supremes	1 serv	337	21	16	58	26	1	629
Corn On The Cob	1 serv	140	5	2	0	34	2	20
Dirty Rice	1 serv	166	5	6	10	24	1	762
Green Beans	1 serv	25	0	0	0	5	2	710
Macaroni & Cheese	1 serv	198	7	14	26	12	tr	418
Marinated Cole Slaw	1 serv	136	1	3	0	26	3	454
Potatoes w/o Gravy	1 serv	80	2	1	0	16	1	380
Sandwich Cajun Filet w/o Mayo	1	337	22	11	45	41	3	401
Sandwich Cajun Filet w/ Mayo	1	437	22	22	55	41	3	506
Sandwich Grilled Filet w/ Mayo	1	335	23	16	61	25	2	645
Sandwich Grilled Filet w/o Mayo	1	235	23	5	51	25	2	540
Seasoned Fries	1 serv	344	5	19	13	39	4	480
Southern Style Breast	1 serv	261	16	16	76	12	tr	702
Southern Style Leg	1 serv	254	19	15	94	11	tr	446
Southern Style Thigh	1 serv	308	16	21	78	14	tr	630
Southern Style Wing	1 serv	337	17	21	86	19	tr	684
Sweet Biscuit Bo Berry	1	320	4	18	tr	37	1	560
Sweet Biscuit Cinnamon	1	320	4	18	tr	37	1	560

BOSTON MARKET

DESSERTS

Apple Pie	1 slice	420	3	20	0	56	2	650
Brownie Chocolate Chip Fudge	1	580	9	23	90	81	3	390
Chocolate Cake	1 serv	600	5	32	65	75	2	210
Cookie Chocolate Chip	1	370	4	19	20	49	2	340
Cornbread	1 piece	180	2	5	10	31	0	320

MAIN MENU SELECTIONS

Broccoli w/ Garlic Butter	1 serv	80	3	6	0	6	3	230
Butternut Squash	1 serv	140	2	5	10	25	2	35
Carver Boston Chicken	1	700	44	29	90	68	3	1560
Carver Boston Meatloaf	1	940	49	45	155	96	6	2080
Carver Boston Sirloin Dip	1	1000	67	51	200	70	3	1690

FOOD	PORTION	CALS	PROT	FAT	CHOL	CARB	FIBER	SOD
Carver Boston Turkey	1	770	66	27	125	68	3	1810
Carver Boston Turkey Dip	1	770	66	27	125	67	3	1890
Carver Half Boston Chicken	1	340	24	15	65	29	1	710
Carver Half Boston Sirloin Dip	1	500	33	25	100	35	1	850
Carver Half Boston Turkey	1	390	33	14	60	34	2	910
Cinnamon Apples	1 serv	210	0	3	0	47	3	15
Cranberry Walnut Relish	1 serv	140	1	2	0	30	2	0
Creamed Spinach	1 serv	280	9	23	70	12	4	580
Dip Spinach Artichoke	1 serv	100	3	8	15	3	1	220
Family Meals Boneless Turkey Breast	1 serv (5 oz)	180	38	3	70	0	0	620
Family Meals Raosted Turkey	1 serv (5 oz)	180	38	3	72	0	0	635
Family Meals Rotisserie Chicken	1 serv (6 oz)	290	39	14	175	4	0	710
Family Meals Sprial Sliced Ham	1 serv (8 oz)	450	40	26	140	13	0	2230
Family Meals Whole Turkey	1 serv (6.7 oz)	310	40	18	135	0	0	940
Fresh Vegetable Stuffing	1 serv	190	3	8	0	25	2	580
Garden Fresh Coleslaw	1 serv	170	2	9	10	21	2	270
Garlic Dill New Potatoes	1 serv	140	3	3	0	24	3	120
Green Bean Casserole	1 serv	60	2	2	5	9	2	620
Green Beans	1 serv	60	2	4	0	7	3	180
Individual Meal ¼ White Rotisserie Chicken	1 serv	290	45	11	170	4	0	780
Individual Meal Award Winning Roasted Sirloin	1 serv	290	39	15	125	0	0	440
Individual Meal Meatloaf	1 serv	480	29	33	125	23	2	970
Individual Meals 1 Thigh & 1 Drumstick	1 serv	300	32	17	180	6	0	630
Individual Meals ¼ White Rotisserie Chicken No Skin	1 serv	210	42	2	135	6	0	640
Individual Meals 3 Piece Dark	1 serv	380	45	19	250	7	0	880
Individual Meals 3 Piece Dark Skinless	1 serv	240	37	8	205	7	0	650

FOOD	PORTION	CALS	PROT	FAT	CHOL	CARB	FIBER	SOD
Individual Meals Roasted Turkey	1 serv	180	38	3	72	0	0	635
Macaroni & Cheese	1 serv	330	14	12	30	39	1	1290
Mashed Potatoes	1 serv	210	4	9	25	29	3	660
Pot Pie Pastry Topped Chicken	1	780	29	47	125	60	4	930
Poultry Gravy	1 serv (4 oz)	15	1	1	0	4	0	570
Seasonal Fresh Fruit Salad	1 serv	60	1	0	0	15	1	20
Spinach w/ Garlic Butter Sauce	1 serv	130	5	9	20	9	5	200
Squash Casserole	1 serv	320	9	24	50	21	3	1380
Steamed Fresh Vegetables	1 serv	60	2	2	0	8	3	40
Sweet Corn	1 serv	170	6	4	0	37	2	95
Sweet Potato Casserole	1 serv	460	4	17	20	77	3	210
SALADS								
Entree Caesar	1 serv	500	13	45	45	12	3	1190
Entree Caesar w/o Dressing	1 serv	140	11	8	15	8	2	280
Entree Market Chopped	1 serv	580	10	48	10	30	9	1990
Entree Market Chopped w/o Dressing	1 serv	210	10	9	10	28	9	280
Side Caesar	1 serv	400	5	40	30	7	2	980
Side Caesar w/o Dressing	1 serv	40	3	2	5	3	1	75
Side Market Chopped	1 serv	440	4	43	5	12	3	1790
Side Market Chopped w/o Dressing	1 serv	80	3	4	5	10	3	85
SOUPS								
Chicken Noodle	1 serv	170	13	5	60	17	1	210
Chicken Tortilla w/ Toppings	1 serv	340	12	22	45	24	1	1310
Tortilla Soup w/o Toppings	1 serv	980	5	5	15	7	1	900

BOSTON PIZZA
CHILDREN'S MENU SELECTIONS

FOOD	PORTION	CALS	PROT	FAT	CHOL	CARB	FIBER	SOD
Baked Salmon w/ Ceasar Salad	1 serv	330	23	14	–	13	tr	330
Bug N' Cheese	1 serv	500	21	13	–	73	3	710
Chicken Fingers w/ Fries	1 serv	390	26	19	–	28	2	570
Pizza Pint Size	1	390	19	7	–	64	tr	520

FOOD	PORTION	CALS	PROT	FAT	CHOL	CARB	FIBER	SOD
Quesadilla Bacon Double Cheeseburger w/ Caesar Salad	1 serv	540	26	27	–	49	3	1660
Reduced Size Fruit Cup	1 serv	80	0	0	0	18	tr	0
Sandwich Grilled Chicken w/ Garden Greens	1 serv	600	10	38	–	45	3	1000
Sandwich Grilled Chicken w/ Garden Greens	1 serv	780	34	52	–	47	2	810
Super Spaghetti	1 serv	440	12	13	–	68	5	690
Wrap Ham & Cheese w/ Fries	1 serv	550	16	28	–	60	4	790
DESSERTS								
Blondie Maple	1	850	7	43	–	111	1	350
Blondie Maple Bite Size	1	430	4	21	–	58	tr	170
Brownie Chocolate Addiction	1	490	5	13	–	92	2	170
Brownie Chocolate Addiction Bite Size	1	200	2	7	–	35	1	90
Cheesecake New York	1 slice	620	11	33	–	80	0	440
Cheesecake Vanilla Bean	1 slice	770	9	52	–	70	1	320
Chocolate Explosion	1 serv	890	11	50	–	103	4	510
Tarte Au Sucre	1 serv	310	4	21	–	71	1	9500
MAIN MENU SELECTIONS								
Angus Beef Sirloin Steak w/ Spaghetti	1 serv	1260	72	70	–	83	8	1560
Baked 3 Cheese Penne	1 half order	460	21	14	–	62	4	1030
Baked Seven Cheese Ravioli	1 half order	310	17	14	–	28	2	1000
Baked Shrimp & Feta Penne	1 half order	480	28	19	–	54	4	690
Boston's Lasagne	1 half order	340	18	10	–	45	3	860
Boston's Smokey Mountain Spaghetti	1 order	1290	59	47	–	161	13	2650
Chicken & Mushroom Fettuccini	1 half order	710	23	38	–	72	4	680
Chicken Parmesan w/ Seasonal Vegetables	1 serv	1060	47	74	–	55	9	1190
Fries	1 serv	430	7	25	–	45	5	640
Garlic Mashed Potatoes	1 serv	730	6	60	–	42	5	1800
Garlic Toast	1 slice	150	3	6	–	20	1	330
Homestyle Lasagna	1 order	590	39	33	–	37	4	1910

FOOD	PORTION	CALS	PROT	FAT	CHOL	CARB	FIBER	SOD
Jambalaya Fettuccini	1 half order	860	33	51	–	71	6	2170
Lemon Baked Salmon w/ Fries	1 serv	1150	50	74	–	61	9	2330
Mama Meata Penne	1 half order	940	35	62	–	66	7	1890
Mushroom Chicken w/ Garlic Mashed Potatoes	1 serv	1030	68	62	–	53	9	1450
Pad Thai w/ Chicken	1 serv	2110	77	47	–	356	21	30
Pad Thai w/ Shrimp	1 serv	2090	77	45	–	358	22	390
Pollo Pomodoro Spaghetti	1 serv	520	26	14	–	73	7	1060
Salmon Filet Lemon Baked	1 serv	430	51	13	–	33	10	250
Scallop & Prawn Fettuccini	1 half order	710	21	41	–	67	5	660
Seasoned Vegetables	1 serv	70	0	0	–	10	4	760
Shrimp Skewers Lime & Parmesan	1 serv	190	15	7	–	20	3	1020
Sicilan Penne	1 half order	720	20	48	–	55	5	740
Sirloin Steak w/ Prawns & Fries	1 serv	1480	78	104	–	58	9	2140
Slow Roasted Pork Back Ribs w/ Fries	1 serv	1680	68	123	–	78	8	2080
Spaghetti w/ Alfredo Sauce	1 half order	440	15	11	–	70	3	710
Spaghetti w/ Bolognese	1 half order	400	15	5	–	73	5	670
Spaghetti w/ Creamy Tomato Sauce	1 half order	410	14	11	–	66	4	410
Spaghetti w/ Pomodoro Sauce	1 half order	450	13	14	–	68	5	720
Spicy Italian Penne	1 half order	980	30	61	–	81	5	1440
Starter Baked Raviolo Bites	1 serv	450	20	22	–	45	4	1410
Starter Basket Garlic Twist	1 serv	1140	32	39	–	165	tr	2910
Starter Basket Three Cheese Toast	1 serv	730	33	34	–	72	0	1580
Starter Boston's Poutine	1 serv	740	23	45	–	53	7	1860
Starter Bruschetta Sun Dried Tomato	1 serv	470	10	21	–	59	5	1130
Starter Cactus Cuts Potatoes & Dip	1 serv	1150	15	89	–	72	7	1430
Starter Chicken Fingers	1 serv	360	46	14	–	12	0	520
Starter Chicken Fingers Buffalo Style	1 serv	370	46	14	–	14	1	2080
Starter Cracked Pepper Dry Ribs	1 serv	380	69	41	–	3	1	1880

FOOD	PORTION	CALS	PROT	FAT	CHOL	CARB	FIBER	SOD
Starter Nachos Cactus w/ Cactus Dip	1 serv	1830	59	128	–	111	12	3160
Starter Nachos Spicy Chicken w/ Sour Cream & Salsa	1 serv	1430	73	72	–	126	12	2330
Starter Nachos Taco Beef w/ Sour Cream & Salsa	1 serv	1560	73	86	–	129	13	2180
Starter Nachos w/ Sour Cream & Salsa	1 serv	1320	53	71	–	126	12	1790
Starter Panzerotti Roll	1	820	41	32	–	94	3	1370
Starter Pizza Bread Bandera w/ Santa Fe Ranch Dip	1 serv	960	32	54	–	89	tr	1880
Starter Pizza Bread w/o Sauce	1 serv	500	15	12	–	84	0	660
Starter Potato Skins	1 serv	650	22	46	–	39	tr	1390
Starter Quesadilla Southwest w/ Sour Cream & Salsa	1 serv	770	55	27	–	77	4	1740
Starter Quesadilla Oven Roasted Chicken	1 serv	900	43	39	–	96	6	1850
Starter Shrimp Stuffed Mushroom Caps	1 serv	490	23	41	–	12	2	1150
Starter Team Platter w/ Dips & Sauces	1 serv	3030	153	205	–	144	12	3930
Starter Thai Chicken Bites	1 serv	540	46	15	–	55	2	1540
Starter Wings Breaded BBQ	1 serv	930	72	52	–	28	tr	3770
Starter Wings Breaded Honey Garlic	1 serv	940	72	52	–	31	0	3470
Starter Wings Breaded Mild	1 serv	880	72	52	–	17	0	3380
Starter Wings Breaded Teriyaki	1 serv	940	73	52	–	30	tr	3720
Starter Wings Breaded Thai	1 serv	1110	73	52	–	73	2	4720
Starter Wings Oven Roasted BBQ	1 serv	670	54	42	–	10	tr	410
Starter Wings Oven Roasted Honey Garlic	1 serv	700	54	42	–	26	2	125
Starter Wings Oven Roasted Hot	1 serv	620	53	42	–	9	tr	1060
Starter Wings Oven Roasted Teriyaki	1 serv	670	54	42	–	20	tr	360

FOOD	PORTION	CALS	PROT	FAT	CHOL	CARB	FIBER	SOD
Starter Wings Oven Roasted Thai Chili	1 serv	770	52	40	–	50	1	1030
The Ribber w/ Spaghetti	1 serv	970	49	43	–	96	5	1540
Tortellini w/ Alfredo Sauce	1 half order	340	12	15	–	37	1	880
Tortellini w/ Bolognese	1 half order	300	13	9	–	40	3	840
Tortellini w/ Creamy Tomato Sauce	1 half order	310	11	14	–	33	2	580
Tortellini w/ Pomodoro Sauce	1 half order	340	10	18	–	35	3	880
Veal Parmesan w/ Spaghetti	1 serv	1020	44	72	–	106	9	1920
PIZZA								
Bacon Double Cheeseburger Individual	1 pie	1140	73	54	–	94	2	2600
Bacon Double Cheeseburger Slice	1 med	280	18	12	–	25	tr	660
BBQ Chicken Individual	1 pie	730	37	24	–	93	1	1270
BBQ Chicken Slice	1 med	190	10	6	–	25	0	350
Boston Royal Individual	1 pie	840	53	27	–	98	3	1520
Boston Royal Slice	1 med	210	13	6	–	26	tr	410
Californian Slice	1 med	280	11	15	–	24	0	280
Clubhouse Individual	1 pie	1040	44	56	–	94	3	1070
Deluxe Individual	1 pie	850	55	29	–	94	2	1550
Deluxe Slice	1 med	220	14	7	–	25	tr	420
Great White North Individual	1 pie	960	63	39	–	91	1	1600
Great White North Slice	1 med	240	16	9	–	24	0	400
Hawaiian Individual	1 pie	780	49	20	–	101	2	1150
Hawaiian Slice	1 med	210	13	5	–	27	0	320
Indy California	1 (11.3 oz)	440	16	12	–	69	7	490
La Quebecoise Individual	1 pie	770	42	27	–	93	3	1650
La Quebecoise Slice	1 med	200	11	7	–	25	tr	460
Meateor Individual	1 pie	950	63	37	–	91	1	1640
Meateor Slice	1 med	260	17	10	–	25	0	460
Pepperoni Individual	1 pie	750	40	27	–	89	2	1650
Pepperoni Slice	1 med	200	10	7	–	24	0	450
Pepperoni & Mushroom Individual	1 pie	750	41	27	–	90	2	1650
Pepperoni & Mushroom Slice	1 med	200	10	7	–	24	tr	460
Popeye Individual	1 pie	720	41	22	–	93	2	1170

FOOD	PORTION	CALS	PROT	FAT	CHOL	CARB	FIBER	SOD
Popeye Slice	1 med	200	11	7	–	25	tr	320
Rustic Italian Individual	1 pie	950	49	39	–	102	3	4270
Rustic Italian Slice	1 med	260	13	10	–	28	tr	1250
Spicy Perogy Individual	1 pie	980	46	45	–	99	2	1090
Spicy Perogy Slice	1 med	280	13	13	–	28	0	330
Szechuan Individual	1 pie	750	39	17	–	99	1	800
Szechuan Slice	1 med	200	10	4	–	27	0	210
Tandoori Individual	1 pie	730	40	24	–	90	2	940
Tandoori Slice	1 med	200	11	6	–	25	tr	260
Thai Chicken Individual	1 pie	840	45	28	–	108	4	1090
Thai Chicken Slice	1 med	240	12	8	–	30	1	300
The Basic Individual	1 pie	620	34	16	–	88	1	1140
The Basic Slice	1 med	160	9	4	–	24	0	310
Tropical Chicken Individual	1 pie	970	59	39	–	97	tr	1690
Tropical Chicken Slice	1 med	260	15	10	–	26	0	450
Tuscan Individual	1 pie	940	50	37	–	106	5	1650
Tuscan Slice	1 med	250	13	10	–	29	1	460
Ultimate Pepperoni Individual	1 pie	870	46	37	–	89	2	2010
Ultimate Pepperoni Slice	1 med	230	12	9	–	24	tr	550
Vegetarian Individual	1 pie	680	37	16	–	101	4	1160
Vegetarian Slice	1 med	180	9	4	–	26	1	320
Zorba The Greek Individual	1 pie	800	43	29	–	97	4	1400
Zorba The Greek Slice	1 med	210	11	8	–	26	1	390
SALAD DRESSINGS AND TOPPINGS								
House Dressing	1 serv (2 oz)	270	1	28	–	4	tr	210
Ketchup	1 serv (2 oz)	60	1	1	–	15	tr	460
Salsa	1 serv (2 oz)	20	1	1	–	3	tr	350
Sour Cream	1 serv (2 oz)	100	2	9	–	3	0	0
SALADS								
Chipotle Chicken & Bacon	1 serv	630	28	41	–	40	6	1040
Crispy Chicken Pecan	1 serv	1100	62	86	–	25	6	1310
Entree Caesar	1 serv	500	13	38	–	29	4	920
Entree Spinach	1 serv	450	13	41	–	9	3	890
Garden Greens w/ House Dressing	1 serv	310	3	29	–	13	4	230
Garden Greens w/ Low Fat Raspberry Vinagrette	1 serv	130	2	6	–	19	3	160
Side Caesar	1 serv	170	5	11	–	13	1	300
Starter Spinach	1 serv	250	9	22	–	6	2	510

FOOD	PORTION	CALS	PROT	FAT	CHOL	CARB	FIBER	SOD
Taco Salad Beef w/o Sour Cream & Salsa	1 serv	610	31	33	–	50	6	830
Taco Salad Chicken w/o Sour Cream & Salsa	1 serv	480	31	19	–	48	6	990
Thai Chicken Salad	1 serv	1060	61	40	–	117	12	1020
SANDWICHES								
Beef Dip w/ Fries & Au Jus	1 serv	1340	77	62	–	118	5	3330
Boston Cheesesteak w/ Caesar Salad & Au Jus	1 serv	1300	86	66	–	90	3	3350
Boston Brute w/ Caesar Salad & Au Jus	1 serv	820	40	30	–	99	4	2660
Buffalo Chicken w/ Fries	1 serv	1220	55	53	–	130	7	4200
Chicken Parmesan w/ Fries	1 serv	1370	53	81	–	107	7	1810
Ciabatta Chicken w/ Caesar Salad	1 serv	920	40	53	–	73	4	1130
New York Steak w/ Garden Greens & Au Jus	1 serv	660	43	39	–	32	2	870
Stromboli Bacon Double Cheeseburger w/ Caesar Salad	1 serv	910	34	38	–	111	3	4230
Stromboli Chicken Santa Fe w/ Caesar Salad	1 serv	750	33	22	–	106	4	940
Stromboli Smoked Ham & Chicken w/ Caesar Salad	1 serv	880	52	31	–	99	1	820
Wrap Thai Chicken	1	570	26	9	–	98	6	1260
SOUPS								
Baked French Onion	1 serv	330	17	14	–	40	3	2480
Clam Chowder	1 serv	260	9	14	–	18	0	910

BROWN'S CHICKEN & PASTA

FOOD	PORTION	CALS	PROT	FAT	CHOL	CARB	FIBER	SOD
Breadsticks Garlic	1	50	1	1	tr	9	–	53
Breast	3 oz	284	26	15	67	12	–	529
Cheezy Potatoes	1 serv (12 oz)	188	7	11	19	16	1	580
Coleslaw	3 oz	131	2	10	6	9	–	211
Corn Fritters	3 oz	415	5	25	4	42	–	552
Corn On Cob	1 ear (3 in)	126	3	3	1	22	–	23
French Fries	3 oz	503	5	22	1	44	–	235
Gizzard	3 oz	387	24	20	88	26	–	795
Leg	3 oz	287	26	16	52	9	–	542

FOOD	PORTION	CALS	PROT	FAT	CHOL	CARB	FIBER	SOD
Liver	3 oz	341	23	19	147	19	–	704
Mostaccioli Meatless Sauce	1 serv (12 oz)	792	24	10	0	146	–	842
Mostaccioli w/ Meat Sauce	1 serv (12 oz)	835	27	14	17	144	–	898
Mushrooms	3 oz	289	6	16	1	30	–	671
Potato Salad	3 oz	94	2	4	11	13	–	639
Ravioli Meatless Sauce	1 serv (12 oz)	822	27	16	0	140	–	878
Ravioli w/ Meat Sauce	1 serv (12 oz)	865	30	20	17	138	–	934
Shrimp	3 oz	277	13	10	31	34	–	778
Spaghetti w/ Meat Sauce	1 serv (12 oz)	835	27	14	17	144	–	898
Spaghetti w/ Meatless Sauce	1 serv (12 oz)	792	24	10	0	146	–	842
Thigh	3 oz	355	21	24	63	13	–	574
Wing	3 oz	385	23	25	81	17	–	654

BRUEGGER'S BAGELS
BAGELS

FOOD	PORTION	CALS	PROT	FAT	CHOL	CARB	FIBER	SOD
Asiago Parmesan	1	330	14	4	5	62	4	640
Baked Apple	1	370	12	3	0	77	5	660
Blueberry	1	330	11	2	0	67	4	530
Chocolate Chip	1	350	12	5	0	64	4	570
Cinnamon Sugar	1	330	11	2	0	69	4	510
Cranberry Orange	1	330	11	2	0	68	4	510
Everything	1	320	12	2	0	64	4	740
Garlic	1	320	12	2	0	65	4	560
Honey Grain	1	330	13	3	0	65	5	510
Jalapeno Bagel	1	320	12	2	0	64	4	560
Multi-Grain	1	350	12	4	0	68	6	540
Onion	1	320	12	2	0	64	4	560
Plain	1	320	12	2	0	64	4	560
Poppy	1	320	12	3	0	64	4	560
Pumpernickel	1	330	12	3	0	67	12	620
Pumpkin	1	330	11	2	0	68	6	500
Rosemary Olive Oil	1	350	12	7	0	64	4	540
Salt	1	320	12	2	0	64	4	1610
Sesame	1	360	13	3	0	68	4	660

FOOD	PORTION	CALS	PROT	FAT	CHOL	CARB	FIBER	SOD
Sourdough	1	340	13	2	0	68	4	640
Square Asiago Parmesan	1	360	15	5	5	66	4	740
Square Everything	1	320	12	2	0	64	4	740
Square Plain	1	350	13	3	0	70	4	670
Square Sesame	1	360	13	3	0	68	4	660
Sun Dried Tomato	1	320	12	2	0	64	4	640
Whole Wheat	1	390	16	6	0	73	9	680
DESSERTS								
Brownie Chocolate Chunk	1	330	4	18	55	40	2	150
Cake Lemon Pound	1 slice	320	5	13	75	48	tr	170
Cookie Chocolate Chip	1	500	5	22	40	71	3	300
Cookie Oatmeal Raisin	1	460	5	19	40	71	3	240
Cookie Peanut Butter	1	480	8	23	40	63	2	300
Cookie Triple Chocolate Chunk	1	560	6	28	35	71	3	350
Cookie White Chocolate Macadamia	1	580	6	31	35	70	1	360
Luscious Lemon Bar	1	300	3	16	95	36	0	120
Marshmallow Chew	1	280	2	6	10	55	0	330
Muffin Blueberry	1	450	8	19	65	64	3	290
Muffin Chocolate	1	460	6	24	30	57	3	250
Oreo Dream Bar	1	470	5	28	60	49	2	270
Pecan Chocolate Chunk	1 slice	310	3	19	40	32	1	160
Raspberry Sammies	1 slice	340	3	16	45	44	1	170
Seven Layer Bar	1	650	10	43	10	58	5	280
Toffee Almond Bar	1	400	4	19	50	53	1	340
SALADS								
Caesar w/ Dressing	1 serv	270	9	17	40	22	2	900
Tossed Chicken Caesar w/ Dressing	1 serv	370	27	20	85	23	2	1420
Tossed Mandarin Medley	1 serv	340	8	17	20	36	4	660
Tossed Sesame Chicken	1 serv	480	22	28	45	30	2	780
SANDWICHES								
BLT w/ Mayo	1	570	20	23	35	72	5	1060
Chicken Breast	1	660	47	11	95	87	5	780
Chicken Fajita	1	530	30	11	80	81	6	1040
Chicken Salad w/ Mayo	1	630	28	26	80	73	5	1080
Cranberry Gobbler	1	620	32	21	55	78	5	1430
Cuban Chicken	1	680	44	25	85	74	4	2180
Denver Egg	1	460	30	18	205	74	5	1150

FOOD	PORTION	CALS	PROT	FAT	CHOL	CARB	FIBER	SOD
Egg Cheese	1	420	23	18	195	71	4	1090
Egg Cheese Sausage	1	640	32	38	235	72	5	1130
Egg Cheese Bacon	1	460	28	23	210	65	4	980
Egg Cheese Ham	1	460	31	18	210	73	4	1270
Ham	1	460	27	7	30	76	5	2110
Herby Turkey	1	560	30	14	45	78	5	1310
Leonardo Da Veggie	1	480	21	12	30	74	5	870
Radishy Roast Beef	1	560	35	18	60	73	5	1270
Roadhouse Chicken	1	710	50	19	100	84	4	1600
Roast Beef	1	730	30	36	65	71	5	1280
Santa Fe Turkey	1	490	30	9	50	75	5	1450
Smoked Salmon	1	490	28	10	45	74	5	770
Softwich BLT w/ Mayo	1	600	22	25	40	73	5	1220
Softwich Chicken Breast	1	630	47	11	95	81	5	800
Softwich Chicken Fajita	1	570	39	10	20	81	6	1180
Softwich Chicken Salad	1	670	32	27	95	76	5	1220
Softwich Cranberry Gobbler	1	730	40	28	80	80	5	1750
Softwich Cuban Chicken	1	810	56	32	125	77	4	2740
Softwich Garden Veggie	1	380	15	3	0	76	6	680
Softwich Garden Veggie	1	380	15	3	0	76	6	680
Softwich Ham	1	510	29	6	40	85	5	1770
Softwich Herby Turkey	1	580	33	14	50	80	5	1490
Softwich Hummus	1	540	20	13	0	85	11	930
Softwich Leonardo De Veggie	1	550	25	15	40	79	6	1160
Softwich Mediterranean	1	790	30	33	45	90	11	1280
Softwich Peanut Chicken	1	590	36	12	60	82	5	1810
Softwich Radishy Roast Beef	1	670	43	26	90	75	5	1540
Softwich Roadhouse Chicken	1	670	50	19	100	74	4	1620
Softwich Roast Beef	1	750	33	40	75	72	5	1350
Softwich Roasted Turkey	1	550	32	15	45	74	5	1450
Softwich Smoked Salmon	1	520	30	11	50	76	5	800
Softwich Supreme Club w/o Mayo	1	880	55	39	120	79	5	2780
Softwich Tuna Salad	1	720	26	34	45	76	5	1170
Softwich Western Wheat	1	820	30	58	225	76	8	1480
Supreme Club w/o Mayo	1	470	28	9	35	72	5	1460

FOOD	PORTION	CALS	PROT	FAT	CHOL	CARB	FIBER	SOD
Tuna Salad	1	620	23	27	35	73	5	990
Turkey	1	510	26	14	35	70	5	1290
Wrap Classic w/ Bacon	1	520	36	45	405	52	4	1120
Wrap Classic w/ Ham	1	510	40	41	420	54	4	1630
Wrap Classic w/ Sausage	1	660	38	60	435	52	4	1210
Wrap Rio Grande Sausage	1	510	27	47	400	53	4	960
Wrap Rio Grande Bacon	1	560	34	49	415	55	4	1380
Wrap Rio Grande Ham	1	630	31	34	400	55	4	1450
Wrap Sesame Chicken Salad	1	770	31	36	45	80	5	1100
Wrap Tossed Chicken Caesar	1	660	36	28	85	73	5	1740
Wrap Tossed Mandarin Medley Salad	1	630	17	25	20	87	7	980
SOUPS								
Chicken Pot Pie	1 cup	250	10	19	80	12	2	1100
Chicken Spaeztle	1 cup	120	9	5	25	12	1	1050
Chicken Wild Rice	1 cup	260	2	19	75	16	1	1170
Creamy Tomato	1 cup	150	5	9	15	16	3	820
Hearty Mushroom Barley	1 cup	110	5	2	0	18	4	790
Italian Wedding	1 cup	160	8	8	20	15	2	680
Minestrone	1 cup	120	7	2	0	21	5	780
Moroccan Stew	1 cup	140	4	3	0	26	4	330
New England Clam	1 cup	300	10	18	55	23	1	840
Sweet Potato Cheddar	1 cup	200	6	11	20	20	2	580
TOPPINGS								
Cream Cheese Bacon Scallion	1 scoop (1.5 oz)	140	3	12	40	5	0	150
Cream Cheese Cucumber Dill	1 scoop (1.5 oz)	140	3	13	35	3	0	120
Cream Cheese Garden Veggie	1 scoop (1.5 oz)	130	3	11	35	5	1	140
Cream Cheese Honey Walnut	1 scoop (1.5 oz)	150	3	12	35	8	tr	125
Cream Cheese Jalapeno	1 scoop (1.5 oz)	140	3	13	45	4	0	150
Cream Cheese Light Garden Veggie	1 scoop (1.5 oz)	90	6	6	25	3	0	105
Cream Cheese Light Herb Garlic	1 scoop (1.5 oz)	100	6	6	25	4	0	125

FOOD	PORTION	CALS	PROT	FAT	CHOL	CARB	FIBER	SOD
Cream Cheese Light Plain	1 scoop (1.5 oz)	100	3	6	25	4	tr	125
Cream Cheese Olive Pimento	1 scoop (1.5 oz)	140	3	13	45	3	0	130
Cream Cheese Onion & Chive	1 scoop (1.5 oz)	140	3	13	35	3	0	105
Cream Cheese Plain	1 scoop (1.5 oz)	130	3	11	40	6	tr	125
Cream Cheese Pumpkin	1 scoop (1.5 oz)	120	3	11	45	4	0	135
Cream Cheese Strawberry	1 scoop (1.5 oz)	140	3	13	30	4	0	100
Cream Cheese Wildberry	1 scoop (1.5 oz)	140	3	12	40	5	0	120
Hummus	1 scoop (2 oz)	110	5	6	0	10	0	120

BURGER KING
BEVERAGES

FOOD	PORTION	CALS	PROT	FAT	CHOL	CARB	FIBER	SOD
Apple Juice	1 (6.67 oz)	90	0	0	0	23	–	15
BK Joe Regular	1 sm	5	1	0	0	1	–	15
BK Joe Turbo	1 sm (12 oz)	10	1	0	0	1	–	20
Chocolate Milk 1% Low Fat	1 (9 oz)	180	9	3	15	31	1	140
Coke Classic	1 sm (16 oz)	140	0	0	0	39	–	0
Diet Coke	1 sm (16 oz)	0	0	0	0	0	0	15
Dr Pepper	1 sm (16 oz)	140	0	0	0	39	–	35
Iced Coffee Mocha BK Joe	1 (16 oz)	380	6	10	40	66	1	290
Icee Coco Cola	1 sm (16 oz)	110	0	0	0	31	–	10
Icee Minute Maid Cherry	1 sm (16 oz)	110	0	0	0	31	–	5
Milk 1% Low Fat	1	110	8	3	10	13	0	130
Minute Maid Orange Juice	8 oz	140	2	0	0	33	–	20
Shake Chocolate	1 sm (16 oz)	470	8	14	55	75	1	320
Shake Oreo Sundae Chocolate	1 sm (16 oz)	680	9	24	55	105	2	480
Shake Oreo Sundae Strawberry	1 sm (16 oz)	660	9	23	55	103	1	380
Shake Oreo Sundae Vanilla	1 sm (16 oz)	610	9	24	60	87	1	400
Shake Strawberry	1 sm (16 oz)	460	7	14	55	73	0	240
Shake Vanilla	1 sm (16 oz)	400	8	15	60	57	0	240
Sprite	1 sm (16 oz)	140	0	0	0	39	–	30
Water Nestle Pure Life	1 bottle (16 oz)	0	0	0	0	0	0	0

FOOD	PORTION	CALS	PROT	FAT	CHOL	CARB	FIBER	SOD
BREAKFAST SELECTIONS								
Biscuit Bacon Egg & Cheese	1	410	16	25	150	31	1	1320
Biscuit Ham Egg & Cheese	1	390	16	22	145	31	1	1410
Biscuit Sausage	1	390	12	26	35	28	1	1020
Biscuit Sausage Egg & Cheese	1	530	20	37	175	31	1	1490
Croissan'wich Bacon Egg & Cheese	1	340	15	20	155	26	tr	890
Croissan'wich Double w/ Bacon Egg & Cheese	1	430	21	27	175	27	tr	1250
Croissan'wich Double w/ Sausage Bacon Egg & Cheese	1	550	25	39	200	27	1	1420
Croissan'wich Double w/ Sausage Egg & Cheese	1	680	29	51	220	26	1	1590
Croissan'wich Double w/ Ham Bacon Egg & Cheese	1	420	24	24	180	27	1	1600
Croissan'wich Double w/ Ham Egg & Cheese	1	420	27	23	185	27	1	2210
Croissan'wich Double w/ Ham Sausage Egg & Cheese	1	550	28	37	205	27	1	2040
Croissan'wich Egg & Cheese	1	300	12	17	145	26	tr	740
Croissan'wich Ham Egg & Cheese	1	340	18	18	160	26	1	1230
Croissan'wich Sausage Egg & Cheese	1	470	19	32	180	26	tr	1060
Croissan'wich w/ Sausage & Cheese	1	370	14	25	50	23	tr	810
French Toast Sticks	3 pieces	240	4	13	0	26	1	260
Hash Browns	1 sm	260	2	17	0	25	2	500
Hash Browns	1 lg	620	5	40	0	60	6	1200
Omelet Sandwich Enormous	1	730	37	45	330	44	2	1940
Omelet Sandwich Ham	1	290	13	13	85	33	1	870
DESSERTS								
Cini-minis	1 serv	390	7	18	20	51	2	560
Dutch Apple Pie	1 serv	300	2	13	0	45	1	270
Hershey Sundae Pie	1	310	3	19	10	32	1	220

FOOD	PORTION	CALS	PROT	FAT	CHOL	CARB	FIBER	SOD
MAIN MENU SELECTIONS								
BK Chicken Fries	6 pieces	260	12	15	35	18	2	650
BK Stacker Double	1	610	34	39	125	32	1	1100
BK Stacker Quad	1	1000	62	68	240	34	1	1800
BK Stacker Triple	1	800	48	54	185	33	1	1450
BK Veggie Burger	1	420	23	16	10	46	7	1100
Cheeseburger	1	330	17	16	55	31	1	780
Cheeseburger Double	1	500	30	29	105	31	1	1030
Chicken Sandwich Original	1	660	24	40	70	52	4	1440
Chicken Sandwich Tendercrisp	1	790	33	44	70	68	5	1640
Chicken Sandwich Tendergrill	1	510	37	19	75	49	4	1180
Chicken Tenders	5 pieces	210	12	12	35	13	0	600
Chick'n Crisp Spicy Sandwich	1	480	15	31	45	36	1	870
Double Cheeseburger	1	410	25	21	85	30	1	600
French Fries No Salt Added	1 sm	230	2	13	0	26	2	240
French Fries Salted	1 sm	230	2	13	0	26	2	380
French Fries Salted	1 lg	500	5	28	0	57	5	820
Hamburger	1	290	15	12	40	30	1	560
Onion Rings	1 sm	140	2	7	0	18	2	210
Onion Rings	1 lg	440	6	22	0	53	5	620
Sandwich BK Big Fish	1	640	24	32	65	67	3	1450
The Angus Steak Burger	1	640	33	33	185	55	3	1260
Whopper	1	670	28	39	95	51	3	1020
Whopper Double	1	900	47	57	175	51	3	1090
Whopper Double w/ Cheese	1	990	52	64	195	52	3	1520
Whopper Jr.	1	370	15	21	50	31	2	570
Whopper Jr. w/ Cheese	1	410	18	24	60	32	2	780
Whopper Triple	1	1130	67	74	255	51	3	1160
Whopper Triple w/ Cheese	1	1230	71	82	275	52	3	1590
Whopper w/ Cheese	1	760	33	47	115	52	3	1450
SALAD DRESSINGS AND TOPPINGS								
Breakfast Syrup	1 serv (1 oz)	80	0	0	0	21	0	20
Croutons Garlic Parmesan	1 serv	60	1	2	0	9	0	120
Dipping Sauce Barbecue	1 serv (1 oz)	40	0	0	0	11	0	310
Dipping Sauce Honey Mustard	1 serv (1 oz)	90	0	6	10	8	0	180

FOOD	PORTION	CALS	PROT	FAT	CHOL	CARB	FIBER	SOD
Dipping Sauce Ranch	1 serv (1 oz)	140	1	15	5	1	0	95
Dipping Sauce Sweet And Sour	1 serv (1 oz)	40	0	0	0	11	0	55
Dressing Ken's Creamy Caesar	1 serv (2 oz)	210	3	21	25	4	0	610
Dressing Ken's Fat Free Ranch	1 serv (2 oz)	60	0	0	0	15	2	740
Dressing Ken's Honey Mustard	1 serv (2 oz)	270	1	23	20	15	0	520
Dressing Ken's Ranch	1 serv (2 oz)	190	1	20	20	2	0	560
Jam Grape	1 serv	30	0	0	0	7	0	0
Jam Strawberry	1 serv	30	0	0	0	7	0	0
Ketchup	1 pkg	10	0	0	0	3	0	125
Mayonnaise	1 pkg	80	0	9	10	1	0	75
SALADS								
Chicken Garden Tendercrisp	1	410	29	22	70	26	5	1080
Chicken Garden Tendergrill w/o Dressing or Croutons	1	240	33	9	80	8	4	720
Side Garden w/o Dressing	1	15	1	0	0	3	1	0

CAPTAIN D'S SEAFOOD

FOOD	PORTION	CALS	PROT	FAT	CHOL	CARB	FIBER	SOD
Baked Chicken Dinner	1 serv	350	30	5	60	49	5	880
Baked Fish Dinner	1 serv	390	36	5	10	49	5	750
Baked Potato	1 serv	190	4	0	0	44	4	15
Baked Salmon Dinner	1 serv	470	40	8	30	58	5	940
Carb Counter Chicken Dinner	1 serv	320	27	15	70	19	6	1010
Carb Counter Fish Dinner	1 serv	350	33	15	70	19	6	880
Cole Slaw	1 serv	150	3	6	5	22	1	150
Corn On The Cob	1 serv	150	5	3	0	34	2	20
Fresh Steamed Broccoli	1 serv	25	3	1	0	5	3	25
Green Beans	1 serv	90	2	3	5	15	4	505
Rice Pilaf	1 serv	160	4	1	0	35	1	625
Shrimp Scampi Dinner	1 serv	370	29	5	170	50	5	340
Side Salad w/o Dressing	1	30	2	1	0	6	2	20
Tuscan Style Vegetables	1 serv	30	1	0	0	7	2	10

CARIBOU COFFEE

FOOD	PORTION	CALS	PROT	FAT	CHOL	CARB	FIBER	SOD
Black Forest Mocha	1 med	553	12	19	–	83	–	–
Black Forest Wild Drink	1 med	553	12	19	–	86	–	–

FOOD	PORTION	CALS	PROT	FAT	CHOL	CARB	FIBER	SOD
Cappuccino	1 med (16 oz)	113	11	1	–	15	–	–
Cappuccino 2%	1 med (16 oz)	162	11	7	–	17	–	–
Caramel Hirise	1 med (16 oz)	414	11	13	–	59	–	–
Chai Latte 2%	1 med (16 oz)	286	8	5	–	50	–	–
Chai Skim	1 med (16 oz)	236	8	–	–	48	–	–
Cooler Caramel	1 med (12 oz)	450	3	10	–	83	–	–
Cooler Chocolate	1 med (12 oz)	257	4	3	–	54	–	–
Cooler Coffee	1 med (16 oz)	230	4	3	–	48	–	–
Cooler Espresso	1 med (16 oz)	193	3	2	–	40	–	–
Cooler Mint Oreo	1 med (12 oz)	614	10	19	–	108	–	–
Cooler Vanilla	1 med (16 oz)	257	3	4	–	52	–	–
Glacier Gum	2 pieces	5	0	0	0	2	–	–
Hot Apple Blast	1 med	379	–	8	–	76	–	–
Latte 2%	1 med (16 oz)	171	11	6	–	17	–	–
Latte Skim	1 med (16 oz)	121	12	1	–	17	–	–
Latte Skinny Bou Low Cal	1 med	120	12	1	–	17	–	–
Lite White Berry	1 med (16 oz)	311	9	5	–	57	–	–
Mint Condition	1 med (16 oz)	520	10	19	–	75	–	–
Mints All Flavors	3 pieces	5	0	0	0	1	–	–
Mocha 2%	1 med (16 oz)	347	10	16	–	41	–	–
Mocha Skim	1 med (16 oz)	302	13	12	–	34	–	–
Mocha Turtle	1 med (16 oz)	559	10	19	–	82	–	–

FOOD	PORTION	CALS	PROT	FAT	CHOL	CARB	FIBER	SOD
Smoothie Passion Green Tea	1 med (16 oz)	252	2	tr	–	61	–	–
Smoothie Raspberry	1 med (12 oz)	293	2	tr	–	70	–	–
Smoothie Strawberry Banana	1 med (16 oz)	253	2	tr	–	61	–	–
Smoothie Wild Berry	1 med (16 oz)	235	2	tr	–	56	–	–

CARL'S JR.
BEVERAGES

FOOD	PORTION	CALS	PROT	FAT	CHOL	CARB	FIBER	SOD
Malt Chocolate	1 (15 oz)	780	17	35	105	98	1	360
Malt Oreo Cookie	1 (15 oz)	790	18	39	105	91	1	420
Malt Strawberry	1 (15 oz)	770	17	35	105	97	0	310
Malt Vanilla	1 (15 oz)	760	17	35	105	99	0	300
Shake Chocolate	1 (14 oz)	710	14	33	100	85	1	290
Shake Oreo Cookie	1 (14 oz)	720	16	37	100	79	1	350
Shake Strawberry	1 (14 oz)	700	14	33	100	84	0	240
Shake Vanilla	1 (14 oz)	710	14	33	100	86	0	230

BREAKFAST SELECTIONS

FOOD	PORTION	CALS	PROT	FAT	CHOL	CARB	FIBER	SOD
Breakfast Burger	1	830	37	47	275	65	3	1580
Burrito Bacon & Egg	1	570	30	33	515	37	1	990
Burrito Loaded Breakfast	1	820	38	51	595	52	2	1530
Burrito Steak & Egg	1	660	40	36	545	44	2	1690
French Toast Dips w/o Syrup	5	430	9	18	0	58	1	530
Hash Brown Nuggets	1 serv	330	3	21	0	32	3	460
Sandwich Sourdough Breakfast	1 serv	460	28	21	280	39	2	1050
Sunrise Croissant Sandwich	1	560	20	41	290	27	1	970

DESSERTS

FOOD	PORTION	CALS	PROT	FAT	CHOL	CARB	FIBER	SOD
Cheesecake Strawberry Swirl	1 serv	290	6	17	55	30	0	230
Chocolate Cake	1 serv	300	3	12	30	48	1	350
Cookie Chocolate Chip	1	350	3	18	20	46	1	330

MAIN MENU SELECTIONS

FOOD	PORTION	CALS	PROT	FAT	CHOL	CARB	FIBER	SOD
Burger Jalapeno	1	720	27	45	90	50	3	1320
Burger Teriyaki	1	660	28	34	80	61	3	1070
Cheeseburger Double Western Bacon	1	970	62	52	155	71	3	1820

FOOD	PORTION	CALS	PROT	FAT	CHOL	CARB	FIBER	SOD
Cheeseburger Western Bacon	1	710	32	33	85	70	3	1480
Chicken Breast Strips	3	420	23	25	50	28	1	1210
Chicken Stars	4	170	9	11	25	10	1	320
CrissCut Fries	1 serv	410	5	24	0	43	4	950
Famous Star w/ Cheese	1	660	27	39	85	53	3	1260
Fish & Chips	1 serv	630	26	28	10	68	3	990
French Fries	1 sm	290	5	14	0	37	3	180
Fried Zucchini	1 serv	320	6	19	0	31	0	850
Hamburger Big	1	470	24	17	60	54	3	1000
Hamburger Kid's	1	460	24	17	60	53	2	1060
Onion Rings	1 serv	430	6	21	0	53	2	550
Sandwich Bacon Swiss Crispy Chicken	1	720	35	35	85	64	3	1750
Sandwich Carl's Catch Fish	1	660	22	31	30	75	3	1290
Sandwich Charbroiled Chicken Club	1	550	40	25	95	43	4	1410
Sandwich Charbroiled Santa Fe Chicken	1	610	37	32	100	43	4	1540
Sandwich Charbroiled BBQ Chicken	1	360	34	5	60	48	4	1150
Sandwich Spicy Chicken	1	560	15	30	40	59	2	1480
Six Dollar Burger The Bacon Cheese	1	1070	46	76	170	50	3	1010
Six Dollar Burger The Guacamole Bacon	1	1140	43	86	160	54	6	2010
Six Dollar Burger The Jalapeno	1	1030	39	74	150	52	3	2050
Six Dollar Burger The Low Carb	1	490	33	37	130	6	2	1290
Six Dollar Burger The Original	1	1010	40	68	150	60	3	1980
Six Dollar Burger The Western Bacon	1	1130	47	66	150	83	4	2540
Super Star w/ Cheese	1	930	47	59	160	54	3	1600
SALAD DRESSINGS								
Blue Cheese	1 serv (2 oz)	320	2	34	20	1	0	410
House	1 serv (2 oz)	220	1	22	20	2	0	440
Low Fat Balsamic	1 serv (2 oz)	35	0	15	0	5	0	480
Thousand Island	1 serv (2 oz)	240	0	23	20	7	0	460

FOOD	PORTION	CALS	PROT	FAT	CHOL	CARB	FIBER	SOD
SALADS								
Charbroiled Chicken	1	260	34	7	75	16	5	710
Side	1	50	3	3	5	5	2	60
CARVEL								
Brown Bonnet	1	370	3	21	55	40	0	105
Cake Ice Cream	1 slice	270	4	14	35	33	1	135
Carvelanche Cake Mix	1 reg (16 oz)	720	13	27	85	106	0	540
Carvelanche Cookies & Cream	1 reg (16 oz)	550	7	30	120	64	0	280
Carvelanche Triple Fudge Cake Mix	1 reg (16 oz)	900	16	41	65	134	4	300
Chipsters	1	330	4	16	40	44	4	220
Cone Cake Chocolate	1 sm	260	6	13	35	32	1	135
Cone Cake Chocolate	1 lg	600	13	30	80	71	3	310
Cone Cake Vanilla	1 sm	280	4	16	75	31	0	135
Cone Cake Vanilla	1 lg	650	9	36	180	68	0	300
Cone Sugar Chocolate	1 sm	300	7	13	40	40	1	160
Cone Sugar Vanilla	1 sm	320	5	15	75	39	0	160
Cone Waffle Chocolate	1 sm	330	7	13	47	47	2	160
Cone Waffle Chocolate	1 lg	660	15	30	80	86	3	340
Cone Waffle Vanilla	1 sm	350	5	16	75	46	1	160
Cone Waffle Vanilla	1 lg	710	10	36	180	83	1	330
Dashers Banana Barge	1	940	17	46	110	121	7	250
Dashers Bananas Foster	1	600	6	24	100	90	2	350
Dashers Fudge Brownie	1	810	9	42	120	98	4	400
Dashers Mint Chocolate Chip	1	720	8	39	110	85	2	350
Dashers Peanut Butter Cup	1	1090	20	63	55	97	4	630
Dashers Strawberry Shortcake	1	590	8	29	100	78	2	170
Flying Saucer 98% Fat Free Chocolate	1	180	5	3	0	34	1	160
Flying Saucer Chocolate	1	230	4	10	20	33	1	125
Flying Saucer Deluxe Sprinkles	1	330	4	15	40	47	1	120
Flying Saucer Vanilla	1	240	4	11	45	33	1	170
Flying Saucers 98% Fat Free Vanilla	1	180	5	3	0	35	1	170
Ice Cream Chocolate	1 sm (4 oz)	250	6	13	35	29	0	130
Ice Cream Vanilla	1 sm (4 oz)	240	3	14	70	25	0	115

FOOD	PORTION	CALS	PROT	FAT	CHOL	CARB	FIBER	SOD
Ice Cream No Fat Chocolate	1 sm (4 oz)	160	3	0	0	37	0	55
Ice Cream No Fat Vanilla	1 sm (4 oz)	160	5	0	0	33	0	75
Sherbet All Flavors	1 sm (4 oz)	180	1	2	5	39	0	70
Sinful Love Bar	1	460	4	29	25	47	5	220
Sprinkle Cup	1	230	2	15	45	28	1	75
Sundae Bittersweet Fudge	1 reg	690	8	38	77	77	1	280
Sundae Caramel	1 reg	670	8	34	145	81	0	360
Sundae Hot Fudge	1 reg	670	8	38	145	73	1	280
Sundae Strawberry	1 reg	580	7	33	145	63	1	210
Sundae Mini Chocolate Syrup	1	200	2	9	45	27	0	85
Thick Shake Chocolate	1 reg (16 oz)	650	14	27	70	93	2	320
Thick Shake Vanilla	1 reg (16 oz)	610	10	28	135	81	0	260
Thinny Thin Classic Sundae No Fat Strawberry	1 reg	320	8	0	0	69	1	150
Thinny Thin Classic Sundae No Fat Fudge	1 reg	380	8	2	0	81	0	180
Thinny Thin Minature Sundae No Fat	1	190	4	0	0	45	0	95
Thinny Thin Minature Sundae No Sugar Added	1	200	5	3	15	42	0	125
Thinny Thin No Fat Carvelanche Strawberry	1 (16 oz)	430	12	0	0	91	1	160
Thinny Thin No Fat Chocolate	1 sm	160	3	0	0	37	0	55
Thinny Thin No Fat Vanilla	1 sm	160	5	0	0	33	0	75
Thinny Thin No Sugar Added Vanilla	1 sm	180	7	3	20	34	0	115
Thinny Thin Parfait No Fat	1	190	4	0	0	42	0	95
Thinny Thin Shake No Fat Chocolate	1 (16 oz)	440	5	0	0	104	0	190
Thinny Thin Shake No Fat Mocha	1 (16 oz)	440	10	0	0	97	0	230
Thinny Thin Shake No Fat Vanilla	1 (16 oz)	300	9	0	0	62	0	135

CHEVY'S

FOOD	PORTION	CALS	PROT	FAT	CHOL	CARB	FIBER	SOD
Black Beans	1 serv	59	3	0	–	11	–	–
Catch Of The Day w/ San Antonio Vegetables Salsa & Tomalito	1 serv	428	47	16	–	16	–	–

FOOD	PORTION	CALS	PROT	FAT	CHOL	CARB	FIBER	SOD
Chicken Fajitas w/ San Antonio Vegetables & Tomalito	1 serv	285	39	6	–	13	–	–
Fish Tacos w/ Taco Dressing Lettuce & Pico De Gallo	1 serv	483	16	18	–	56	–	–
Grilled Chicken Salad w/ Salsa Vinaigrette	1 serv	533	38	18	–	53	–	–
Guacamole	1 serv (2 oz)	103	0	10	–	3	–	–
Mexican Rice	1 serv	211	3	3	–	39	–	–
Mixed Green Salad w/ Salsa Vinaigrette	1 serv	358	11	16	–	42	–	–
Salsa	1 serv (5 oz)	40	1	0	0	8	–	–
Shrimp Fajitas w/ San Antonio Vegetables & Tomalito	1 serv	286	13	7	–	32	–	–
Sour Cream	1 serv	121	2	12	–	2	–	–
Tortilla Corn	1	80	0	1	–	17	–	–
Tortilla El Machino	1	167	3	4	–	27	–	–
Veggie Burrito w/ San Antonio Vegetables Pico De Gallo & Ranchero Sauce	1 serv	430	7	19	–	49	–	–
Veggie Fajitas w/ San Antonio Vegetables & Tomalito	1 serv	345	0	28	–	16	–	–

CHICK-FIL-A
BEVERAGES

FOOD	PORTION	CALS	PROT	FAT	CHOL	CARB	FIBER	SOD
Coca-Cola Classic	1 sm	110	0	0	0	28	0	10
Diet Coke	1 sm	0	0	0	0	0	0	10
Diet Lemonade	1 sm	25	0	0	0	5	0	5
Ice Tea Sweetened	1 sm	80	0	0	0	19	0	0
Iced Tea Unsweetened	1 sm	0	0	0	0	0	0	0
Lemonade	1 sm	170	0	1	0	41	0	10

BREAKFAST SELECTIONS

FOOD	PORTION	CALS	PROT	FAT	CHOL	CARB	FIBER	SOD
Bagel Chicken Egg & Cheese	1	500	31	20	290	49	3	1260
Bagel Wheat	1	220	7	3	0	41	2	350
Biscuit Bacon	1	300	6	14	5	38	1	790
Biscuit Bacon & Egg	1	390	13	20	250	38	1	860
Biscuit Bacon Egg Cheese	1	440	16	24	265	30	1	1090

FOOD	PORTION	CALS	PROT	FAT	CHOL	CARB	FIBER	SOD
Biscuit Buttered	1	270	4	12	0	38	1	660
Biscuit Chicken	1	420	18	19	35	44	2	1270
Biscuit Chicken w/ Cheese	1	470	21	23	50	45	2	1500
Biscuit Egg	1	350	11	16	240	38	1	740
Biscuit Egg Cheese	1	400	14	21	255	38	1	970
Biscuit Sausage	1	410	9	23	20	42	1	740
Biscuit Sausage Egg	1	500	15	29	265	43	1	810
Biscuit Sausage Egg Cheese	1	550	18	33	280	43	1	1040
Biscuit w/ Gravy	1	330	8	15	5	44	1	930
Burrito Chicken	1	420	23	19	270	39	2	960
Burrito Sausage	1	460	20	24	270	40	2	750
Chick-N-Minis	1 serv	270	14	11	50	28	1	640
Hashbrowns	1 serv	260	2	17	5	25	3	380
DESSERTS								
Cheesecake	1 slice	340	6	21	90	30	2	270
Fudge Nut Brownie	1	330	4	15	20	45	2	210
Icedream Cone	1 sm	160	4	4	15	28	0	80
Lemon Pie	1 slice	390	6	13	30	63	1	300
MAIN MENU SELECTIONS								
Carrot & Raisin Salad	1 sm	170	1	6	10	28	2	110
Chicken Filet	1	230	23	11	60	10	0	990
Chicken Filet Chargrilled	1	100	21	2	65	1	0	610
Chick-N-Strips	4	290	29	13	65	14	1	730
Cole Slaw	1 sm	260	2	21	25	17	2	220
Cool Wrap Chargrilled Chicken	1	390	29	7	65	54	3	1020
Cool Wrap Chicken Caesar	1	460	36	10	80	52	3	1350
Cool Wrap Spicy Chicken	1	380	30	6	60	52	3	1090
Fruit Cup	1 serv	60	1	0	0	16	2	0
Hearty Breast of Chicken Soup	1 cup	140	8	4	23	18	1	900
Nuggets	8	260	26	12	70	12	tr	1090
Polynesian Sauce	1 pkg	110	0	6	0	13	0	210
Sandwich Chargrilled Chicken	1	270	28	4	65	33	3	940
Sandwich Chicken	1	410	28	16	60	38	1	1300
Sandwich Chicken Deluxe	1	420	28	16	60	39	2	1300
Sandwich Chicken Salad On Wheat Bread	1	350	20	15	65	32	5	880
Waffle Potato Fries	1 sm	270	3	13	0	34	4	115

FOOD	PORTION	CALS	PROT	FAT	CHOL	CARB	FIBER	SOD
SALAD DRESSINGS AND SAUCES								
Barbecue Sauce	1 pkg	45	0	0	0	11	0	180
Blue Cheese	2 tbsp	150	1	16	20	1	0	300
Buffalo Sauce	1 pkg	15	0	2	0	1	0	410
Buttermilk Ranch	2 tbsp	160	0	16	5	1	0	270
Buttermilk Ranch Sauce	1 pkg	110	0	12	5	1	0	200
Caesar	2 tbsp	160	1	17	30	1	0	240
Fat Free Honey Mustard	2 tbsp	60	0	0	0	14	0	200
Honey Mustard	1 pkg	45	0	0	0	10	0	130
Honey Roasted BBQ Sauce	1 pkg	60	0	6	5	2	0	90
Light Italian	2 tbsp	15	0	1	0	2	0	570
Raspberry Vinaigrette Reduced Fat	2 tbsp	80	0	2	0	15	0	240
Spicy	2 tbsp	140	0	14	5	2	0	130
Thousand Island	2 tbsp	150	0	14	10	5	0	250
SALADS								
Chargrilled Chicken Garden Salad	1 serv	180	22	6	65	9	3	620
Chick-N-Strips Salad	1 serv	390	34	18	80	22	4	860
Croutons Garlic & Butter	1 pkg	50	tr	3	0	6	0	90
Honey Roasted Sunflower Kernels	1 pkg	80	3	7	0	3	1	38
Side Salad	1 serv	60	3	3	10	4	2	75
Southwest Chargrilled Salad	1 serv	240	25	8	60	17	5	770
Tortilla Strips	1 pkg	70	2	4	0	9	1	53

CHILI'S
CHILDREN'S MENU SELECTIONS

FOOD	PORTION	CALS	PROT	FAT	CHOL	CARB	FIBER	SOD
Corn Dog	1	250	5	17	–	18	1	260
Grilled Chicken Platter	1 serv	140	26	3	–	3	tr	790
Little Chicken Crispers	1 serv	590	34	42	–	19	0	1300
Little Mouth Burger	1 serv	280	20	15	–	14	1	300
Little Mouth Cheeseburger	1 serv	350	24	21	–	14	1	600
Macaroni & Cheese	1 serv	510	16	18	–	69	3	940
Pepper Pal Pasta w/ Alfredo	1 serv	410	15	19	–	47	2	1680
Pepper Pal Pasta w/ Marinara	1 serv	290	7	5	–	52	2	1510
Pizza	1	570	23	24	–	67	3	1130
Rib Basket	1 serv	370	20	24	–	16	1	1960

FOOD	PORTION	CALS	PROT	FAT	CHOL	CARB	FIBER	SOD
Sandwich Grilled Cheese	1 serv	420	16	27	–	26	1	1200
Sandwich Grilled Chicken	1 serv	140	19	3	–	10	1	620
DESSERTS								
Cheesecake	1 serv	760	11	44	–	75	2	470
Chocolate Chip Paradise Pie w/ Vanilla Ice Cream	1 serv	1600	19	78	–	215	6	950
Frosty Chocolate Shake w/ Chocolate Sprinkles	1 serv	850	13	36	–	123	1	330
Molten Chocolate Cake w/ Vanilla Ice Cream	1 serv	1270	14	62	–	172	6	1060
MAIN MENU SELECTIONS								
Awesome Blossom	1 serv	2710	24	203	–	194	15	6360
Baby Back Ribs & Chicken	1 serv	1460	75	67	–	163	12	4870
Black Bean Burger	1 serv	650	38	12	–	96	26	1540
Boneless Buffalo Wings	1 serv	1250	56	80	–	55	4	4320
Boneless Shanghai Wings	1 serv	1260	59	71	–	97	5	3030
Bottomless Tostada Chips	1 basket	400	3	36	–	18	3	1540
Burger Bacon	1 serv	1080	55	71	–	54	3	1660
Burger BBQ Ranch	1 serv	1110	56	71	–	60	3	1920
Burger Chipotle Bleu Cheese Bacon	1 serv	1090	51	71	–	57	3	2070
Burger Ground Peppercorn	1 serv	1050	44	68	–	61	3	1410
Burger Mushroom Swiss	1 serv	1100	53	71	–	60	4	1590
Burger Oldtimer	1 serv	800	43	44	–	54	3	1190
Chicken Crispers	1 serv	1870	67	129	–	132	8	3020
Chicken Tacos	1 serv	1200	60	41	–	143	13	4620
Cinnamon Apples	1 serv	210	0	8	–	35	5	80
Citrus Fire Chicken & Shrimp	1 serv	760	62	27	–	68	6	2990
Classic Nachos	1 serv	1570	67	115	–	66	15	2980
Country Fried Steak	1 serv	1890	99	107	–	148	7	2750
Fried Cheese w/ Marinara Sauce	1 serv	1210	42	89	–	82	3	2470
Garlic Toast	1 piece	200	3	12	–	18	1	310
Grilled Baby Back Ribs	1 serv	1370	45	82	–	112	12	4410
Grilled Salmon w/ Garlic & Herbs	1 serv	700	48	33	–	53	5	1420
Guiltless Grill Chicken Pita	1 serv	550	36	9	–	70	13	2110
Guiltless Grill Chicken Platter	1 serv	580	38	9	–	89	5	2780

FOOD	PORTION	CALS	PROT	FAT	CHOL	CARB	FIBER	SOD
Guiltless Grill Chicken Sandwich	1 serv	490	39	8	–	63	11	2720
Guiltless Grill Salmon	1 serv	480	54	14	–	31	10	1080
Guiltless Grill Tomato Basil Pasta	1 serv	650	19	14	–	107	7	2560
Homestyle Fries	1 serv	520	5	31	–	53	5	260
Kettle Black Beans	1 serv	140	8	1	–	23	6	770
Loaded Mashed Potatoes	1 serv	560	14	37	–	42	3	1050
Margarita Grilled Chicken	1 serv	690	49	14	–	85	9	2980
Monterey Chicken	1 serv	1170	72	71	–	70	8	3530
Pasta Cajun Chicken	1 serv	1460	76	75	–	118	5	5800
Pasta Grilled Shrimp Alfredo	1 serv	1340	66	72	–	102	5	5120
Pasta Tomato Basil Chicken	1 serv	860	45	26	–	111	5	3980
Pita Chicken Caesar	1 serv	650	36	41	–	31	4	1540
Pita Chicken Fajita	1 serv	450	43	17	–	35	3	1750
Pita Steak Fajita	1 serv	580	36	33	–	32	3	1770
Quesadillas Fajita Chicken	1 serv	1720	93	82	–	150	15	5000
Quesadillas Fajita Combo	1 serv	1840	97	94	–	148	14	5290
Quesadillas Fajita Steak	1 serv	1970	102	106	–	147	14	5580
Ribeye Cajun	1 serv	870	40	76	–	3	1	730
Ribeye Flame Grilled	1 serv	960	40	87	–	1	0	1090
Rice	1 serv	210	4	2	–	45	1	1020
Sandwich Cajun Chicken	1 serv	820	45	43	–	66	4	2220
Sandwich Chicken Ranch	1 serv	1150	45	70	–	82	3	2830
Sandwich Chili's Cheesesteak	1 serv	1010	61	55	–	72	4	2510
Sandwich Grilled Chicken	1 serv	840	48	47	–	57	2	1950
Sandwich Smoked Turkey	1 serv	930	43	57	–	65	4	2920
Sauteed Mushrooms Onions & Bell Peppers	1 serv	120	3	10	–	6	2	360
Seasonal Grilled Veggies	1 serv	90	3	6	–	7	3	90
Seasonal Steamed Veggie w/ Parmesan Cheese	1 serv	60	4	1	–	8	3	110
Sirloin Chili's Classic	1 serv	530	36	41	–	1	0	890
Sirloin Honey BBQ	1 serv	800	48	56	–	19	1	1180
Skillet Queso	1 serv	670	35	53	–	12	3	2380
Southwestern Eggrolls	1 serv	810	29	51	–	59	10	1250
Steamed Broccoli	1 serv	80	3	6	–	6	3	280
Sweet Corn On The Cob	1 serv	180	6	2	–	55	3	100

FOOD	PORTION	CALS	PROT	FAT	CHOL	CARB	FIBER	SOD
Triple Play	1 serv	2330	91	177	–	96	9	5360
Wings Over Buffalo	1 serv	1140	54	100	–	4	0	2540
SALAD DRESSINGS AND SAUCES								
Dressing Asian Sesame Ginger	1 serv (2 oz)	250	1	22	–	11	0	520
Dressing Avocado Ranch	1 serv (2 oz)	150	3	15	–	3	1	240
Dressing Bleu Cheese	1 serv (2 oz)	330	2	35	–	1	0	420
Dressing Caesar	1 serv (2 oz)	350	2	37	–	3	0	530
Dressing Chipotle Ranch	1 serv (2 oz)	170	3	18	–	2	0	280
Dressing Citrus Balsamic Vinaigrette	1 serv (2 oz)	350	0	35	–	8	0	310
Dressing Creamy Cilantro	1 serv (2 oz)	300	1	32	–	2	0	450
Dressing Honey Lime	1 serv (2 oz)	270	1	22	–	17	0	340
Dressing Honey Mustard	1 serv (2 oz)	260	1	28	–	2	0	510
Dressing Ranch	1 serv (2 oz)	240	4	25	–	3	0	370
Dressing Thousand Island	1 serv (2 oz)	270	1	26	–	9	0	600
Dressing Low Fat Ranch	1 serv (2 oz)	110	1	6	–	12	0	480
Dressing No Fat Balsamic Vinaigrette	1 serv (2 oz)	50	0	0	0	9	0	530
Dressing No Fat Honey Mustard	1 serv (2 oz)	90	0	1	–	14	1	650
Sauce Peanut Dipping	1 serv (2 oz)	190	4	13	–	15	1	430
Sauce Picante Salsa	1 serv (2 oz)	40	2	0	0	4	1	530
Sauce Sesame Dipping	1 serv (2 oz)	70	2	0	0	11	1	1030
SALADS								
Boneless Buffalo Chicken	1 serv	870	44	55	–	50	7	2320
Chicken Caesar w/ Dressing	1 serv	1010	38	76	–	39	7	1910
Crispy Chicken	1 serv	810	39	47	–	59	8	1650
Dinner Caesar w/ Dressing	1 serv	430	8	34	–	20	4	690
Dinner House	1 serv	140	6	7	–	12	2	190
Grilled Caribbean	1 serv	440	33	10	–	51	6	1410
Lettuce Wraps	1 serv	330	7	21	–	29	6	890
Lime Grilled Shrimp Caesar w/ Dressing	1 serv	980	31	77	–	39	7	1900
Quesadilla Explosion	1 serv	850	56	45	–	60	11	2230
Southwestern Cobb	1 serv	650	43	32	–	49	8	2090
SOUPS								
Broccoli Cheese	1 cup	160	7	9	–	12	2	760
Chicken Enchilada	1 cup	220	13	14	–	11	2	650

FOOD	PORTION	CALS	PROT	FAT	CHOL	CARB	FIBER	SOD
Chicken Noodle	1 cup	50	2	1	–	7	1	540
Chicken Tortilla	1 cup	140	8	7	–	10	2	840
Chili w/ Cheese	1 cup	500	30	35	–	19	3	1710
New England Clam Chowder	1 cup	470	17	33	–	27	3	970
Potato	1 cup	220	8	16	–	12	1	630
Southwestern Vegetable	1 cup	110	5	5	–	13	2	620

CHIPOTLE

FOOD	PORTION	CALS	PROT	FAT	CHOL	CARB	FIBER	SOD
Barbacoa	1 serv (4 oz)	228	27	13	59	1	0	544
Black Beans	1 serv (4 oz)	130	9	1	0	22	12	318
Carnitas	1 serv (4 oz)	227	29	12	66	0	0	873
Cheese	1 serv (1 oz)	110	7	9	30	tr	0	180
Chicken	1 serv (4 oz)	219	29	11	96	0	0	431
Chips	1 serv (4 oz)	490	7	19	0	71	5	130
Crispy Taco Shells	3	180	3	7	0	26	2	30
Fajita Vegetables	1 serv (3 oz)	100	1	8	0	6	1	640
Flour Tortilla	1 (6 in)	300	9	8	0	48	6	630
Flour Tortilla	1 (13 in)	330	9	8	0	55	5	710
Guacamole	1 serv (4 oz)	170	2	15	0	8	5	370
Lettuce	1 serv (1 oz)	5	tr	0	0	tr	tr	0
Pinto Beans	1 serv (4 oz)	138	9	1	0	23	10	374
Rice	1 serv (3.5 oz)	168	3	5	0	28	tr	427
Salsa Corn	1 serv (4 oz)	100	3	1	0	22	3	540
Salsa Tomato	1 serv (4 oz)	25	1	0	0	6	1	560
Sour Cream	1 serv (2 oz)	120	2	10	40	2	0	30
Steak	1 serv (4 oz)	230	29	12	51	2	0	306
Tomatillo Green	1 serv (2 oz)	15	1	tr	0	3	1	227
Tomatillo Red	1 serv (2 oz)	28	1	1	0	4	1	493
Vinaigrette	1 serv (2 oz)	282	0	26	17	11	0	1525

CHURCH'S CHICKEN
DESSERTS

FOOD	PORTION	CALS	PROT	FAT	CHOL	CARB	FIBER	SOD
Pie Apple	1 pie (3 oz)	280	2	11	5	39	1	250
Pie Edward's Double Lemon	1 pie (3 oz)	300	5	14	25	39	0	160
Pie Edward's Strawberry Cream Cheese	1 pie (2.8 oz)	280	4	15	15	32	2	130

MAIN MENU SELECTIONS

FOOD	PORTION	CALS	PROT	FAT	CHOL	CARB	FIBER	SOD
Biscuit Honey Butter	1	240	3	12	<5	28	1	540

FOOD	PORTION	CALS	PROT	FAT	CHOL	CARB	FIBER	SOD
Cajun Rice	1 reg	130	1	7	5	16	tr	260
Chicken Fried Steak w/ White Gravy	1 serv (7.5 oz)	610	24	43	70	31	2	1465
Cole Slaw	1 reg	150	1	10	5	15	2	170
Corn On The Cob	1 ear	140	4	3	0	24	9	15
Country Fried Steak w/ White Gravy	1 serv (5.8 oz)	470	21	28	65	36	1	1620
Crunchy Tenders	1 (2 oz)	120	12	6	35	6	tr	440
French Fries	1 reg	290	3	14	0	38	4	320
Jalapeno Cheese Bombers	4 (4 oz)	240	8	10	30	29	3	970
Macaroni & Cheese	1 reg	210	8	11	15	23	1	690
Mashed Potatoes & Gravy	1 reg	70	2	2	tr	12	1	480
Okra	1 reg	350	3	22	0	36	5	590
Original Breast	1	200	22	11	80	3	1	450
Original Leg	1	110	10	6	55	3	0	280
Original Thigh	1	330	21	23	110	8	1	680
Original Wing	1	300	27	19	120	7	3	540
Sandwich Bigger Better Chicken w/ Cheese	1	510	20	27	50	46	4	1070
Sandwich Country Fried Steak	1	490	13	32	30	38	2	880
Sandwich Spicy Fish	1	320	10	20	25	25	2	560
Spicy Breast	1	320	21	20	75	12	1	760
Spicy Crunchy Tenders	1 (2 oz)	135	11	7	25	7	4	480
Spicy Fish Fillet	1 piece (2.3 oz)	160	7	9	25	13	1	350
Spicy Leg	1	180	12	11	65	8	1	470
Spicy Thigh	1	480	22	35	135	20	2	1035
Spicy Wing	1	430	29	27	125	17	2	1020
Sweet Corn Nuggets	1 reg	600	7	29	0	72	5	1260
Whole Jalapeno Peppers	2	10	0	0	0	2	1	390
SAUCES								
BBQ	1 pkg	30	0	0	0	7	0	180
Creamy Jalapeno	1 pkg	100	0	11	10	1	0	140
Honey	1 pkg	27	0	0	0	7	0	0
Honey Mustard	1 pkg	110	0	11	10	4	0	130
Hot Sauce	1 pkg	0	0	0	0	0	0	210
Ketchup	1 pkg	18	0	0	0	5	0	190
Purple Pepper	1 pkg	45	0	0	0	12	0	26
Ranch	1 pkg	130	0	13	10	1	0	320
Sweet & Sour	1 pkg	30	0	0	0	8	0	120

FOOD	PORTION	CALS	PROT	FAT	CHOL	CARB	FIBER	SOD
CICI'S								
EXTRAS								
Apple Pizza	1 slice	149	3	4	0	26	1	193
Brownie	1	143	1	6	0	22	1	96
Cinnamon Roll	1	139	2	6	0	20	1	99
Garlic Bread	1 slice	99	4	5	5	10	tr	120
PIZZA								
Buffet 12 Inch Alfredo	1 slice	139	8	5	10	18	1	199
Buffet 12 Inch Bacon Cheddar	1 slice	145	6	5	13	18	3	312
Buffet 12 Inch Bar-B-Que	1 slice	172	8	6	12	21	2	311
Buffet 12 Inch Beef	1 slice	170	9	7	20	18	1	281
Buffet 12 Inch Cheese	1 slice	152	7	5	9	20	1	305
Buffet 12 Inch Ham & Pineapple	1 slice	141	7	4	10	19	1	319
Buffet 12 Inch Ole	1 slice	108	5	4	7	13	2	261
Buffet 12 Inch Pepperoni	1 slice	175	8	7	13	21	2	384
Buffet 12 Inch Pepperoni & Jalapeno	1 slice	163	8	6	11	20	2	394
Buffet 12 Inch Sausage	1 slice	197	8	7	11	19	1	358
Buffet 12 Inch Spinach Alfredo	1 slice	151	7	5	11	20	2	215
Buffet 12 Inch Zesty Ham & Cheese	1 slice	153	6	6	9	18	1	271
Buffet 12 Inch Zesty Pepperoni	1 slice	157	6	7	7	18	1	302
Buffet 12 Inch Zesty Tomato Alfredo	1 slice	136	6	5	10	18	2	202
Buffet 12 Inch Zesty Veggie	1 slice	124	5	4	4	17	1	224
To-Go 15 Inch Bar-B-Que	1 slice	289	13	10	17	36	2	446
To-Go 15 Inch Cheese	1 slice	223	11	8	17	28	3	428
To-Go 15 Inch Ham & Pineapple	1 slice	225	11	8	21	27	2	394
To-Go 15 Inch Ole	1 slice	169	7	4	8	26	3	350
To-Go 15 Inch Pepperoni	1 slice	240	11	10	21	27	3	504
To-Go 15 Inch Spinach Alfredo	1 slice	243	11	8	18	32	3	347
To-Go 15 Inch Zesty Pepperoni	1 slice	246	10	12	12	26	2	475
To-Go 15 Inch Zesty Veggie	1 slice	213	9	9	7	25	2	394

FOOD	PORTION	CALS	PROT	FAT	CHOL	CARB	FIBER	SOD
CINNABON								
BAKED SELECTIONS								
Caramel Pecanbon	1	1100	16	56	63	141	8	600
Cinnabon Bites	6	520	8	16	10	78	2	530
Cinnabon Classic	1	813	15	32	67	117	4	801
Cinnabon Stix	1	379	6	21	16	41	1	413
Cinnamon Filled Churro	1	281	5	11	–	39	–	–
Minibon	1	339	6	13	27	49	2	337
BEVERAGES								
Caramelatta Chill	1 (16 oz)	520	12	19	75	76	0	250
Chillatta Cappuccino	1 (16 oz)	330	5	11	35	56	1	120
Chillatta Caramel	1 (16 oz)	480	8	18	65	72	0	270
Chillatta Chocolate Mocha	1 (16 oz)	460	8	14	45	72	3	270
Chillatta Mango	1 (16 oz)	340	6	11	40	57	0	105
Chillatta Strawberry	1 (16 oz)	330	5	11	40	54	0	105
Chillatta Strawberry Banana	1 (16 oz)	350	5	11	40	58	0	105
Chillatta Tropical Blast	1 (16 oz)	330	2	7	20	69	–	50
Mochalatta Chill	1 (16 oz)	450	11	18	60	66	1	310
COLD STONE CREAMERY								
Waffle Cone Dipped	1	310	4	15	5	46	2	70
Waffle Cone Dipped w/ Candy	1	390	5	20	5	55	2	55
Waffle Cone Or Bowl	1	160	3	4	5	29	0	70
FROZEN YOGURT								
Cheesecake	1 serv (6 oz)	170	9	0	<5	49	0	140
Low Fat Chocolate	1 serv (6 oz)	230	11	2	<5	48	3	140
Nonfat Coffee	1 serv (6 oz)	220	10	0	<5	45	0	150
Nonfat Sweet Cream	1 serv (6 oz)	220	9	0	<5	45	0	150
ICE CREAM								
Amaretto	1 serv (6 oz)	390	6	24	95	40	0	95
Banana	1 serv (6 oz)	370	6	22	85	40	0	85
Black Cherry	1 serv (6 oz)	390	6	22	90	43	0	90
Butter Pecan	1 serv (6 oz)	390	6	24	95	40	0	95
Cake A Cheesecake Named Desire	1 slice (5 oz)	410	4	19	50	57	0	250
Cake Butterfinger Bonanza	1 slice (5 oz)	450	7	22	50	58	tr	270
Cake Celebration Sensation	1 slice (4.5 oz)	350	4	17	50	46	tr	230

FOOD	PORTION	CALS	PROT	FAT	CHOL	CARB	FIBER	SOD
Cake Chocolate Chipper	1 slice (4.6 oz)	450	6	28	50	50	3	200
Cake Coffeehouse Crunch	1 slice (5 oz)	530	6	31	45	59	2	270
Cake Cookie Dough Delirium	1 slice (4.8 oz)	420	5	21	55	53	tr	230
Cake Cookies & Creamery	1 slice (4.5 oz)	390	6	20	50	48	1	290
Cake Midnight Delight	1 slice (5.3 oz)	510	7	28	50	61	4	230
Cake MMMMMM Chip	1 slice (4.5 oz)	380	5	20	45	46	2	230
Cake Peanut Butter Playground	1 slice (5 oz)	490	7	29	45	54	4	240
Cake Raspberry Truffle Temptation	1 slice (5 oz)	480	5	27	50	57	4	200
Cake Snicker's Supreme	1 slice (5 oz)	510	7	29	50	57	3	240
Cake Strawberry Passion	1 slice (5 oz)	380	4	19	50	50	1	260
Cake Zebra Stripes	1 slice (4.8 oz)	400	5	22	55	46	1	210
Cake Batter	1 serv (6 oz)	410	6	23	85	50	0	210
Candy Cane	1 serv (6 oz)	420	6	24	85	48	0	90
Caramel Latte	1 serv (6 oz)	400	6	22	85	47	0	125
Carrot Cake Batter	1 serv (6 oz)	450	6	24	80	54	0	230
Cheesecake	1 serv (6 oz)	390	6	22	85	44	0	90
Chocolate	1 serv (6 oz)	390	7	24	90	39	1	115
Cinnamon	1 serv (6 oz)	400	6	24	95	41	tr	95
Coconut	1 serv (6 oz)	390	6	23	90	39	0	90
Coffee	1 serv (6 oz)	400	6	24	95	40	0	95
Cookie Batter	1 serv (6 oz)	450	6	24	80	53	0	280
Cotton Candy	1 serv (6 oz)	390	6	23	90	41	0	90
Dark Chocolate Peppermint	1 serv (6 oz)	410	7	23	90	41	2	90
Egg Nog	1 serv (6 oz)	400	6	22	90	46	0	95
Expresso	1 serv (6 oz)	350	6	21	85	36	0	85
French Vanilla	1 serv (6 oz)	400	6	23	120	45	0	95
Irish Cream	1 serv (6 oz)	390	6	24	95	40	0	95
Macadamia Nut	1 serv (6 oz)	390	6	24	95	40	0	95

FOOD	PORTION	CALS	PROT	FAT	CHOL	CARB	FIBER	SOD
Mango	1 serv (6 oz)	370	6	22	85	40	0	85
Mint	1 serv (6 oz)	400	6	23	90	43	0	90
Mocha	1 serv (6 oz)	390	7	24	90	40	1	115
Oatmeal Batter	1 serv (6 oz)	400	6	23	90	44	0	130
Orange Dreamsicle	1 serv (6 oz)	380	6	22	90	41	0	90
Peanut Butter	1 serv (6 oz)	440	9	29	85	39	tr	150
Pecan Praline	1 serv (6 oz)	400	6	22	85	44	0	110
Pistachio	1 serv (6 oz)	390	6	24	95	40	0	100
Pumpkin	1 serv (6 oz)	390	6	22	90	42	0	100
Raspberry	1 serv	390	6	22	90	43	0	90
Sinless Sans Fat Sweet Cream	1 serv (6 oz)	160	7	0	<5	41	tr	135
Strawberry	1 serv (6 oz)	380	6	22	90	41	0	90
Sweet Cream	1 serv (6 oz)	390	6	24	95	95	0	95
Vanilla Bean	1 serv (6 oz)	400	6	23	90	39	0	90
White Chocolate	1 serv (6 oz)	390	6	23	90	40	0	90
MIX-INS AND TOPPINGS								
Almond Joy	1 piece	180	1	9	0	20	2	50
Apple Pie Filling	0.75 oz	60	0	0	0	16	1	25
Banana	½	60	1	0	0	14	1	0
Black Cherries	0.75 oz	80	0	0	0	19	0	30
Blackberries	0.75 oz	10	0	0	0	2	1	0
Blueberries	0.75 oz	10	0	0	0	2	0	0
Brownies	1 piece	180	2	6	5	29	1	190
Butterfinger	½ bar	140	4	6	0	20	1	60
Butterscotch Fat Free	1 oz	80	1	0	0	19	0	85
Caramel	1 oz	100	0	0	0	22	0	65
Caramel Topping Fat Free	1 oz	110	0	0	0	24	0	85
Cashews	1 oz	170	5	14	0	9	1	190
Chocolate Chips	1 oz	130	2	7	0	15	0	55
Cinnamon	⅛ tsp	15	0	0	0	4	3	0
Coconut	1 oz	80	0	5	0	7	1	40
Cookie Dough	1 piece	180	2	8	10	25	1	85
Fudge	1 oz	100	tr	3	0	17	0	45
Fudge Topping Fat Free	1 oz	80	tr	0	0	20	0	15
Granola	1 oz	120	2	2	0	23	2	30
Gumballs	1 oz	120	0	0	0	34	0	0
Gummi Bears	1 oz	120	0	0	0	30	0	15
Heath Candy	1 bar	110	1	7	0	12	0	75
Honey	1 oz	90	0	0	0	25	0	0

FOOD	PORTION	CALS	PROT	FAT	CHOL	CARB	FIBER	SOD
Kit Kat	½ bar	100	1	5	0	13	0	15
M&M's	1 oz	170	2	7	<5	25	1	20
M&M's Peanut	1 oz	150	3	8	<5	18	1	30
Macadamia Nuts	1 oz	180	2	19	0	3	2	65
Maraschino Cherry	1	5	0	0	0	1	0	0
Marshmallow Creme	1 oz	100	0	0	0	24	0	20
Marshmallows	1 oz	100	1	0	0	24	0	10
Nestle Crunch	½ bar	130	2	7	<5	16	1	35
Nilla Wafers	3	70	1	3	5	11	0	50
Oreo Cookies	2	120	2	5	0	17	1	170
Peach Pie Filling	1 oz	60	0	0	0	16	1	25
Peanut Butter	0.75 oz	150	6	13	0	5	1	115
Peanuts	1 oz	200	9	17	0	7	3	150
Pecan Pralines	1 oz	210	2	21	0	5	2	230
Pecans	1 oz	140	1	14	0	3	1	150
Pie Crust Graham Cracker	1 oz	110	2	3	0	19	1	160
Pie Crust Oreo	1 oz	180	0	8	0	19	0	190
Pistachio Nuts	1 oz	210	5	18	0	10	4	0
Raisins	1 oz	80	1	0	0	20	1	0
Raspberries	0.75 oz	15	1	0	0	4	1	0
Reese's Peanut Butter Cup	1 piece	190	4	11	0	19	1	110
Reese's Pieces	1 oz	170	5	7	0	21	1	50
Roasted Almonds	1 oz	190	6	17	0	5	3	230
Sliced Almonds	1 oz	210	7	20	0	6	4	0
Snickers	½ bar	170	3	9	<5	21	1	95
Sprinkles Chocolate	1 oz	25	0	0	0	6	0	0
Sprinkles Rainbow	1 oz	25	0	0	0	6	0	0
Strawberries	0.75 oz	20	0	0	0	7	1	0
Toasted Coconut	1 oz	180	2	14	0	13	1	10
Twix	1 cup	150	1	7	0	20	0	60
Walnuts	1 oz	130	3	12	0	4	1	0
Whip Topping	1 serv	45	tr	3	0	5	0	15
White Chocolate Chips	1 oz	160	2	9	<5	18	0	45
Whoppers	1 oz	100	tr	4	0	16	0	70
Yellow Sponge Cake	1 piece	70	1	1	25	15	0	60
York Peppermint Patties	2 pieces	120	1	2	0	24	1	5
SORBET								
Sinless Lemon	1 serv (6 oz)	180	0	0	0	48	0	20
Sinless Raspberry	1 serv (6 oz)	200	0	0	0	50	0	20
Sinless Tangerine	1 serv (6 oz)	200	tr	0	0	52	0	15

FOOD	PORTION	CALS	PROT	FAT	CHOL	CARB	FIBER	SOD
COSI								
BEVERAGES								
Arctic Double Chai	1 tall (12 oz)	621	7	25	72	96	1	382
Arctic Latte	1 tall (12 oz)	396	5	12	37	71	0	150
Arctic Mocha	1 tall (12 oz)	623	4	11	0	155	0	246
Arctic Raspberry Chai	1 tall (12 oz)	300	2	8	26	55	0	49
Arctic Thai as prep	1 tall (12 oz)	432	4	9	27	86	0	121
Caramel Mocha	1 tall (9 oz)	344	6	20	78	35	1	99
Chai Tea Latte	1 tall (8 oz)	109	4	4	16	15	0	62
Hot Chocolate	1 tall (12 oz)	436	10	29	111	38	1	162
Kefir Blueberry	1 (12 oz)	278	21	3	15	42	4	190
Lemonade	1 (15 oz)	112	0	0	0	26	0	9
Lemonade Strawberry	1 tall (12 oz)	290	0	0	55	72	1	0
Smoothie Mango Mania	1 tall (12 oz)	186	tr	0	33	44	tr	3
Smoothie Peach	1 tall (12 oz)	186	tr	0	33	44	tr	3
Smoothie Strawberry Banana	1 tall (12 oz)	186	tr	0	33	44	tr	3
Smores Latte	1 tall (11 oz)	401	10	20	71	47	1	232
Wildberry Blast	1 tall (12 oz)	186	tr	0	33	44	tr	3
BREAKFAST SELECTIONS								
Bagel Asiago Cheese	1 (6 oz)	327	9	1	3	68	2	132
Bagel Cinnamon Raisin	1 (6 oz)	438	10	1	3	90	5	133
Bagel Cranberry Orange	1 (6 oz)	372	9	1	3	80	2	131
Bagel Everything	1 (5.5 oz)	353	10	3	3	71	3	819
Bagel Plain	1 (5.5 oz)	326	9	1	0	68	2	122
Bagel Poppy Seed	1 (5.5 oz)	346	10	3	3	69	3	132
Cream Cheese Honey Pecan	1 serv (2 oz)	159	2	14	53	7	0	221
Cream Cheese Plain	1 serv (2 oz)	182	4	18	51	2	0	182
Cream Cheese Plain Low Fat	1 serv (2 oz)	121	6	12	40	2	0	304
Cream Cheese Veggie Low Fat	1 serv (2 oz)	113	4	9	28	2	0	246
Croissant Almond	1	340	7	16	35	42	2	280
Croissant Butter	1	330	7	17	45	38	1	350
Croissant Chocolate	1	370	8	18	35	45	2	300
Fruit Salad	1 serv	216	4	1	0	54	5	46
Granola Cereal	1 serv	564	14	12	16	107	8	371
Granola Parfait Peach	1 serv	389	13	6	13	74	3	257
Granola Parfait Strawberry	1 serv	426	13	6	13	84	4	257

FOOD	PORTION	CALS	PROT	FAT	CHOL	CARB	FIBER	SOD
Muffin Banana Nut	1	480	9	22	80	63	3	350
Muffin Blueberry	1	440	8	19	70	60	2	490
Muffin Carrot Raisin	1	470	8	22	85	62	3	420
Muffin Corn	1	450	7	25	75	50	3	690
Muffin Lowfat Bran	1	351	8	6	40	70	8	432
Scones Blueberry	1	410	8	17	50	60	2	380
DESSERTS								
Apple Tart	1 serv	396	5	6	10	83	4	73
Blondie Brownie	1	570	6	36	65	57	2	460
Cheesecake	1 serv	567	7	33	62	62	0	364
Cheesecake Brownie	1 serv	470	5	28	95	55	1	260
Cinnamon Apple Pie	1 serv	960	10	40	73	147	4	636
Cookie Chocolate Chunk	1	480	8	20	40	72	0	460
Cookie Oatmeal Raisin	1	440	8	14	40	76	0	380
Ice Cream Double Scoop	1 serv	225	4	14	38	22	0	52
Sundae	1 med	408	6	24	76	43	1	74
SALAD DRESSINGS								
Caesar	1 serv (2 oz)	301	2	32	77	2	0	193
Cosi Vinaigrette	1 serv (2 oz)	357	0	39	0	2	0	169
Fat Free Balsamic Vinaigrette	1 serv (2 oz)	45	0	0	0	11	0	290
Lowfat Ginger Soy	1 serv (2 oz)	74	1	2	0	13	1	414
Pepperanch	1 serv (2 oz)	262	2	28	17	2	0	296
Reduced Fat Roasted Shallot Sherry Vinaigrette	1 serv (2 oz)	85	0	5	0	3	0	45
Roasted Shallot Sherry Vinaigrette	1 serv (2 oz)	308	0	31	0	8	0	120
SALADS								
Bombay Chicken No Dressing	1 serv	176	27	3	50	13	4	600
Caesar No Dressing	1 serv	182	8	8	>5	20	2	416
Caesar w/ Grilled Chicken No Dressing	1 serv	340	33	10	72	21	3	741
Cosi Cobb No Dressing	1 serv	419	43	28	135	8	4	1252
Greek No Dressing	1 serv	236	11	17	30	9	4	922
Mixed Greens No Dressing	1 serv	46	3	1	0	9	4	35
Shanghai Chicken No Dressing	1 serv	221	26	9	61	16	5	261
Signature No Dressing	1 serv	375	15	21	38	40	7	629

FOOD	PORTION	CALS	PROT	FAT	CHOL	CARB	FIBER	SOD
SANDWICHES								
Buffalo Blue	1	649	44	30	130	57	5	1742
Cosi Club	1	729	37	35	81	59	4	1775
Green Market	1	555	23	17	16	74	7	1110
Grilled Chicken T.B.M.	1	791	48	43	95	60	6	1123
Hummus & Fresh Veggies	1	432	13	8	0	77	8	1126
Italiano	1	834	43	47	107	58	4	2682
Melts Bacon Turkey Cheddar	1	682	45	25	98	74	4	1780
Melts Chicken TBM	1	926	64	47	182	68	8	2205
Melts Grilled Chicken Parmesan	1	701	50	27	116	64	8	1970
Melts Pesto Chicken	1	809	54	39	150	64	7	1765
Melts Tomato Basil & Mozzarella	1	666	31	34	79	67	7	1788
Melts Tuna	1	1012	64	60	122	56	4	1948
Polpette Rustica	1	553	27	23	38	60	5	1651
Roasted Turkey & Brie	1	772	41	36	111	71	3	1660
Sesame Ginger Chicken	1	508	38	11	81	70	6	1374
Shrimp Salad	1	471	25	17	112	55	4	1631
Smoked Ham & Brie	1	639	33	25	90	69	3	2251
T.B.M.	1	729	26	42	21	61	6	1004
Tandoori Chicken	1	633	40	26	67	58	4	1637
Tuna Cheddar	1	956	60	55	109	55	4	1857
Turkey Light	1	476	30	9	51	73	4	1299
Turkey Rustica	1	619	37	27	101	60	4	1673
Tuscan Pesto Chicken	1	571	43	22	108	58	6	1192
Vegi Muffaletta	1	824	24	51	24	24	4	2929
Wasabi Roast Beef	1	626	31	28	78	64	5	2374
SOUPS								
Cajun Gumbo	1 serv (10 oz)	251	10	18	29	14	1	1529
Chicken Gumbo	1 serv (6 oz)	151	6	11	17	9	1	917
Chicken Noodle	1 serv (10 oz)	116	10	4	11	11	1	818
Grilled Chicken Corn Chowder	1 serv (10 oz)	305	16	16	72	24	2	1037
Lentil	1 serv (10 oz)	199	13	3	0	32	7	1159

FOOD	PORTION	CALS	PROT	FAT	CHOL	CARB	FIBER	SOD
Minestone	1 serv (10 oz)	174	8	3	6	28	4	995
New England Clam Chowder	1 serv (10 oz)	440	22	29	133	24	1	625
Three Bean Chili	1 serv (10 oz)	162	9	1	0	34	10	937

DAIRY QUEEN
FOOD SELECTIONS

FOOD	PORTION	CALS	PROT	FAT	CHOL	CARB	FIBER	SOD
Chicken Strip Basket	4 pieces	520	32	49	40	92	7	2090
Chili Cheese Dog	1	330	14	21	45	22	2	1090
DQ Homestyle Bacon Double Cheeseburger	1	610	41	36	130	31	2	1380
DQ Homestyle Burger	1	290	17	12	45	29	2	630
DQ Homestyle Cheeseburger	1	340	20	17	55	29	2	850
DQ Homestyle Double Cheeseburger	1	540	35	31	115	30	2	1130
DQ Ultimate Burger	1	670	40	43	135	29	2	1210
French Fries	1 sm	300	3	12	0	45	3	640
Grillburger 1/2 Lb	1	800	47	50	130	41	2	1230
Grillburger 1/2 Lb w/ Cheese	1	930	56	60	160	41	2	1380
Grillburger 1/4 Lb FlameThrower	1	850	34	64	130	38	1	1590
Grillburger Bacon Cheddar	1	710	36	45	105	40	1	1430
Grillburger California	1	630	26	42	75	37	1	820
Grillburger Classic	1	540	27	30	65	41	2	990
Grillburger Classic w/ Cheese	1	610	31	36	85	41	2	1110
Grillburger Mushroom Swiss	1	700	30	47	90	37	1	890
Hot Dog	1	240	9	14	25	19	1	730
Onion Rings	1 reg	470	6	30	0	45	3	740
Salad Crispy Chicken No Dressing	1 serv	350	21	20	40	21	6	620
Salad Grilled Chicken No Dressing	1 serv	240	26	10	65	17	4	950
Sandwich Crispy Chicken	1	590	21	34	40	50	5	1100
Sandwich Gilled Chicken	1	340	22	16	55	26	2	1000

FOOD	PORTION	CALS	PROT	FAT	CHOL	CARB	FIBER	SOD
Side Salad	1 serv	60	3	3	5	6	2	60
ICE CREAM								
Banana Split	1	510	8	12	30	96	3	180
Blizzard Banana Split	1 sm	460	10	14	40	73	tr	210
Blizzard Chocolate Chip Cookie Dough	1 sm	720	12	28	50	105	0	370
Blizzard Oreo Cookies	1 sm	570	11	21	40	83	tr	430
Blizzard Reese's Peanut Butter Cup	1 sm	600	14	21	40	87	0	220
Blizzard Strawberry Cheesecake	1 sm	530	10	21	85	76	tr	320
Brownie Earthquake	1	740	10	27	50	112	0	350
Buster Bar	1	500	11	28	15	45	2	230
Cake 8 Inch Round	1/8 cake	370	7	13	25	56	tr	280
Cake Blizzard Oreo Cookie	1/8 cake	490	8	20	30	67	1	250
Cake Blizzard Reese's Peanut Butter Cup	1/8 cake	490	6	20	30	67	1	190
Cone Chocolate	1 sm	240	6	8	20	37	0	115
Cone Vanilla	1 sm	230	6	7	20	38	0	115
Cone Dipped	1 sm	340	6	17	20	42	1	130
Dilly Bar Chocolate	1	220	3	13	15	25	0	85
DQ Fudge Bar No Sugar Added	1	50	4	0	0	13	0	70
DQ Sandwich	1	200	4	6	10	31	1	140
DQ Soft Serve Chocolate	1/2 cup	150	4	5	15	22	0	75
DQ Soft Serve Vanilla	1/2 cup	140	3	5	15	22	0	70
DQ Vanilla Orange Bar No Sugar Added	1	60	2	0	0	17	0	40
Malt Chocolate	1 sm	640	15	16	55	111	1	340
MooLatte Cappuccino	1 (16 oz)	490	7	18	30	68	0	170
MooLatte Caramel	1 (16 oz)	630	9	20	35	96	0	250
MooLatte French Vanilla	1 (16 oz)	570	7	18	30	87	0	170
MooLatte Mocha	1 (16 oz)	590	8	23	30	80	1	210
Peanut Buster Parfait	1	730	16	31	35	99	2	400
Shake Chocolate	1 sm	560	13	15	50	93	1	280
Slush Arctic Rush	1 sm	220	0	0	0	56	0	20
Starkiss	1	80	0	0	0	21	0	10
Sundae Chocolate	1 sm	280	5	7	20	49	0	140
Sundae Strawberry	1 sm	240	5	7	20	40	0	110

FOOD	PORTION	CALS	PROT	FAT	CHOL	CARB	FIBER	SOD
SALAD DRESSINGS								
Blue Cheese	1 serv (2 oz)	210	2	20	5	4	0	700
Honey Mustard	1 serv (2 oz)	260	1	21	20	18	0	370
Italian Fat Free	1 serv (2 oz)	10	0	0	0	3	0	390
Ranch	1 serv (2 oz)	310	1	33	25	3	0	390
D'ANGELO								
CHILDREN'S MENU SELECTIONS								
D'Lite Turkey	1	217	19	3	14	30	3	369
Sub Cheeseburger	1	294	15	13	43	28	3	459
Sub Ham & Cheese	1	227	14	5	30	32	1	997
Sub Kidz Tuna	1	438	15	29	18	30	1	614
Sub Meatball	1	330	15	15	37	37	4	812
SALAD DRESSINGS								
Bleu Cheese	1 serv	152	1	15	15	3	0	283
Caesar	1 serv	397	6	43	43	6	0	1191
Caesar Fat Free	1 serv	57	0	0	0	9	0	1673
Creamy Italian	1 serv	340	0	37	0	9	0	851
Greek w/ Feta Cheese	1 serv	227	0	26	14	6	0	765
Honey Mustard	1 serv	150	0	142	0	7	0	210
Olive Oil Vinaigrette	1 serv	170	0	17	0	9	0	652
Ranch Lite	1 serv	240	2	19	20	6	1	961
SALADS								
Antipasto	1 serv	284	16	18	40	17	6	1109
Caesar w/ Dressing	1 serv	474	15	39	40	25	4	1208
Chicken Caesar w/ Dressing	1 serv	533	35	38	99	19	4	1654
Chicken Stir Fry w/o Dressing	1 serv	168	25	3	59	11	4	590
Cobb w/o Dressing	1 serv	292	27	17	76	11	4	636
Greek	1 serv	290	11	23	50	17	4	1098
Lobster w/o Dressing	1 serv	376	26	26	86	12	4	589
Roast Beef w/o Dressing	1 serv	131	19	3	42	10	4	208
Steak Tip Caesar	1 serv	661	32	50	95	21	3	1627
Tossed Garden w/o Dressing	1 serv	49	3	1	0	11	4	22
Turkey w/o Dressing	1 serv	157	26	2	22	10	4	86
SANDWICHES								
D'Lite Chicken Caesar Salad	1	374	34	7	68	43	4	2002

FOOD	PORTION	CALS	PROT	FAT	CHOL	CARB	FIBER	SOD
D'Lite Chicken Stir Fry	1	426	37	6	73	57	7	1241
D'Lite Classic Veggie	1	362	15	7	13	63	8	839
D'Lite Fresh Veggie	1	348	13	7	13	62	7	651
D'Lite Grilled Chicken Breast	1	388	31	7	67	52	6	953
D'Lite Roast Beef	1	338	25	5	42	51	6	727
D'Lite Turkey	1	347	28	4	19	51	6	595
D'Lite Turkey Cranberry	1	444	28	4	19	75	6	595
Pokket Big Papi	1	469	39	11	84	53	3	2536
Pokket BLT & Cheese	1	397	22	17	50	38	3	1266
Pokket Caesar Salad	1	616	20	39	40	54	3	1518
Pokket Capacola & Cheese	1	362	26	13	60	35	2	1547
Pokket Cheese	1	519	29	27	74	41	2	1765
Pokket Cheeseburger	1	459	27	25	85	31	2	811
Pokket Chicken Caesar Salad	1	674	40	39	99	47	3	1964
Pokket Chicken Club	1	526	34	28	87	36	2	1088
Pokket Chicken Honey Dijon	1	508	41	20	111	40	2	1165
Pokket Chicken Salad	1	623	27	42	71	34	2	639
Pokket Chicken Stir Fry	1	380	35	9	79	39	2	1276
Pokket Classic Vegetable	1	368	19	13	33	46	4	934
Pokket Classic Veggie No Cheese	1	212	9	1	0	44	4	331
Pokket Greek	1	790	16	61	50	49	4	1892
Pokket Grilled Chicken	1	303	29	5	67	35	2	739
Pokket Ham	1	229	17	3	33	35	2	1050
Pokket Ham & Cheese	1	326	22	10	53	38	2	1493
Pokket Ham & Salami	1	386	23	17	56	34	12	1301
Pokket Hamburger	1	399	24	20	72	29	2	343
Pokket Italian	1	525	28	30	80	36	2	1678
Pokket Lobster	1	530	29	31	84	34	2	897
Pokket Meatball	1	574	26	31	73	52	4	1765
Pokket Mortadella & Cheese	1	410	21	21	56	35	2	1114
Pokket Number 9	1	407	31	18	76	31	2	685
Pokket Pastrami	1	438	24	25	91	33	1	1643
Pokket Pepperoni	1	407	21	20	47	35	3	1147
Pokket Roast Beef	1	247	23	3	42	33	2	511
Pokket Salad	1	196	8	1	0	40	4	340

FOOD	PORTION	CALS	PROT	FAT	CHOL	CARB	FIBER	SOD
Pokket Salami & Cheese	1	509	25	30	75	33	2	1590
Pokket Seafood Salad	1	449	14	22	11	50	3	1182
Pokket Steak	1	305	25	12	59	24	1	324
Pokket Steak & Cheese	1	377	29	17	74	26	1	665
Pokket Steak Bomb	1	631	43	32	102	44	3	1794
Pokket Steak Tip	1	452	27	16	54	45	2	1189
Pokket Tuna	1	664	24	49	32	33	2	825
Pokket Turkey	1	256	26	2	19	33	2	379
Pokket Turkey Club	1	332	34	7	54	32	2	610
Sub Big Papi	1 sm	525	40	15	83	60	7	2700
Sub BLT & Cheese	1 sm	463	23	19	50	51	6	1437
Sub Capicola & Cheese	1 sm	408	25	13	50	48	5	1482
Sub Cheese	1 sm	589	30	28	74	55	5	1939
Sub Cheeseburger	1 sm	526	29	26	86	44	5	774
Sub Chicken Club	1	593	35	29	87	49	5	1260
Sub Chicken Honey Dijon	1	575	42	22	111	53	5	1338
Sub Chicken Salad	1 sm	692	29	44	71	48	5	813
Sub Chicken Stir Fry	1 sm	449	37	11	79	53	6	1449
Sub Classic Veggie	1 sm	462	21	15	34	64	8	1162
Sub Grilled Chicken	1 sm	369	30	7	67	48	5	911
Sub Ham	1 sm	302	18	5	33	49	2	1226
Sub Ham & Cheese	1 sm	395	24	11	53	52	2	1667
Sub Ham & Salami	1 sm	456	25	19	56	48	2	1475
Sub Hamburger	1 sm	466	25	22	73	42	5	503
Sub Italian	1 sm	614	30	31	80	54	3	1893
Sub Lobster	1 sm	598	30	33	84	48	5	1089
Sub Meatball	1 sm	644	28	33	73	66	7	1939
Sub Meatballs & Cheese	1 sm	750	36	41	94	67	7	2204
Sub Mortadella & Cheese	1 sm	479	23	23	56	49	5	1288
Sub Number 9	1 sm	450	31	19	74	41	4	802
Sub Pastrami	1 sm	613	34	34	118	47	5	1875
Sub Pepperoni	1 sm	603	28	33	72	49	7	1836
Sub Roast Beef	1 sm	320	25	5	42	48	5	687
Sub Salad	1 sm	281	10	3	0	57	8	522
Sub Salami & Cheese	1 sm	579	27	32	75	47	5	1764
Sub Seafood Salad	1 sm	498	14	23	10	61	6	1208
Sub Steak	1 sm	373	27	14	59	37	4	491
Sub Steak & Cheese	1 sm	446	31	19	74	40	4	832
Sub Steak Bomb	1 sm	670	43	33	102	52	6	1904
Sub Steak Tip	1 sm	545	29	18	54	63	3	1413

FOOD	PORTION	CALS	PROT	FAT	CHOL	CARB	FIBER	SOD
Sub Toasted Italian Bistro	1 sm	585	29	31	81	49	5	1912
Sub Toasted Pastrami Reuben	1 sm	750	30	47	104	55	7	2226
Sub Toasted Roast Beef & Cheddar	1 sm	564	35	26	88	51	5	1117
Sub Toasted Spicy Meatball	1 sm	933	61	57	102	71	9	2560
Sub Toasted Tuna & Swiss	1 sm	796	32	54	55	49	5	1027
Sub Toasted Turkey & Ham	1 sm	532	33	24	66	49	5	1507
Sub Toasted Turkey Thanksgiving	1 sm	705	32	20	21	80	6	1315
Sub Tuna	1	685	24	46	29	47	2	952
Sub Turkey Club	1 sm	401	33	9	48	49	3	806
Wrap Big Papi	1	593	41	23	83	56	4	2859
Wrap BLT & Cheese	1	544	24	26	50	54	4	1542
Wrap Buffalo Chicken Salad	1	823	40	44	101	67	4	2917
Wrap Caesar Salad	1	711	20	44	40	65	5	1679
Wrap Capacola & Cheese	1	494	25	20	50	53	4	1589
Wrap Cheese	1	675	30	35	74	59	4	2046
Wrap Cheeseburger	1	609	30	33	86	48	3	879
Wrap Chicken Caesar Salad	1	830	42	47	99	65	5	2246
Wrap Chicken Cobb	1	931	36	55	102	71	6	1790
Wrap Chicken Filet & Bacon	1	639	38	28	87	58	2	1078
Wrap Chicken Honey Dijon	1	672	60	29	110	43	5	1466
Wrap Chicken Salad	1	782	29	51	71	53	4	922
Wrap Chicken Stir Fry	1	535	37	17	79	57	4	1557
Wrap Classic Veggie	1	486	24	13	34	68	5	936
Wrap Greek	1	765	15	61	50	44	4	1723
Wrap Grilled Chicken	1	422	34	6	67	59	4	733
Wrap Ham & Cheese	1	435	26	10	53	60	3	1481
Wrap Ham & Salami	1	513	57	18	63	30	3	1449
Wrap Hamburger	1	509	28	21	74	50	3	340
Wrap Italian	1	631	32	29	80	59	3	1667
Wrap Lobster	1	749	33	43	86	57	3	954
Wrap Meatball	1	687	31	31	73	75	5	1755
Wrap Mortadella & Cheese	1	522	25	21	56	58	3	1103
Wrap Number 9	1	517	32	24	74	44	3	885
Wrap Pastrami	1	550	28	25	91	55	2	1632
Wrap Peppercorn Steak	1	702	41	40	110	45	3	1745
Wrap Pepperoni	1	519	25	21	47	57	4	1136

FOOD	PORTION	CALS	PROT	FAT	CHOL	CARB	FIBER	SOD
Wrap Roast Beef	1	448	26	13	42	58	4	881
Wrap Salad	1	324	13	2	0	66	6	337
Wrap Salami & Cheese	1	605	29	29	72	56	3	1510
Wrap Seafood Salad	1	541	17	22	10	69	3	1024
Wrap Steak	1	392	28	13	59	41	2	316
Wrap Steak & Cheese	1	464	33	18	74	43	2	657
Wrap Steak Bomb	1	670	43	33	102	52	6	1904
Wrap Steak Tip	1	432	26	16	54	41	2	1029
Wrap Tuna	1	731	27	44	29	56	3	769
Wrap Turkey	1	369	30	3	19	55	3	369
Wrap Turkey Club	1	415	34	8	48	52	3	590
SOUPS								
Beef Stew	1 sm	220	12	8	30	23	2	819
Broccoli & Cheddar Cheese	1 sm	270	9	21	60	11	2	859
Chicken Noodle	1 sm	110	6	3	25	14	1	829
Hearty Vegetable	1 sm	40	2	0	0	7	2	270
Italian Wedding	1 sm	120	6	6	15	11	2	919
Lobster Bisque	1 sm	360	8	29	105	16	1	819
New England Clam Chowder	1 sm	320	9	18	60	31	1	699
Portuguese Kale	1 sm	130	8	4	10	16	3	629

DELTACO
BEVERAGES

FOOD	PORTION	CALS	PROT	FAT	CHOL	CARB	FIBER	SOD
Barq's Root Beer	1 sm	278	0	0	0	75	0	60
Classic Coke	1 sm	248	0	0	0	68	0	15
Diet Coke	1 sm	2	0	0	0	0	0	25
Iced Tea	1 sm	0	0	0	0	1	0	10
Light Lemonade Minute Maid	1 sm	13	0	0	0	3	0	13
Milk 2% Low Fat	1 serv	152	10	6	24	15	0	125
Mr Pibb Xtra	1 sm	243	0	0	0	65	0	35
Orange Juice	1 serv	140	1	0	0	34	1	0
Shake Chocolate	1 (15 oz)	680	16	18	45	117	1	350
Shake Strawberry	1 (15 oz)	540	14	8	40	100	1	280
Shake Vanilla	1 (15 oz)	550	16	10	50	97	0	320
Sprite	1 sm	243	0	0	0	65	0	55
BREAKFAST SELECTIONS								
Burrito Breakfast	1	250	10	11	160	24	1	520
Burrito Egg & Cheese	1	450	23	24	530	39	3	740

FOOD	PORTION	CALS	PROT	FAT	CHOL	CARB	FIBER	SOD
Burrito Macho Bacon & Egg	1	1030	40	60	790	82	6	1760
Burrito Steak & Egg	1	580	33	34	560	41	3	1270
Hash Brown Sticks	5 pieces	250	0	19	0	20	0	200
Quesadilla Bacon & Egg	1	450	21	23	260	40	2	920
Side of Bacon	2 strips	50	3	4	10	0	0	170
MAIN MENU SELECTIONS								
Beans 'n Cheese Cup	1 serv	260	16	3	5	44	16	1810
Bun Taco	1	440	24	21	65	37	4	830
Burrito Del Beef	1	550	31	30	90	42	3	1090
Burrito Del Classic Chicken	1	560	24	36	70	41	3	1100
Burrito Del Combo	1	530	28	22	55	61	11	1680
Burrito Deluxe Combo	1	570	29	26	60	64	12	1700
Burrito Deluxe Del Beef	1	590	32	33	95	45	4	1110
Burrito Green Bean & Cheese	1	280	11	8	15	36	6	1030
Burrito Green Half Pound	1	430	20	12	20	59	13	1690
Burrito Macho Beef	1	1170	60	62	190	89	7	2190
Burrito Macho Chicken	1	930	47	33	100	111	16	2990
Burrito Macho Combo	1	1050	49	44	115	113	17	2760
Burrito Red Bean & Cheese	1	270	11	8	15	36	6	1020
Burrito Red Half Pound	1	430	20	12	20	65	13	1670
Burrito Spicy Chicken	1	480	23	16	40	66	8	1850
Burrito Works Chicken	1	520	26	23	65	57	4	1620
Burrito Works Steak	1	590	27	31	70	56	5	1820
Burrito Works Veggie	1	490	18	18	25	69	9	1660
Burritos Crispy Fish	1	497	17	21	48	59	2	1117
Cheeseburger	1	330	16	13	35	37	3	870
Cheeseburger Double Del	1	560	26	35	85	35	4	960
Cheeseburger Double Del Bacon	1	610	29	39	95	35	4	1130
Chips & Salsa	1 sm	156	2	7	0	22	1	290
Del Cheeseburger	1	430	16	25	45	35	4	710
Fries	1 sm	350	3	23	0	34	3	270
Fries Chili Cheese	1 serv	670	17	46	45	51	5	880
Fries Deluxe Chili Cheese	1 serv	710	17	49	50	53	6	880
Hamburger	1	280	13	9	25	37	3	640
Nachos	1 serv	380	5	24	5	40	2	630
Nachos Macho	1 serv	1100	31	63	55	113	15	2640
Quesadilla Cheddar	1	500	23	27	75	39	2	860

FOOD	PORTION	CALS	PROT	FAT	CHOL	CARB	FIBER	SOD
Quesadilla Spicy Jack	1	490	23	28	75	38	2	920
Quesadilla Spicy Jack Chicken	1	570	32	30	105	40	2	1300
Quesadillas Chicken Cheddar	1	580	33	31	104	41	2	1240
Rice Cup	1 serv	140	3	2	2	27	1	910
Taco	1	160	7	10	20	11	1	150
Taco Big Fat	1	320	16	11	35	39	3	680
Taco Big Fat Chicken	1	340	18	13	45	38	3	840
Taco Big Fat Steak	1	390	18	19	45	38	3	960
Taco Carne Asada	1	237	9	8	25	22	2	481
Taco Crispy Fish	1	290	7	16	20	30	2	460
Taco Del Carbon Chicken	1	170	12	5	30	19	2	530
Taco Del Carbon Steak	1	220	12	11	30	19	2	680
Taco Macho	1	504	13	37	107	19	5	833
Taco Soft	1	160	8	8	20	16	1	330
Taco Soft Chicken	1	210	11	12	30	16	1	520
SALADS								
Deluxe Chicken Salad	1 serv	740	33	34	70	77	15	2610
Taco Salad	1 serv	350	10	30	45	10	2	390
Taco Salad Deluxe	1	780	33	40	80	76	14	2250

DENNY'S
BEVERAGES

FOOD	PORTION	CALS	PROT	FAT	CHOL	CARB	FIBER	SOD
Apple Juice	1 reg	126	0	0	0	33	0	24
Cappuccino French Vanilla	8 oz	100	3	2	0	28	1	220
Cappuccino Original	8 oz	100	2	3	0	17	0	100
Grapefruit	1 serv (10 oz)	162	0	0	0	41	0	43
Malted Milk Shake Chocolate Or Vanilla	12 oz	583	12	26	100	82	tr	278
Orange Juice	10 oz	126	2	0	0	31	0	31
Tomato Juice	1 serv (10 oz)	56	2	0	0	11	2	921

BREAKFAST SELECTIONS

FOOD	PORTION	CALS	PROT	FAT	CHOL	CARB	FIBER	SOD
All American Slam	1 serv	816	45	67	828	3	1	1826
Applesauce	1 serv	60	0	0	0	15	1	13
Belgian Waffle	1	619	22	45	274	28	0	1638
Breakfast Dagwood	1 serv	1446	82	90	765	81	1	4003
Cantaloupe	¼	32	1	0	0	8	1	16
Chicken Fajita Skillet	1 serv	855	26	49	515	30	11	1863

FOOD	PORTION	CALS	PROT	FAT	CHOL	CARB	FIBER	SOD
Corned Beef Hash Slam	1 serv	668	32	55	535	11	1	816
Country Fish Potatoes	1 serv	394	3	20	9	23	10	938
Egg	1	120	6	10	210	tr	0	120
English Muffin Dry	1	125	5	1	0	24	1	198
French Slam	1 serv	1119	45	77	705	71	3	2265
Grand Slam Slugger	1 serv	927	34	55	476	74	3	2399
Grapefruit	½	60	1	0	0	16	6	0
Grapes	1 serv	55	1	1	0	15	1	0
Grits	1 serv	80	2	0	0	18	0	520
Ham & Cheddar Omelette	1 serv	595	41	47	783	5	0	1200
Ham & Cheese Omelette w/ Eggbeaters	1 serv	468	37	32	58	5	0	1351
Ham Slice	1	94	15	3	23	2	0	761
Hash Browns	1 serv	197	2	12	0	20	2	446
Honeydew	¼	31	1	0	0	8	1	22
Lumberjack Slam w/ Hash Browns	1 serv	1035	51	58	589	73	3	4462
Meat Lover's Skillet	1 serv	1031	39	74	528	27	10	2374
Moon Over My Hammy	1 serv	841	54	51	580	42	2	2699
Oatmeal	1 serv	100	5	2	0	18	3	175
Oatmeal Deluxe	1 serv	460	13	6	11	95	7	87
Original Grand Slam	1 serv	665	26	49	515	33	2	1106
Ready To Eat Cereal	1 serv	100	2	0	0	23	1	276
Sausage	4 links	354	16	32	64	0	0	944
Scram Slam	1 serv	827	45	68	801	8	1	1937
Senior Omelette	1 serv	429	25	20	515	8	2	755
T-Bone Steak & Eggs	1 serv	991	73	77	657	1	1	1003
Toast Dry	1 slice	92	3	1	0	17	1	166
Ultimate Omelette	1 serv	611	34	50	756	11	3	1007
CHILDREN'S MENU SELECTIONS								
Burgerlicious w/ Cheese	1 serv	341	15	20	40	24	1	560
Frenchtastic Slam	1 serv	452	19	33	311	22	1	664
Junior Shrimps Ahoy!	1 serv	411	13	18	66	50	4	792
Oreo Blender Blaster	1 serv	580	11	29	87	72	1	194
Pizza Party	1 serv	400	18	15	10	47	7	1090
Smiley-Face Hotcakes w/ Meat	1 serv	463	14	22	38	63	2	1410
Smiley-Face Hotcakes w/o Meat	1 serv	344	7	9	13	62	2	1014

FOOD	PORTION	CALS	PROT	FAT	CHOL	CARB	FIBER	SOD
DESSERTS								
Banana Split	1	894	15	43	78	121	6	177
Carrot Cake	1 serv	799	9	45	125	99	2	630
Cheesecake	1 serv	580	8	38	174	51	0	380
Chocolate Topping	1 serv	317	2	25	0	27	0	83
Chocolate Peanut Butter Pie	1 serv	653	15	39	27	64	3	319
Double Scoop Sundae	1 serv	375	6	27	74	29	0	86
Float Rootbeer or Coke	12 oz	280	3	10	39	47	0	109
Milkshake Vanilla or Chocolate	12 oz	560	11	26	100	76	tr	272
Oreo Blender Blaster	1 serv	895	16	46	135	112	2	280
Single Scoop Sundae	1 serv	188	3	14	37	14	0	43
MAIN MENU SELECTIONS								
Albacore Tuna Melt	1 serv	640	30	39	109	42	3	1436
Applesauce	1 serv	60	0	0	0	15	1	13
Bacon Lettuce & Tomato	1	610	15	38	35	50	2	862
BBQ Chicken Sandwich	1 serv	1089	48	62	103	86	5	1872
Buffalo Chicken Sandwich	1 serv	708	37	28	74	80	5	1733
Buffalo Chicken Strips	5 pieces	734	48	42	96	43	0	1673
Buffalo Wings	12 pieces	856	92	54	500	1	1	5552
Burger Bacon Cheddar	1	875	53	52	163	58	5	1672
Burger BBQ	1 serv	953	52	52	136	72	4	2130
Burger Boca	1 serv	601	32	27	14	64	9	1446
Burger Classic	1	694	40	35	100	56	4	785
Burger Classic w/ Cheese	1	852	49	48	140	57	4	1385
Burger Mushroom Swiss	1 serv	880	51	49	137	63	5	1619
Chicken Strips	5 pieces	720	47	33	95	56	0	1666
Chicken Ranch Melt	1 serv	758	44	45	105	44	3	2195
Club Sandwich	1	718	32	38	75	62	3	1666
Coleslaw	1 serv	274	2	30	37	14	2	568
Country Fried Steak	1 serv	644	28	48	89	30	11	2149
French Fries Unsalted	1 serv	423	6	20	0	57	5	221
Fried Shrimp & Shrimp Scampi	1 serv	346	27	20	241	15	1	1104
Grilled Cheese Sandwich	1	510	19	30	54	40	3	1360
Grilled Chicken Sandwich	1	469	35	14	77	53	4	1392
Ham & Swiss On Rye	1	417	32	16	57	39	5	1763
Hoagie Chicken Melt	1	751	46	44	93	43	2	1834
Hoagie Philly Melt	1 serv	874	47	50	114	58	5	2444

FOOD	PORTION	CALS	PROT	FAT	CHOL	CARB	FIBER	SOD
Mozzarella Sticks	8 pieces	710	36	41	48	49	6	5220
Onion Rings	1 serv	381	5	23	6	38	1	1003
Patty Melt	1	798	45	51	127	37	4	1285
Pot Roast Dinner w/ Gravy	1 serv	292	42	11	87	5	0	927
Roast Turkey & Stuffing w/ Gravy	1 serv	388	46	3	116	38	2	2467
Sampler	1 serv	1405	47	80	75	124	4	5305
Senior Chicken Strip Dinner	1 serv	285	19	10	37	31	0	969
Senior Club	1 serv	540	29	31	89	34	3	1499
Senior Country Fried Steak	1 serv	341	14	23	44	18	6	1464
Senior French Slam	1 serv	820	28	65	432	40	1	777
Senior Fried Shrimp Dinner	1 serv	129	12	5	66	13	1	645
Senior Grilled Chicken Breast	1 serv	200	25	5	67	15	1	824
Shrimp Scampi Skillet Dinner	1 serv	289	25	19	192	3	tr	766
Sirloin Steak Dinner	1 serv	337	18	28	687	1	1	344
Smoothered Cheese Fries	1 serv	767	27	48	78	69	0	875
The Super Bird Sandwich	1	620	35	32	60	48	2	1880
Turkey Breast On Multigrain w/o Mayo	1	277	23	4	15	41	5	1607
SALAD DRESSINGS AND TOPPINGS								
BBQ Sauce	1.5 oz	47	0	1	0	11	0	595
Bleu Cheese	1 oz	163	1	18	20	1	0	205
Blueberry Topping	1 serv	71	0	0	0	17	0	10
Caesar	1 oz	133	1	14	2	1	0	380
Cherry Topping	1 serv	57	0	0	0	14	0	3
Cream Cheese	1 oz	100	2	10	31	1	0	6
French	1 oz	106	0	10	7	3	0	274
Fudge Topping	1 serv	201	1	10	3	30	1	96
Honey Mustard	1 serv	160	0	15	20	20	0	123
Low Calorie Italian	1 oz	15	0	1	0	3	0	390
Marinara Sauce	1 serv	48	1	2	0	7	1	206
Ranch	1 oz	129	0	14	8	1	0	189
Ranch Fat Free	1 serv	25	0	tr	0	6	0	300
Sour Cream	1.5 oz	91	1	9	19	2	0	23
Strawberry Topping	1 serv	77	1	1	0	17	1	8
Syrup	3 tbsp	143	0	0	0	36	0	26
Syrup Sugar Free	1 serv	23	0	0	0	9	0	71
Tartar Sauce	1 serv	225	0	23	15	3	0	157

FOOD	PORTION	CALS	PROT	FAT	CHOL	CARB	FIBER	SOD
Thousand Island	1 oz	118	0	11	15	5	0	170
Whipped Margarine	1 serv	87	0	10	0	0	0	117
Whipped Cream	2 tbsp	23	0	2	7	2	0	3
SALADS								
Garden Salad w/ Albacore Tuna	1 serv	444	35	29	81	12	4	824
Garden Salad w/ Fried Chicken Strips	1 serv	438	33	26	78	26	4	1030
Garden Salad w/ Grilled Chicken Breast	1 serv	264	32	11	89	10	4	714
Grilled Chicken Caesar Salad w/ Dressing	1 serv	600	37	41	101	19	4	1792
Side Caesar w/ Dressing	1 serv	362	11	26	23	20	3	913
Side Garden Salad w/o Dressing	1 serv	113	3	4	0	16	3	147
SOUPS								
Chicken Noodle	1 serv	60	2	2	10	8	0	640
Clam Chowder	1 serv	624	7	42	5	55	4	1474
Cream Of Broccoli	1 serv	574	6	43	0	41	2	1174
Vegetable Beef	1 serv	79	6	1	5	11	2	820

DESERT MOON CAFE
CHILDREN'S MENU SELECTIONS

FOOD	PORTION	CALS	PROT	FAT	CHOL	CARB	FIBER	SOD
Burrito Bean & Cheese	1 serv	650	22	26	30	83	6	1450
Kids Nachos	1 serv	500	13	23	25	59	2	570
Kids Taco w/ Chicken	1	280	15	7	30	38	2	590
Kids Taco w/ Steak	1	290	15	8	30	38	2	590
Kidsadilla	1 serv	630	23	30	50	70	1	1220
MAIN MENU SELECTIONS								
Alamo Burger	1	810	51	51	160	35	3	730
Burrito Adobe Moon w/ Chicken	1	730	35	28	65	85	4	1230
Burrito Adobe Moon w/ Steak	1	750	35	31	70	85	4	1230
Burrito Black Bean w/ Chicken	1	770	41	25	85	98	5	1190
Burrito Black Bean w/ Steak	1	790	40	27	85	98	5	1190
Burrito Full Moon w/ Chicken	1	620	36	24	70	66	7	1310
Burrito Full Moon w/ Steak	1	640	36	26	75	66	7	1300

FOOD	PORTION	CALS	PROT	FAT	CHOL	CARB	FIBER	SOD
Burrito Get It Smothered	1	120	7	9	30	4	0	540
Burrito Harvest Wrap w/ Chicken	1	620	32	30	65	57	6	1250
Burrito Harvest Wrap w/ Steak	1	300	32	33	70	57	6	1240
Enchilada Mesa	1	710	37	27	105	74	4	1370
Enchilada Queso	1	730	43	26	105	74	4	1650
Enchilada Shrimp	1	830	32	28	110	110	4	2620
Fajita Platter w/ Chicken	1 serv	1160	61	51	165	109	13	2280
Fajita Platter w/ Shrimp	1 serv	1060	44	49	175	109	13	2900
Fajita Platter w/ Steak	1	1190	61	55	165	109	13	2270
Hell Canyon Chili	1 serv	260	15	14	45	20	3	580
Mucho Nachos	1 serv	800	27	47	80	71	5	970
Mucho Nachos w/ Chicken	1 serv	900	45	49	130	71	5	1010
Mucho Nachos w/ Steak	1 serv	920	44	52	130	71	5	1010
Pizza Texas BBQ	1	330	44	37	125	68	2	1320
Quesadilla Baja Chicken	1	650	41	32	150	53	2	1180
Quesadilla Coyote w/ Chicken	1	660	41	32	105	53	2	1140
Quesadilla Coyote w/ Steak	1	680	41	35	105	53	2	1130
Quesadilla Sonoran	1	660	24	39	50	60	5	1220
Rice Bowl Black Bean w/ Chicken	1 serv	790	41	14	75	123	4	1290
Rice Bowl Black Bean w/ Steak	1 serv	820	41	17	80	123	4	1290
Rice Bowl Chili w/ Chicken	1 serv	760	40	17	90	109	2	1440
Rice Bowl Chili w/ Steak	1 serv	790	39	20	95	109	2	1430
Rice Bowl Shrimp Creole	1 serv	910	61	19	300	124	3	4060
Shrimp Dippers	1 serv	430	21	15	85	50	4	1660
Soup Black Bean	1 serv	360	21	7	15	55	10	250
Soup Tortilla	1 serv	330	11	13	15	45	5	1950
Taco Acapulco Shrimp	1	230	7	9	35	30	2	340
Taco Classic w/ Chicken	1	190	14	6	35	17	2	370
Taco Classic w/ Steak	1	200	14	7	35	17	2	370
Taco Fajita w/ Chicken	1	200	14	6	35	19	2	420
Taco Fajita w/ Steak	1	210	14	8	35	19	2	410
SALAD DRESSINGS AND SAUCES								
BBQ Sauce	1 serv (1 oz)	50	0	1	0	12	0	100
Buffalo Wing Sauce	1 serv (1 oz)	45	0	5	0	1	0	530

FOOD	PORTION	CALS	PROT	FAT	CHOL	CARB	FIBER	SOD
Dressing Bleu Cheese	1 serv (2 oz)	300	2	32	30	2	0	590
Dressing Creamy Caesar	1 serv (2 oz)	320	2	36	30	0	0	550
Dressing Honey Dijon Fat Free	1 serv (2 oz)	80	2	0	0	17	2	470
Dressing Lite Ranch	1 serv (2 oz)	150	2	13	10	4	0	640
Dressing Lite Raspberry Vinaigrette	1 serv (2 oz)	150	0	11	0	6	0	240
Dressing Poblano	1 serv (1 oz)	150	1	16	10	2	1	35
Guacamole	1 serv (2 oz)	100	1	9	0	4	3	95
Pepper Cream Sauce	1 serv (2 oz)	100	1	9	30	4	0	260
Pico De Gallo	1 serv (2 oz)	15	1	0	0	3	1	125
Salsa Black Bean	1 serv (2 oz)	20	1	0	0	4	1	55
Salsa Fruit	1 serv (2 oz)	60	1	2	0	12	0	0
Salsa Mild Tomato	1 serv (2 oz)	15	1	0	0	3	1	100
Salsa Rattlesnake	1 serv (2 oz)	15	0	0	0	3	1	130
SALADS W/O TORTILLA BOWL								
Caesar	1 serv	530	17	47	50	15	4	1220
Caesar w/ Chicken	1 serv	640	36	49	100	15	4	1260
Caesar w/ Shrimp	1 serv	570	25	48	110	15	4	1680
Chopped Chicken	1 serv	520	32	35	95	21	5	670
Taco w/ Chicken	1 serv	310	30	15	95	15	3	460
Taco w/ Steak	1 serv	340	30	17	95	15	3	450

DONATOS PIZZA

PIZZA

FOOD	PORTION	CALS	PROT	FAT	CHOL	CARB	FIBER	SOD
Dessert Apple	¼ pie	722	12	20	21	137	15	926
Dessert Cherry	¼ pie	818	12	20	20	149	13	924
Original Chicken Vegy Medley	¼ pie	500	28	19	80	56	11	1768
Original Chicken Vegy Medley No Cheese	¼ pie	392	21	10	56	54	11	1536
Original Hawaiian No Cheese	¼ pie	411	17	13	46	58	11	1379
Original Mariachi Beef	¼ pie	613	31	30	81	56	11	2324
Original Mariachi Chicken	¼ pie	580	35	25	94	56	11	2480
Original Serious Meat	¼ pie	817	45	47	136	68	10	2535
SALAD DRESSINGS								
Italian Lite	1 serv (1.5 oz)	20	0	1	0	2	0	780

FOOD	PORTION	CALS	PROT	FAT	CHOL	CARB	FIBER	SOD
SIDE ORDERS								
Breadsticks	2	220	5	5	0	29	0	330
Chicken Wings Hot	5	449	41	29	286	6	tr	1766
Three Cheese Garlic Bread	1 bun	605	24	28	38	66	3	689
SUBS								
Grilled Chicken	1 serv	786	31	43	71	68	3	1184
Steak & Cheese	1 serv	929	43	52	111	107	3	907

DUNKIN' DONUTS
BAGELS AND CREAM CHEESE

FOOD	PORTION	CALS	PROT	FAT	CHOL	CARB	FIBER	SOD
Bagel Blueberry	1	330	10	3	0	66	2	600
Bagel Cinnamon Raisin	1	330	10	3	0	65	3	430
Bagel Everything	1	370	14	6	0	67	3	650
Bagel Harvest	1	350	13	6	0	61	7	500
Bagel Onion	1	320	12	4	0	61	3	610
Bagel Plain	1	320	12	3	0	62	2	650
Bagel Poppyseed	1	370	14	7	0	65	3	650
Bagel Reduced Carb w/ Cheese	1	380	25	12	20	45	14	780
Bagel Salsa	1	310	13	3	0	60	2	790
Bagel Salt	1	370	12	3	0	62	2	4520
Bagel Sesame	1	380	14	8	0	64	3	650
Bagel Wheat	1	330	12	4	0	62	4	610
Cream Cheese Chive	2 oz	170	4	17	45	4	2	230
Cream Cheese Garden Vegetable	2 oz	170	2	15	45	4	0	340
Cream Cheese Lite	2 oz	110	4	9	30	6	0	230
Cream Cheese Plain	2 oz	190	4	17	55	4	0	190
Cream Cheese Salmon	2 oz	170	4	17	45	2	0	180
Cream Cheese Strawberry	2 oz	190	4	17	45	9	0	150
BAKED SELECTIONS								
Apple Fritter	1	300	4	14	0	41	1	360
Biscuit	1	250	5	13	0	29	1	780
Bismark Chocolate Iced	1	340	3	15	0	50	1	290
Coffee Roll	1	270	4	14	0	33	1	340
Coffee Roll Chocolate Frosted	1	290	4	15	0	36	1	340
Coffee Roll Maple Frosted	1	290	4	14	0	36	1	340
Coffee Roll Vanilla Frosted	1	290	4	14	0	36	1	340
Cookie Chocolate Chunk	2	220	3	11	35	28	1	105

FOOD	PORTION	CALS	PROT	FAT	CHOL	CARB	FIBER	SOD
Cookie Chocolate Chunk w/ Walnuts	2	230	3	12	35	27	1	110
Cookie Oatmeal Raisin Pecan	2	220	3	10	30	29	1	110
Cookie White Chocolate Chunk	2	230	3	12	35	28	1	120
Croissant Plain	1	330	5	18	5	37	0	270
Danish Apple	1	330	4	20	30	32	1	260
Danish Cheese	1	340	4	22	35	30	1	270
Danish Strawberry Cheese	1	320	4	20	30	31	1	260
Donut Apple Crumb	1	230	3	10	0	34	1	270
Donut Apple Crumb Cake	1	290	3	15	15	41	1	320
Donut Apple N' Spice	1	200	3	8	0	29	1	270
Donut Bavarian Kreme	1	210	3	9	0	30	1	270
Donut Black Raspberry	1	210	3	8	0	32	1	280
Donut Blueberry	1	290	3	16	10	35	1	400
Donut Blueberry Crumb	1	240	3	10	0	36	1	260
Donut Boston Kreme	1	240	3	9	0	36	1	280
Donut Bow Tie	1	300	4	17	0	34	1	340
Donut Chocolate Coconut	1	300	4	19	0	31	1	370
Donut Chocolate Frosted	1	360	4	20	25	40	1	350
Donut Chocolate Glazed	1	290	3	16	0	33	1	370
Donut Chocolate Kreme Filled	1	270	3	13	0	35	1	260
Donut Cinnamon	1	330	4	20	25	34	1	340
Donut Double Chocolate	1	310	3	17	0	37	2	370
Donut Frosted Lemon	1	240	2	14	0	28	0	150
Donut Glazed	1	180	3	8	0	25	1	250
Donut Glazed Gingerbread	1	260	3	11	20	35	1	320
Donut Glazed Lemon	1	240	2	14	0	28	0	150
Donut Jelly Filled	1	210	3	8	0	32	1	280
Donut Lemon Burst	1	300	3	14	0	35	3	300
Donut Maple Frosted	1	210	3	9	0	30	1	260
Donut Marble Frosted	1	200	3	9	0	29	1	260
Donut Old Fashioned	1	300	4	19	25	28	1	330
Donut Powdered	1	330	4	19	25	36	1	330
Donut Strawberry	1	210	3	8	0	32	1	260
Donut Strawberry Frosted	1	210	3	9	0	30	1	260
Donut Sugar Raised	1	170	3	8	0	22	1	250
Donut Vanilla Kreme Filled	1	270	3	13	0	36	1	250

FOOD	PORTION	CALS	PROT	FAT	CHOL	CARB	FIBER	SOD
Donut Whole Wheat Glazed	1	310	4	19	0	32	2	380
Eclair	1	270	3	11	0	39	1	290
English Muffin	1	160	6	2	0	31	2	340
French Cruller	1	150	2	8	20	17	1	105
Fritter Glazed	1	260	4	14	0	31	1	330
Muffin Banana Walnut	1	540	10	25	65	69	3	520
Muffin Blueberry	1	470	8	17	60	73	2	500
Muffin Chocolate Chip	1	630	10	26	70	89	2	560
Muffin Coffee Cake	1	580	9	19	65	78	1	520•
Muffin Corn	1	510	8	18	75	77	1	860
Muffin Cranberry Orange	1	440	8	17	65	66	3	480
Muffin Honey Bran Raisin	1	480	8	15	60	79	5	480
Muffin Reduced Fat Blueberry	1	400	8	5	60	78	3	490
Munchkins Chocolate Glazed	3	200	2	10	0	26	1	250
Munchkins Cinnamon	4	270	3	19	25	31	1	210
Munchkins Glazed	3	280	3	13	20	38	1	190
Munchkins Jelly Filled	5	210	3	9	0	30	1	240
Munchkins Lemon Filled	4	170	2	8	0	23	0	190
Munchkins Plain	4	270	3	16	25	27	1	240
Munchkins Powdered	4	270	3	14	25	31	1	210
Munchkins Sugar Raised	7	220	4	12	0	26	1	290
Stick Cinnamon	1	450	4	30	35	42	1	310
Stick Glazed	1	490	4	29	35	51	1	310
Stick Glazed Chocolate	1	470	4	29	0	49	2	490
Stick Jelly	1	530	4	29	35	61	1	320
Stick Plain	1	420	4	29	35	35	1	310
Stick Powdered	1	450	4	29	35	42	1	310
BEVERAGES								
Cappuccino	1 (10 oz)	60	4	5	20	7	0	70
Cappuccino w/ Soy Milk	1 (10 oz)	70	4	3	0	6	1	80
Cappuccino w/ Soy Milk Sugar	1 (10 oz)	120	4	3	0	20	1	80
Cappuccino w/ Sugar	1 (10 oz)	130	4	4	15	21	0	65
Coffee Blueberry	1 (10 oz)	20	1	0	0	4	0	65
Coffee Caramel	1 (10 oz)	20	1	0	0	4	0	65
Coffee Chocolate	1 (10 oz)	20	1	0	0	4	0	60
Coffee Cinnamon	1 (10 oz)	20	1	0	0	4	0	65

FOOD	PORTION	CALS	PROT	FAT	CHOL	CARB	FIBER	SOD
Coffee Coconut	1 (10 oz)	20	1	0	0	4	0	65
Coffee French Vanilla	1 (10 oz)	20	1	0	0	4	0	60
Coffee Hazelnut	1 (10 oz)	20	1	0	0	4	0	60
Coffee Marshmallow	1 (10 oz)	20	0	0	0	4	0	65
Coffee Regular	1 (10 oz)	15	1	0	0	3	0	60
Coffee Toasted Almond	1 (10 oz)	20	1	0	0	4	0	65
Coffee w/ Cream	1 (10 oz)	70	1	6	20	3	0	65
Coffee w/ Cream Sugar	1 (10 oz)	120	1	6	20	15	0	65
Coffee w/ Milk	1 (10 oz)	35	2	1	5	4	0	70
Coffee w/ Milk Sugar	1 (10 oz)	80	2	1	5	16	0	70
Coffee w/ Skim Milk	1 (10 oz)	25	2	0	0	4	0	70
Coffee w/ Skim Milk Sugar	1 (10 oz)	70	2	0	0	16	0	70
Coffee w/ Sugar	1 (10 oz)	60	1	0	0	15	0	60
Coolatta Lemonade	1 (16 oz)	240	0	0	0	59	0	35
Coolatta Strawberry Fruit	1 (16 oz)	290	0	0	0	72	1	30
Coolatta Tropicana Orange	1	370	1	0	0	92	3	50
Coolatta Vanilla Bean	1 (16 oz)	440	1	17	0	70	1	95
Coolatta Coffee w/ 2% Milk	1 (16 oz)	190	4	2	10	41	0	80
Coolatta Coffee w/ Cream	1 (16 oz)	350	3	22	75	40	0	65
Coolatta Coffee w/ Milk	1 (16 oz)	210	4	4	15	42	0	80
Coolatta Coffee w/ Skim Milk	1 (16 oz)	170	4	0	0	41	0	80
Dunkaccino	1 (10 oz)	230	2	10	5	35	0	210
Expresso	1 (2 oz)	0	0	0	0	1	0	5
Expresso w/ Sugar	1 (2 oz)	30	0	0	0	7	0	5
Hot Chocolate	1 (10 oz)	220	2	8	0	38	2	280
Iced Coffee	1 (16 oz)	15	1	0	0	3	0	70
Iced Coffee w/ Cream	1 (16 oz)	70	2	6	20	4	0	75
Iced Coffee w/ Cream Sugar	1 (16 oz)	120	2	6	20	16	0	75
Iced Coffee w/ Milk	1 (16 oz)	35	2	1	5	4	0	80
Iced Coffee w/ Milk Sugar	1 (16 oz)	80	2	1	5	16	0	80
Iced Coffee w/ Skim Milk	1 (16 oz)	25	2	0	0	4	0	75
Iced Coffee w/ Skim Milk Sugar	1 (16 oz)	70	2	0	0	16	0	75
Iced Coffee w/ Sugar	1 (16 oz)	60	1	0	0	15	0	70
Iced Latte	1 (16 oz)	120	6	7	25	11	0	105
Iced Latte Caramel Creme	1 (16 oz)	260	8	9	20	40	0	125
Iced Latte Caramel Swirl	1 (16 oz)	240	8	7	25	37	0	150
Iced Latte Caramel Swirl w/ Skim Milk	1 (16 oz)	180	8	0	0	36	0	150

FOOD	PORTION	CALS	PROT	FAT	CHOL	CARB	FIBER	SOD
Iced Latte Lite	1 (16 oz)	80	7	0	0	13	0	110
Iced Latte Mocha Almond	1 (16 oz)	290	8	10	20	46	1	115
Iced Latte Mocha Swirl	1 (16 oz)	240	7	8	25	38	1	125
Iced Latte Mocha Swirl w/ Skim Milk	1 (16 oz)	180	7	1	0	37	1	115
Iced Latte w/ Skim Milk	1 (16 oz)	70	7	0	0	11	0	110
Iced Latte w/ Skim Milk Sugar	1 (16 oz)	120	7	0	0	23	0	110
Iced Latte w/ Sugar	1 (16 oz)	170	6	7	25	23	0	110
Latte	1 (10 oz)	120	6	6	25	10	0	95
Latte Caramel Creme	1 (10 oz)	260	8	9	20	40	0	125
Latte Caramel Swirl	1 (10 oz)	230	8	6	25	36	0	140
Latte Caramel Swirl w/ Soy Milk	1 (10 oz)	210	8	4	0	34	1	160
Latte Lite	1 (10 oz)	70	8	0	0	11	0	90
Latte Mocha Almond	1 (10 oz)	290	8	10	20	46	1	115
Latte Mocha Swirl	1 (10 oz)	230	6	7	25	37	1	110
Latte Mocha Swirl w/ Soy Milk	1 (10 oz)	210	7	5	0	35	2	130
Latte w/ Soy Milk	1 (10 oz)	90	6	4	0	8	1	110
Latte w/ Soy Milk Sugar	1 (10 oz)	150	6	4	0	22	1	110
Latte w/ Sugar	1 (10 oz)	160	6	6	25	22	0	95
Smoothie Mango Passion Fruits	1 (16 oz)	360	7	3	10	79	2	120
Smoothie Strawberry Banana	1 (16 oz)	360	7	3	10	79	2	79
Smoothie Wildberry	1 (16 oz)	360	7	3	10	79	1	120
Tea Regular or Decaffeinated	1 (10 oz)	0	0	0	0	1	0	0
Tea w/ Milk	1 (10 oz)	25	1	1	5	2	0	15
Tea w/ Milk Sugar	1 (10 oz)	70	1	1	5	14	0	15
Tea w/ Skim Milk	1 (10 oz)	25	2	0	0	4	0	70
Tea w/ Skim Milk Sugar	1 (10 oz)	60	1	0	0	14	0	15
Tea w/ Sugar	1 (10 oz)	50	0	0	0	13	0	0
Turbo Ice	1 (16 oz)	120	1	7	20	14	0	25
Vanilla Chai	1 (10 oz)	230	1	8	5	40	0	50
SANDWICHES								
Bagel Bacon Egg Cheese	1	540	18	18	200	69	2	1400
Bagel Egg Cheese	1	470	20	15	190	65	2	1120
Bagel Ham Egg Cheese	1	510	26	16	200	65	2	1390

FOOD	PORTION	CALS	PROT	FAT	CHOL	CARB	FIBER	SOD
Bagel Sausage Egg Cheese	1	660	28	35	225	63	3	1450
Biscuit Egg Cheese	1	410	14	25	190	32	1	1250
Biscuit Sausage Egg Cheese	1	610	23	43	235	32	1	1760
Croissant Bacon Egg Cheese	1	520	16	33	205	40	0	940
Croissant Egg Cheese	1	550	20	34	320	41	0	950
Croissant Ham Egg Cheese	1	520	20	32	215	40	0	1010
Croissant Sausage Egg Cheese	1	490	22	51	230	40	0	1080
English Muffin Bacon Egg Cheese	1	360	17	16	200	36	1	1300
English Muffin Egg Cheese	1	280	15	9	140	34	1	1010
English Muffin Ham Egg Cheese	1	310	21	10	160	34	1	1270
English Muffin Sausage Egg Cheese	1	530	23	32	235	37	1	1610
Panini Meatball	1	480	22	19	40	56	3	1180
Panini Southwestern Chicken	1	420	23	10	45	57	3	970
Panini Steak	1	450	30	12	45	56	3	1630

EDDIE'S PIZZA

FOOD	PORTION	CALS	PROT	FAT	CHOL	CARB	FIBER	SOD
Bar Pie	1 pie	350	37	11	41	27	8	676
Bar Pie No Fat Cheese	1 pie	270	39	1	10	27	8	616

EINSTEIN BROS BAGELS
BAGELS AND BREADS

FOOD	PORTION	CALS	PROT	FAT	CHOL	CARB	FIBER	SOD
Bagel Asiago Cheese	1	360	13	3	5	71	2	570
Bagel Cranberry Special	1	350	10	1	0	78	3	490
Bagel Egg	1	340	11	3	35	69	2	510
Bagel Honey Whole Wheat	1	320	10	1	0	71	3	470
Bagel Jalapeno	1	330	11	1	0	71	2	510
Bagel Lucky Green	1	320	11	1	0	71	2	520
Bagel Mango	1	360	10	1	0	80	2	490
Bagel Marble Rye	1	340	11	2	0	73	3	690
Bagel Potato	1	350	10	5	0	69	2	590
Bagel Power	1	410	13	5	0	81	4	310
Bagel Power w/ Peanut Butter	1	750	27	34	0	92	7	780
Bagel Pumpkin	1	330	10	2	0	72	3	470

FOOD	PORTION	CALS	PROT	FAT	CHOL	CARB	FIBER	SOD
Bagel Roasted Red Pepper & Pesto	1	410	17	7	15	73	2	710
Bagel Six Cheese	1	390	16	6	15	72	2	650
Bagel Spicy Nacho	1	450	17	9	20	77	3	890
Bagel Spinach Florentine	1	410	17	7	20	72	3	620
Bagel Twist	1	220	8	4	5	39	1	510
Bread Ciabatta	1 serv	320	12	3	0	64	3	460
Chocolate Chip	1	370	11	3	0	76	3	500
Chopped Garlic	1	380	13	3	0	79	4	600
Chopped Onion	1	330	11	1	0	71	2	500
Cinnamon Raisin Swirl	1	350	11	1	0	78	2	490
Cinnamon Sugar	1	330	10	1	0	74	2	490
Dark Pumpernickel	1	320	11	1	0	68	3	730
Everything	1	340	13	2	0	75	2	820
Focaccia Cheese Pizza	1 serv	500	25	11	35	75	3	1010
Focaccia Margherita	1 serv	400	14	17	5	76	3	580
Nutty Banana	1	360	11	3	0	74	2	510
Plain	1	320	11	1	0	71	2	520
Poppy Dip'd	1	350	12	2	0	74	2	680
Roll Challah	1	300	11	5	40	55	2	270
Salt	1	330	11	1	0	73	2	1790
Sesame Dip'd	1	380	11	5	0	75	3	680
Sun Dried Tomato	1	320	11	1	0	69	3	520
Wild Blueberry	1	350	11	1	0	77	3	510
BEVERAGES								
Cafe Latte	1 reg	140	9	5	20	13	0	140
Chai 2% Milk	1 reg	210	4	2	10	41	0	75
SANDWICHES								
Bagel New York Lox	1	660	26	27	85	79	3	1150
Bagel Tasty Turkey	1	570	31	15	80	83	4	1420
Bagel The Veg Out	1	490	17	13	30	77	3	850
Bagel Turkey Pastrami	1	440	31	2	40	76	3	1610
SPREADS								
Cream Cheese Maple Walnut Raisin	2 tbsp	60	1	5	15	4	0	45
Cream Cheese Plain	2 tbsp	60	1	7	20	1	0	65
Cream Cheese Plain Reduced Fat	2 tbsp	60	1	5	15	2	0	85
Cream Cheese Smoked Salmon	2 tbsp	60	1	5	15	3	0	115

FOOD	PORTION	CALS	PROT	FAT	CHOL	CARB	FIBER	SOD
Cream Cheese Strawberry	2 tbsp	70	1	5	15	5	0	50
Cream Cheese Sun Dried Tomato & Basil	2 tbsp	60	1	5	15	2	0	50
Fruit Spread Apricot	1 serv	75	0	0	0	19	0	8
Hummus	1 serv	110	3	7	0	9	2	390
Peanut Butter	2 tbsp	190	7	15	0	8	2	140

EL POLLO LOCO
DESSERTS

FOOD	PORTION	CALS	PROT	FAT	CHOL	CARB	FIBER	SOD
Caramel Flan	1 serv (5.5 oz)	290	5	12	50	41	0	135
Churros	2	300	3	18	25	32	2	210
Cone Vanilla	1	330	8	8	35	55	0	180
Soft Serve Vanilla	1 cup (5 oz)	300	8	8	35	48	0	170

MAIN MENU SELECTIONS

FOOD	PORTION	CALS	PROT	FAT	CHOL	CARB	FIBER	SOD
BBQ Black Beans	1 serv (6 oz)	200	7	3	0	38	4	520
Bowl The Original Pollo	1 serv	540	37	4	70	85	11	1590
Burrito BRC	1 (7.5 oz)	390	14	10	15	61	6	880
Burrito Classic Chicken	1 (10.3 oz)	500	30	14	95	63	6	1230
Burrito Twice Grilled	1 (15 oz)	830	66	37	215	58	5	2230
Burrito Ultimate Grilled	1 (13.6 oz)	650	38	20	100	80	8	1690
Chicken Breast	1 (4.3 oz)	220	36	9	140	0	0	620
Chicken Breast Skinless	1 (4 oz)	180	35	4	0	0	0	580
Chicken Leg	1 (1.8 oz)	90	12	4	70	0	0	170
Chicken Thigh	1 (3.1 oz)	220	21	15	180	0	0	320
Chicken Wing	1 (1.3 oz)	90	11	5	60	0	0	290
Cole Slaw	1 serv (6 oz)	120	1	9	5	8	2	200
Corn Cobbette	1 (5 oz)	90	2	1	0	19	2	0
French Fries	1 serv (5.5 oz)	440	6	21	0	57	6	910
Fresh Vegetables w/ Margarine	1 serv (4.1 oz)	60	2	3	0	8	3	65
Fresh Vegetables w/o Margarine	1 serv (4 oz)	35	2	0	0	8	3	35
Gravy	1 serv (1 oz)	10	0	0	0	2	0	150
Loco Nachos	1 serv	170	3	14	10	7	1	210
Macaroni & Cheese	1 serv (5.5 oz)	280	11	17	55	28	6	770
Mashed Potatoes	1 serv (5 oz)	100	2	1	0	20	2	350
Pinto Beans	1 serv (6 oz)	140	9	0	0	25	7	330

FOOD	PORTION	CALS	PROT	FAT	CHOL	CARB	FIBER	SOD
Quesadilla Cheese	1 (4.5 oz)	420	19	23	60	35	2	810
Refried Beans w/ Cheese	1 serv (6.3 oz)	270	14	7	10	36	10	730
Skinless Breast Meal	1 serv	310	35	12	105	17	5	780
Soup Chicken Tortilla w/o Tortilla Strips	1 serv (10 oz)	140	15	6	50	8	2	1040
Spanish Rice	1 serv (4.5 oz)	160	3	1	0	34	1	420
Taco Al Carbon	1 (3.1 oz)	150	11	5	40	17	1	290
Taco Soft Chicken	1 (4.5 oz)	270	17	13	75	19	2	700
Taquito Chicken	1	190	10	9	25	18	1	330
Tortilla Chips	1 serv (1.5 oz)	210	3	10	0	28	3	300
Tortilla Corn 6 Inches	2	120	2	2	0	24	2	60
Tortilla Flour 6.5 Inches	2	210	5	7	0	30	2	370
SALAD DRESSINGS AND TOPPINGS								
Creamy Cilantro	1 serv (1.5 oz)	220	1	23	20	1	0	300
Creamy Cilantro Light	1 pkg	70	1	5	5	6	0	400
Guacamole	1 serv (1 oz)	45	tr	4	0	4	tr	135
Hot Sauce Jalapeno	1 pkg	5	0	0	0	1	0	110
Jack & Poblano Queso	1 serv (1.8 oz)	100	3	8	<5	4	0	340
Ketchup	1 pkg	10	0	0	0	2	0	100
Light Italian	1 pkg	20	0	1	0	2	0	770
Pico De Gallo Medium	1 serv (1 oz)	10	0	1	0	1	0	190
Ranch	1 pkg	230	1	24	10	2	0	390
Salsa Avocado Hot	1 serv (1 oz)	30	0	3	0	1	tr	200
Salsa Chipotle Hot	1 serv (1 oz)	5	0	0	0	1	0	180
Salsa House Mild	1 serv (1 oz)	5	0	0	0	1	0	105
Sour Cream	1 serv (1 oz)	60	1	5	20	1	0	15
Thousand Island	1 pkg	220	0	21	20	6	0	350
SALADS								
Caesar Pollo	1 (11.4 oz)	520	27	38	100	17	4	980
Ceasar Pollo w/o Dressing	1 (9.4 oz)	220	25	7	75	15	4	580
Garden	1 (4.8 oz)	120	5	4	15	9	2	290
Tostada Chicken	1 (17.3 oz)	840	40	40	100	76	7	1390
Tostada Chicken w/o Shell	1 (14.7 oz)	410	33	11	100	42	5	1100

FOOD	PORTION	CALS	PROT	FAT	CHOL	CARB	FIBER	SOD
FAZOLI'S								
BEVERAGES								
Lemon Ice All Flavors	1	360	0	0	0	90	0	20
Lemon Ice Original	1 reg	180	0	0	0	45	0	15
Lemon Ice Strawberry	1	320	0	0	0	81	0	60
CHILDREN'S MENU SELECTIONS								
Fettuccine Alfredo	1 serv	290	9	5	5	50	2	420
Meat Lasagna	1 serv	260	14	13	35	21	2	880
Ravioli w/ Marinara	1 serv	290	13	7	30	43	3	580
Spaghetti w/ Meat Sauce	1 serv	300	11	4	5	53	4	520
Spaghetti w/ Meatballs	1 serv	270	9	2	0	53	4	390
Spaghetti w/ Meatballs	1 serv	350	14	7	20	55	4	620
Ziti w/ Meat Sauce	1 serv	190	9	6	15	25	3	710
DESSERTS								
Cheesecake Original	1 slice	290	6	22	95	17	0	220
Cheesecake Turtle	1 slice	450	6	28	75	43	2	340
Cookie Chocolate Chunk	1	510	5	26	75	68	3	350
MAIN MENU SELECTIONS								
Breadstick	1	100	3	2	0	20	0	160
Breadstick Garlic	1	150	3	7	0	20	1	290
Fettuccine Alfredo	1 sm	520	16	12	15	83	4	1060
Fettuccine w/ Marinara	1 serv	450	15	3	0	88	7	770
Fettuccine w/ Meat Sauce	1 serv	500	20	7	10	87	7	1020
Oven Baked Chicken Parmesan	1 serv	960	56	33	115	117	9	2350
Oven Baked Meat Lasagna	1 serv	510	27	25	70	43	5	1710
Oven Baked Rigatoni Romano	1 serv	1090	11	54	135	101	11	3180
Oven Baked Spaghetti	1 serv	680	32	22	65	90	7	1480
Oven Baked Spaghetti w/ Meatballs	1 serv	940	46	40	120	100	9	2370
Panini Four Cheese & Tomato	1	510	28	22	60	53	3	960
Panini Grilled Chicken	1	540	35	18	80	56	3	1360
Panini Smoked Turkey	1	620	35	29	95	54	3	2110
Penne w/ Alfredo	1 serv	520	16	12	15	83	4	1060
Penne w/ Marinara	1 serv	450	15	3	0	88	7	770
Penne w/ Meat Sauce	1 serv	500	20	7	10	87	7	1020
Pizza Slice Cheese	1	270	13	11	25	31	2	700
Pizza Slice Pepperoni	1	310	14	14	30	31	2	850

FOOD	PORTION	CALS	PROT	FAT	CHOL	CARB	FIBER	SOD
Platter Ultimate Sampler	1	980	43	29	70	134	11	2780
Platters Classic Sampler	1	810	34	25	55	110	8	2130
Ravioli w/ Marinara	1 serv	500	22	15	80	71	7	1210
Ravioli w/ Meat Sauce	1 serv	300	15	8	30	42	3	660
Ravioli w/ Meat Sauce	1 serv	550	26	20	90	71	7	1460
Spaghetti w/ Alfredo	1 serv	520	16	12	15	83	4	1060
Spaghetti w/ Marinara	1 sm	450	15	3	0	88	7	770
Spaghetti w/ Meat Sauce	1 sm	500	20	7	10	87	7	1020
Submarinos Club	half	973	37	34	75	65	3	2870
Submarinos Ham n' Swiss	1	680	34	30	60	65	3	2440
Submarinos Italian Beef	half	660	46	24	90	68	3	2320
Submarinos Original	half	940	35	58	95	68	4	3040
Topping Broccoli	1 serv	25	3	0	0	5	3	10
Topping Broccoli & Tomatoes	1 serv	30	3	0	0	6	3	10
Topping Garlic Shrimp	1 serv	160	10	12	45	3	1	440
Topping Italian Sausage	1 serv	240	10	21	45	3	1	770
Topping Meatballs	1 serv	160	13	18	55	6	1	700
Topping Peppery Chicken	1 serv	70	14	1	35	1	0	330
Ziti w/ Meat Sauce	1 serv	480	23	15	40	65	6	1430
SALAD DRESSINGS								
Caesar	1 serv	220	1	25	45	1	0	350
Fat Free Honey Mustard	1 serv	60	0	0	0	15	1	350
Fat Free Italian	1 serv	25	0	0	0	6	0	390
Honey French	1 serv	220	0	18	0	14	0	310
Italian	1 serv	160	0	14	0	7	0	760
Ranch	1 serv	220	1	24	10	2	0	470
Ranch Lite	1 serv	120	1	12	5	2	0	350
SALADS								
Chicken & Fruit	1	220	23	2	55	28	4	700
Chicken & Pasta Caesar	1	440	35	15	65	41	4	1320
Chicken BLT Ranch	1	270	31	10	80	13	4	1060
Parmesan Chicken	1	360	31	15	65	31	4	850
Side Caesar	1	40	4	2	5	4	2	70
Side Garden	1	25	2	0	0	4	3	30
Side Pasta	1 serv	320	11	12	5	41	1	620

FRESHENS
PRETZELS

FOOD	PORTION	CALS	PROT	FAT	CHOL	CARB	FIBER	SOD
Bites	1 serv (3 oz)	255	7	3	0	48	2	390
Gourmet	1 (6 oz)	510	14	6	0	98	4	780

FOOD	PORTION	CALS	PROT	FAT	CHOL	CARB	FIBER	SOD
SMOOTHIES								
Berry Berry	1 serv (21 oz)	280	–	tr	tr	–	–	–
Blueberry Breeze	1 serv (21 oz)	396	–	1	14	–	–	–
Caribbean Craze	1 serv (21 oz)	315	–	tr	tr	–	–	–
Cayman Cooler	1 serv (21 oz)	320	–	tr	tr	–	–	–
Club Trim	1 serv (21 oz)	291	–	0	0	–	–	–
Fitness Fuel	1 serv (21 oz)	521	–	5	24	–	–	–
Immune Support	1 serv (21 oz)	377	–	3	10	–	–	–
Jamaican Jammer	1 serv (21 oz)	378	–	1	14	–	–	–
Maui Mango	1 serv (21 oz)	354	–	tr	tr	–	–	–
Mocha Coffee	1 serv (21 oz)	385	–	3	15	–	–	–
Mystic Mango	1 serv (21 oz)	407	–	3	10	–	–	–
Orange Shooter	1 serv (21 oz)	330	–	3	10	–	–	–
Orange Sunrise	1 serv (21 oz)	367	–	3	10	–	–	–
Peach Sunset	1 serv (21 oz)	388	–	tr	tr	–	–	–
Peachy Pineapple	1 serv (21 oz)	415	–	1	14	–	–	–
Peanut Butter Chocolate	1 serv (21 oz)	312	–	20	45	–	–	–
Pina Colada	1 serv (21 oz)	451	–	4	14	–	–	–
Pineapple Passion	1 serv (21 oz)	389	–	4	tr	–	–	–
Raspberry Royale	1 serv (21 oz)	346	–	tr	tr	–	–	–

FOOD	PORTION	CALS	PROT	FAT	CHOL	CARB	FIBER	SOD
Rockin' Raspberry	1 serv (21 oz)	332	–	tr	14	–	–	–
Strawberry Shooter	1 serv (21 oz)	251	–	tr	tr	–	–	–
Strawberry Squeeze	1 serv (21 oz)	313	–	1	14	–	–	–
Vanilla Coffee	1 serv (21 oz)	438	–	3	15	–	–	–
Vanilla Fudge	1 serv (21 oz)	275	–	17	45	–	–	–

FRUITFULL
BREADS

FOOD	PORTION	CALS	PROT	FAT	CHOL	CARB	FIBER	SOD
Almond Cherry	½ slice	226	3	11	23	29	1	279
Apple Spice	½ slice	186	2	7	19	29	1	124
Banana	½ slice	165	3	6	22	24	1	177
Cappuccino Chocolate Chip	½ slice	229	3	13	25	27	1	161
Carrot	½ slice	190	3	9	24	24	0	177
Chocolate	½ slice	120	2	0	0	26	2	155
Lemon Blueberry	½ slice	120	3	0	0	27	1	181
Old Fashion Pound Cake	½ slice	227	3	13	51	25	0	181
Orange Cranberry	½ slice	130	3	0	0	28	0	200
Pumpkin	½ slice	150	4	0	0	32	0	150
Sweet Potato	½ slice	176	2	6	19	28	1	204
Zucchini	½ slice	190	3	9	22	24	1	215

DIPS

FOOD	PORTION	CALS	PROT	FAT	CHOL	CARB	FIBER	SOD
Banana Cream	1 serv (4.5 oz)	250	2	15	5	26	–	35
Banana Split	1 serv (4.5 oz)	290	2	16	10	34	–	40
Cherry Cream	1 serv (4.5 oz)	280	3	15	15	33	–	45
Coconut Cream	1 serv (4.5 oz)	300	3	15	10	37	–	50
Mud Pie	1 serv (4.5 oz)	380	2	24	15	34	–	75
Strawberry Cream	1 serv (4.5 oz)	270	3	16	10	28	–	50

FROZEN BARS

FOOD	PORTION	CALS	PROT	FAT	CHOL	CARB	FIBER	SOD
Cream Banana	1	110	1	3	20	18	–	25

FOOD	PORTION	CALS	PROT	FAT	CHOL	CARB	FIBER	SOD
Cream Coconut	1	130	2	5	15	18	–	25
Cream Peaches 'n' Cream	1	150	2	5	25	24	–	50
Cream Pina Colada	1	90	1	3	10	16	–	20
Cream Raspberry Cream	1	110	2	3	10	18	–	20
Cream Strawberry Cream	1	110	2	3	15	20	–	25
Happy Indulgence Berry Cobbler	1	200	2	8	20	31	–	80
Happy Indulgence Key Lime Pie	1	220	3	8	35	33	–	65
Happy Indulgence Peach Cobbler	1	170	3	8	20	23	–	120
Juice Fuzzy Navel	1	70	0	0	0	18	–	10
Juice Green Tea Melon	1	90	0	0	0	21	–	25
Juice Guava	1	70	0	0	0	17	–	20
Juice Lemon	1	90	0	0	0	24	–	10
Juice Lime	1	80	0	0	0	20	–	10
Juice Passionate Cherry	1	80	0	0	0	20	–	25
Juice Pineapple	1	80	0	0	0	20	–	5
Juice Raspberry	1	70	0	0	0	18	–	5
Juice Strawberry	1	70	0	0	0	18	–	5
Juice Tamarind	1	90	0	0	0	21	–	20
Juice Tropical Splash	1	80	0	0	0	19	–	25
Juice Watermelon	1	60	0	0	0	13	–	5
Yogurt Blueberry	1	120	3	0	0	28	–	90
Yogurt Chocolate	1	160	6	0	0	33	–	65
Yogurt Vanilla	1	140	5	0	0	32	–	85
SMOOTHIES								
Berry Berry Best	1 (4 oz)	160	2	2	5	34	–	20
Make Mine Mango	4 oz	160	1	0	0	38	–	0
Strawberry Ana Banana	4 oz	120	15	1	0	26	–	25
SNACKS								
All About Almonds	1 pkg (1 oz)	170	6	15	0	5	4	0
Buzzworthy Banana	1 pkg (1.1 oz)	140	3	8	0	17	2	35
Calypso Cashews	1 pkg (1.1 oz)	170	4	13	1	7	1	75
Chocolate Twisted Bliss	1 pkg (1.4 oz)	190	3	8	6	27	1	210
Debbie Loves Fruit	1 pkg (1 oz)	110	0	2	0	23	1	20

FOOD	PORTION	CALS	PROT	FAT	CHOL	CARB	FIBER	SOD
Got Nuts?	1 pkg (1.1 oz)	180	6	13	1	9	2	55
Hit The Road Jack	1 pkg (1.1 oz)	130	3	6	0	19	2	10
Honey I Ate The Peanuts	1 pkg (1 oz)	160	7	12	0	8	1	115
Jamaican Me Crazy Cranberry Mix	1 pkg (1.1 oz)	100	0	0	0	24	2	10
Judy's Apple Crisps	1 pkg (1 oz)	140	0	7	0	20	2	15
Nacho Chips They're Mine	1 pkg (1.1 oz)	120	2	2	1	25	0	240
Nature Lover's Choice	1 pkg (1.1 oz)	140	4	7	0	15	2	5
Power Pistachios	1 pkg (1.1 oz)	100	4	9	0	14	2	130
Reggae Rice Crackers	1 pkg (1.1 oz)	120	2	0	0	26	0	200
Rockin' Raisins	1 pkg (1.4 oz)	170	3	7	4	28	1	20
Rocky Mountain Munch	1 pkg (1.1 oz)	120	1	4	0	22	1	20
Sour Wiggle Giggle	1 pkg (1.5 oz)	150	9	0	0	9	0	35
Soy Glad You're Healthy	1 pkg (1.1 oz)	160	9	10	0	9	4	100
Survivor Snacks	1 pkg (1.1 oz)	140	4	8	0	15	2	0
Swinging Sesame Stix	1 pkg (1.1 oz)	180	4	13	0	12	2	320
Tammy's Flax Snacks	1 pkg (1.1 oz)	170	5	13	0	10	3	150
Whassup Wasabi!	1 pkg (1.1 oz)	150	5	7	0	17	2	300
Yogurt Twisted Bliss	1 pkg (1.4 oz)	190	1	8	0	28	1	200
You've Got Trail	1 pkg (1.1 oz)	150	4	8	0	17	2	15
Yummy Gummy In My Tummy	1 pkg (1.4 oz)	150	2	0	0	33	0	10
Zydeco Cajun Mix	1 pkg (1.1 oz)	108	4	11	1	15	1	350

FOOD	PORTION	CALS	PROT	FAT	CHOL	CARB	FIBER	SOD
GODFATHER'S PIZZA								
Breadstick	1	80	2	2	0	14	1	71
Golden All Meat Combo	1 med slice	300	14	14	30	27	1	670
Golden Apple Dessert	1/6 sm	202	4	5	0	37	1	200
Golden Bacon Cheeseburger	1 med slice	270	13	12	25	26	1	630
Golden Cheese	1 med slice	220	10	8	15	26	1	370
Golden Cherry Dessert	1/6 sm	206	4	5	0	38	1	19
Golden Cinnamon Streusel	1/6 sm	226	4	6	0	39	1	205
Golden Combo	1 med slice	290	13	13	25	28	2	650
Golden Hawaiian	1 med slice	240	11	8	15	29	1	460
Golden Hot Stuff	1 med slice	290	13	14	25	27	1	650
Golden Humble Pie	1 med slice	310	13	15	30	27	1	590
Golden M&M Streusel Dessert	1/6 sm	249	5	7	1	42	1	208
Golden Pepperoni	1 med slice	260	11	11	20	26	1	490
Golden Super Combo	1 med slice	320	28	15	35	13	2	740
Golden Super Hawaiian	1 med slice	250	11	10	20	27	1	480
Golden Super Taco	1 med slice	330	15	17	40	28	2	650
Golden Taco	1 med slice	300	15	14	35	27	2	620
Golden Veggie	1 med slice	230	10	8	15	27	2	420
Monkey Bread	1/6	120	3	2	0	23	1	130
Original All Meat Combo	1 med slice	370	18	16	35	35	2	860
Original Bacon Cheeseburger	1 med slice	330	16	13	35	35	2	810
Original Cheese	1 med slice	260	12	7	15	34	1	450
Original Combo	1 med slice	350	17	14	30	37	3	850
Original Hawaiian	1 med slice	280	13	8	20	38	1	550
Original Hot Stuff	1 med slice	360	17	6	35	35	2	840
Original Humble Pie	1 med slice	380	16	18	35	35	2	750
Original Pepperoni	1 med slice	290	13	10	20	34	1	580
Original Super Combo	1 med slice	390	19	17	40	37	3	940
Original Super Hawaiian	1 med slice	280	13	8	20	37	1	550
Original Super Taco	1 med slice	390	19	18	45	36	2	850
Original Taco	1 med slice	360	18	16	40	36	2	810
Original Veggie	1 med slice	270	12	9	15	36	2	520
Potato Wedges	1 serv (4 oz)	192	3	9	0	24	4	342
Thin All Meat Combo	1 med slice	280	13	15	30	20	1	570
Thin Bacon Cheeseburger	1 med slice	250	11	13	30	20	1	530
Thin Cheese	1 med slice	180	8	8	15	16	1	260

FOOD	PORTION	CALS	PROT	FAT	CHOL	CARB	FIBER	SOD
Thin Combo	1 med slice	250	11	13	25	18	1	540
Thin Hawaiian	1 med slice	200	9	9	15	19	1	350
Thin Hot Stuff	1 med slice	270	12	15	30	20	1	550
Thin Humble Pie	1 med slice	270	11	16	30	17	1	480
Thin Pepperoni	1 med slice	220	9	11	20	16	1	220
Thin Super Combo	1 med slice	300	14	16	35	21	2	640
Thin Super Hawaiian	1 med slice	230	10	11	20	21	1	380
Thin Super Taco	1 med slice	310	14	18	10	21	2	550
Thin Taco	1 med slice	260	13	15	35	17	1	510
Thin Veggie	1 med slice	190	8	9	15	18	1	300

HARDEE'S
BEVERAGES

FOOD	PORTION	CALS	PROT	FAT	CHOL	CARB	FIBER	SOD
Barq's Root Beer	1 sm (20 oz)	290	0	0	0	79	0	90
Cherry Coke	1 sm (20 oz)	260	0	0	0	70	0	10
Coca-Cola	1 sm (20 oz)	260	0	0	0	71	0	40
Coffee Black	1 sm (12 oz)	5	0	0	0	1	0	5
Diet Coke	1 sm (20 oz)	0	0	0	0	0	0	40
Dr Pepper	1 sm (20 oz)	260	0	0	0	68	0	90
Hi-C Fruit Punch	1 sm (20 oz)	260	0	0	0	70	0	22
Hi-C Orange	1 sm (20 oz)	280	0	0	0	76	0	90
Lemonade Minute Maid	1 sm (20 oz)	250	0	0	0	70	0	100
Mello Yellow	1 sm (20 oz)	265	0	0	0	72	0	20
Milk 2%	1 (10 oz)	150	14	3	15	18	0	180
Orange Juice	1 serv (10 oz)	150	1	0	0	37	0	0
Shake Chocolate	1 (16 oz)	700	15	34	100	85	1	290
Shake Strawberry	1 (16 oz)	700	14	33	100	86	0	240
Shake Vanilla	1 (16 oz)	710	14	33	100	87	0	240
Sprite	1 sm	260	0	0	0	68	0	85

BREAKFAST SELECTIONS

FOOD	PORTION	CALS	PROT	FAT	CHOL	CARB	FIBER	SOD
Big Country Breakfast Platter Bacon	1 serv	980	28	56	435	90	3	2080
Big Country Breakfast Platter Breaded Pork Chop	1 serv	1220	48	68	465	102	4	2230
Big Country Breakfast Platter Chicken	1 serv	1140	44	61	480	105	4	2580
Big Country Breakfast Platter Country Ham	1 serv	970	33	53	460	90	3	2600

FOOD	PORTION	CALS	PROT	FAT	CHOL	CARB	FIBER	SOD
Big Country Breakfast Platter Country Steak	1 serv	1150	36	68	455	98	4	2260
Big Country Breakfast Platter Grilled Pork Chop	1 serv	1130	42	61	465	92	3	2430
Big Country Breakfast Platter Sausage	1 serv	1060	30	64	455	91	4	2140
Biscuit Bacon	1 serv	430	8	28	10	35	0	1110
Biscuit Bacon Egg Cheese	1	560	16	38	225	37	0	1360
Biscuit Breaded Pork Chop	1 serv	690	29	42	40	48	1	1330
Biscuit Chicken Fillet	1 serv	600	24	34	55	50	1	1680
Biscuit Cinnamon 'N' Raisin	1	280	3	12	0	40	0	650
Biscuit Country Ham	1	440	14	26	35	36	0	1710
Biscuit Country Steak	1 serv	620	16	41	35	44	0	1360
Biscuit Country Steak & Egg	1 serv	690	22	47	235	44	0	1800
Biscuit Egg	1 serv	450	11	29	205	35	0	940
Biscuit Ham Egg Cheese	1	560	23	35	245	37	0	1800
Biscuit Loaded Omelet	1 serv	640	21	44	245	37	0	1610
Biscuit Made From Scratch	1	370	5	23	0	35	0	890
Biscuit 'N' Gravy	1	530	8	34	10	47	0	1550
Biscuit Sausage	1	530	11	36	30	36	0	1240
Biscuit Sausage Egg	1	610	17	44	235	36	0	1290
Breakfast Bowl Loaded Biscuit 'N' Gravy	1 serv	770	20	54	245	49	1	1950
Breakfast Bowl Low Carb	1 serv	620	36	50	325	6	2	325
Burrito Loaded Breakfast	1	780	40	51	495	38	2	1620
Burrito Steak 'N' Egg Breakfast	1	470	26	22	255	38	1	1280
Folded Egg	1 serv	80	6	6	205	1	0	50
Frisco Breakfast Sandwich	1	410	27	17	245	39	2	870
Grits	1 serv	110	2	5	0	16	0	480
Hash Rounds	1 sm	260	3	16	0	25	2	360
Loaded Omelet	1	270	16	21	245	2	0	620
Pancake Platter	1 serv	300	8	5	25	55	2	830
Scrambled Egg	1 serv	160	12	12	405	1	0	100
Sunrise Croissant	1	210	4	10	5	26	0	200
Sunrise Croissant w/ Bacon	1	450	19	29	240	28	0	900
Sunrise Croissant w/ Ham	1	430	23	26	250	28	0	1050
Sunrise Croissant w/ Sausage	1	550	22	38	265	29	0	1030

FOOD	PORTION	CALS	PROT	FAT	CHOL	CARB	FIBER	SOD
CHILDREN'S MENU SELECTIONS								
French Fries	1 serv	250	4	12	0	32	3	150
Kids Meal Cheeseburger	1 serv	600	21	27	45	68	4	930
Kids Meal Chicken Strips	1 serv	500	19	25	35	50	3	1050
Kids Meal Hamburger	1 serv	560	18	24	35	67	6	710
DESSERTS								
Apple Turnover	1	290	2	15	5	36	1	350
Cone Single Scoop	1	285	6	13	47	37	0	140
Cookie Chocolate Chip	1	290	4	11	20	44	0	270
Ice Cream Bowl Single Scoop	1 serv	235	5	13	47	27	0	85
Peach Cobbler	1 serv	280	1	7	0	56	1	230
MAIN MENU SELECTIONS								
Burger Six Dollar	1	1060	40	72	150	60	3	1860
Cheeseburger	1	350	17	16	45	36	1	780
Cheeseburger	1	680	29	39	90	52	2	1450
Cheeseburger Double	1	510	28	26	90	38	1	1120
Chicken Strips	3 pieces	380	22	21	55	27	1	1360
Cole Slaw	1 serv	170	1	10	10	20	2	140
Crispy Curls	1 sm	340	4	17	0	43	4	840
French Fries	1 sm	390	6	19	0	51	4	240
Fried Chicken Breast	1 piece	370	29	15	75	29	0	1190
Fried Chicken Leg	1 piece	170	13	7	45	15	0	570
Fried Chicken Thigh	1 piece	330	19	15	60	30	0	1000
Fried Chicken Wing	1 piece	200	10	8	30	23	0	740
Grilled Onions	1 serv	35	0	3	0	2	0	0
Hamburger	1	310	14	12	35	36	1	560
Hamburger Double	1	420	23	19	70	37	1	670
Hot Dog	1	420	16	30	55	22	1	1200
Hot Ham 'N' Cheese	1	420	30	18	55	39	2	1600
Hot Ham 'N' Cheese Big	1	520	40	24	85	40	2	2190
Mashed Potatoes	1 sm	90	1	2	0	17	0	410
Roast Beef Big	1	470	29	23	60	38	2	1290
Roast Beef Regular	1	330	19	16	40	29	2	860
Sandwich Big Chicken Fillet	1	850	42	42	95	76	3	1900
Sandwich Charbroiled Chicken Club	1	560	39	30	100	33	3	1430
Sandwich Fish Supreme	1	500	17	27	60	38	1	1030
Thickburger	1	850	30	57	105	54	3	1470
Thickburger Bacon Cheese	1	910	33	63	115	50	3	1490

FOOD	PORTION	CALS	PROT	FAT	CHOL	CARB	FIBER	SOD
Thickburger Double	1	1240	52	90	195	55	3	2090
Thickburger Double Bacon Cheese	1	1300	55	96	205	51	3	2110
Thickburger Low Carb	1	420	30	32	115	5	2	1010
Thickburger Monster	1	1410	60	107	229	47	2	2740
Thickburger Mushroom 'N Swiss	1	720	35	42	100	48	2	1570
SAUCES AND TOPPINGS								
Au Jus Sauce	1 serv (3 oz)	10	0	0	0	2	0	320
Chicken Gravy	1 serv (1.5 oz)	20	0	1	0	3	0	220
Dipping Sauce BBQ	1 serv (0.5 oz)	15	0	0	0	3	0	130
Dipping Sauce Honey Mustard	1 serv (1 oz)	110	0	9	10	6	0	220
Dipping Sauce Ranch Dressing	1 serv (1 oz)	160	0	16	15	2	0	240
Dipping Sauce Sweet N Sour	1 serv (1 oz)	45	0	0	0	10	0	85
Gravy Biscuit	1 serv (5 oz)	160	3	11	10	12	0	660
Horseradish Sauce	1 pkg	25	0	2	5	1	0	35
Hot Sauce	1 pkg	0	0	0	0	0	0	210
Jam Grape	1 serv	10	0	0	0	2	0	0
Jam Strawberry	1 serv	35	0	0	0	9	0	0
Ketchup	1 pkg	10	0	0	0	2	0	105
Mayonnaise	1 pkg	90	0	9	5	1	0	70
Pancake Syrup	1 serv (1 oz)	90	0	0	0	21	0	0

HUNGRY HOWIE'S PIZZA
OTHER MENU SELECTIONS

FOOD	PORTION	CALS	PROT	FAT	CHOL	CARB	FIBER	SOD
Cajun Bread	¼ bread	300	9	9	2	46	1	239
Chicken Tenders	2	140	13	5	30	11	0	460
Cinnamon Bread	¼ bread	313	9	9	2	59	1	239
Howie Bread	¼ bread	300	9	9	2	46	1	239
Howie Wings	5	180	14	13	60	0	0	760
Sub Deluxe Italian	½ sub	506	24	18	44	61	2	1005
Sub Ham & Cheese	½ sub	475	26	15	44	61	2	1020
Sub Pizza	½ sub	689	30	34	86	67	3	1722
Sub Pizza Special	½ sub	606	29	24	65	68	3	1584
Sub Steak & Cheese	½ sub	491	27	15	47	64	2	914

FOOD	PORTION	CALS	PROT	FAT	CHOL	CARB	FIBER	SOD
Sub Turkey	½ sub	466	25	13	38	63	2	1108
Sub Turkey Club	½ sub	556	42	15	42	63	2	1065
Sub Vegetarian	½ sub	530	22	21	39	64	3	895
Three Cheeser Bread	¼ bread	370	15	14	17	47	1	384
PIZZA								
Cheese Slice	1 extra lg	395	23	9	25	42	2	882
Cheese Slice	1 lg	208	12	5	13	25	1	464
Cheese Slice	1 sm	161	10	4	11	20	1	370
Cheese Slice	1 med	191	11	6	11	23	1	437
Cheese Slice Thin	1 med	111	7	5	11	10	tr	256
Cheese Slice Thin	1 lg	124	8	6	13	11	1	323
Medium Topping Anchovies	1 serv	44	7	3	16	0	0	736
Medium Topping Bacon	1 serv	32	6	1	1	tr	0	–
Medium Topping Banana Peppers	1 serv	6	tr	0	0	1	0	162
Medium Topping Beef	1 serv	30	2	2	6	tr	tr	96
Medium Topping Black Olives	1 serv	7	0	tr	2	tr	tr	47
Medium Topping Ham	1 serv	7	1	tr	4	0	0	81
Medium Topping Mushrooms	1 serv	2	tr	0	0	tr	tr	0
Medium Topping Pepperoni	1 serv	22	1	2	6	0	0	75
Medium Topping Pineapple	1 serv	5	1	0	0	2	1	0
Medium Topping Sausage	1 serv	27	2	2	4	tr	tr	121
SALAD DRESSINGS AND SAUCES								
Dressing Blue Cheese	1 serv (1 oz)	150	1	16	20	1	0	300
Dressing Creamy Italian	1 serv (1 oz)	120	0	12	0	2	0	210
Dressing Fat Free Italian	1 serv (1.5 oz)	25	0	0	0	5	0	390
Dressing Fat Free Ranch	1 serv (1.5 oz)	45	0	0	0	10	1	540
Dressing French Style	1 serv (1 oz)	30	0	0	0	7	0	170
Dressing Greek	1 serv (1 oz)	110	0	11	0	2	0	70
Dressing Italian	1 serv (1 oz)	80	0	8	0	2	0	560
Dressing Ranch	1 serv (1 oz)	180	0	19	3	1	0	250
Dressing Thousand Island	1 serv (1 oz)	140	0	14	20	4	0	240
Sauce Dipping	1 serv (3 oz)	45	3	1	0	9	1	380

FOOD	PORTION	CALS	PROT	FAT	CHOL	CARB	FIBER	SOD
SALADS								
Antipasto	1 sm	115	9	7	28	3	2	554
Chef	1 sm	114	9	7	28	4	2	396
Garden	1 sm	20	1	tr	0	3	2	10
Greek	1 sm	126	7	7	29	8	2	581
IHOP								
Pancake Buckwheat	1 (1.7 oz)	110	3	4	50	15	1	280
Pancake Buttermilk	1 (1.7 oz)	110	3	3	30	17	tr	450
Pancake Harvest Grain 'N Nut	1 (2.25 oz)	180	5	9	40	20	2	410
IN-N-OUT BURGER								
BEVERAGES								
Coca-Cola	1 (16 oz)	198	0	0	0	54	0	12
Coffee Black	1 (10 oz)	5	0	0	0	1	0	3
Diet Coca-Cola	1 (16 oz)	0	0	0	0	0	0	20
Dr Pepper	1 (16 oz)	180	0	0	0	52	0	60
Iced Tea	1 (16 oz)	0	0	0	0	0	0	0
Lemonade	1 (16 oz)	180	0	0	0	40	0	20
Milk	1 (10 oz)	108	12	6	30	18	0	190
Root Beer	1 (16 oz)	222	0	0	0	60	0	48
Seven-Up	1 (16 oz)	200	0	0	0	54	0	60
Shake Chocolate	1 (15 oz)	690	9	36	95	83	0	350
Shake Strawberry	1 (15 oz)	690	9	33	85	91	0	280
Shake Vanilla	1 (15 oz)	680	9	37	90	78	0	390
MAIN MENU SELECTIONS								
Cheeseburger w/ Onions	1	480	22	27	60	39	3	1000
Cheeseburger w/ Onions Lettuce Bun	1	330	18	25	60	11	3	720
Cheeseburger w/ Onions Mustard Ketchup No Spread	1	400	22	18	60	41	3	1080
French Fries	1 serv (4.4 oz)	400	7	18	0	54	2	245
Hamburger Double Double w/ Onions	1	670	37	41	120	39	3	1446
Hamburger Double Double w/ Onions Lettuce Bun	1	520	33	39	120	11	3	1160

FOOD	PORTION	CALS	PROT	FAT	CHOL	CARB	FIBER	SOD
Hamburger Double Double w/ Onions Mustard Ketchup No Spread	1	590	37	32	115	41	3	1520
Hamburger w/ Onions	1	390	16	19	40	39	3	650
Hamburger w/ Onions Lettuce Bun	1	240	13	17	40	11	3	370
Hamburger w/ Onions Mustard Ketchup No Spread	1	310	16	10	35	41	3	730

IVAR'S SEAFOOD BARS

FOOD	PORTION	CALS	PROT	FAT	CHOL	CARB	FIBER	SOD
Chicken	3 pieces (4.5 oz)	250	22	11	–	14	–	6
Chowder Salmon	1 cup	220	4	13	–	22	2	510
Chowder White	1 cup	330	17	19	–	24	4	1115
Clams	1 serv (5 oz)	400	17	21	–	33	1	–
Cocktail Sauce	¼ cup	50	1	0	0	12	1	730
Fish	3 pieces	220	22	9	–	12	1	7
French Fries	1 serv (3.5 oz)	300	4	16	–	34	2	1
Oysters	5	290	17	14	–	22	1	–
Prawns	1 serv (5 oz)	290	20	15	–	18	tr	17
Salmon Fried	3 pieces (4.5 oz)	210	24	9	–	9	1	–
Scallops	1 serv (5 oz)	240	22	9	–	14	tr	–
Tartar Sauce	2 tbsp	140	0	15	–	1	0	250

JACK IN THE BOX
BEVERAGES

FOOD	PORTION	CALS	PROT	FAT	CHOL	CARB	FIBER	SOD
Barq's Root Beer	1 (20 oz)	180	0	0	0	50	0	40
Chocolate Milk Low Fat Chug	1 (3.5 oz)	200	11	3	5	34	1	230
Coca Cola Classic	1 (20 oz)	170	0	0	0	46	0	0
Coffee Regular & Decafe	1 (11 oz)	5	0	0	0	1	0	5
Diet Coke	1 (20 oz)	0	0	0	0	0	0	15
Dr Pepper	1 (20 oz)	150	0	0	0	42	0	50
Fanta Orange	1 (20 oz)	150	0	0	0	41	0	50
Fanta Strawberry	1 (20 oz)	150	0	0	0	41	0	10

FOOD	PORTION	CALS	PROT	FAT	CHOL	CARB	FIBER	SOD
Iced Tea	1 (20 oz)	5	0	0	0	2	0	20
Lemonade	1 (20 oz)	160	0	0	0	42	0	65
Orange Juice	1 (10 oz)	140	2	0	0	32	2	25
Reduced Fat Milk Chug	1 (3.5 oz)	130	10	5	25	13	0	130
Shake Chocolate	1 (16 oz)	880	14	45	135	107	1	330
Shake Oreo	1 (16 oz)	910	14	49	135	102	1	420
Shake Strawberry	1 (16 oz)	880	13	44	135	105	0	290
Shake Vanilla	1 (16 oz)	790	13	44	135	83	0	280
Sprite	1 (20 oz)	160	0	0	0	42	0	40
BREAKFAST SELECTIONS								
Biscuit Bacon Egg Cheese	1	430	17	25	220	34	1	1100
Biscuit Chicken	1	450	15	24	30	42	2	980
Biscuit Sausage	1	440	12	29	35	32	2	870
Biscuit Sausage Egg Cheese	1	740	27	55	280	35	2	1430
Biscuit Spicy Chicken	1	460	21	22	40	44	2	1020
Breakfast Sandwich Ciabatta	1	710	36	30	440	63	3	1730
Breakfast Sandwich Ultimate	1	570	34	27	445	49	2	1700
Breakfast Jack	1	290	17	12	220	39	1	760
Breakfast Jack Bacon	1	300	16	14	215	29	1	730
Breakfast Jack Sausage	1	450	20	28	245	29	1	840
Burrito Hearty Breakfast	1	480	25	29	350	29	2	1210
Burrito Sirloin Steak & Egg w/o Salsa	1	790	37	48	450	52	6	1320
Croissant Sausage	1	580	21	39	255	37	2	770
Croissant Supreme	1	450	20	25	235	36	1	860
French Toast Sticks	4 (4.2 oz)	470	7	23	25	58	4	450
French Toast Sticks Blueberry	4	450	8	20	0	59	3	550
Hash Brown	1 serv	150	1	10	0	13	2	230
Sandwich Extreme Sausage	1	670	29	48	290	31	2	1300
DESSERTS								
Cake Chocolate Overload	1 serv (3.2 oz)	300	4	7	40	57	2	350
Cheesecake	1 serv (3.6 oz)	310	7	16	55	34	0	220
MAIN MENU SELECTIONS								
Bacon Cheddar Potato Wedges	1 serv (9 oz)	720	21	48	45	52	4	1360

FOOD	PORTION	CALS	PROT	FAT	CHOL	CARB	FIBER	SOD
Cheeseburger Bacon Ultimate	1	1090	46	77	140	53	2	2040
Cheeseburger Junior Bacon	1	430	20	25	60	30	1	820
Cheeseburger Sourdough Ultimate	1	950	38	73	125	36	2	1360
Cheeseburger Ultimate	1	1010	40	71	125	53	2	1580
Chicken Fajita Pita	1	280	21	9	60	30	2	1110
Chicken Sandwich	1	400	15	21	35	38	2	730
Chicken Strips Crispy	4	500	35	25	80	36	3	1260
Chicken Strips Grilled	4 (5 oz)	180	37	2	125	3	0	700
Ciabatta Chipotle w/ Grilled Chicken	1	690	44	28	105	65	4	1850
Ciabatta Chipotle w/ Spicy Crispy Chicken	1	750	37	34	80	75	5	1650
Ciabatta Sirloin Steak 'N' Cheddar	1	770	43	38	110	65	4	1310
Ciabatta Burger Bacon 'N Cheese	1	1120	45	76	135	66	4	1670
Ciabatta Burger Single Bacon 'N' Cheese	1	870	31	54	90	66	4	1550
Club Sourdough Grilled Chicken	1	530	36	28	85	34	3	1430
Curly Fries Seasoned	1 sm (3 oz)	270	4	15	0	30	3	590
Dipping Sauce Barbeque	1 serv (1 oz)	45	0	0	0	11	0	330
Egg Rolls	1	130	5	6	5	15	2	310
Fish & Chips	1 serv (7.6 oz)	570	17	30	35	58	4	1100
Fries Natural Cut	1 sm	340	5	17	0	41	5	620
Fruit Cup	1 serv	90	1	0	0	22	2	20
Hamburger	1	310	16	14	40	30	1	600
Hamburger Deluxe	1	370	17	21	45	31	2	560
Hamburger Deluxe w/ Cheese	1	460	21	28	70	33	2	930
Hamburger w/ Cheese	1	350	18	17	50	31	1	790
Jack's Spicy Chicken	1 serv	620	25	31	50	61	4	1100
Jack's Spicy Chicken w/ Cheese	1	700	29	37	70	62	4	1410
Jumbo Jack	1	600	21	35	45	51	3	940
Jumbo Jack w/ Cheese	1	690	25	42	70	54	3	1310
Mozzarella Cheese Sticks	3	240	11	12	25	21	1	420

FOOD	PORTION	CALS	PROT	FAT	CHOL	CARB	FIBER	SOD
Onion Rings	8 (4.2 oz)	500	6	30	0	51	3	420
Sampler Trio	1 serv	750	35	39	85	65	5	1760
Sandwich Bacon Chicken	1	440	19	24	40	39	2	970
Sirloin Burger w/ American Cheese & Red Onion	1	1120	54	73	190	63	4	2620
Sirloin Burger w/ Swiss & Grilled Onions	1	1070	53	71	180	61	4	1850
Sirloin Steak Melt	1	640	36	40	100	34	2	1490
Sourdough Jack	1	710	27	51	75	36	3	1230
Spicy Chicken Bites	1 serv	290	18	14	45	21	3	660
Stuffed Jalapeno	3 (2.5 oz)	230	7	13	20	22	2	690
Taco Monster Beef	1	240	8	14	20	20	3	390
Taco Regular Beef	1	160	5	8	15	15	2	270
SALAD DRESSINGS AND TOPPINGS								
Asian Sesame	1 serv (2.5 oz)	230	1	17	0	20	0	780
Dipping Sauce Buttermilk House	1 serv (0.9 oz)	130	0	13	10	3	0	210
Dipping Sauce Frank's Red Hot Buffalo	1 serv (1 oz)	10	0	0	0	2	0	840
Dipping Sauce Sweet & Sour	1 serv (1 oz)	45	0	0	0	11	0	160
Dipping Sauce Teriyaki	1 serv (1 oz)	60	1	0	0	13	0	460
Dipping Sauce Zesty Marinara	1 serv (0.8 oz)	15	0	0	0	4	0	200
Dressing Bacon Ranch	1 serv (2.5 oz)	320	2	33	35	4	0	810
Dressing Creamy Southwest	1 serv (2.5 oz)	270	1	27	30	4	0	1060
Low Fat Balsamic	1 serv (2.5 oz)	40	0	2	0	6	0	600
Mayo Onion Sauce	1 serv (0.5 oz)	90	1	10	5	4	0	590
Ranch	1 serv (2.5 oz)	390	1	41	30	4	0	590
Ranch Lite	1 serv (2.5 oz)	190	1	18	25	3	0	700
Soy Sauce	1 serv (0.3 oz)	5	1	0	0	1	0	480
Syrup Log Cabin	1 serv (2 oz)	190	0	0	0	49	0	35

FOOD	PORTION	CALS	PROT	FAT	CHOL	CARB	FIBER	SOD
Taco Sauce	1 serv (0.3 oz)	0	0	0	0	0	0	80
Tartar Sauce	1 serv (1.5 oz)	210	0	22	20	2	0	370
SALADS								
Asian w/ Crispy Chicken w/o Dressing	1 (13.8 oz)	330	21	13	40	34	7	650
Asian w/ Grilled Chicken w/o Dressing	1 (12.8 oz)	160	22	2	65	18	5	380
Chicken Club w/ Crispy Chicken w/o Dressing	1 (14 oz)	480	33	27	80	26	6	1060
Chicken Club w/ Grilled Chicken w/o Dressing	1 (13 oz)	320	34	16	105	11	4	780
Side w/o Dressing	1 (4.3 oz)	50	3	3	10	5	2	60
Southwest Crispy Chicken w/o Dressing	1 (16 oz)	480	30	23	70	44	9	1040
Southwest w/ Grilled Chicken w/o Dressing	1 (15 oz)	320	31	12	90	27	7	760
JAMBA JUICE								
Acai Supercharger Original	1 (24 oz)	420	7	5	0	86	5	85
Aloha Pineapple Original	1 (26 oz)	500	8	2	5	117	4	30
Banana Berry Original	1 (25 oz)	480	5	1	0	112	4	115
Berry Fulfilling Original	1 (24 oz)	290	9	1	5	62	8	320
Berry Lime Sublime Original	1 (26 oz)	460	3	2	5	106	5	35
Caribbean Passion Original	1 (26 oz)	440	4	2	5	102	4	60
Chocolate Moo'd Original	1 (24 oz)	680	18	8	30	138	2	420
Citrus Squeeze Original	1 (26 oz)	470	5	2	5	110	4	35
Coldbuster Original	1 (25 oz)	430	5	3	5	100	5	35
Grape Escape Original	1 (24 oz)	300	3	0	0	74	5	20
Mango Mantra Original	1 (25 oz)	310	10	1	5	71	6	310
Mango-A-Go-Go Original	1 (24 oz)	440	3	2	5	104	4	50
Matcha Green Tea Blast Original	1 (24 oz)	440	10	1	0	97	1	230
Matcha Green Tea Mist Original	1 (24 oz)	280	9	0	0	60	1	270
Mega Mango Original	1 (24 oz)	330	2	1	0	80	5	30
Mighty Cherry Charger Original	1 (24 oz)	490	18	1	0	103	3	210

FOOD	PORTION	CALS	PROT	FAT	CHOL	CARB	FIBER	SOD
Orange Berry Blitz Original	1 (26 oz)	410	5	3	5	94	5	35
Orange Dream Machine Original	1 (24 oz)	540	18	3	10	111	tr	310
Orange-A-Peel Original	1 (25 oz)	440	8	2	5	102	5	160
Passion Berry Breeze Original	1 (24 oz)	270	8	1	0	60	5	270
Peach Pleasure Original	1 (25 oz)	460	4	2	5	108	4	60
Peanut Butter Moo'd Original	1 (24 oz)	840	25	21	15	139	7	480
Peenya Kowlada Original	1 (26 oz)	690	9	5	10	152	3	180
Protein Berry Pizazz Original	1 (24 oz)	440	20	2	0	92	5	240
Raspberry Rainbow Original	1 (24 oz)	300	2	1	0	73	6	30
Razzmatazz Original	1 (26 oz)	480	3	2	5	112	4	70
Strawberries Wild Original	1 (25 oz)	450	6	1	5	105	4	180
Strawberry Nirvana Original	1 (25 oz)	280	9	1	5	64	7	320
Strawberry Surf Rider Original	1 (25 oz)	490	3	2	0	119	4	10
Strawberry Whirl Original	1 (24 oz)	310	2	1	0	76	6	25

KENTUCKY FRIED CHICKEN
BEVERAGES

FOOD	PORTION	CALS	PROT	FAT	CHOL	CARB	FIBER	SOD
Diet Pepsi	1 med (14 oz)	0	0	0	0	0	0	45
Mountain Dew	1 med (14 oz)	190	0	0	0	54	0	90
Pepsi	1 med (14 oz)	180	0	0	0	47	0	45

DESSERTS

FOOD	PORTION	CALS	PROT	FAT	CHOL	CARB	FIBER	SOD
Cake Double Chocolate Chip	1 slice	330	4	16	50	41	1	260
Cookie Sweet Life Chocolate Chip	1 (1.2 oz)	160	2	7	10	23	1	95
Cookie Sweet Life Oatmeal Raisin	1 (1.2 oz)	150	2	5	5	24	1	135
Cookie Sweet Life Sugar	1 (1.2 oz)	160	2	6	5	23	0	120
Lil' Bucket Chocolate Cream	1	280	3	13	0	38	3	230
Lil' Bucket Lemon Creme	1 serv	410	7	15	0	61	2	270

FOOD	PORTION	CALS	PROT	FAT	CHOL	CARB	FIBER	SOD
Lil' Bucket Strawberry ShortCake	1 serv	210	2	7	10	33	1	125
Pie Mini's Apple	3 (4 oz)	370	2	20	0	44	2	260
Teddy Graham Cinnamon Snacks	1 serv	90	1	3	0	15	1	95
MAIN MENU SELECTIONS								
Baked Beans	1 serv	220	8	1	0	45	7	730
Biscuit	1 (2 oz)	220	4	11	0	24	1	640
Bowl Chicken & Biscuit	1	870	29	44	60	88	7	2420
Bowl Mashed Potato w/ Gravy	1	740	27	36	60	80	7	2350
Bowl Rice w/ Gravy	1	620	26	28	60	67	6	2150
Chicken Pot Pie	1 (15 oz)	770	33	40	115	70	5	1680
Cole Slaw	1 serv	180	1	10	5	22	3	270
Corn On The Cob	1 ear (3 in)	70	2	2	0	13	3	5
Crispy Strips	2 (3.5 oz)	240	20	13	50	11	0	800
Extra Crispy Breast	1 (5.7 oz)	440	34	27	105	15	0	970
Extra Crispy Drumstick	1 (2 oz)	160	12	10	55	6	0	370
Extra Crispy Thigh	1 (4 oz)	370	18	28	85	12	0	850
Extra Crispy Whole Wing	1 (1.8 oz)	170	13	11	55	6	1	350
Green Beans	1 serv	50	2	2	5	7	2	570
KFC Snacker	1	290	15	13	30	29	2	680
KFC Snacker Buffalo	1	260	15	8	25	31	1	860
KFC Snacker Fish	1	330	17	15	60	31	1	710
KFC Snacker Fish w/o Sauce	1	290	17	12	60	29	1	610
KFC Snacker Honey BBQ	1	210	14	3	40	32	2	530
KFC Snacker Ultimate Cheese	1	280	15	11	25	30	1	780
Macaroni & Cheese	1 serv	180	8	8	15	18	0	800
Mashed Potatoes w/ Gravy	1 serv	140	2	5	0	20	1	560
Mashed Potatoes w/o Gravy	1 serv	110	2	4	0	17	1	320
Original Breast	1 (5.6 oz)	360	37	21	115	7	0	1020
Original Recipe Breast	1 (5.6 oz)	360	37	21	115	7	0	1020
Original Recipe Breast w/o Skin Or Breading	1 (3.8 oz)	140	29	2	65	1	0	520
Original Recipe Drumstick	1 (2 oz)	130	12	8	65	2	0	350
Original Recipe Thigh	1 (4.4 oz)	330	20	24	110	8	0	870

FOOD	PORTION	CALS	PROT	FAT	CHOL	CARB	FIBER	SOD
Original Recipe Whole Wing	1 (1.6 oz)	130	11	8	50	4	0	350
Popcorn Chicken	1 reg (4 oz)	400	21	26	60	22	3	1160
Potato Salad	1 serv	180	2	9	5	22	2	470
Potato Wedges	1 serv	260	4	13	0	33	3	740
Sandwich Crispy Twister	1	550	26	28	55	49	3	1500
Sandwich Double Crunch	1	470	27	23	55	38	2	1190
Sandwich Honey BBQ	1	280	22	4	60	40	3	780
Sandwich Tender Roast	1	380	37	13	80	29	2	1180
Sandwich Tender Roast w/o Sauce	1	300	37	5	70	28	2	1060
Seasoned Rice	1 serv	180	4	1	0	32	2	630
Twister Oven Roasted	1	420	28	17	60	40	3	1250
Twister Oven Roasted w/o Sauce	1	330	28	7	50	39	3	1120
Wings Fiery Buffalo	5	380	21	24	105	19	2	1480
Wings Honey BBQ	5	390	21	24	105	23	3	930
Wings Hot	5	350	20	24	105	14	2	740
Wings Hot & Spicy	5	400	21	24	105	24	2	760
Wings Teriyaki	5	480	22	25	105	40	2	830
Wings Boneless Fiery Buffalo	5	420	28	20	65	33	3	2260
Wings Boneless Honey BBQ	5	450	28	20	65	41	4	1880
Wings Boneless Sweet & Spicy	5	440	27	19	65	38	3	1700
Wings Boneless Teriyaki	5	500	28	21	65	50	3	1730
SALAD DRESSINGS								
Creamy Parmesan Caesar	1 serv (2 oz)	260	2	26	15	4	0	540
Golden Italian Light	1 serv (1.5 oz)	45	0	3	0	6	0	660
Ranch	1 serv (2 oz)	200	1	20	25	3	0	470
Ranch Fat Free	1 serv (1.5 oz)	35	1	0	0	8	0	410
SALADS								
Crispy BLT w/o Dressing	1 (12 oz)	330	28	17	65	18	4	1130
Crispy Caesar w/o Dressing & Croutons	1 (11 oz)	350	29	19	70	16	3	1080

FOOD	PORTION	CALS	PROT	FAT	CHOL	CARB	FIBER	SOD
Croutons Parmesan Garlic	1 pkg	60	2	3	0	8	0	135
Roasted BLT w/o Dressing	1 (12 oz)	200	29	6	65	8	4	880
Roasted Caesar w/o Dressing & Croutons	1 (11 oz)	220	30	8	70	6	3	830
Side Caesar w/o Dressing & Croutons	1 (3 oz)	50	4	3	10	2	1	135
Side House w/o Dressing	1 (3 oz)	15	1	0	0	2	1	10

KOO-KOO-ROO

FOOD	PORTION	CALS	PROT	FAT	CHOL	CARB	FIBER	SOD
Rotisserie Half Chicken	1 serv	655	80	34	254	2	tr	1188
Sandwich BBQ Chicken	1	562	45	12	113	71	3	1398
Sandwich Chicken Caesar	1	781	56	36	138	63	2	1775
Sandwich Original Chicken	1	661	41	29	116	63	3	1144
Traditional Turkey Dinner	1 serv	692	42	29	127	67	8	3719
Turkey Pot Pie	1 serv	883	37	44	98	83	6	1287
Turkey Sandwich Hand Carved	1	599	46	32	122	31	5	786
Wrap Chipotle Chicken	1	924	42	43	123	89	6	2449

KRISPY KREME
BEVERAGES

FOOD	PORTION	CALS	PROT	FAT	CHOL	CARB	FIBER	SOD
Chiller Kremey Berries & Kreme	1 (12 oz)	620	3	28	30	92	tr	220
Chillers Fruity Orange You Glad	1 (12 oz)	180	0	0	0	43	0	10
Chillers Fruity Very Berry	1 (12 oz)	170	0	0	0	43	0	10
Chillers Kremey Chocolate Chocolate	1 (12 oz)	970	4	29	30	104	2	320
Chillers Kremey Lemon Sherbert	1 (12 oz)	630	3	28	30	95	tr	220
Chillers Kremey Lotta Latte	1 (12 oz)	670	4	28	30	49	tr	380
Chillers Kremey Mocha Dream	1 (12 oz)	670	3	28	30	105	1	320
Chillers Kremey Oranges & Kreme	1 (12 oz)	630	3	28	30	92	tr	220

DOUGHNUTS

FOOD	PORTION	CALS	PROT	FAT	CHOL	CARB	FIBER	SOD
Apple Fritter	1	380	4	20	5	47	2	220
Caramel Kreme Crunch	1	380	4	19	10	40	tr	170
Chocolate Iced w/ Sprinkles	1	270	3	12	5	38	tr	100
Chocolate Iced Cake	1	280	3	14	20	36	tr	320

FOOD	PORTION	CALS	PROT	FAT	CHOL	CARB	FIBER	SOD
Chocolate Iced Custard Filled	1	300	3	17	5	36	tr	150
Chocolate Iced Glazed	1	250	3	12	5	33	tr	100
Chocolate Iced Kreme Filled	1	350	3	20	5	39	tr	140
Cinnamon Apple Filled	1	290	3	16	5	32	tr	150
Cinnamon Bun	1	260	3	16	5	28	tr	125
Cinnamon Twist	1	240	3	15	5	23	tr	130
Dulce De Leche	1	300	3	18	5	31	tr	160
Glazed Lemon Filled	1	290	3	16	5	36	tr	135
Glazed Raspberry Filled	1	300	3	16	5	36	tr	125
Glazed Sour Cream	1	300	2	13	20	43	tr	250
Glazed Chocolate Cake	1	300	3	15	20	42	2	250
Glazed Cinnamon	1	210	2	12	5	24	tr	100
Glazed Creme Filled	1	340	3	20	5	39	tr	140
Glazed Cruller	1	240	2	14	15	26	tr	240
Glazed Cruller Chocolate	1	290	2	15	15	37	tr	240
Glazed Pumpkin Spice	1	300	2	14	20	42	tr	250
Holes Glazed Blueberry	4	220	3	12	20	27	tr	280
Holes Glazed Cake	4	210	2	10	15	29	tr	240
Holes Glazed Chocolate Cake	4	210	2	10	15	29	tr	240
Holes Glazed Original	4	200	2	11	5	25	tr	90
Holes Glazed Pumpkin Spice	4	210	2	10	15	29	tr	240
Maple Iced Glazed	1	240	2	12	5	32	tr	100
New York Cheesecake	1	340	4	20	15	34	tr	200
Original Glazed	1	200	2	12	5	22	tr	95
Powdered Strawberry Filled	1	290	3	16	5	33	tr	135
Powdered Cake	1	290	3	14	20	37	tr	320
Sugar	1	200	2	12	5	21	0	95
Traditional Cake	1	230	3	13	20	25	tr	320

KRYSTAL
BEVERAGES

FOOD	PORTION	CALS	PROT	FAT	CHOL	CARB	FIBER	SOD
Coca-Cola Classic	1 sm (16 oz)	129	0	0	0	40	0	9
Diet Coke	1 sm (16 oz)	tr	0	0	0	tr	0	15
Sprite	1 sm (16 oz)	126	0	0	0	39	0	33

FOOD	PORTION	CALS	PROT	FAT	CHOL	CARB	FIBER	SOD
BREAKFAST SELECTIONS								
Biscuit Bacon Egg & Cheese	1	390	11	23	40	33	0	1090
Biscuit Chik	1	360	13	15	20	40	0	1030
Country Breakfast	1 serv	660	24	42	590	46	8	1450
Kryspers	1 serv	190	1	13	10	17	2	340
Krystal Sunriser	1	240	12	14	255	14	2	460
Scrambler	1 serv	440	20	26	255	33	3	840
DESSERTS								
Fried Apple Turnover	1	220	3	10	<5	31	2	300
Lemon Icebox Pie	1 serv	260	5	9	25	41	2	180
MAIN MENU SELECTIONS								
Chik'n Bites	1 sm	310	17	19	55	16	1	790
Fries	1 med	470	4	20	20	53	7	90
Fries Chili Cheese	1 serv	540	13	28	45	59	5	800
Krystal	1	160	7	7	20	17	1	260
Krystal Bacon Cheese	1	190	10	10	25	16	2	430
Krystal Cheese	1	180	9	9	25	17	2	430
Krystal Chik	1	240	11	11	25	24	2	640
Krystal Chili	1 serv	200	13	7	25	22	7	1130
Krystal Double	1	260	13	13	40	24	2	550
Krystal Double Cheese	1	310	16	16	65	26	tr	800
Pup	1	170	6	9	25	15	1	500
Pup Chili Cheese	1	210	9	12	40	17	2	510
Pup Corn	1	260	6	19	50	19	1	490

LONG JOHN SILVER'S

FOOD	PORTION	CALS	PROT	FAT	CHOL	CARB	FIBER	SOD
BEVERAGES								
Coca-Cola	1 sm	150	0	0	0	37	0	10
Diet Coke	1 sm	0	0	0	0	0	0	15
Sprite	1 sm	140	0	0	0	36	0	30
DESSERTS								
Pie Chocolate Cream	1 pie	310	5	44	15	24	1	170
Pie Pecan	1 pie	370	4	15	40	55	2	190
Pie Pineapple Cream	1 pie	290	4	13	15	39	1	210
MAIN MENU SELECTIONS								
Baked Cod	1 piece	120	22	5	90	0	1	240
Battered Chicken	1 piece	140	8	8	20	9	0	400
Battered Fish	1 piece	230	11	13	30	16	0	700
Battered Shrimp	1 piece	45	2	3	15	3	0	125
Breaded Clams	1 serv	240	8	13	10	22	1	1110

FOOD	PORTION	CALS	PROT	FAT	CHOL	CARB	FIBER	SOD
Cheesesticks	3 pieces	140	4	8	10	12	1	320
Clam Chowder	1 bowl	220	9	10	25	23	tr	810
Corn Cobbette	1 piece	90	3	3	0	14	3	0
Crumblies	1 serv	170	1	12	0	14	1	420
Crunchy Shrimp	21 pieces	330	12	18	105	31	2	700
Fries	1 reg	230	3	10	0	34	3	350
Hushpuppy	1 piece	60	1	3	0	9	1	200
Rice	1 serv	180	3	4	0	34	3	540
Sandwich Chicken	1	360	13	15	25	41	3	810
Sandwich Fish	1	440	17	20	35	48	3	1120
Sandwich Ultimate Fish	1	500	20	28	50	48	3	1310
Slaw	1 serv	200	1	15	20	15	3	340

MAGGIE MOO'S

FOOD	PORTION	CALS	PROT	FAT	CHOL	CARB	FIBER	SOD
Ice Cream Fat Free	½ cup	80	3	0	0	18	0	50
Ice Cream Low Carb Sugar Added	½ cup	100	2	6	30	11	0	60
Ice Cream Udderly Cream	½ cup	180	3	11	45	18	0	40
Sorbet	½ cup	90	0	0	0	22	0	5

MANHATTAN BAGEL

FOOD	PORTION	CALS	PROT	FAT	CHOL	CARB	FIBER	SOD
Blueberry	1	260	9	tr	0	54	2	560
Cheddar Cheese	1	270	11	4	10	48	2	560
Cinnamon Raisin	1	280	10	tr	0	57	3	560
Egg	1	270	10	2	0	53	2	710
Everything	1	290	11	3	0	54	3	2000
Garlic	1	270	10	tr	0	55	2	560
Jalapeno Cheddar	1	260	16	2	0	53	2	310
Marble	1	260	10	tr	0	52	3	540
Oat Bran	1	260	10	1	0	53	3	470
Oat Bran Raisin Walnut	1	270	10	3	0	54	3	450
Onion	1	270	10	tr	0	55	2	560
Plain	1	260	10	tr	0	52	2	560
Poppy	1	300	11	4	0	54	5	560
Pumpernickel	1	250	10	1	0	52	3	530
Salt	1	260	10	tr	0	53	2	7100
Sesame	1	310	11	5	0	55	3	560
Spinach	1	270	10	tr	0	54	3	580
Sun-Dried Tomato	1	260	10	1	0	53	3	340
Whole Wheat	1	260	10	tr	0	52	3	470

FOOD	PORTION	CALS	PROT	FAT	CHOL	CARB	FIBER	SOD
MARBLE SLAB CREAMERY								
Cone Honey Wheat	1	130	3	3	15	24	tr	10
Cone Sugar	1	130	2	3	15	23	0	10
Cone Vanilla Cinnamon	1	130	2	3	15	24	tr	10
Frozen Yogurt Nonfat	½ cup	100	3	1	0	22	1	55
Frozen Yogurt Nonfat No Sugar Added	½ cup	90	4	1	0	17	1	85
Sorbet	½ cup	90	0	0	0	22	0	5
MAUI WOWI								
SMOOTHIES								
Fresh Fruit Banana Banana	1 (12 oz)	210	2	1	0	50	2	55
Fresh Fruit Black Raspberry	1 (12 oz)	240	2	0	0	59	0	40
Fresh Fruit Kiwi Lemon Lime	1 (12 oz)	180	3	0	0	42	0	35
Fresh Fruit Lemon Wave	1 (12 oz)	415	tr	tr	0	108	tr	1
Fresh Fruit Mango Orange Banana	1 (12 oz)	240	3	1	0	57	tr	35
Fresh Fruit Passion Papaya	1 (12 oz)	220	2	1	0	54	tr	50
Fresh Fruit Pina Colada	1 (12 oz)	240	3	3	0	57	0	70
MAX & ERMA'S								
Black Bean Roll Up	1 serv	577	29	10	14	95	10	1203
Caribbean Chicken Lunch Portion	1 serv	536	28	20	97	59	3	1151
Fruit Smoothie	1	124	1	tr	0	29	1	4
Garlic Breadstick	1	156	4	6	0	21	0	293
Hula Bowl w/ Fat Free Honey Mustard Dressing w/o Breadsticks	1 serv	823	46	7	131	79	6	1554
Salad Baby Greens w/o Breadstick	1 serv	119	1	11	0	6	2	259
Salad Shrimp Stack	1 serv	322	20	12	178	116	3	823
Salad Dressing Bleu Cheese	2 tbsp	201	1	21	19	tr	0	169
Salad Dressing French Fat Free	2 tbsp	126	tr	tr	0	31	2	1034
Salad Dressing Honey Mustard Fat Free	2 tbsp	60	0	0	0	14	0	360
Salad Dressing Italian	2 tbsp	110	0	12	0	1	0	180
Salad Dressing Ranch	2 tbsp	120	1	13	11	1	0	90

FOOD	PORTION	CALS	PROT	FAT	CHOL	CARB	FIBER	SOD
Salad Dressing Tex Mex Low Fat	2 tbsp	23	3	tr	2	2	tr	129

McALISTER'S DELI
CHILDREN'S MENU SELECTIONS

FOOD	PORTION	CALS	PROT	FAT	CHOL	CARB	FIBER	SOD
Kid's Nacho	1 serv	734	12	43	17	74	3	679
Mac's Dog	1	307	10	19	35	24	1	827
Pita Pizza	1	503	24	21	46	54	3	887
Sandwich Ham & Cheese	1	455	26	22	75	39	4	1819
Sandwich PB&J	1	714	23	32	0	86	7	644
Sandwich Toasted Cheese	1	620	30	38	107	40	4	2031
Sandwich Turkey & Cheese	1	451	26	21	79	39	4	1670

DESSERTS

FOOD	PORTION	CALS	PROT	FAT	CHOL	CARB	FIBER	SOD
Brownie Chocolate	1 (3.5 oz)	424	6	18	0	59	3	311
Brownie Delight	1 (11 oz)	917	13	48	108	111	4	519
Chocolate Loving Spoon Cake	1 (4 oz)	538	6	35	69	54	2	486
Ice Cream Vanilla Bean	1 scoop (5 oz)	160	3	10	40	19	0	70
Kentucky Pie	1 slice (12 oz)	807	14	64	211	110	1	393
New York Cheesecake	1 slice (5 oz)	505	7	35	92	37	2	239
Sundae Topping Caramel	2 tbsp	100	1	0	0	20	0	110
Sundae Topping Chocolate	1 tbsp	110	1	0	0	21	0	20

MAIN MENU SELECTIONS

FOOD	PORTION	CALS	PROT	FAT	CHOL	CARB	FIBER	SOD
Appetizers Chips & Salsa	1 serv (5 oz)	87	3	5	0	9	0	128
Appetizers Dip Cheese & Chili	1 serv (5 oz)	572	10	35	17	54	3	598
Appetizers Dip Cheese & Veggie Chili	1 serv (5 oz)	552	9	31	9	58	5	583
Appetizers Nacho Basket	1 serv (6 oz)	579	10	33	17	61	3	832
Appetizers Nacho Chili	1 serv (6 oz)	564	12	37	26	46	4	713
Appetizers Nacho Veggie Chili	1 serv (6 oz)	537	11	31	14	52	6	693
Chicken Cordon Bleu	1 serv	810	59	39	156	53	2	2862
Chili Vegetarian	1 serv (8 oz)	133	8	1	0	28	15	987
Cole Slaw	1 serv (4 oz)	190	1	15	15	14	7	215
Fruit Cup	1 serv (4 oz)	98	1	0	0	12	2	12
Giant Spud Cheese	1 (27 oz)	930	55	48	60	139	19	60

FOOD	PORTION	CALS	PROT	FAT	CHOL	CARB	FIBER	SOD
Giant Spud Grilled Chicken	1 (27 oz)	839	52	25	–	99	19	88
Giant Spud Just A Spud	1 (26 oz)	604	20	4	0	123	18	63
Giant Spud Ole	1 (30 oz)	1252	68	60	120	110	18	770
Giant Spud Ole w/ Chili	1 (33 oz)	1512	69	78	99	134	21	1255
Giant Spud Ole w/ Veggie Chili	1 (33 oz)	1457	67	67	76	146	24	1214
Giant Spud Veggie	1 (28 oz)	668	29	18	0	99	18	347
Macaroni & Cheese	1 serv (4 oz)	200	8	7	20	17	1	580
Mashed Potatoes	1 serv (4 oz)	136	2	8	2	19	2	347
Meatloaf w/ Gravy	1 serv	340	40	37	189	21	1	752
Open-Faced Roast Beef	1 serv	751	55	21	87	88	6	3099
Pot Roast Spud	1 serv	906	38	30	72	121	17	125
Potato Salad	1 serv (4 oz)	200	3	11	1	22	3	161
Salmon Filet	1 serv	235	46	4	152	3	1	269
Steamed Vegetables	1 serv (4 oz)	43	1	0	0	7	3	52
SALAD DRESSINGS AND SAUCES								
Au Jus	1 serv (4 oz)	10	0	0	0	2	0	60
Comeback Gravy	1 serv (4 oz)	37	1	2	1	6	0	450
Dressing Blue Cheese	2 tbsp	140	0	15	10	1	0	290
Dressing Greek	2 tbsp	90	0	9	0	2	0	250
Dressing Parmesan Peppercorn	2 tbsp	150	0	16	2	2	0	310
Dressing Ranch	2 tbsp	100	0	11	10	1	0	290
Dressing Tomato Basil	2 tbsp	30	0	0	0	6	0	230
Dressing Lite Olive Oil Vinaigrette	2 tbsp	60	0	6	0	3	0	230
Dressing Lite Ranch	2 tbsp	100	0	10	10	1	0	290
Dressing Low Calorie Italian	2 tbsp	25	0	2	0	2	0	410
SALADS								
Caesar w/ Salmon	1 (17 oz)	800	34	53	109	42	5	1680
Chicken Fiesta	1 (20 oz)	493	38	22	92	34	8	991
Chicken Grill	1 (21 oz)	840	57	15	131	47	4	3164
Garden	1 (15 oz)	264	17	17	38	21	4	1312
Garden w/ Chicken Salad	1 (18 oz)	537	30	45	34	14	5	1333
Garden w/ Salmon	1 (17 oz)	315	28	10	76	28	6	883
Garden w/ Tuna Salad	1 (18 oz)	373	31	18	15	21	5	1361

FOOD	PORTION	CALS	PROT	FAT	CHOL	CARB	FIBER	SOD
Greek Chicken	1 (19 oz)	584	38	32	65	32	7	2161
Side Caesar	1 (6 oz)	328	5	24	16	19	1	679
Side Garden	1 (8 oz)	138	8	9	19	11	2	867
Taco	1 (26 oz)	641	38	40	86	33	11	1680
Taco w/ Veggie Chili	1 (26 oz)	641	38	40	64	33	15	1639
SANDWICHES								
BLT	1	654	28	38	56	50	6	2015
Chicken Salad	1	677	15	43	59	58	2	967
Deli Corned Beef On Wheat	1	369	34	9	76	39	4	1879
Deli Ham On Wheat	1	350	24	9	43	43	5	1854
Deli Pastrami On Wheat	1	371	33	10	75	36	4	1385
Deli Roast Beef On Wheat	1	398	27	12	29	49	5	1937
Deli Salami On Wheat	1	565	27	32	100	43	5	2465
Deli Turkey On Wheat	1	342	24	9	51	43	5	1556
French Dip	1	676	44	34	118	50	2	1889
Grilled Chicken Breast	1	751	50	36	120	56	2	1772
Grilled Chicken Club	1	1234	76	64	193	87	7	2733
Ham Melt	1	700	49	34	114	52	4	2303
McAlisters Club	1	1225	66	69	195	86	7	2845
Meatloaf Parmesan	1	708	47	36	140	49	5	1046
Memphian	1	585	41	26	85	48	4	2237
Muffuletta	¼ (8 oz)	615	36	35	67	40	2	2015
New Yorker	1	628	50	25	127	50	4	2119
Orange Cranberry Club	1	954	63	52	171	62	6	2230
Reuben On Rye	1	492	25	30	71	35	2	2175
Roast Beef Melt	1	635	40	32	102	48	4	2170
Salmon	1	608	37	21	76	66	3	1006
Submarine	1	833	50	48	130	53	3	2866
Sweetberry Chicken On Wheatberry	1	701	53	24	102	67	5	1618
Tuna Salad On Wheat	1	452	25	19	15	47	5	941
Turkey Melt	1	700	45	35	124	52	4	2262
Veggie On Pita	1	522	15	36	41	33	2	950
Wrap Greek Chicken	1	630	48	25	53	57	14	2813
Wrap Grill Chicken Caesar	1	533	42	25	40	46	13	2023
SOUPS								
Asiago Cheese Bisque	1 serv (8 oz)	240	5	17	47	17	0	720
Broccoli Cheddar	1 serv (8 oz)	213	8	15	47	13	0	947
Cheddar Potato	1 serv (8 oz)	213	5	13	40	19	1	773
Cheesy Chicken Tortilla	1 serv (8 oz)	150	10	6	30	13	0	1470

FOOD	PORTION	CALS	PROT	FAT	CHOL	CARB	FIBER	SOD
Chicken & Sausage Gumbo	1 serv (8 oz)	150	8	5	20	17	2	1040
Clam Chowder	1 serv (8 oz)	200	8	11	40	09	0	960
Country Vegetable	1 serv (8 oz)	93	3	1	0	17	3	973
Country Potato	1 serv (8 oz)	173	4	8	20	23	0	760
French Onion	1 serv (8 oz)	80	1	1	7	11	1	144
Red Beans & Rice	1 serv (8 oz)	107	9	3	7	25	11	760
Southwest Roasted Corn	1 serv (8 oz)	90	4	4	0	20	3	893

McDONALD'S
BEVERAGES

FOOD	PORTION	CALS	PROT	FAT	CHOL	CARB	FIBER	SOD
Apple Juice	1 box (6.8 oz)	90	0	0	0	23	0	15
Chocolate Milk 1% Low Fat	8 oz	170	9	3	5	26	1	150
Coca-Cola Classic	1 sm (16 oz)	150	0	0	0	40	0	10
Coffee	1 sm (12 oz)	0	0	0	0	0	0	0
Diet Coke	1 sm (16 oz)	0	0	0	0	0	0	20
Half & Half Creamer	1 pkg	20	0	2	10	0	0	1
Hi-C Orange Lavaburst	1 sm (16 oz)	160	0	0	0	44	0	5
Ice Coffee Hazelnut	1 sm (16 oz)	130	1	5	20	21	0	40
Iced Coffee Caramel	1 sm (16 oz)	130	1	5	20	21	1	80
Iced Coffee Regular	1 sm (16 oz)	140	1	5	20	22	0	40
Iced Coffee Vanilla	1 sm (16 oz)	130	1	5	20	21	0	40
Iced Tea	1 sm (16 oz)	0	0	0	0	0	0	10
Milk Lowfat 1%	1 pkg	100	8	3	10	12	0	125
Orange Juice	1 sm (12 oz)	140	2	0	0	33	0	5
Powerade Mountain Blast	1 sm (16 oz)	100	0	0	0	27	0	85
Shake Triple Thick Chocolate	1 sm (12 oz)	440	10	10	40	76	1	190
Shake Triple Thick Strawberry	1 sm (12 oz)	420	10	10	40	73	0	130
Shake Triple Thick Vanilla	1 sm (16 oz)	420	9	10	40	72	0	140
Sprite	1 sm (16 oz)	150	0	0	0	39	0	40

BREAKFAST SELECTIONS

FOOD	PORTION	CALS	PROT	FAT	CHOL	CARB	FIBER	SOD
Big Breakfast Regular Biscuit	1 serv	720	27	46	555	49	3	1500
Biscuit	1 reg	250	4	11	0	32	2	700
Biscuit Regular Bacon Egg Cheese	1	450	18	25	245	36	2	1360
Biscuit Regular Sausage	1	410	11	27	30	33	2	1040

FOOD	PORTION	CALS	PROT	FAT	CHOL	CARB	FIBER	SOD
Biscuit Regular Sausage w/ Egg	1	500	17	32	250	35	2	1130
Burrito Sausage	1	300	12	16	130	26	1	830
Deluxe Breakfast Regular Biscuit w/o Syrup & Margarine	1 serv	1070	36	55	575	109	6	2090
English Muffin	1	160	5	3	0	27	2	280
Hash Browns	1 serv	140	1	8	0	15	2	290
Hotcake Syrup	1 pkg (2 oz)	180	0	0	0	45	0	20
Hotcakes & Sausage w/o Syrup & Margarine	1 serv	520	15	24	50	61	3	930
Hotcakes w/o Syrup & Margarine	1 serv	350	8	9	20	60	3	590
McGriddles Bacon Egg Cheese	1	460	19	21	245	48	2	1360
McGriddles Sausage	1	420	11	22	35	44	2	1030
McGriddles Sausage Egg & Cheese	1	560	20	32	265	48	2	1360
McMuffin Sausage	1	370	14	22	45	29	2	850
McMuffin Sausage w/ Egg	1	250	21	27	285	30	2	920
McSkillet Burrito w/ Sausage	1	610	27	36	410	44	3	1390
McSkillet Burrito w/ Steak	1	570	32	30	430	44	3	1470
Sausage Patty	1	170	7	15	30	1	0	340
Scrambled Eggs	2	170	15	11	520	1	0	180
DESSERTS								
Apple Dippers	1 pkg	35	0	0	0	8	0	0
Apple Pie Baked	1	270	3	12	0	36	4	190
Carmel Dip Low Fat	1 pkg	70	0	1	5	15	0	35
Cinnamon Melts	1 serv	460	6	19	15	66	3	370
Cookie Chocolate Chip	1	180	2	7	10	22	1	90
Cookie Oatmeal	1 (1.1 oz)	150	2	6	10	22	1	135
Cookie Sugar	1 (1.1 oz)	150	2	6	5	21	0	110
Cookies McDonaldland	1 pkg (2 oz)	250	4	8	0	42	1	270
Cookies McDonaldland Chocolate Chip	1 pkg	270	3	11	35	39	1	170
Fruit 'n Yogurt Parfait	1 serv	160	4	2	5	31	1	85
Ice Cream Cone Reduced Fat Vanilla	1	150	4	4	15	24	0	60
Kiddie Cone	1	45	1	1	5	8	0	20

FOOD	PORTION	CALS	PROT	FAT	CHOL	CARB	FIBER	SOD
McFlurry Oreo	1 (12 oz)	560	14	16	50	88	0	250
McFlurry w/ M&M's	1 (12 oz)	620	14	20	55	96	1	190
Peanuts For Sundae	1 serv	45	2	4	0	2	1	0
Sundae Hot Caramel	1	340	7	7	30	60	1	160
Sundae Hot Fudge	1	330	8	10	25	54	2	180
Sundae Strawberry	1	280	6	6	25	49	1	95
MAIN MENU SELECTIONS								
Apple Sauce Strawberry	1 serv	90	0	0	0	23	tr	0
Big Mac	1	540	25	29	75	45	3	1040
Big N' Tasty	1	460	24	24	70	37	3	720
Big N' Tasty w/ Cheese	1	510	27	28	85	38	3	960
Cheeseburger	1	300	15	12	40	33	2	750
Cheeseburger Double	1	440	25	23	80	34	2	1150
Cheesy Tots	6 pieces	210	7	12	20	20	2	650
Chicken McNuggets	4 pieces	170	10	10	25	10	0	450
Chicken Selects	3 pieces	380	23	20	55	28	0	930
Filet-O-Fish	1	380	15	18	35	38	2	660
French Fries	1 sm	250	2	13	0	30	3	140
French Fries	1 lg	570	6	30	0	70	7	330
Hamburger	1	250	12	9	25	31	2	520
McChicken	1	360	14	16	40	40	1	790
McRib	1	500	22	26	70	44	3	980
Onion Rings	1 sm	140	2	7	0	18	2	210
Quarter Pounder	1	410	24	19	65	37	3	730
Quarter Pounder Double w/ Cheese	1	740	48	42	155	40	3	1380
Quarter Pounder w/ Cheese	1	510	29	26	90	40	3	1190
Sandwich Chicken Classic Crispy	1	500	27	17	50	61	3	1330
Sandwich Chicken Classic Grilled	1	420	32	10	70	51	3	1190
Sandwich Club Chicken Crispy	1	660	39	28	80	63	4	1860
Sandwich Club Chicken Grilled	1	570	44	21	100	52	4	1720
Sandwich Ranch BLT Chicken Crispy	1	600	35	23	70	64	3	1900
Sandwich Ranch BLT Chicken Grilled	1	520	40	16	90	53	3	1760

FOOD	PORTION	CALS	PROT	FAT	CHOL	CARB	FIBER	SOD
Snack Wrap Grilled w/ Chipotle BBQ	1	260	18	8	45	28	1	820
Snack Wrap Grilled w/ Honey Mustard	1	260	18	9	45	27	1	800
Snack Wrap Grilled w/ Ranch	1	270	18	10	45	26	1	830
Snack Wrap w/ Chipotle BBQ	1	320	14	14	25	35	2	780
Snack Wrap w/ Honey Mustard	1	320	14	15	30	34	1	750
Snack Wrap w/ Ranch	1	140	14	16	30	32	2	780
SALAD DRESSINGS AND SAUCES								
Dipping Sauce Buffalo	1 serv (1 oz)	80	0	8	5	2	0	350
Dipping Sauce Zesty Onion Ring	1 serv (1 oz)	150	0	15	15	3	tr	210
Dressing Ken's Light Italian	1 pkg (2 oz)	120	0	11	0	5	0	440
Dressing Newman's Own Creamy Caesar	1 pkg (2 oz)	170	2	18	20	4	0	500
Dressing Newman's Own Creamy Southwest	1 pkg (1.5 oz)	100	1	6	20	11	0	340
Dressing Newman's Own Low Fat Balsamic Vinaigrette	1 pkg (1.5 oz)	40	0	3	0	4	0	730
Dressing Newman's Own Low Fat Family Recipe Italian	1 pkg (1.5 oz)	60	1	3	0	8	0	730
Dressing Newman's Own Low Fat Sesame Ginger	1 pkg (1.5 oz)	90	1	3	0	15	0	740
Dressing Newman's Own Ranch	1 pkg (2 oz)	170	1	15	20	9	0	530
Honey	1 pkg (0.5 oz)	50	0	0	0	12	0	0
Ketchup	1 pkg	15	0	0	0	3	0	110
Sauce Barbeque	1 pkg (1 oz)	50	0	0	0	12	0	260
Sauce Creamy Ranch	1 pkg (1.5 oz)	200	0	22	10	2	0	320
Sauce Hot Mustard	1 pkg (1 oz)	60	1	3	5	9	2	250
Sauce Southwestern Chipotle Barbeque	1 pkg (1.5 oz)	70	0	0	0	18	1	260

FOOD	PORTION	CALS	PROT	FAT	CHOL	CARB	FIBER	SOD
Sauce Spicy Buffalo	1 pkg (1.5 oz)	60	0	7	0	1	2	960
Sauce Sweet 'N Sour	1 pkg (1 oz)	50	0	0	0	12	0	150
Sauce Tangy Honey Mustard	1 pkg (1.5 oz)	70	1	3	5	13	0	170
SALADS								
Asian w/ Crispy Chicken w/o Dressing	1 serv	380	27	17	45	33	5	1030
Asian w/ Grilled Chicken w/o Dressing	1 serv	300	32	10	65	23	5	890
Asian w/o Chicken & Dressing	1 serv	150	8	7	0	15	5	35
Bacon Ranch w/ Crispy Chicken	1 serv	350	28	16	70	23	3	1150
Bacon Ranch w/ Grilled Chicken w/o Dressing	1 serv	260	33	9	90	12	3	1010
Bacon Ranch w/o Chicken	1 serv	140	9	7	25	10	3	300
Caesar w/ Crispy Chicken	1 serv	300	25	13	55	22	3	1020
Caesar w/ Grilled Chicken	1 serv	220	30	6	75	12	3	890
Caesar w/o Chicken	1 serv	90	7	4	10	9	3	180
Croutons Butter Garlic	1 pkg	60	2	2	0	10	1	140
Fruit & Walnut Snack Size	1 serv	210	4	8	5	31	2	60
Side Salad	1 serv	20	1	0	0	4	1	10
Southwest w/ Crispy Chicken w/o Dressing	1 serv	400	25	16	50	41	7	1110
Southwest w/ Grilled Chicken	1 serv	320	30	9	70	30	7	970
Southwest w/o Chicken & Dressing	1 serv	140	6	5	10	20	6	150

MIMIS CAFE
BEVERAGES

FOOD	PORTION	CALS	PROT	FAT	CHOL	CARB	FIBER	SOD
Cappuccino	1 serv	86	4	5	17	7	0	72
Cappuccino Iced	1 serv	86	4	5	17	7	0	72
Espresso	1 serv	8	0	0	0	1	0	13
Hot Chocolate w/ Whipped Cream	1 serv	986	8	17	3	193	8	800
Mocha Iced	1 serv	376	6	11	17	70	2	102
Mocha Latte	1 serv	376	6	11	17	70	2	146

FOOD	PORTION	CALS	PROT	FAT	CHOL	CARB	FIBER	SOD
CHILDREN'S MENU SELECTIONS								
Chicken Fingers	1 serv	408	30	21	67	21	1	686
Grilled Cheese	1 serv	273	13	19	50	14	0	499
Macaroni & Cheese	1 serv	353	12	13	19	48	2	652
Mini Burger	1 serv	554	25	28	66	48	3	686
Mini Corn Dogs	1 serv	460	7	32	35	35	0	672
Pancakes Chocolate Chip	1 serv	563	11	29	73	71	3	747
Pancakes Mimi Mouse	1 serv	477	11	18	63	69	1	985
PB&J Soldiers	1 serv	730	18	40	0	78	4	728
Pepperoni Pizzadillas	1 serv	617	31	38	86	39	3	1600
Scrambled Eggs & Bacon	1 serv	216	18	16	441	1	0	449
Spaghetti	1 serv	343	13	5	–	62	5	711
Turkey Dinner	1 serv	337	11	16	69	25	3	1110
DESSERTS								
Apple Crisp Cinnamon	1 serv	898	7	37	25	141	4	427
Bread Pudding	1 serv	819	18	55	329	69	1	730
Brownie Triple Chocolate	1 serv	1950	25	87	303	280	6	1073
Cheesecake New York Style	1 serv	1075	19	42	373	85	4	744
Pie Bananas Foster Mud	1 serv	1245	14	73	218	138	4	477
Pie Pecan Chocolate Chip	1 serv	1879	21	111	231	220	12	1064
MAIN MENU SELECTIONS								
Appetizer Dip Spinach & Artichoke	1 serv	2459	90	138	262	191	11	4320
Appetizer Fried Chicken Tenders	1 serv	800	60	33	134	60	3	1730
Appetizer Fried Dill Pickles	1 serv	972	16	42	12	132	12	3740
Appetizer Jazz Fest	1 serv	1252	43	72	122	108	8	2085
Appetizer Zucchini Parmesan	1 serv	626	22	28	26	73	7	1111
Blackened Soul w/ Shrimp Creole	1 serv	852	78	34	334	59	9	2312
Broil Flat Iron Steak	1 serv	1026	68	58	164	58	9	1751
Burger Half Pound	1	684	42	34	132	48	3	668
Cafe Fish & Chips	1 serv	1290	69	57	121	119	10	2166
Cajun Blackened Salmon	1 serv	919	57	55	220	55	9	1915
Cheeseburger BBQ Ranch	1	999	58	57	192	62	3	1433
Cheeseburger Half Pound	1	855	53	48	177	49	3	932
Chicken Cordon Bleu	1 serv	1360	100	81	306	51	5	3007
Chicken Feta Penne	1 serv	1879	57	99	253	158	12	1756
Ciabatta Chicken	1	1251	70	72	213	81	4	1846

FOOD	PORTION	CALS	PROT	FAT	CHOL	CARB	FIBER	SOD
Ciabatta Meatloaf	1	1036	41	61	171	83	3	2017
Ciabatta Turkey Pesto	1	1248	45	73	172	83	6	1672
Club Cafe	1	1132	42	63	175	73	4	1438
Country Fried Steak	1 serv	1061	42	56	156	107	9	1418
Crab Cake Dinner	1 serv	1662	59	100	646	129	9	3732
Diablo Center Cut Pork Chops	1 serv	1094	54	73	219	55	8	2179
Dip Classic Beef	1	521	49	15	108	43	5	3928
Fillet Of Soul	1 serv	636	45	26	163	56	7	1316
French Quarter	1	1480	66	105	214	68	7	1917
Garlic Shrimp Spaghettini	1 serv	860	37	20	261	109	7	1073
Grilled Beef Liver	1 serv	1003	75	45	937	75	10	1457
Grilled Chicken Tuscan Style	1 serv	880	58	36	181	80	12	1529
Habachi Salmon	1 serv	846	49	40	119	75	8	274
Mimi's Meatloaf	1 serv	910	43	53	291	68	8	2650
Mimis Pot Roast	1 serv	1291	88	78	323	57	8	2252
Original Patty Melt	1	976	56	56	177	62	6	1261
Parmesan Crusted Chicken Breast	1 serv	1820	91	54	194	211	15	1466
Pasta Jambalaya	1 serv	1223	74	44	295	113	8	1727
Pot Pie Chicken	1 serv	1403	70	87	388	86	11	2416
Reuben West Coast	1	2015	62	138	226	120	11	3798
Sandwich 5 Way Grilled Cheese	1	703	39	39	92	49	2	1150
Sandwich Albacore & Avocado	1	993	33	71	94	58	9	960
Sandwich Bacon Lettuce & Tomato	1	586	24	34	56	48	7	1545
Sandwich Fresh Roasted Turkey Breast	1	532	20	27	134	28	1	546
Sandwich Turkey Walnut Salad On Raisin Bread	1	549	7	42	54	36	3	447
Sandwich Veggie Stack	1	836	27	43	48	93	6	1807
Slow Roasted Turkey Breast	1 serv	851	25	41	154	72	11	2086
Small Bites Black & Blue Quesadilla	1 serv	1241	73	80	216	60	7	2403
Small Bites Chicken & Fruit	1 serv	460	73	9	193	21	3	192
Small Bites Citrus Salmon	1 serv	699	44	43	119	37	10	368
Small Bites Crab Cakes	1 serv	412	18	25	212	27	2	1089

FOOD	PORTION	CALS	PROT	FAT	CHOL	CARB	FIBER	SOD
Small Bites Smokey Chicken Enchiladas	1 serv	1154	61	72	179	68	8	1922
Small Bites Sweet & Sour Coconut Shrimp	1 serv	608	22	50	120	79	4	767
Small Bites Thai Chicken Wrap	1 serv	1004	51	41	96	106	7	1522
Top Sirloin 12 oz	1 serv	947	79	48	237	49	7	1076
SALAD DRESSINGS								
Balsamic Vinaigrette	1 serv	316	0	32	0	8	0	337
Blue Cheese	1 serv	298	2	31	30	1	0	241
Caesar	1 serv	273	1	29	22	2	0	451
Chinese Sesame	1 serv	263	0	25	0	11	0	307
Dijon Vinaigrette	1 serv	296	0	32	0	3	0	335
Honey Mustard	1 serv	243	1	22	10	11	0	423
Non Fat French	1 serv	65	1	0	0	16	1	222
Ranch	1 serv	194	1	20	18	2	0	321
Thousand Island	1 serv	232	0	23	19	6	0	439
SALADS								
Asian Chopped	1 serv	751	81	22	193	55	14	347
Blue Cheese & Walnut	1 serv	728	26	53	53	45	10	1097
Caesar Blackened Chicken	1 serv	570	59	17	132	41	6	1565
Chopped Cobb	1 serv	524	35	32	329	18	4	1516
Fried Chicken	1 serv	764	23	67	272	16	3	469
Zesty Chicken Tostada	1 serv	1046	47	57	134	89	15	1184
SOUPS								
Broccoli Cheddar	1 serv	270	12	10	51	18	2	916
Chicken Gumbo	1 serv	235	7	12	17	25	2	1112
Clam Chowder	1 serv	240	10	14	49	21	2	657
Corn Chowder	1 serv	196	3	9	20	28	3	722
Cream Of Chicken	1 serv	337	0	29	32	19	1	1083
French Market Onion	1 serv	207	10	12	16	16	2	1269
Red Bean & Andouille Sausage	1 serv	256	13	10	29	30	5	706
Split Pea	1 serv	194	14	3	11	29	11	636
Vegetarian Vegetable	1 serv	60	2	0	0	12	2	1561
MRS. FIELDS								
Brownie Double Fudge	1 (2.7 oz)	360	4	19	80	59	2	240
Brownie Frosted Fudge	1 (3.7 oz)	440	4	21	80	62	2	265
Brownie Pecan Fudge	1 (2.7 oz)	340	4	21	70	40	2	220

FOOD	PORTION	CALS	PROT	FAT	CHOL	CARB	FIBER	SOD
Brownie Pecan Pie	1 (2.7 oz)	340	5	20	70	40	2	220
Brownie Walnut Fudge	1 (2.7 oz)	380	5	23	80	45	tr	240
Bundt Cake Banana Walnut	1 piece (2.9 oz)	350	6	21	40	35	3	300
Bundt Cake Banana Walnut w/ Chocolate Chips	1 piece (2.9 oz)	370	6	22	35	39	3	240
Bundt Cake Blueberry	1 piece (2.9 oz)	270	4	12	50	36	1	330
Bundt Cake Raspberry	1 piece (2.9 oz)	270	4	12	50	36	tr	330
Bundt Cake White w/ Chocolate Chips	1 piece (2.9 oz)	350	4	17	50	45	tr	330
Cookie Butter Toffee	1 (2.3 oz)	290	3	13	55	40	tr	190
Cookie Cinnamon Sugar	1 (2.3 oz)	300	3	12	50	41	tr	250
Cookie Coconut Macadamia	1 (2.3 oz)	280	3	13	20	39	tr	220
Cookie Debra's Special	1 (2.3 oz)	280	4	12	40	39	2	180
Cookie Milk Chocolate	1 (2.3 oz)	280	3	13	40	38	tr	180
Cookie Milk Chocolate & Walnuts	1 (2.3 oz)	320	4	17	40	37	1	180
Cookie Milk Chocolate Macadamia	1 (2.3 oz)	320	4	18	40	36	tr	180
Cookie Oatmeal Chocolate Chip	1 (2.3 oz)	280	3	13	35	40	1	140
Cookie Oatmeal Raisin & Walnuts	1 (2.3 oz)	280	4	12	40	39	2	180
Cookie Peanut Butter	1 (2.3 oz)	310	5	16	45	34	tr	260
Cookie Peanut Butter w/ Milk Chocolate Chips	1 (2.3 oz)	300	5	17	40	35	tr	160
Cookie Semi-Sweet Chocolate	1 (2.3 oz)	280	2	14	30	40	1	160
Cookie Semi-Sweet Chocolate & Walnuts	1 (2.3 oz)	310	3	16	35	38	2	170
Cookie White Chunk Macadamia	1 (2.3 oz)	310	4	17	35	37	tr	170
Jumbo Cookie Snickerdoodle	1 (5 oz)	640	7	29	110	90	2	540
Nibbler Cookies	2 (0.9 oz)	110	1	5	15	15	0	90
Nibbler Cookies Chewy Chocolate Fudge	2 (0.9 oz)	110	1	5	10	15	tr	130

FOOD	PORTION	CALS	PROT	FAT	CHOL	CARB	FIBER	SOD
Nibbler Cookies Cinnamon Sugar	2 (0.9 oz)	120	1	5	15	17	0	90
Nibbler Cookies Debra's Special	2 (0.9 oz)	100	1	5	10	13	0	80
Nibbler Cookies M&M	2 (0.9 oz)	110	1	5	15	16	0	55
Nibbler Cookies Milk Chocolate	2 (0.9 oz)	110	1	5	15	15	tr	70
Nibbler Cookies Milk Chocolate w/ Walnuts	2 (0.9 oz)	120	1	6	10	14	tr	65
Nibbler Cookies Peanut Butter	2 (0.9 oz)	110	2	6	15	13	0	95
Nibbler Cookies Semi-Sweet Chocolate	2 (0.9 oz)	110	1	5	10	15	tr	60
Nibbler Cookies Triple Chocolate	2 (0.9 oz)	110	1	6	15	15	tr	65
Nibbler Cookies White Chunk Macadamia	2 (0.9 oz)	120	1	7	10	13	tr	60

NEWPORT CREAMERY

FOOD	PORTION	CALS	PROT	FAT	CHOL	CARB	FIBER	SOD
Ice Cream Chocolate No Sugar Added	½ cup	110	–	3	10	22	–	–
Ice Cream Vanilla No Sugar Added	½ cup	100	–	3	15	19	–	–
Vanilla Yogurt	½ cup	120	–	3	10	20	–	–
Vanilla Yogurt Nonfat	½ cup	100	–	0	0	22	–	–

OLD SPAGHETTI FACTORY
CHILDREN'S MENU SELECTIONS

FOOD	PORTION	CALS	PROT	FAT	CHOL	CARB	FIBER	SOD
Grilled Cheese Sandwich	1 serv	360	11	22	25	28	1	990
Macaroni & Cheese	1 serv	350	11	9	10	57	2	780
Spaghetti w/ Tomato Sauce	1 serv	300	9	4	0	56	4	680
Spaghetti w/ Tomato Sauce & Meatballs	1 serv	440	20	13	40	59	4	1030

DESSERTS

FOOD	PORTION	CALS	PROT	FAT	CHOL	CARB	FIBER	SOD
Caramel Turtle Pie	1 serv	660	7	29	45	93	0	420
Mud Pie	1 serv	680	9	32	45	90	3	350
New York Cheese Cake w/ Strawberry Topping	1 serv	690	10	40	180	72	1	400

MAIN MENU SELECTIONS

FOOD	PORTION	CALS	PROT	FAT	CHOL	CARB	FIBER	SOD
Baked Chicken	1 dinner serv	880	58	47	165	55	4	2100

FOOD	PORTION	CALS	PROT	FAT	CHOL	CARB	FIBER	SOD
Chicken Marsala	1 dinner serv	960	81	44	250	55	4	980
Fettuccine Alfredo	1 dinner serv	1130	31	83	260	71	4	1200
Fettuccine Chicken	1 dinner serv	960	43	56	220	74	6	770
Lasagne	1 dinner serv	630	45	33	110	36	4	1820
Parmigiana Chicken	1 dinner serv	840	46	34	80	84	5	2150
Parmigiana Eggplant	1 dinner serv	670	23	32	130	75	8	1550
Pot Pourri	1 dinner serv	710	26	30	95	84	6	1240
Ravioli Spinach & Cheese	1 dinner serv	480	24	15	70	59	4	1280
Salmon Tuscany	1 dinner serv	680	52	43	175	21	1	1620
Sandwich Meatball	1	860	49	41	140	74	4	2800
Sandwich Sausage	1	730	40	40	105	53	4	2450
Sandwich Tuscan Chicken	1	1060	76	60	175	53	4	1110
Seafood Cheddar Melt	1 serv	790	40	42	165	65	4	1850
Spaghetti w/ Clam Sauce	1 dinner serv	690	22	28	125	84	5	850
Spaghetti w/ Clam Sauce & Mizithra	1 dinner serv	960	39	54	180	81	5	1270
Spaghetti w/ Meat & Clam Sauces	1 dinner serv	980	22	17	70	84	6	980
Spaghetti w/ Meat Sauce	1 dinner serv	470	21	5	15	83	6	1110
Spaghetti w/ Meat Sauce & Mizithra	1 dinner serv	850	38	42	125	80	5	1400
Spaghetti w/ Meat Sauce & Sausage	1 dinner serv	830	43	35	105	85	6	2150
Spaghetti w/ Meatballs	1 dinner serv	840	47	33	130	86	5	1430
Spaghetti w/ Mizithra	1 dinner serv	1010	37	64	180	74	4	1150
Spaghetti w/ Mushroom & Clam Sauces	1 dinner serv	830	18	18	65	83	5	830

FOOD	PORTION	CALS	PROT	FAT	CHOL	CARB	FIBER	SOD
Spaghetti w/ Mushroom & Meat Sauces	1 dinner serv	460	17	6	10	83	6	960
Spaghetti w/ Mushroom Sauce	1 dinner serv	460	14	7	0	83	6	810
Spaghetti w/ Mushroom Sauce & Mizithra	1 dinner serv	850	34	43	120	80	5	1250
Spaghetti w/ Tomato & Mizithra	1 dinner serv	840	34	42	120	81	5	1360
Spaghetti w/ Tomato & Meat Sauces	1 dinner serv	460	17	5	10	84	6	1060
Spaghetti w/ Tomato Sauce	1 dinner serv	440	14	5	0	84	7	1020
Spaghetti w/ Tomato Sauce & Clam Sauce	1 dinner serv	560	18	17	65	84	6	940
Starter Sausage	1 serv	690	31	56	140	7	tr	1790
Tortellini Mortadella & Chicken	1 dinner serv	930	25	56	205	82	2	1440

ON THE BORDER
CHILDREN'S MENU SELECTIONS

FOOD	PORTION	CALS	PROT	FAT	CHOL	CARB	FIBER	SOD
Border Chicken Strips	1 serv	570	23	36	–	36	2	1940
Corn Dog	1	320	5	21	–	11	1	760
Crispy Taco Mexican Dinner Beef	1 serv	740	35	31	–	77	18	2180
Crispy Taco Mexican Dinner Chicken	1 serv	740	31	28	–	85	17	2480
Hamburger	1	390	22	23	–	23	1	290
Nachos Bean & Cheese	1 serv	980	47	57	–	71	18	1850
Nachos Cheese	1 serv	670	31	47	–	28	3	760
Quesadillas Chicken	1 serv	720	33	48	–	36	1	1230
Sandwich Grilled Chicken	1	630	42	21	–	63	2	1490
Soft Taco Mexican Dinner Beef	1 serv	840	36	35	–	91	17	2760
Soft Taco Mexican Dinner Chicken	1 serv	750	32	27	–	89	15	2770
Sundae w/ Chocolate Syrup	1 serv	300	1	13	–	40	4	90
Sundae w/ Strawberry Puree	1 serv	340	4	13	–	52	0	70

FOOD	PORTION	CALS	PROT	FAT	CHOL	CARB	FIBER	SOD
DESSERTS								
Border Brownie Sundae	1	440	7	25	–	51	1	130
Chocolate Turtle Empanadas	1 serv	1280	11	81	–	131	4	440
Dulce De Leche Cheesecake	1 serv	1160	15	72	–	122	2	800
Kahlua Ice Cream Pie	1 serv	850	10	44	–	100	5	470
Sizzling Apple Crisp	1 serv	960	11	36	–	157	5	350
Sopapillas	1 serv	1230	13	56	–	136	1	1320
Vanilla Ice Cream	1 scoop	180	3	10	–	19	0	60
MAIN MENU SELECTIONS								
Bacon Wrapped Shrimp	1 serv	730	36	62	–	6	1	1940
Baja Chicken	1 serv	610	56	43	–	50	8	2510
Bandera Sirloin	1 serv	640	43	43	–	13	3	2900
Beans Black	1 serv	180	8	7	–	19	6	690
Beans Refried	1 serv	290	15	11	–	36	13	960
Black Bean & Corn Relish	1 serv	80	1	4	–	6	1	160
Border Chimichanga Fajita Chicken w/ Onions & Mushrooms	1 serv	1230	34	93	–	51	3	1820
Border Chimichanga Ground Beef	1 serv	1310	41	98	–	49	4	2210
Border Chimichanga Spicy Chicken	1 serv	1160	33	85	–	46	2	2230
Border Sampler	1 serv	1940	103	120	–	110	17	4200
Bordurrito Big Beef w/ Side Salad	1 serv	1600	46	103	–	119	9	2790
Bordurrito Big Chicken w/ Side Salad	1 serv	1420	42	57	–	121	8	2600
Burrito Beef	1 serv	1080	65	57	–	71	5	2210
Burrito Chicken	1 serv	880	31	56	–	55	4	2350
Burrito Three Sauce Fajita Chicken	1 serv	870	51	45	–	59	3	2890
Burrito Three Sauce Fajita Steak	1 serv	1050	54	61	–	57	4	3080
Carne Asada & Shrimp	1 serv	1040	69	74	–	22	4	2780
Cheese Chile Relleno	1	880	28	61	–	60	1	1630
Cheesy Pepper Jack Mashed Potatoes	1 serv	380	10	27	–	26	2	660
Chicken Flautas Appetizer	1 serv	970	38	66	–	50	7	2020

FOOD	PORTION	CALS	PROT	FAT	CHOL	CARB	FIBER	SOD
Chile Con Queso	1 cup	250	15	18	–	8	1	1210
Chile Con Queso	1 bowl	390	25	29	–	14	1	1930
Corona Extra Dinner	1 serv	2040	77	128	–	136	13	4280
Crispy Taco Beef	1	330	18	20	–	19	4	610
Crispy Taco Chicken	1	240	12	12	–	16	2	620
Crispy Taco Veggie	1	250	6	16	–	20	3	160
Dos XX Fish Tacos	1 serv	1590	40	113	–	100	5	2880
Empanadas Beef	1	440	13	31	–	26	2	580
Empanadas Chicken	1	390	11	26	–	25	1	590
Empanadas Chicken	1 serv	1090	34	74	–	68	3	2030
Empanadas Ground Beef	1 serv	1150	37	81	–	68	5	1930
Enchilada Beef	1	340	19	17	–	27	6	790
Enchilada Cheese & Onion	1	410	20	24	–	27	5	750
Enchilada Chicken	1	350	11	23	–	21	3	680
Fajitas 7 Pepper Steak	1 serv	910	56	62	–	30	7	3370
Fajitas Blackened Chicken w/ Portobello Mushrooms	1 serv	640	70	29	–	27	6	4000
Fajitas Carnitas	1 serv	830	50	62	–	19	6	2470
Fajitas Grilled Vegetables w/ Portobello Mushrooms	1 serv	390	7	28	–	30	7	2340
Fajitas Jalapeno BBQ Chicken	1 serv	760	62	32	–	53	4	4330
Fajitas Mesquite Grilled Chicken	1 serv	440	48	18	–	20	4	1870
Fajitas Mesquite Grilled Steak	1 serv	620	42	41	–	18	3	2120
Fajitas Monterey Ranch Chicken	1 serv	840	69	21	–	21	17	3130
Fajitas Shrimp	1 serv	750	28	63	–	18	3	2500
Fajitas Ultimate	1 serv	1230	58	102	–	20	4	3230
Fajitas Chicken Con Queso	1 skillet	1130	86	82	–	7	1	2420
Firecracker Stuffed Jalapenos	1 serv	980	58	56	–	70	4	4730
French Fries	1 serv	390	4	25	–	40	3	1320
Grande Fajita Nachos Beef	1 serv	1970	98	127	–	109	28	3780
Grande Fajita Nachos Chicken	1 serv	1890	110	113	–	109	28	3790
Grande Fajita Nachos Combo	1 serv	1940	104	121	–	109	28	3790
Guacamole	1 serv	130	2	10	–	9	6	400

FOOD	PORTION	CALS	PROT	FAT	CHOL	CARB	FIBER	SOD
Guacamole Live	1 serv	570	10	50	–	33	31	1170
Margarita Chicken	1 serv	290	36	11	–	21	2	1140
Mexican Rice	1 serv	220	3	6	–	33	2	910
Mexican Shrimp Scampi	1 serv	740	33	64	–	8	2	1510
Pico Chicken & Shrimp	1 serv	730	65	51	–	9	1	2410
Quesadillas Combo Fajita	1 serv	1450	81	96	–	59	6	2890
Quesadillas Double Stacked Club	1 serv	1860	101	123	–	88	15	3440
Quesadillas Fajita Chicken	1 serv	1430	93	91	–	59	6	3030
Quesadillas Fajita Steak	1 serv	1530	81	107	–	59	6	3040
Quesadillas Spinach & Mushroom	1 serv	1420	55	105	–	66	9	2320
Ranchiladas	1 serv	1360	84	86	–	53	9	1940
Red Chili Ribeye	1 serv	900	46	72	–	12	3	4430
Salmon Mexican	1 serv	650	41	50	–	4	1	890
Sandwich Chicken Blackened w/ French Fries	1 serv	1510	73	93	–	101	10	6560
Sandwich Chicken Grilled w/ French Fries	1 serv	1430	64	92	–	101	8	5690
Sauteed Shrimp	4	170	16	10	–	1	0	380
Shaken Margarita Shrimp Cocktail	1 serv	280	25	13	–	22	4	1280
Shaken Margarita Shrimp Cocktail w/ Tortilla Chips	1 serv	780	31	40	–	57	4	2440
Soft Taco Beef	1	340	19	19	–	23	2	900
Soft Taco Chicken	1	250	13	11	–	20	1	910
Soft Taco Veggie	1	210	8	9	–	24	2	340
Superior Dinner	1 serv	1350	62	85	–	80	13	2810
Tamale	1	310	12	17	–	26	3	870
Tortilla Soup	1 bowl	350	14	22	–	24	5	1540
Tortillas Corn	3	230	6	4	–	43	5	100
Tortillas Flour	3	300	7	9	–	45	0	750
Tres Enchilada Dinner Beef	1 serv	1010	56	52	–	00	17	2350
Tres Enchilada Dinner Cheese	1 serv	1210	60	73	–	80	14	2240
Tres Enchilada Dinner Chicken	1 serv	1040	34	68	–	64	10	2030
Ultimate Loaded Queso	1 serv	900	49	59	–	46	16	2980
Vegetables Grilled	1 serv	50	2	1	–	8	3	190
Vegetables Sauteed	1 serv	70	2	4	–	9	3	210

FOOD	PORTION	CALS	PROT	FAT	CHOL	CARB	FIBER	SOD
SALAD DRESSINGS AND SAUCES								
Chili Con Carne Sauce	1 serv (2 oz)	70	4	3	–	6	1	360
Chipotle Mayonnaise	1 serv (1 oz)	190	0	21	–	1	0	490
Dressing Chipotle Honey Mustard	1 serv (2 oz)	310	0	29	–	11	0	380
Dressing Ranch	1 serv (2 oz)	220	1	23	–	2	0	440
Dressing Smoked Jalapeno Vinaigrette	1 serv (2 oz)	230	0	22	–	8	0	760
Dressing Sweet Pepper Vinaigrette	1 serv (2 oz)	270	1	25	–	10	0	380
Dressing Fat Free Balsamic Vinaigrette	1 serv (2 oz)	50	0	0	0	10	0	610
Dressing Lo Fat Ranch	1 serv (2 oz)	110	1	6	–	11	0	460
Parrila Butter	1 serv (1 oz)	120	0	13	–	1	–	250
Pico De Gallo	1 scoop	20	0	1	–	2	1	120
Ranchero Sauce	1 serv (2 oz)	18	0	1	–	3	0	150
Salsa	1 serv (2 oz)	25	0	1	–	3	2	160
Sour Cream	1 serv (2 oz)	140	1	14	–	2	0	240
SALADS								
Chopped Chicken w/ Dressing	1 serv	1330	81	89	–	54	10	2770
Fiesta Blackened Chicken w/ Dressing	1 serv	1150	65	75	–	54	8	3310
Fiesta Chicken w/ Dressing	1 serv	1140	66	74	–	52	7	2640
Grande Taco Beef	1 serv	1450	54	102	–	78	13	2410
Grande Taco Chicken	1 serv	1280	43	89	–	74	10	2300
House	1 serv	170	6	10	–	15	4	110
Sizzling Fajita Chicken	1 serv	760	58	48	–	23	7	2080
Sizzling Fajita Steak	1 serv	910	57	65	–	24	8	2330
PACIUGO GELATO								
Milk Base Amarena Black Cherry Swirl	1 scoop (3.5 oz)	160	4	4	15	30	tr	50
Milk Base Banana Creme Pie	1 scoop (3.5 oz)	80	2	2	13	14	tr	35
Milk Base Cheesecake	1 scoop (3.5 oz)	90	3	4	18	12	tr	55
Milk Base Chocolate	1 scoop (3.5 oz)	80	3	3	8	14	tr	48
Milk Base Chocolate Cookies'N Milk	1 scoop (3.5 oz)	90	3	3	8	16	tr	63

FOOD	PORTION	CALS	PROT	FAT	CHOL	CARB	FIBER	SOD
Milk Base Coconut	1 scoop (3.5 oz)	80	2	3	8	13	tr	30
Milk Base Coffee	1 scoop (3.5 oz)	75	2	3	8	12	tr	30
Milk Base Fiordilatte	1 scoop (3.5 oz)	75	2	2	8	13	tr	30
Milk Base French Vanilla Bean	1 scoop (3.5 oz)	80	2	3	20	13	tr	30
Milk Base Green Tea	1 scoop (3.5 oz)	70	2	2	8	12	tr	30
Milk Base Hazelnut	1 scoop (3.5 oz)	85	3	4	8	11	tr	30
Milk Base Lemon Custard	1 scoop (3.5 oz)	75	3	3	30	12	tr	30
Milk Base Mascarpone Chocolate Rum	1 scoop (3.5 oz)	95	3	5	15	11	tr	35
Milk Base Pannacotta Wedding Cake	1 scoop (3.5 oz)	75	2	2	8	13	tr	28
Milk Base Peppermint	1 scoop (3.5 oz)	75	2	2	8	14	1	30
Milk Base Rose	1 scoop (3.5 oz)	70	8	2	8	12	tr	30
Milk Base Tiramisu	1 scoop (3.5 oz)	80	2	3	28	12	tr	30
Milk Base Zabajone	1 scoop (3.5 oz)	80	3	3	30	12	tr	30
No Sugar Added Chocolate	1 scoop (3.5 oz)	28	2	1	3	9	1	313
No Sugar Added Mint	1 scoop (3.5 oz)	25	1	1	3	9	1	23
No Sugar Added Mocha	1 scoop (3.5 oz)	28	2	1	3	9	1	22
No Sugar Added Strawberry Milk	1 scoop (3.5 oz)	23	1	1	1	8	1	19
Soy Banana	1 scoop (3.5 oz)	40	tr	2	0	6	1	3
Soy Blueberry	1 scoop (3.5 oz)	40	tr	2	0	6	1	3
Soy Chocolate	1 scoop (3.5 oz)	38	tr	2	0	5	1	9

FOOD	PORTION	CALS	PROT	FAT	CHOL	CARB	FIBER	SOD
Soy Coffee	1 scoop (3.5 oz)	35	tr	2	0	5	1	3
Soy Hazelnut	1 scoop (3.5 oz)	35	tr	2	0	5	1	3
Soy Strawberry	1 scoop (3.5 oz)	38	tr	2	0	6	1	3
Soy Wild Berries	1 scoop (3.5 oz)	40	tr	2	0	6	1	3
Water Base Blackberry	1 scoop (3.5 oz)	28	0	0	0	7	tr	0
Water Base Ginger Lemon	1 scoop (3.5 oz)	25	0	0	0	7	tr	0
Water Base Green Apple	1 scoop (3.5 oz)	28	0	0	0	7	tr	0
Water Base Lemon Sage	1 scoop (3.5 oz)	25	0	0	0	7	tr	0
Water Base Lychee	1 scoop (3.5 oz)	25	0	0	0	6	tr	0
Water Base Orange Vidalia	1 scoop (3.5 oz)	25	0	0	0	7	0	0
Water Base Passion Fruit	1 scoop (3.5 oz)	23	0	0	0	6	0	0
Water Base Pineapple	1 scoop (3.5 oz)	28	0	0	0	7	tr	0
Water Base Strawberry Port	1 scoop (3.5 oz)	25	0	0	0	6	tr	0
Water Base Watermelon	1 scoop (3.5 oz)	25	0	0	0	7	tr	0

PANDA EXPRESS
MAIN MENU SELECTIONS

FOOD	PORTION	CALS	PROT	FAT	CHOL	CARB	FIBER	SOD
BBQ Pork	1 serv	350	32	19	85	13	tr	970
Beef & Broccoli	1 serv	150	11	8	15	9	1	730
Beef w/ String Beans	1 serv	170	12	9	20	11	2	640
Black Pepper Chicken	1 serv	180	13	10	40	10	2	630
Chicken w/ Mushrooms	1 serv	130	11	7	50	7	2	590
Chicken w/ Potato	1 serv	220	12	11	55	17	1	910
Chicken w/ String Beans	1 serv	170	11	8	30	12	3	560
Egg Roll Chicken	1 (3 oz)	190	8	8	25	21	3	450
Fried Shrimp	6 pieces	260	12	12	65	26	tr	730

FOOD	PORTION	CALS	PROT	FAT	CHOL	CARB	FIBER	SOD
Mandarin Chicken	1 serv	250	34	9	125	8	2	960
Mixed Vegetables	1 serv	70	3	3	0	8	1	420
Orange Chicken	1 serv	480	21	21	80	50	2	820
Spicy Chicken w/ Peanuts	1 serv	200	18	7	70	17	4	800
Spring Roll Veggie	1 (1.7 oz)	80	2	3	0	14	tr	270
Steamed Rice	1 serv	330	7	1	0	74	2	20
String Beans w/ Fried Tofu	1 serv	180	10	11	0	11	3	650
Sweet & Sour Chicken	1 serv	310	18	14	50	28	2	330
Sweet & Sour Pork	1 serv	410	19	30	55	17	3	350
Vegetable Chow Mein	1 serv	330	10	11	0	48	4	810
Vegetable Fried Rice	1 serv	390	9	12	85	61	2	740
SAUCES								
Hot	2 tsp	10	0	1	0	2	0	130
Hot Mustard	1 serv	18	0	0	0	1	0	90
Mandarin	1 serv	70	tr	0	0	16	0	670
Soy	1 tbsp	16	2	0	0	2	0	660
Sweet & Sour	1 serv	60	tr	0	0	15	0	120
PINKBERRY								
Frozen Yogurt Coffee	½ cup	90	4	0	5	24	0	50
Frozen Yogurt Green Tea	½ cup	50	3	0	5	10	0	50
Frozen Yogurt Original	½ cup	70	3	0	5	14	0	55
PIZZA HUT								
APPETIZERS								
Breadstick	1	150	4	6	0	20	tr	220
Breadstick Cheese	1	200	7	10	15	21	tr	340
Hot Wings	2 pieces	110	11	6	70	1	0	450
Mild Wings	2 pieces	110	11	7	70	tr	0	320
BEVERAGES								
Diet Pepsi	1 med (14 oz)	0	0	0	0	0	0	45
Mt. Dew	1 med (14 oz)	190	0	0	0	54	0	60
Pepsi	1 med (14 oz)	180	0	0	0	47	0	45
DESSERTS								
Apple Pizza	1 slice	260	4	4	0	53	1	250
Cherry Pizza	1 slice	240	4	4	0	47	1	250
Cinnamon Sticks	2	170	4	5	0	27	tr	170

FOOD	PORTION	CALS	PROT	FAT	CHOL	CARB	FIBER	SOD
PIZZA								
Fit 'N Delicious Diced Chicken Mushroom Jalapeno	1 med slice	170	10	5	15	22	2	690
Fit 'N Delicious Diced Chicken Red Onion Green Pepper	1 med slice	170	10	5	15	23	2	460
Fit 'N Delicious Diced Red Tomato Mushroom Jalapeno	1 med slice	150	6	4	10	22	2	590
Fit 'N Delicious Green Pepper Red Onion Diced Red Tomato	1 med slice	150	6	4	10	24	2	360
Fit 'N Delicious Ham Pineapple Diced Red Tomato	1 med slice	160	8	4	15	24	2	470
Fit 'N Delicious Ham Red Onion Mushroom	1 med slice	160	8	5.	15	22	2	470
Hand Tossed Cheese	1 med slice	240	12	8	25	30	2	520
Hand Tossed Chicken Supreme	1 med slice	230	14	6	25	30	2	550
Hand Tossed Ham	1 med slice	220	12	6	20	29	2	550
Hand Tossed Meat Lover's	1 med slice	300	15	13	35	29	2	760
Hand Tossed Pepperoni	1 med slice	250	12	9	25	29	2	570
Hand Tossed Pepperoni Lover's	1 med slice	300	15	13	40	30	2	710
Hand Tossed Super Supreme	1 med slice	300	15	13	35	31	2	780
Hand Tossed Supreme	1 med slice	270	13	11	25	30	2	660
Hand Tossed Veggie Lover's	1 med slice	220	10	6	15	31	2	490
Pan Cheese	1 med slice	280	11	13	25	29	1	500
Pan Chicken Supreme	1 med slice	280	13	12	25	30	2	530
Pan Ham	1 med slice	260	11	11	20	29	1	540
Pan Meat Lover's	1 med slice	340	15	19	35	29	2	750
Pan Pepperoni	1 med slice	290	11	15	25	29	2	560
Pan Pepperoni Lover's	1 med slice	340	15	19	40	29	2	700
Pan Super Supreme	1 med slice	340	14	18	35	30	2	760
Pan Supreme	1 med slice	320	13	16	25	30	2	650
Pan Veggie Lover's	1 med slice	260	10	12	15	30	2	470

FOOD	PORTION	CALS	PROT	FAT	CHOL	CARB	FIBER	SOD
Personal Pan Cheese	1 pie	630	27	27	60	71	4	1240
Personal Pan Chicken Supreme	1 pie	620	21	23	55	73	4	1310
Personal Pan Meat Lover's	1 pie	800	36	41	90	71	5	1910
Personal Pan Pepperoni	1 pie	660	27	30	60	70	4	1370
Personal Pan Pepperoni Lover's	1 pie	800	35	42	95	71	4	1760
Personal Pan Super Supreme	1 pie	790	35	40	85	74	6	1940
Personal Pan Supreme	1 pie	750	32	36	70	73	6	1980
Personal Pan Veggie Lover's	1 pie	580	22	23	40	73	5	1190
Stuffed Crust Cheese	1 lg slice	360	18	13	40	43	2	820
Stuffed Crust Chicken Supreme	1 lg slice	380	20	13	40	44	3	1020
Stuffed Crust Ham	1 lg slice	340	18	11	40	43	2	960
Stuffed Crust Meat Lover's	1 lg slice	450	21	21	55	43	3	1250
Stuffed Crust Pepperoni	1 lg slice	370	18	15	45	42	2	970
Stuffed Crust Pepperoni Lover's	1 lg slice	420	21	19	55	43	3	1120
Stuffed Crust Super Supreme	1 lg slice	440	21	20	50	45	3	1270
Stuffed Crust Supreme	1 lg slice	400	20	16	45	44	3	1070
Stuffed Crust Veggie Lover's	1 lg slice	360	16	14	35	45	3	980
Thin'N Crispy Cheese	1 med slice	200	10	8	25	21	1	490
Thin'N Crispy Chicken Supreme	1 med slice	200	12	7	25	22	1	520
Thin'N Crispy Ham	1 med slice	180	9	6	20	21	1	530
Thin'N Crispy Meat Lover's	1 med slice	270	13	14	35	21	2	740
Thin'N Crispy Pepperoni	1 med slice	210	10	10	25	21	1	550
Thin'N Crispy Pepperoni Lover's	1 med slice	260	13	14	40	21	2	690
Thin'N Crispy Super Supreme	1 med slice	260	13	13	35	23	2	760
Thin'N Crispy Veggie Lover's	1 med slice	180	8	7	15	23	2	480
XL Full House Cheese	1 slice	280	12	12	25	30	3	760
XL Full House Chicken Supreme	1 slice	270	13	10	25	31	3	770

FOOD	PORTION	CALS	PROT	FAT	CHOL	CARB	FIBER	SOD
XL Full House Ham	1 slice	260	12	10	25	30	3	790
XL Full House Meat Lover's	1 slice	380	17	21	45	30	3	1120
XL Full House Pepperoni	1 slice	290	12	13	25	30	3	810
XL Full House Pepperoni Lover's	1 slice	310	12	15	30	30	3	880
XL Full House Super Supreme	1 slice	330	15	16	35	32	3	1000
XL Full House Supreme	1 slice	310	13	15	30	31	3	890
XL Full House Veggie Lover's	1 slice	280	10	11	20	32	3	740
SALAD DRESSINGS AND SAUCES								
Dipping Cup White Icing	1 serv	170	0	0	0	46	0	0
Dipping Sauce Breadstick	1 serv	45	2	0	0	9	2	380
Dipping Sauce Wing Blue Cheese	1 serv	230	2	24	25	2	0	550
Dipping Sauce Wing Ranch	1 serv	210	tr	22	10	4	0	340
Dressing Caesar	2 tbsp	150	tr	16	5	1	0	280
Dressing French	2 tbsp	140	0	11	0	11	0	220
Dressing Italian	2 tbsp	140	0	15	0	2	0	360
Dressing Ranch	2 tbsp	100	tr	10	5	1	0	240
Dressing Thousand Island	2 tbsp	110	0	9	10	6	0	300
Dressing Lite Italian	2 tbsp	60	0	5	0	5	0	410
Dressing Lite Ranch	1 tbsp	70	tr	7	10	0	0	200

POLLO TROPICAL
DESSERTS

FOOD	PORTION	CALS	PROT	FAT	CHOL	CARB	FIBER	SOD
Flan	1 serv (4 oz)	390	9	13	110	59	1	200
Key Lime	1 serv (3.9 oz)	210	8	9	90	26	0	550
Tres Leches	1 serv (5.4 oz)	410	9	9	70	76	0	210
MAIN MENU SELECTIONS								
Balsamic Tomato	1 sm	176	2	2	0	14	2	1278
Balsamic Tomato	1 combo	88	1	1	0	7	1	639
Bananas Tropical	1 serv	437	4	11	0	89	9	0
Beef Skewers	1 (1 oz)	77	7	5	26	1	tr	121
Black Beans	1 combo	90	6	3	0	18	7	382
Black Beans	1 sm	203	14	6	0	41	16	859
Boiled Yuca	1 combo	188	0	0	0	51	4	490

FOOD	PORTION	CALS	PROT	FAT	CHOL	CARB	FIBER	SOD
Boiled Yuca	1 sm	251	0	0	0	68	5	653
Caesar Salad	1 sm	207	4	18	25	6	1	368
Caesar Salad	1 combo	130	3	11	16	4	1	233
Chicken Boneless Breast	2 pieces	240	52	3	160	0	0	341
Chicken ¼ Dark Meat	1 serv	291	32	18	156	0	0	506
Chicken ¼ Dark Meat No Skin	1 serv	191	25	10	111	0	0	265
Chicken ¼ White Meat	1 serv	323	43	16	171	0	0	711
Chicken ¼ White Meat No Skin	1 serv	204	36	6	120	0	0	452
Chicken Caesar Salad	1 serv	669	58	41	207	13	3	1089
Corn	1 combo	121	3	4	0	19	5	20
French Fries	1 sm	311	4	15	0	40	4	111
Ribs	¼ rack (2 oz)	200	14	15	51	1	0	338
Ribs	½ rack (4 oz)	400	28	31	102	2	0	677
Roast Pork	1 serv	392	48	23	143	0	0	316
Sandwich Chicken Caesar	1	881	70	34	203	71	5	1417
Sandwich Grilled Chicken	1	827	65	24	168	84	6	1109
Sandwich Roast Pork	1	773	53	26	119	83	5	1323
Steak & Chicken Dark Meat	1 serv	437	46	28	205	2	tr	736
TropiChop Chicken w/ Yellow Rice & Vegetables	1 serv	341	23	5	53	50	2	776
TropiChop Chicken w/ White Rice & Black Beans	1 serv	564	31	10	53	95	11	1514
TropiChop Grilled Chicken Deluxe	1 serv	409	37	6	94	52	3	862
TropiChop Pork w/ White Rice & Black Beans	1 serv	714	38	23	72	97	12	1660
TropiChop Pork w/ Yellow Rice & Vegetables	1 serv	480	35	21	72	91	5	1420
TropiChop Ropa Vieja	1 serv	618	28	17	65	98	13	2001
TropiChop Shrimp Creole	1 serv	506	27	11	185	75	3	1497
TropiChop Vegetarian	1 serv	580	17	13	0	109	16	1194
TropiChop Max Chicken w/ Yellow Rice & Vegetables	1 serv	864	74	21	202	93	4	1793
TropiChop Max Chicken w/ White Rice & Black Beans	1 serv	1117	83	27	202	144	16	2595

FOOD	PORTION	CALS	PROT	FAT	CHOL	CARB	FIBER	SOD
TropiChop Max Grilled Chicken Deluxe	1 serv	753	72	11	187	91	5	1557
TropiChop Max Pork w/ White Rice & Black Beans	1 serv	1273	71	50	158	147	18	2650
TropiChop Max Pork w/ Yellow Rice & Vegetables	1 serv	1020	62	43	158	96	6	1847
TropiChop Max Ropa Vieja	1 serv	1160	51	41	145	161	20	3673
TropiChop Max Shrimp Creole	1 serv	102	54	29	384	129	7	2950
TropiChop Max Vegetarian	1 serv	950	26	21	0	177	26	1822
White Rice	1 combo	203	3	3	0	40	1	418
White Rice	1 sm	339	6	6	0	66	2	697
Wrap Chicken Ceasar	1	901	49	48	161	64	4	1336
Wrap Chicken Classic	1	694	43	26	115	68	5	717
Wrap Curry Chicken	1	930	40	43	97	94	6	631
Wrap Steak	1	993	32	48	74	106	6	1467
Yellow Rice w/ Vegetables	1 combo	163	4	3	0	31	1	414
Yellow Rice w/ Vegetables	1 sm	245	6	4	0	47	2	622
Yucatan Fries	1 serv	497	2	24	0	69	3	226
SALAD DRESSINGS AND SAUCES								
BBQ Sauce	1 serv (1.8 oz)	83	0	0	0	20	0	612
BBQ Sauce Guava	1 serv (1.8 oz)	83	0	0	0	22	0	25
Dressing Caesar	1 serv (1 oz)	161	2	17	24	1	0	255
Guacamole Sauce	1 serv (1.8 oz)	75	0	6	0	3	3	33
Mojo Sauce	1 serv (0.9 oz)	97	tr	tr	0	3	tr	196
Mustard Curry Sauce	1 serv (1.8 oz)	265	0	30	0	0	0	25
Salsa	1 serv (1.8 oz)	8	0	0	0	2	0	157
SOUPS								
Caribbean Chicken	1 sm (8 oz)	121	9	2	14	21	3	631
Tropical Shrimp	1 sm (8 oz)	134	10	3	59	18	0	1198
POPEYE'S								
Buttermilk Biscuit	1	240	3	14	0	25	1	500
Cajun Rice	1 reg	180	8	7	60	23	2	440

FOOD	PORTION	CALS	PROT	FAT	CHOL	CARB	FIBER	SOD
Coleslaw	1 serv	230	1	17	15	20	9	260
Collard Greens	1 serv	50	2	2	5	7	3	500
Corn On The Cob	1	220	7	4	0	48	4	25
Etouffee Chicken	1 serv	223	8	6	20	35	2	420
Etouffee Crawfish	1 serv	200	8	7	48	26	2	530
French Fries	1 serv	261	3	12	7	34	3	632
Fried Catfish	1 serv	300	16	18	55	19	0	820
Fried Crawfish	1 serv	370	17	21	185	27	tr	830
Green Beans	1 serv	40	2	1	5	6	2	480
Jambalaya Chicken Sausage	1 serv	257	9	13	32	26	1	370
Mashed Potatoes & Gravy	1 serv	120	3	4	5	18	2	570
Mashed Potatoes No Gravy	1 serv	100	1	3	0	17	tr	380
Mild Breast	1	510	43	30	195	18	0	1380
Mild Breast Skinless	1	280	38	11	145	7	0	960
Mild Leg	1	200	17	12	110	7	0	500
Mild Leg Skinless	1	110	15	5	100	2	0	370
Mild Strips	2	280	21	12	55	21	tr	1260
Mild Strips No Breading	2	200	21	8	50	12	0	920
Mild Thigh	1	390	25	27	150	12	0	890
Mild Thigh Skinless	1	210	19	14	125	6	0	690
Mild Wing	1	220	14	14	90	10	0	510
Mild Wing Skinless	1	130	12	7	70	4	tr	470
Naked Chicken Strips	3	170	29	5	80	2	0	790
Popcorn Shrimp	1 serv	280	10	17	95	22	tr	710
Red Beans & Rice	1 reg	340	7	19	20	33	16	700
Sandwich Catfish Fully Dressed	1	640	23	35	45	59	5	1330
Sandwich Deluxe Tame w/ Mayo	1	728	31	39	71	63	3	1500
Sandwich Deluxe Tame w/o Mayo	1	530	31	17	55	63	3	1340
Sandwich Shrimp Fully Dressed	1	740	20	40	100	741	8	1860
Smothered Chicken	1 serv	210	10	8	23	24	1	743
Spicy Breast	1	530	46	31	185	13	1	1090
Spicy Breast Skinless	1	290	39	12	135	7	tr	730
Spicy Leg	1	190	17	11	85	5	0	420
Spicy Leg Skinless	1	120	14	8	70	2	0	260
Spicy Strips	2	310	21	14	55	24	tr	1370

FOOD	PORTION	CALS	PROT	FAT	CHOL	CARB	FIBER	SOD
Spicy Strips No Breading	2	190	19	7	55	11	0	880
Spicy Thigh	1	390	23	29	145	10	0	690
Spicy Thigh Skinless	1	200	21	13	125	2	0	450
Spicy Wing	1	220	14	15	85	7	0	370
Spicy Wing Skinless	1	140	13	9	80	5	tr	310
Turnover Cinnamon Apple	1	250	3	10	5	37	2	290

QUIZNO'S
COOKIES

FOOD	PORTION	CALS	PROT	FAT	CHOL	CARB	FIBER	SOD
Dark Chocolate Chunk	1	380	5	15	25	58	1	300
Double Chocolate Chip	1	370	5	15	0	58	3	230
Oatmeal Raisin	1	340	5	11	25	59	2	290
Snickerdoodle	1	400	3	16	20	59	0	280

SANDWICHES

FOOD	PORTION	CALS	PROT	FAT	CHOL	CARB	FIBER	SOD
Breakfast Bacon Egg Cheddar	1	380	21	21	175	36	4	1030
Breakfast Black Angus Steak & Cheddar	1 sm	330	26	13	180	36	3	950
Breakfast Egg & cheddar	1	240	12	11	145	35	3	540
Breakfast Garden Vegetable Cheddar	1	250	13	11	145	38	4	540
Breakfast Ham Egg Cheddar	1	290	19	12	165	37	4	1010
Deli Honey Ham & Swiss	1	260	17	4	25	38	4	1020
Deli Oven Roasted Turkey & Cheese	1	250	15	4	20	39	4	1010
Deli Roast Beef & Cheddar	1	230	13	4	10	37	4	450
Deli Tuna Melt	1	500	14	33	40	37	4	630
Sammie Alpine Chicken	1	200	13	6	25	24	1	520
Sammie Balsamic Chicken	1	170	11	4	15	24	1	410
Sammie Black Angus Steak	1	180	11	4	15	24	1	480
Sammie Bristro Steak Melt	1	180	11	4	15	25	1	490
Sammie Italiano	1	240	10	11	25	24	1	710
Sammie Sonoma Turkey	1	160	8	4	10	25	1	580
Sub Baja Chicken w/ Bacon	1 sm	320	25	9	45	37	4	920
Sub Black Angus Steak On Rosemay Parmesan	1 sm	380	30	8	55	46	5	1140
Sub Chicken Carbonara w/ Bacon	1 sm	360	26	10	45	42	3	1010
Sub Classic Club w/ Bacon	1 sm	320	21	9	35	39	5	1270

FOOD	PORTION	CALS	PROT	FAT	CHOL	CARB	FIBER	SOD
Sub Classic Italian	1 sm	360	18	15	45	38	4	1220
Sub Honey Bacon Club	1 sm	320	21	9	35	39	5	1270
Sub Honey Burbon Chicken	1 sm	260	28	4	35	38	4	700
Sub Honey Mustard Chicken w/ Bacon	1 sm	330	25	9	45	38	4	950
Sub Mesquite Chicken w/ Bacon	1 sm	330	25	9	45	38	4	930
Sub Prime Rib Cheesesteak	1 sm	360	24	11	45	40	4	920
Sub Prime Rib & Peppercorn	1 sm	380	30	8	55	46	5	1140
Sub Steakhouse Beef Dip	1 sm	260	13	6	15	37	4	1070
Sub The Traditional	1 sm	260	16	5	20	39	5	920
Sub Turkey Bacon Guacamole	1 sm	360	21	12	30	43	6	1390
Sub Turkey Ranch & Swiss	1 sm	250	16	4	20	39	5	970
Sub Tuscan Turkey On Rosemary Parmesan	1 sm	300	17	5	20	47	4	1070
Sub Veggie	1 sm	270	10	8	0	41	6	770
SOUPS								
Bread Bowl Country French	1 serv	720	28	22	45	100	5	1730
Bread Bowls Chili	1 serv	730	31	22	50	104	8	1680
Broccoli Cheese	1 cup	150	7	10	25	10	2	800
Chicken Noodle	1 cup	130	6	3	30	18	0	1290
Chili	1 cup	140	9	7	30	12	4	620

RANCH 1

FOOD	PORTION	CALS	PROT	FAT	CHOL	CARB	FIBER	SOD
Baked Potato w/ Broccoli	1 serv	510	12	1	0	117	12	50
Chicken Tenders	1 serv	370	52	15	140	7	0	620
Fajita Grilled Chicken	1	330	22	16	50	25	4	560
Platter Grilled Chicken & Vegetables	1 serv	790	54	7	105	129	16	270
Sandwich American Rancher	1	390	25	10	50	51	3	780
Sandwich Grilled Chicken Philly	1	450	28	14	50	53	3	500
Sandwich Ranch Classic	1	370	26	5	50	53	3	550
Sandwich Spicy Grilled Chicken	1	420	23	11	35	58	3	620
Sandwich Club	1	470	29	16	60	53	3	750

FOOD	PORTION	CALS	PROT	FAT	CHOL	CARB	FIBER	SOD
RED MANGO								
Blenders Blueberry Moon	1 cup	150	3	2	0	33	1	115
Blenders Captain Berry	1 cup	140	4	1	0	31	2	135
Blenders Green Tea Blueberry	1 cup	130	3	0	0	29	1	115
Blenders Green Tea Honeydew	1 cup	130	3	0	0	29	0	125
Blenders Mango Island	1 cup	150	3	2	0	31	1	115
Blenders Pina Colada	1 cup	160	4	3	0	30	1	120
Blenders Tri-Berry	1 cup	130	3	0	0	30	2	115
Blenders Watermelon Breeze	1 cup	130	3	0	0	29	0	115
Frozen Yogurt All Flavors	½ cup	90	3	0	0	19	0	130
RITA'S								
Cream Ice	1 reg	312	1	4	1	70	1	61
Cream Ice Kids	1 serv	193	0	2	1	44	0	38
Custard	1 reg	385	7	21	125	43	1	210
Custard Kids	1 serv	285	5	15	93	32	1	155
Gelati w/ Chocolate Custard	1 reg	351	4	11	65	60	1	116
Gelati w/ Vanilla Custard	1 reg	120	4	13	85	59	0	150
Gelati w/ Cream Ice w/ Chocolate Custard	1 reg	368	5	13	66	60	1	133
Gelati w/ Cream Ice w/ Vanilla Custard	1 reg	392	5	15	86	61	0	173
Ice	1 reg	263	0	0	0	69	0	23
Ice Kids	1 serv	165	0	0	0	43	0	13
Misto w/ Chocolate Custard	1 reg	409	3	7	35	90	1	83
Misto w/ Vanilla Custard	1 reg	420	3	7	45	90	0	104
Misto w/ Cream Ice w/ Chocolate Custard	1 reg	463	3	11	37	90	1	131
Misto w/ Cream Ice w/ Vanilla Custard	1 reg	473	3	12	47	90	0	151
Sugar Free Gelati w/ Chocolate Custard	1 reg	268	4	11	65	45	1	118
Sugar Free Gelati w/ Vanilla Custard	1 reg	288	4	13	85	45	0	155
Sugar Free Ice	1 reg	160	0	0	0	39	0	29
Sugar Free Ice Kids	1 serv	63	0	0	8	24	0	18

FOOD	PORTION	CALS	PROT	FAT	CHOL	CARB	FIBER	SOD
Sugar Free Misto w/ Chocolate Custard	1 reg	233	3	7	36	56	1	91
Sugar Free Misto w/ Vanilla Custard	1 reg	245	3	8	46	57	0	111

ROBEKS
FREEZES AND SHAKES

FOOD	PORTION	CALS	PROT	FAT	CHOL	CARB	FIBER	SOD
800 Lb Gorilla	12 oz	375	26	9	27	50	2	216
Freeze Lemon	12 oz	279	2	2	9	60	0	24
Freeze Orange	12 oz	242	9	0	0	56	1	144
Shake Bananasplit	12 oz	302	11	0	0	69	2	168
Shake P-Nut Power	12 oz	422	17	18	0	52	4	288

SMOOTHIES

FOOD	PORTION	CALS	PROT	FAT	CHOL	CARB	FIBER	SOD
Acai Energizer	12 oz	167	2	1	3	36	2	48
Awesome Acai	12 oz	183	34	1	3	42	2	48
Banzai Blueberry	12 oz	175	31	1	3	38	3	24
Berry Brilliance	12 oz	194	30	1	3	45	2	24
Big Wednesday	12 oz	172	1	1	3	40	1	0
Cardio Cooler	12 oz	215	9	1	3	44	3	24
Citrus Stinger	12 oz	194	56	1	3	40	2	24
Cranberry Quest	12 oz	173	24	0	3	40	1	24
Dr. Robeks	12 oz	181	3	1	3	40	3	0
Guava Lava	12 oz	180	20	1	3	42	2	0
Hummingbird	12 oz	185	2	1	3	44	1	0
Infinite Orange	12 oz	181	4	0	0	42	3	48
Mahalo Mango	12 oz	174	2	1	3	42	1	24
Malibu Peach	12 oz	153	3	0	0	36	1	48
Outrageous Raspberry	12 oz	174	2	1	3	39	2	0
Passionfruit Cove	12 oz	168	2	1	3	38	1	24
Pina Koolada	12 oz	261	39	8	3	46	3	48
Polar Pineapple	12 oz	164	13	1	3	38	1	0
Pomegranate Passion	12 oz	196	4	0	0	48	1	72
Pomegranate Power	12 oz	211	3	0	3	50	1	24
Pro Arobek	12 oz	265	15	1	3	54	3	24
Raspberry Romance	12 oz	172	4	0	3	42	2	48
Robeks MuscleMax	12 oz	202	11	1	15	38	2	24
Robeks Rejuvenator	12 oz	193	5	1	3	43	2	24
South Pacific Squeeze	12 oz	188	2	1	3	42	3	0
Strawnana Berry	12 oz	179	3	0	0	44	2	48
Venice Burner	12 oz	231	9	1	3	46	4	24
Zen Berry	12 oz	190	3	1	0	45	5	24

FOOD	PORTION	CALS	PROT	FAT	CHOL	CARB	FIBER	SOD
RUBIO'S								
MAIN MENU SELECTIONS								
Black Beans	1 serv	220	12	3	5	37	12	840
Carne Asada	1 serv	1430	54	87	170	114	19	2680
Chips	1 serv	430	5	22	0	56	7	480
Grilled Grande Bowl Asada Black Beans	1 serv	770	41	37	85	70	11	2350
Grilled Grande Bowl Asada Pinto	1 serv	760	38	37	85	70	12	2230
Grilled Grande Bowl Chicken Black Beans	1 serv	710	44	31	75	69	11	1930
Grilled Grande Bowl Chicken Pinto	1 serv	700	38	32	75	69	12	1810
Guacamole	1 sm	170	2	16	0	8	5	75
Nachos Grande	1 serv	1270	37	79	120	112	19	1790
Nachos Grande w/ Chicken	1 serv	1380	56	82	160	112	19	2280
Pinto Beans	1 serv	190	4	3	5	44	16	600
Roasted Chipotle	1 serv (1.5 oz)	10	0	0	0	2	1	200
Salsa Picante	1 serv (1.5 oz)	30	1	2	0	3	2	290
Taquitos	3	310	16	11	45	37	5	310
SALADS AND SALAD DRESSINGS								
Grilled Chicken Chopped Salad	1 serv	540	33	33	75	33	5	1480
HealthMex Chicken	1 serv	220	22	4	40	27	2	890
Low Carb Chicken	1 serv	480	37	34	95	11	5	980
Serrano Grape Dressing	1 serv (1.3 oz)	10	0	0	0	2	0	160
SALADWORKS								
SALAD DRESSINGS								
Balsamic Vinaigrette	1 serv (2 oz)	192	0	17	0	9	0	–
Blue Cheese	1 serv (2 oz)	192	3	18	13	3	0	–
Creamy Italian	1 serv (2 oz)	232	1	22	11	5	0	–
Dijon Honey	1 serv	272	0	25	11	00	0	–
Fat Free Balsamic w/ Sundried Tomatoes	1 serv (2 oz)	28	0	0	0	2	0	–
French	1 serv (2 oz)	266	0	22	14	16	0	–
Herbal Ranch	1 serv (2 oz)	198	1	19	25	5	0	–

FOOD	PORTION	CALS	PROT	FAT	CHOL	CARB	FIBER	SOD
Italian Vinaigrette	1 serv (2 oz)	255	0	26	0	5	0	–
Lowfat Ranch	1 serv (2 oz)	34	1	1	19	4	0	–
Oriental Sesame	1 serv (2 oz)	147	1	6	0	21	0	–
Royal Caesar	1 serv (2 oz)	266	1	27	14	4	0	–
Russian	1 serv (2 oz)	221	1	21	14	8	0	–
SALADS								
B.L.T.	1 serv	262	19	24	54	9	4	–
Bently	1 serv	340	28	19	171	7	3	–
Caesar	1 serv	283	15	12	240	32	4	–
Caesar Chicken	1 serv	423	41	15	313	32	4	–
Caesar Shrimp	1 serv	350	30	12	380	32	4	–
Fiesta	1 serv	460	38	23	102	26	6	–
Garden	1 serv	58	4	1	0	12	5	–
Mandarin Chicken	1 serv	589	44	15	109	63	6	–
Newport	1 serv	184	23	7	189	8	4	–
Nicoise	1 serv	407	29	11	253	50	6	–
Spinach	1 serv	433	22	25	265	29	2	–
Tivoli	1 serv	563	32	27	61	50	5	–
Turkey Club	1 serv	720	50	19	60	90	6	–
SAMURAI SAM'S **BOWLS**								
Low Carb	1 reg	230	33	4	80	16	5	210
Spicy Beef 'N Broccoli Brown Rice	1 reg	580	26	14	50	85	7	1160
Spicy Beef 'N Broccoli	1 reg	620	26	13	50	97	3	1160
Sumo Brown Rice	1	1022	81	23	214	111	9	1513
Sumo White Rice	1	1083	81	21	214	128	3	1509
Sweet & Sour Dark Chicken	1 reg	610	32	10	85	96	6	200
Sweet & Sour Dark Chicken Brown Rice	1 reg	570	32	12	85	84	9	200
Sweet & Sour White Chicken	1 reg	580	37	5	80	96	6	210
Sweet & Sour White Chicken Brown Rice	1 reg	540	37	6	80	85	9	210
Teriyaki Dark Chicken	1 reg	540	31	10	85	79	2	500
Teriyaki Dark Chicken Brown Rice	1 reg	500	31	11	85	68	12	510
Teriyaki Dark Chicken & Shrimp	1 reg	492	29	6	140	78	2	563

FOOD	PORTION	CALS	PROT	FAT	CHOL	CARB	FIBER	SOD
Teriyaki Dark Chicken & Shrimp Brown Rice	1 reg	451	29	7	290	67	5	565
Teriyaki Dark Chicken & Steak	1 reg	540	27	9	65	83	2	560
Teriyaki Dark Chicken & Steak Brown Rice	1 reg	490	27	10	65	71	5	660
Teriyaki Salmon	1	643	33	3	15	121	3	1223
Teriyaki Shrimp Brown Rice	1 reg	407	28	3	193	65	5	582
Teriyaki Steak	1 reg	530	23	8	50	86	2	810
Teriyaki Steak & Shrimp	1 reg	483	26	5	120	77	2	713
Teriyaki Steak & Shrimp Brown Rice	1 reg	442	25	6	120	66	5	715
Teriyaki Steak Brown Rice	1 reg	490	23	9	50	74	5	510
Teriyaki Veggie	1 reg	363	8	1	0	81	3	393
Teriyaki Veggie Brown Rice	1 reg	323	8	2	0	69	7	395
Teriyaki White Chicken	1 reg	520	37	4	80	79	2	510
Teriyaki White Chicken Brown Rice	1 reg	470	36	5	80	68	5	510
Teriyaki White Chicken & Shrimp	1 reg	478	32	2	127	78	2	567
Teriyaki White Chicken & Shrimp Brown Rice	1 reg	437	32	4	137	67	5	570
Teriyaki White Chicken & Steak	1 reg	520	30	6	65	83	2	660
Teriyaki White Chicken & Steak Brown Rice	1 reg	480	30	7	65	71	5	660
Yakisoba Dark Chicken	1	842	60	24	146	114	6	1154
Yakisoba Dark Chicken & Steak	1	825	54	22	114	113	6	1410
Yakisoba Shrimp	1	677	55	10	330	110	6	1283
Yakisoba Steak	1	809	48	20	83	112	6	1667
Yakisoba Veggie	1	509	19	8	0	110	6	902
Yakisoba White Chicken	1	794	70	14	137	114	6	1169
Yakisoba White Chicken & Steak	1	801	59	17	110	113	6	1410
SALADS AND SIDES								
Crab Rangoon	1 serv	210	7	12	35	20	1	260
Dressing Chinese	1 serv (3.5 oz)	230	0	7	0	44	–	1700
Dressing Chinese Ginger	1 serv (1 oz)	85	0	5	0	9	0	153

FOOD	PORTION	CALS	PROT	FAT	CHOL	CARB	FIBER	SOD
Dressing Oriental	1 serv (1 oz)	70	0	2	0	12	0	180
Egg Roll Grilled Chicken	1	150	7	7	15	17	1	300
Salad Oriental Chicken	1 serv	220	36	4	90	9	3	200
Salad Side	1	10	1	1	0	2	1	5
Salad Toss Sesame Chicken	1	490	41	13	90	57	8	1240
Soup Asian Noodle	1 serv	89	5	2	13	14	1	723
Teriyaki Sauce	1 serv (1 oz)	40	1	0	0	9	0	340
WRAPS								
Teriyaki Dark Chicken	1	670	34	16	75	95	8	1250
Teriyaki Dark Chicken Brown Rice	1	650	34	17	75	90	9	1250
Teriyaki Steak	1	650	27	14	40	101	8	1510
Teriyaki Steak Brown Rice	1	630	27	15	40	95	9	1510
Teriyaki Veggie	1	510	14	8	0	94	8	1130
Teriyaki Veggie Brown Rice	1	490	13	9	0	89	10	1130
Teriyaki White Chicken	1	640	39	11	70	96	8	1260
Teriyaki White Chicken Brown Rice	1	620	39	12	70	90	9	1260
Teriyaki White Chicken & Steak	1	649	33	13	55	95	8	1384
Teriyaki White Chicken & Steak Brown Rice	1	628	33	13	55	89	9	1385

SBARRO
DESSERTS

FOOD	PORTION	CALS	PROT	FAT	CHOL	CARB	FIBER	SOD
Black Forest Cake	1 serv (4.6 oz)	480	3	24	50	59	1	340
Deluxe Carrot Cake	1 serv (5 oz)	540	5	29	65	64	1	400
Deluxe Cheese Cake	1 serv (5.7 oz)	560	9	40	170	42	1	450
Deluxe Milk Chocolate Cake	1 serv (4.3 oz)	490	4	25	30	59	1	310
MAIN MENU SELECTIONS								
Baked Ziti w/ Sauce	1 serv (14 oz)	700	39	41	135	43	4	1220
Calzone Cheese	1 (12 oz)	770	39	28	90	87	3	1410
Chicken Francese	1 serv (11 oz)	640	63	38	175	8	2	590
Chicken Parmigiana	1 serv (11 oz)	520	64	22	175	16	2	750

FOOD	PORTION	CALS	PROT	FAT	CHOL	CARB	FIBER	SOD
Chicken Portofino	1 serv (12 oz)	730	63	48	225	7	1	790
Chicken Vesuvio	1 serv (11 oz)	690	63	43	225	8	1	810
Eggplant Rollatini w/ Cheese	1 serv (11 oz)	580	21	38	50	40	4	900
Garlic Roll	1 (2.2 oz)	170	5	5	0	28	tr	370
Meat Lasagna	1 serv (13 oz)	650	41	37	130	36	3	1130
Meatballs	1 serv (3.7 oz)	140	8	9	30	10	1	880
Mixed Vegetables	1 serv (7 oz)	190	3	15	0	14	4	330
Pasta Milano	1 serv (20 oz)	640	45	32	175	41	6	740
Pasta Rustica	1 serv (14 oz)	600	10	47	70	39	5	2288
Penne Alla Vodka	1 serv (14 oz)	640	23	28	120	67	5	1000
Penne w/ Sausage & Peppers	1 serv (14 oz)	710	35	49	130	33	4	1690
Pizza Cheese	1 slice	460	24	13	30	60	3	1080
Pizza Chicken Vegetable	1 slice	530	24	17	45	69	5	1260
Pizza Fresh Tomato	1 slice	450	20	14	25	60	3	1040
Pizza Mushroom	1 slice	460	19	14	20	62	4	1310
Pizza Pepperoni	1 slice	730	35	37	75	61	3	2200
Pizza Sausage	1 slice	670	35	31	80	60	3	1810
Pizza Sauteed Spinach & Yellow Pepper	1 slice	670	28	24	30	86	5	1470
Pizza Supreme	1 slice	630	31	27	60	63	3	1720
Pizza White	1 slice	570	30	23	55	59	2	1150
Pizza Gourmet Broccoli & Spinach	1 slice	720	29	28	30	88	6	1540
Pizza Gourmet Cheese	1 slice	660	30	21	40	84	4	1460
Pizza Gourmet Ham Pineapple & Bacon	1 slice	680	33	21	45	88	4	1820
Pizza Gourmet Meat Delight	1 slice	780	41	29	80	84	4	2250
Pizza Gourmet Mushroom	1 slice	610	22	20	20	85	5	1600

FOOD	PORTION	CALS	PROT	FAT	CHOL	CARB	FIBER	SOD
Pizza Gourmet Mushroom & Spinach	1 slice	710	29	27	30	87	6	1680
Pizza Gourmet Tomato & Basil	1 slice	700	28	25	40	87	5	1650
Pizza Low Carb Cheese	1 slice	310	34	14	25	18	–	640
Pizza Low Carb Pepperoni	1 slice	420	36	14	60	18	–	940
Pizza Low Carb Sausage Pepperoni	1 slice	560	44	35	95	18	–	1300
Pizza Stuffed Pepperoni	1 slice	960	52	42	115	89	4	3200
Pizza Stuffed Philly Cheesesteak	1 slice	830	38	33	70	94	5	2090
Pizza Stuffed Spinach & Broccoli	1 slice	790	32	34	50	89	5	1610
Sausage & Peppers	1 serv (10 oz)	410	17	30	55	19	4	1340
Spaghetti w/ Chicken Parmasean	1 serv (15 oz)	930	75	36	175	75	6	950
Spaghetti w/ Chicken Francese	1 serv (15 oz)	800	49	37	110	64	5	860
Spaghetti w/ Chicken Vesuvio	1 serv (15 oz)	850	50	41	145	64	4	1100
Spaghetti w/ Meatballs	1 serv (18 oz)	680	19	25	15	96	9	1720
Spaghetti w/ Sauce	1 serv (20 oz)	820	20	28	0	120	10	890
Stromboli Pepperoni	1 (10 oz)	890	39	44	80	82	3	2470
Stromboli Spinach Tomato Broccoli	1 (10 oz)	680	29	24	35	84	5	1420
SALADS								
Caesar	1 serv (8 oz)	80	2	5	5	6	1	200
Cucumber & Tomato	1 serv (8 oz)	130	1	11	0	9	2	85
Fruit Salad	1 serv (12 oz)	130	2	1	0	32	3	15
Greek	1 serv (8 oz)	60	2	5	10	3	tr	130
Mixed Garden	1 serv (8 oz)	35	2	0	0	7	3	15
Pasta Primavera	1 serv (8 oz)	190	4	10	0	21	2	1180
Stringbean & Tomato	1 serv (8 oz)	100	1	7	0	9	2	80

FOOD	PORTION	CALS	PROT	FAT	CHOL	CARB	FIBER	SOD
SEASON 52								
CHILDREN'S MENU SELECTIONS								
Children's Chicken	1 serv	344	57	4	131	21	4	933
Children's Flatbread	1	468	26	18	40	50	1	1216
Children's Pasta	1 serv	177	6	3	2	31	2	522
DESSERTS								
Boston Cream Pie	1 serv	188	3	7	14	30	0	120
Carrot Cake	1 serv	320	4	16	51	42	2	293
Chocolate & Peanut Butter Harlequin	1 serv	330	9	18	41	40	0	89
Fresh Spring Fruit	1 serv	35	1	0	0	8	3	2
Key Lime Pie	1 serv	283	5	13	113	37	0	133
Pecan Pie	1 serv	263	3	15	26	29	2	188
Sorbet w/ Fruit	1 serv	213	1	1	0	50	7	5
Strawberry Shortcake	1 serv	154	2	6	39	22	0	85
Strawberry Mango Cheesecake	1 serv	226	5	14	93	20	1	200
Toasted Almond Amaretto	1 serv	324	5	17	161	38	1	291
FLATBREADS								
Artichoke & Goat Cheese	1	469	19	18	22	59	4	1552
Garlic Chicken	1	474	31	16	57	52	2	1351
Parmesan Crispbread	1	363	24	8	37	50	1	1750
Spicy Shrimp	1	474	28	13	106	61	3	1403
Steak & Mushroom	1	474	26	18	50	52	2	1217
Tomato	1	460	21	17	26	57	3	1391
MAIN MENU SELECTIONS								
Appetizer Goat Cheese Ravioli	1 serv	473	26	23	112	39	2	2581
Appetizer Grilled Artichokes	1 serv	185	9	3	5	32	10	2033
Appetizer Grilled Asparagus	1 serv	186	7	10	19	17	5	1179
Appetizer Roasted Potato Wedges	1 serv	333	9	3	0	68	6	1398
Appetizer Shrimp Cocktail	1 serv	221	37	2	332	14	1	1563
Appetizer Shrimp Stuffed Mushrooms	1 serv	302	32	13	177	15	1	1280
Appetizer Steak Skewers w/ Thai Salad	1 serv	438	37	15	78	39	6	1144
Appetizer Steamed Mussels	1 serv	472	47	9	92	51	4	997

FOOD	PORTION	CALS	PROT	FAT	CHOL	CARB	FIBER	SOD
Cedar Salmon	1 serv	472	39	21	99	32	6	962
Chicken Boccone Pasta	1 serv	434	46	4	82	54	8	2158
Chicken Breast	1 serv	403	58	5	131	31	5	1579
Filet Mignon	1 serv	473	43	17	108	37	5	1213
Grilled Rainbow Trout	1 serv	410	43	12	110	33	5	783
Grilled Scallops	1 serv	471	44	7	71	58	10	1661
Pork Tenderloin	1 serv	392	50	12	130	23	4	1727
Sandwich Chicken Breast	1	472	53	7	115	49	5	958
Sandwich Fresh Fish	1	437	41	6	63	55	6	1165
Sandwich Grilled Steak	1	463	41	13	95	46	4	1081
Sandwich Vegetable Stack	1	461	20	17	26	57	8	1347
Shrimp Stuffed w/ Crab	1 serv	470	52	10	948	43	3	974
Soup Chicken Tortilla	1 serv (8 oz)	181	14	4	29	23	3	946
Soup Vegetable	1 serv (8 oz)	153	5	3	5	27	3	1390
Spring Vegetable Plate	1 serv	465	18	11	1	74	17	1798
Tuna w/o Soy Sauce	1 serv	175	28	1	49	13	2	734
Turkey Skewer	1 serv	404	51	4	110	41	5	2235
Yellowfin Tuna	1 serv	466	60	3	84	49	10	2470
SALADS								
Chicken Cobb	1 entree	474	52	21	125	19	4	1327
Greek	1 entree	478	13	35	51	27	6	1213
Mesclun Greens	1 side	315	5	15	11	37	3	372
Portobello & Romaine	1 entree	270	13	15	34	20	4	1210
Salmon	1 entree	470	37	26	101	22	5	742
Spinach	1 side	272	7	19	5	19	4	507
Spring Greens	1 side	240	5	18	0	16	4	440
Tabbouleh	1 side	417	9	16	0	60	12	1345
Tomato & Blue Cheese Stack	1 side	352	11	25	21	20	5	612

SKIPPERS

MAIN MENU SELECTIONS

FOOD	PORTION	CALS	PROT	FAT	CHOL	CARB	FIBER	SOD
Basket Chicken + Chips & Slaw	1 piece	730	33	25	70	60	0	1650
Grilled Veggies	1 serv	35	2	0	0	8	3	50
Sandwich Fish + Chips & Slaw	1 serv	800	22	34	20	105	4	1780
Sandwich Grilled Chicken + Chips & Slaw	1	1070	57	50	145	92	3	1510

FOOD	PORTION	CALS	PROT	FAT	CHOL	CARB	FIBER	SOD
SALADS								
Green Salad w/o Dressing	1 sm	25	1	0	0	5	2	20
SOUPER SALAD								
DESSERTS								
Blueberry Bread	1 piece	150	3	3	0	29	1	210
Brownies	2 pieces	120	1	5	5	21	0	115
Cornbread	1 piece	170	3	5	0	30	1	350
Cottage Cheese	½ cup	90	13	2	10	5	0	410
Gingerbread	1 piece	180	2	6	0	30	1	290
Peaches	½ cup	70	0	0	0	17	0	10
Pineapple Tidbits	¼ cup	60	0	0	0	15	1	0
Pudding Banana	½ cup	160	2	6	0	26	0	150
Pudding Chocolate	½ cup	170	2	5	0	30	0	115
Soft Serve Cone Chocolate	1	120	1	2	0	22	0	85
Soft Serve Cone Vanilla	1	120	0	3	0	22	0	95
Sponge Cake	4 pieces	80	1	2	5	14	0	160
Strawberry Parfait	½ cup	100	2	2	0	19	0	70
Vanilla Wafers	4	70	1	2	0	13	6	85
Whipped Topping	½ cup	100	0	8	0	8	0	0
PASTA AND PIZZA								
Chicken Alfredo	1 cup	320	19	9	50	40	1	1060
Macaroni & Cheese	1 cup	380	15	18	35	38	1	870
Pizza Slice Cheese	1	70	4	3	5	8	0	125
Pizza Slice Garden	1	80	4	3	5	9	1	125
Pizza Slice Pepperoni	1	90	5	4	10	8	0	190
Pizza Slice Sausage	1	80	4	4	5	9	1	170
Spaghetti & Meatballs	1 cup	280	11	9	15	38	4	700
SALAD DRESSINGS AND SAUCES								
Balsamic Vinegar	1 oz	60	0	0	0	15	0	0
Bleu Cheese	2 oz	220	2	23	25	1	0	310
Caesar	2 oz	280	4	30	30	4	0	840
Chipotle Ranch	2 oz	280	0	28	10	8	0	480
Fat Free French	2 oz	60	0	0	0	18	1	620
Fat Free Italian w/ Cheese	2 oz	30	0	0	0	6	0	680
Green Goddess	2 oz	260	2	24	10	4	0	580
Honey Mustard	2 oz	240	0	26	20	2	0	460
Mayonnaise	2 tbsp	200	0	22	20	20	0	200
Olive Oil	1 oz	240	0	28	0	0	0	0
Peppercorn Ranch	2 oz	220	1	23	20	2	0	360

FOOD	PORTION	CALS	PROT	FAT	CHOL	CARB	FIBER	SOD
Pesto Basil	1 tbsp	45	1	5	0	0	0	100
Ranch	2 oz	220	1	23	20	2	0	360
Reduced Calorie Ranch	2 oz	120	2	11	10	3	0	260
Sauce Alfredo	1½ tbsp	45	2	4	10	2	0	170
Sauce Chipotle Pepper	¼ tsp	0	0	0	0	0	0	30
Sauce Cholula Hot	¼ tsp	0	0	0	0	0	0	5
Sauce Jalapeno Cheese	1 serv (2 oz)	35	1	2	0	5	1	440
Sauce Marinara	1½ tbsp	10	0	0	0	2	0	90
Sauce Meaty Marinara	1½ tbsp	40	1	1	5	2	0	90
Sauce Sriracha Hot	¼ tsp	0	0	0	0	0	0	15
Sour Cream Light	2 tbsp	40	1	3	10	3	0	40
Tangy Oriental	2 oz	160	0	12	0	10	0	760
Thousand Island	1 oz	300	0	30	20	6	0	500
Vinaigrette Cranberry	2 oz	100	0	0	0	24	0	560
Vinaigrette House	2 oz	220	0	22	0	4	0	840
SALADS								
Apple Walnut	1 cup	130	3	11	5	7	1	210
Asian Chicken	1 cup	80	3	3	5	10	2	450
Asian Shrimp	1 cup	100	4	4	20	13	2	470
Buffalo Chicken	1 cup	70	3	6	10	3	1	200
Caesar Shrimp	1 cup	90	4	7	30	3	1	310
Caesar Chicken	1 cup	90	5	7	15	4	1	340
Caesar Chicken Salsa	1 cup	80	4	5	15	4	1	380
California Chicken Salad	⅓ cup	80	5	6	25	4	0	110
Capri	1 cup	50	1	2	0	8	0	540
Chicago Chopped	1 cup	120	4	10	15	3	1	310
Chickpea	⅓ cup	110	3	6	0	11	4	220
Cobb	1 cup	100	4	8	55	2	1	340
Coleslaw Broccoli	⅓ cup	80	1	6	0	6	1	65
Edamame	⅓ cup	70	4	5	0	4	2	50
Fisherman's Kettle Shrimp & Crab	⅓ cup	120	3	8	15	15	1	300
Gazpacho	⅓ cup	30	0	3	0	3	1	100
Green Goddess Crab	1 cup	70	2	5	5	4	1	240
Italian Antipasto	1 cup	70	2	5	5	3	1	320
Mango Berry	1 cup	110	1	6	0	13	1	75
Marinated Mushrooms	⅓ cup	60	1	7	0	1	0	110
Marinated Tomato	1 cup	60	1	2	0	11	1	45
Melon Couscous	⅓ cup	50	1	1	0	10	1	60

FOOD	PORTION	CALS	PROT	FAT	CHOL	CARB	FIBER	SOD
Mustard Potato	⅓ cup	80	1	5	25	7	1	280
Paco's Taco	⅓ cup	100	3	5	0	12	2	200
Pasta De Garden	⅓ cup	80	1	5	0	8	0	210
Pasta Fettuccine	⅓ cup	100	2	5	5	11	1	390
Pasta Primavera	⅓ cup	45	1	3	0	4	0	85
Pasta Thai Chicken	⅓ cup	100	3	5	10	11	1	320
Pasta Tuna Skroodle	⅓ cup	130	3	9	10	10	1	135
Red Potato	⅓ cup	50	1	4	0	5	1	125
Rice Florentine	⅓ cup	90	1	5	0	11	0	105
Roasted Mushrooms & Artichokes w/ Feta Cheese	⅓ cup	40	1	3	0	3	1	90
Roasted Vegetables	⅓ cup	20	0	2	0	2	1	125
Salad Of The Sea	⅓ cup	50	2	2	5	6	0	190
Salmon Medley	1 cup	70	4	2	5	10	1	160
Santa Fe Corn	⅓ cup	100	4	4	0	13	3	310
Shrimp & Crab Louie	1 cup	130	5	10	55	5	1	490
Southwest Chicken Chipotle	1 cup	90	3	7	10	4	1	270
Sweet Garden Slaw	⅓ cup	35	0	2	0	4	1	75
Tropical Tuxedo	⅓ cup	60	1	3	0	7	0	150
Tuna Fish	⅓ cup	70	6	5	15	1	0	220
SOUPS								
Adobe Rice & Chicken	1 (5 oz)	100	3	5	25	10	1	540
Alaskan Salmon Chowder	1 (5 oz)	70	3	2	0	9	1	630
Beef Mushroom Barley	1 (5 oz)	80	4	2	5	11	2	510
Beef Noodle	1 (5 oz)	80	4	3	15	10	1	500
Beef Shellini	1 (5 oz)	90	5	3	10	11	1	460
Beef Stroganoff	1 (5 oz)	120	5	5	15	13	1	820
Black Bean	1 (5 oz)	80	8	2	5	20	11	370
Broccoli Cheese	1 (5 oz)	70	2	2	0	10	1	640
Cajun Gumbo	1 (5 oz)	110	5	4	15	13	1	570
Cauliflower Cheese	1 (5 oz)	70	2	2	0	11	1	650
Cheddar Chicken Broccoli Stew	1 (5 oz)	140	6	6	25	15	2	600
Cherokee Joe Cornbread	1 (5 oz)	70	2	2	0	13	2	950
Chicken Creole	1 (5 oz)	100	5	4	20	12	1	520
Chicken Enchilada	1 (5 oz)	180	6	12	40	13	1	590
Chicken Gumbo	1 (5 oz)	90	4	4	15	10	1	660

FOOD	PORTION	CALS	PROT	FAT	CHOL	CARB	FIBER	SOD
Chicken Mushroom Barley	1 (5 oz)	80	5	3	20	9	1	660
Chicken Noodle	1 (5 oz)	80	5	3	25	9	1	620
Chicken Tetrazini	1 (5 oz)	120	6	5	25	13	1	620
Chicken Tortilla	1 (5 oz)	60	4	2	10	7	1	650
Cream Of Asparagus	1 (5 oz)	140	2	10	15	7	1	710
Cream Of Broccoli	1 (5 oz)	60	2	2	0	9	1	620
Cream Of Cauliflower	1 (5 oz)	60	2	2	0	10	1	630
Cream Of Chicken	1 (5 oz)	100	5	5	20	9	1	610
Cream Of Mushroom	1 (5 oz)	80	2	4	0	10	1	480
Holiday Harvest	1 (5 oz)	90	3	6	25	5	0	480
Marinated Oriental Cucumber	⅓ cup	10	0	0	0	2	0	240
Vegan Split Pea	1 (5 oz)	90	4	1	0	16	5	260
Vegetable Beef	1 (5 oz)	80	4	3	10	11	2	550
Vegetable Cheese	1 (5 oz)	80	2	3	0	12	1	430
Vegetable Lentil	1 (5 oz)	70	5	0	0	16	5	620
Vegetarian Butter Bean	1 (5 oz)	70	6	0	0	21	10	420
Vegetarian Vegetable	1 (5 oz)	50	2	1	0	11	2	320

SOUPLANTATION
BREADS AND MUFFINS

FOOD	PORTION	CALS	PROT	FAT	CHOL	CARB	FIBER	SOD
Focaccia Low Fat Garlic Parmesan	1 piece	100	2	3	0	15	1	170
Muffin French Quarter Praline	1	290	4	15	20	38	2	100

DESSERTS

FOOD	PORTION	CALS	PROT	FAT	CHOL	CARB	FIBER	SOD
Cobbler Apple	½ cup	350	2	10	0	64	1	160
Cobbler Blissful Blueberry	½ cup	380	3	10	0	70	3	230
Cobbler Cherry	½ cup	340	2	10	0	61	2	180
Cobbler Cranberry Apple	½ cup	370	3	10	0	58	3	210
Cobbler Peach	½ cup	360	2	10	0	65	2	220
Cookie Chocolate Chip	1 sm	70	1	3	5	10	0	90
Fat Free Apple Medley	½ cup	70	1	0	0	18	1	5
Fat Free Banana Royale	½ cup	80	1	0	0	20	1	5
Fat Free Frozen Yogurt Chocolate	½ cup	95	3	0	0	21	0	80
Jello Fat Free All Flavors	½ cup	80	1	0	0	20	0	40
Jello Fat Free Sugar Free All Flavors	½ cup	10	1	0	0	0	0	10
Pudding Banana	½ cup	160	4	4	10	27	1	220

FOOD	PORTION	CALS	PROT	FAT	CHOL	CARB	FIBER	SOD
Pudding Vanilla	½ cup	140	4	4	10	24	0	160
Pudding Low Fat Butterscotch	½ cup	140	4	3	10	24	0	160
Pudding Low Fat Chocolate	½ cup	140	4	3	10	23	0	220
Pudding Low Fat Rice	½ cup	110	3	2	10	20	1	50
Soft Serve Reduced Fat Vanilla	½ cup	140	3	4	20	22	0	70
Tapioca Low Fat	½ cup	140	4	3	10	24	0	160
MAIN MENU SELECTIONS								
Alfredo Broccoli w/ Basil	1 cup	380	12	17	40	45	1	790
Alfredo Fettuccine	1 cup	390	15	18	50	41	2	580
Alfredo Four Cheese	1 cup	390	19	13	30	50	3	690
Alfredo Roasted Garlic & Asiago	1 cup	330	13	11	25	45	2	650
Alfredo Roasted Mushroom w/ Rosemary	1 cup	380	19	14	35	44	2	850
Alfredo Southwestern	1 cup	350	10	16	50	42	1	420
Beef Stroganoff	1 cup	340	9	21	75	28	2	590
Carbonara Pasta	1 cup	280	10	8	20	43	2	250
Chili Arizona	1 cup	220	14	8	20	25	7	690
Creamy Herb Chicken	1 cup	310	8	17	80	32	2	360
Creamy Pepper Jack	1 cup	290	6	15	50	35	2	360
Garden Vegetable w/ Italian Sausage	1 cup	300	12	10	20	42	3	540
Garden Vegetable w/ Meatballs	1 cup	270	11	7	10	42	3	460
Greek Mediterranean	1 cup	290	10	8	15	45	2	520
Italian Sausage w/ Red Pepper Puree	1 cup	250	6	10	45	35	2	380
Lemon Cream & Asparagus	1 cup	230	6	9	0	34	1	470
Linguini w/ Clam Sauce	1 cup	380	16	10	40	56	1	890
Low Fat Oriental Green Bean & Noodle	1 cup	240	7	3	0	45	2	780
Macaroni & Cheese	1 cup	260	10	6	15	40	2	480
Nutty Mushroom	1 cup	390	12	20	45	42	2	410
Pasta Florentine	1 cup	360	18	10	15	54	7	920
Penne Arrabbiatta	1 cup	340	18	10	20	43	3	710
Pesto Cilantro Lime	1 cup	370	9	21	20	36	2	760
Roasted Eggplant Marinara	1 cup	340	18	10	20	43	3	700
Smoked Salmon & Dill	1 cup	360	13	16	45	41	2	390

FOOD	PORTION	CALS	PROT	FAT	CHOL	CARB	FIBER	SOD
Tuscany Sausage w/ Capers & Olives	1 cup	240	10	10	15	29	2	920
Vegetable Ragu	1 cup	250	9	5	10	41	3	480
Vegetarian Marinara w/ Basil	1 cup	260	10	4	10	44	3	750
Walnut Pesto	1 cup	310	10	9	10	42	2	610
SALAD DRESSINGS								
Roasted Garlic	2 tbsp	140	1	14	5	2	0	300
Thousand Island	2 tbsp	110	0	11	5	3	0	250
SALADS								
Antipasto w/ Peppered Salami	1 cup	140	5	10	10	6	2	370
Italian White Bean	½ cup	140	6	5	0	19	4	480
Pesto Orzo w/ Pinenuts	1 cup	220	4	17	10	14	2	320
Ragin' Cajun	1 cup	200	7	14	15	12	2	450
Southern Black Eyed Pea	½ cup	130	2	6	0	18	3	220
Southwestern Rice & Beans	½ cup	90	1	3	0	15	3	480
Spicy Southwestern Pasta Low Fat	½ cup	130	5	3	0	21	4	350
Spinach Gorgonzola w/ Spiced Pecans	1 cup	210	5	19	10	5	4	430
Summer Barley w/ Black Beans Low Fat	½ cup	110	4	3	0	19	4	280

SOUTHERN TSUNAMI SUSHI BAR
SALADS

FOOD	PORTION	CALS	PROT	FAT	CHOL	CARB	FIBER	SOD
Calamari	1 serv (4 oz)	148	8	3	307	22	1	1023
Edamame	1 serv (4 oz)	124	1	7	0	9	1	350
Harusame	1 serv (5 oz)	148	2	2	0	33	0	1401
Seabreeze	1 serv (4 oz)	113	0	3	0	23	0	1617
SUSHI								
California Roll	1 (0.8 oz)	31	1	1	0	6	tr	53
Cream Cheese Roll w/ Salmon	1 piece (0.8 oz)	43	2	2	6	5	tr	24
Crunchy Shrimp Roll	1 piece (0.9 oz)	42	2	2	9	5	tr	64
Dragon Roll	1 piece (0.8 oz)	42	2	2	8	6	1	34
Freshwater Eel Roll	1 piece (0.8 oz)	41	2	1	9	5	tr	37

FOOD	PORTION	CALS	PROT	FAT	CHOL	CARB	FIBER	SOD
Green Horseradish	1 tsp	7	0	0	0	1	0	0
Inari	1 piece (1.9 oz)	105	3	2	0	18	0	124
Nigiri Cuttlefish	1 piece (1 oz)	42	2	1	6	9	0	42
Nigiri Egg Cake	1 piece (1.4 oz)	73	2	1	28	13	0	49
Nigiri Fish Roe	1 piece (1.4 oz)	61	6	1	31	9	0	367
Nigiri Fresh Salmon	1 piece (1.3 oz)	68	5	1	8	9	0	29
Nigiri Fresh Water Eel	1 piece (1.6 oz)	108	5	5	32	11	0	82
Nigiri Octopus	1 piece (1.1 oz)	57	2	1	14	9	0	50
Nigiri Sea Eel	1 piece (1.6 oz)	90	4	3	31	11	0	157
Nigiri Shrimp	1 piece (1.1 oz)	44	2	1	9	8	0	28
Nigiri Smoked Salmon	1 piece (1.3 oz)	68	5	1	8	9	0	28
Nigiri Tilapia	1 piece (1.2 oz)	49	2	1	5	8	0	26
Nigiri Tuna	1 piece (1.3 oz)	60	4	0	9	8	0	28
Nigiri Yellowtail	1 piece (1.2 oz)	54	3	1	6	8	0	25
Ocean Crab Roll	1 piece (0.8 oz)	33	2	1	7	5	tr	72
Orange Roll	1 piece (0.8 oz)	32	2	1	5	6	tr	111
Pickled Ginger	1 tbsp	9	0	0	0	2	0	160
Rainbow Roll	1 piece (1 oz)	41	3	1	5	6	tr	57
Sea Eel Roll	1 piece (0.8 oz)	36	1	1	9	6	tr	58
Soy Sauce	1 pkg	16	2	0	0	2	0	660
Spicy Roll Salmon	1 piece (0.8 oz)	40	2	1	4	5	tr	23

FOOD	PORTION	CALS	PROT	FAT	CHOL	CARB	FIBER	SOD
Spicy Roll Shrimp	1 piece (0.8 oz)	31	2	1	9	5	tr	48
Spicy Roll Tuna	1 piece (0.8 oz)	37	2	1	4	5	tr	23
Tempura Roll	1 piece (0.9 oz)	44	2	1	9	7	tr	96
Tofu Roll	1 piece (0.8 oz)	27	1	tr	0	5	tr	17
Tsunami Roll Crab & Fish Roe	1 piece (0.8 oz)	39	2	1	5	6	tr	105

STARBUCKS
BAKED SELECTIONS

FOOD	PORTION	CALS	PROT	FAT	CHOL	CARB	FIBER	SOD
Apple Fritter	1	480	4	22	0	64	1	290
Bagel French Toast	1	280	8	1	0	62	2	400
Bagel Multigrain	1	280	10	3	0	60	4	380
Bagel Plain	1	280	10	0	0	62	2	440
Bar Cranberry Bliss	1	320	3	16	45	41	1	260
Bar Toffee Almond	1	400	4	19	50	53	1	340
Brownie Espresso	1	340	4	19	50	40	2	135
Cinnamon Roll	1	470	6	26	45	56	1	350
Cocoa Crispy Square	1	420	5	17	25	66	1	440
Cookie Chocolate Chunk	1	420	7	20	55	56	6	460
Cookie Coffee Ginger	1	470	6	18	75	70	3	210
Cookie Penguin	1	370	4	18	15	50	tr	280
Cookie Rainbow	1	420	5	19	65	61	1	370
Cookies Mini Black & White	2	240	2	12	40	32	1	160
Croissant Butter	1	370	5	23	65	35	3	310
Dougnut Glazed	1	490	4	23	20	65	1	410
Loaf Banana Nut	1 serv	470	7	24	105	56	2	360
Loaf Iced Lemon	1 serv	500	7	18	140	78	1	440
Loaf Marble	1 serv	410	6	22	130	52	tr	440
Loaf Pumpkin	1 serv	380	5	14	55	59	2	480
Mallorca Sweet Bread	1	420	7	24	20	43	2	560
Muffin Blueberry	1	310	5	11	70	55	1	270
Muffin Pumpkin Cream Cheese	1	490	6	24	85	63	1	470
Muffin Reduced Fat Chocolate	1	290	6	5	75	53	2	460
Muffin Walnut Bran	1	430	8	18	40	62	4	400

FOOD	PORTION	CALS	PROT	FAT	CHOL	CARB	FIBER	SOD
Reduced Fat Coffee Cake Banana Chocolate Chip	1	390	5	8	0	76	3	400
Reduced Fat Coffee Cake Blueberry	1 serv	320	4	6	10	54	1	390
Reduced Fat Coffee Cake Cinnamon Swirl	1 serv	290	4	4	5	52	1	330
Reduced Fat Coffee Cake Pumpkin Chocolate Chip	1	300	5	6	0	58	3	270
Rustic Apple Tart	1	190	1	5	0	37	3	80
Scone Blueberry	1	480	7	22	80	64	2	520
Scone Cran Apple Crumb	1	490	7	20	80	74	4	510
Scone Raspberry	1	470	7	21	80	64	2	510
BEVERAGES								
Apple Juice	1 grande	250	0	0	0	64	0	25
Cafe Americano	1 grande	15	1	0	0	3	0	10
Cafe Au Lait Nonfat Milk	1 grande	70	7	0	5	10	0	90
Caffe Mocha No Whip Nonfat Milk	1 grande	220	13	3	5	42	2	125
Caffe Mocha Whip Nonfat Milk	1 grande	290	13	10	30	44	2	135
Cappuccino Nonfat Milk	1 grande	80	8	0	5	12	0	90
Caramel Macchiato Nonfat Milk	1 grande	190	11	1	10	35	0	135
Caramel Apple Cider Whip	1 grande	380	0	8	25	76	0	30
Caramel Apple Spice No Whip	1 grande	310	0	tr	0	74	0	25
Chocolate Milk Nonfat	1 grande	280	18	3	10	53	2	190
Cinnamon Dolce Creme No Whip Nonfat Milk	1 grande	220	12	0	5	41	0	160
Cinnamon Dolce Whip Nonfat Milk	1 grande	290	13	7	35	43	0	160
Coffe Of The Week Decafe	1 grande	5	1	0	0	0	0	10
Coffee Of The Week	1 grande	5	1	tr	0	0	0	10
Frappuccino Blended Coffee Cafe Vanilla No Whip Soy	1 grande	310	5	3	15	67	0	230
Frappuccino Blended Coffee Cafe Vanilla Whip Nonfat Milk	1 grande	430	6	14	55	70	0	240

FOOD	PORTION	CALS	PROT	FAT	CHOL	CARB	FIBER	SOD
Frappuccino Blended Coffee Cafe Vanilla Whip Soy	1 grande	430	6	14	55	70	0	240
Frappuccino Blended Coffee Caffe Vanilla No Whip Nonfat Milk	1 grande	310	5	3	15	67	0	230
Frappuccino Blended Coffee Caramel No Whip Nonfat Milk	1 grande	270	5	4	15	53	0	230
Frappuccino Blended Coffee Caramel No Whip Soy	1 grande	270	5	4	15	53	0	230
Frappuccino Blended Coffee Caramel Whip Soy	1 grande	380	6	15	55	57	0	240
Frappuccino Blended Coffee Cinnamon Dolce No Whip Nonfat Milk	1 grande	260	5	3	15	52	0	220
Frappuccino Blended Coffee Cinnamon Dolce No Whip Soy	1 grande	260	5	3	15	52	0	220
Frappuccino Blended Coffee Cinnamon Dolce Whip Soy	1 grande	370	6	14	55	55	0	240
Frappuccino Blended Coffee Coffee Whip Nonfat Milk	1 grande	380	6	15	55	57	0	240
Frappuccino Blended Coffee Expresso Nonfat Milk	1 grande	190	4	3	10	38	0	170
Frappuccino Blended Coffee Java Chip No Whip Nonfat Milk	1 grande	340	7	8	15	64	2	230
Frappuccino Blended Coffee Java Chip No Whip Soy	1 grande	190	4	3	10	30	0	170
Frappuccino Blended Coffee Java Chip Whip Nonfat Milk	1 grande	460	7	19	55	67	2	240
Frappuccino Blended Coffee Java Chip Whip Soy	1 grande	460	7	19	55	67	2	240

FOOD	PORTION	CALS	PROT	FAT	CHOL	CARB	FIBER	SOD
Frappuccino Blended Coffee Mocha No Whip Nonfat Milk	1 grande	260	6	4	15	54	0	230
Frappuccino Blended Coffee Mocha No Whip Soy	1 grande	260	6	4	15	54	0	230
Frappuccino Blended Coffee Mocha Whip Nonfat Milk	1 grande	380	6	15	55	57	0	240
Frappuccino Blended Coffee Pumpkin Spice No Whip Nonfat Milk	1 grande	290	6	4	15	59	0	260
Frappuccino Blended Coffee Pumpkin Spice No Whip Soy	1 grande	290	6	4	15	59	0	260
Frappuccino Blended Coffee Pumpkin Spice Whip Nonfat Milk	1 grande	400	7	15	55	62	0	280
Frappuccino Blended Coffee Pumpkin Spice Whip Soy	1 grande	400	7	15	55	62	0	280
Frappuccino Blended Coffee Whip Nonfat Milk	1 grande	370	6	14	55	55	0	240
Frappuccino Blended Coffee White Chocolate Mocha No Whip Nonfat Milk	1 grande	300	6	5	15	59	0	250
Frappuccino Blended Coffee White Chocolate Mocha No Whip Soy	1 grande	300	6	5	15	59	0	250
Frappuccino Blended Coffee White Chocolate Mocha Whip Nonfat Milk	1 grande	410	7	16	55	62	0	270
Frappuccino Blended Coffee White Chocolate Mocha Whip Soy	1 grande	410	7	16	55	62	0	270
Frappuccino Blended Creme Tazo Chai No Whip Nonfat Milk	1 grande	330	10	2	5	67	0	270

FOOD	PORTION	CALS	PROT	FAT	CHOL	CARB	FIBER	SOD
Frappuccino Blended Creme Tazo Chai Whip Nonfat Milk	1 grande	570	12	15	60	95	1	330
Frappuccino Blended Creme Vanilla Bean No Whip Nonfat Milk	1 grande	350	11	3	5	72	0	310
Frappuccino Blended Creme Vanilla Bean Whip Nonfat Milk	1 grande	470	12	14	50	75	0	320
Frappuccino Light Blended Coffee Cafe Vanilla Nonfat Milk	1 grande	190	6	1	0	42	3	240
Frappuccino Light Blended Coffee Caramel	1 grande	160	5	2	5	30	3	230
Frappuccino Light Blended Coffee Cinnamon Dolce Nonfat Milk	1 grande	140	5	1	0	29	3	230
Frappuccino Light Blended Coffee Java Chip Nonfat Milk	1 grande	200	6	5	0	36	4	220
Frappuccino Light Blended Coffee Mocha Nonfat Milk	1 grande	140	6	1	0	29	3	230
Frappuccino Light Blended Coffee Nonfat Milk	1 grande	130	5	1	0	25	3	230
Frappuccino Light Blended Coffee Pumpkin Spice Nonfat Milk	1 grande	150	6	1	0	31	3	240
Frappuccino Light Blended Creme Double Chocolaty Chip Whip Nonfat Milk	1 grande	510	14	19	50	78	2	300
Frappuccino Light Blended Creme Pumpkin Spice No Whip Nonfat Milk	1 grande	360	12	3	5	71	0	350
Frappuccino Light Blended Creme Pumpkin Spice Whip Nonfat Milk	1 grande	470	13	13	50	74	0	360
Frappuccino Light Blended Creme Tazo Green Tea No Whip Nonfat Milk	1 grande	380	11	3	5	78	1	290

FOOD	PORTION	CALS	PROT	FAT	CHOL	CARB	FIBER	SOD
Frappuccino Light Blended Creme Tazo Green Tea Whip Nonfat Milk	1 grande	440	11	13	50	71	0	190
Frappuccino Light Blended Creme Tazo Green Tea Whip Nonfat Milk	1 grande	490	12	14	50	82	1	300
Frappuccino Light Blended Creme White Chocolate No Whip Nonfat Milk	1 grande	480	15	7	10	89	0	410
Frappuccino Light Blended Creme White Chocolate Whip Nonfat Milk	1 grande	610	15	19	60	92	0	420
Frappuccino Light Expresso Nonfat Milk	1 grande	110	5	1	0	20	2	180
Hot Chocolate No Whip Nonfat Milk	1 grande	240	14	3	5	48	2	140
Hot Chocolate Whip Nonfat Milk	1 grande	320	14	10	35	50	2	150
Iced Brewed Coffee	1 grande	90	0	0	0	21	0	5
Iced Cafe Mocha Whip Nonfat Milk	1 grande	290	9	14	45	39	2	90
Iced Caffe Americano	1 grande	15	1	0	0	3	0	10
Iced Caffe Latte Nonfat Milk	1 grande	90	8	0	5	13	0	100
Iced Caffe Mocha No Whip Nonfat Milk	1 grande	170	9	3	5	36	2	80
Iced Caramel Macchiato Nonfat Milk	1 grande	190	10	2	10	34	0	130
Iced Latte Pumpkin Spice No Whip Nonfat Milk	1 grande	220	10	0	5	44	0	170
Iced Latte Pumpkin Spice Whip Nonfat Milk	1 grande	330	11	11	45	48	0	180
Iced Latte Skinny Cinnamon Dolce No Whip Nonfat Milk	1 grande	80	7	0	5	12	0	105
Iced Latte Sugar Free Flavored Syrup Nonfat Milk	1 grande	80	7	0	5	12	0	105
Iced Latte Syrup Flavored Nonfat Milk	1 grande	160	7	0	5	31	0	90

FOOD	PORTION	CALS	PROT	FAT	CHOL	CARB	FIBER	SOD
Iced Latte Vanilla Nonfat Milk	1 grande	160	7	0	5	31	0	90
Iced Peppermint White Chocolate Mocha No Whip Nonfat Milk	1 grande	370	10	6	5	72	0	190
Iced Peppermint White Chocolate Mocha Whip Nonfat Milk	1 grande	490	10	17	45	75	0	190
Iced Tazo Latte Black Tea Nonfat Milk	1 grande	170	8	0	0	35	0	100
Iced Tazo Latte Black Tea Soy	1 grande	200	6	3	0	38	1	90
Iced Tazo Latte Chai Nonfat Milk	1 grande	200	8	0	5	44	0	100
Iced Tazo Latte Green Tea Nonfat Milk	1 grande	220	10	5	0	45	1	120
Iced Tazo Latte Green Tea Soy	1 grande	260	7	4	0	48	2	105
Iced Tazo Latte Red Tea	1 grande	200	6	3	0	38	1	90
Iced Tazo Latte Red Tea Nonfat Milk	1 grande	170	8	0	5	35	0	100
Iced White Chocolate Mocha No Whip Nonfat Milk	1 grande	310	11	6	5	55	0	190
Iced White Chocolate Mocha Whip Nonfat Milk	1 grande	430	11	17	45	59	0	200
Latte Caffe Nonfat Milk	1 grande	130	13	5	5	19	0	150
Latte Cinnamon Dolce No Whip Nonfat Milk	1 grande	210	11	0	5	41	0	135
Latte Cinnamon Dolce w/ Sugar Free Syrup Nonfat Milk	1 grande	130	12	0	5	19	0	170
Latte Cinnamon Dolce Whip Nonfat Milk	1 grande	280	12	7	30	43	0	140
Latte Pumpkin Spice No Whip Nonfat Milk	1 grande	260	14	0	5	50	0	210
Latte Pumpkin Spice Whip Nonfat Milk	1 grande	330	14	7	30	52	0	220
Latte Skinny Caramel No Whip Nonfat Milk	1 grande	130	12	0	5	19	0	170

FOOD	PORTION	CALS	PROT	FAT	CHOL	CARB	FIBER	SOD
Latte Skinny Cinnamon Dolce No Whip Nonfat Milk	1 grande	130	12	0	0	19	0	170
Latte Skinny Cinnamon Dolce No Whip Nonfat Milk	1 grande	130	12	0	0	19	0	170
Latte Skinny Hazelnut No Whip Nonfat Milk	1 grande	130	12	0	0	19	0	170
Latte Skinny Vanilla No Whip Nonfat Milk	1 grande	130	12	0	5	19	0	170
Latte Syrup Flavored Nonfat Milk	1 grande	200	12	0	5	37	0	140
Milk Nonfat	1 grande	180	18	0	10	26	0	220
Peppermint White Chocolate Mocha No Whip Nonfat Milk	1 grande	420	14	6	5	78	0	230
Peppermint White Chocolate Mocha Whip Nonfat Milk	1 grande	490	14	13	35	80	0	240
Pumpkin Spice Creme No Whip Nonfat Milk	1 grande	270	15	0	5	51	0	230
Pumpkin Spice Creme Whip Nonfat Milk	1 grande	340	15	7	35	53	0	240
Shaken Black Iced Tea & Lemonade	1 grande	130	0	0	0	33	0	10
Shaken White Iced Tea Blueberry	1 grande	80	0	0	0	21	0	10
Steamed Apple Juice	1 grande	230	0	0	0	56	0	20
Tazo Black Shaken Iced Tea & Lemonade	1 grande	130	0	0	0	33	0	10
Tazo Chai Latte Iced Tea Soy	1 grande	230	6	3	0	47	1	90
Tazo Chai Latte Nonfat Milk	1 grande	200	8	0	5	44	0	95
Tazo Chai Latte Soy	1 grande	230	5	3	0	47	1	85
Tazo Latte Black Tea Soy	1 grande	190	5	3	0	36	1	75
Tazo Latte Green Tea Soy	1 grande	220	6	3	0	44	2	75
Tazo Latte Black Tea Nonfat Milk	1 grande	170	7	0	5	34	0	90
Tazo Latte Green Tea Nonfat Milk	1 grande	200	8	0	5	42	1	85

FOOD	PORTION	CALS	PROT	FAT	CHOL	CARB	FIBER	SOD
Tazo Latte Red Tea Nonfat Milk	1 grande	170	7	0	5	34	0	90
Tazo Latte Red Tea Soy	1 grande	190	5	3	0	36	1	75
Tazo Shaken Iced Tea Green	1 grande	80	0	0	0	21	0	10
Tazo Shaken Iced Tea Green & Lemonade	1 grande	130	0	0	0	33	0	10
Tazo Shaken Iced Tea Orange Passion	1 grande	70	0	0	0	19	0	10
Tazo Shaken Iced Tea Passion	1 grande	80	0	0	0	21	0	10
Tazo Shaken Iced Tea Passion & Lemonade	1 grande	130	0	0	0	33	0	10
Tazo Tea	1 grande	0	0	0	0	0	0	0
Vanilla Creme Whip Nonfat Milk	1 grande	270	13	7	35	39	0	160
Vanilla Creme No Whip Nonfat Milk	1 grande	200	12	0	5	37	0	160
White Chocolate Mocha No Whip Nonfat Milk	1 grande	360	16	6	10	62	0	260
White Chocolate Mocha Whip Nonfat Milk	1 grande	430	16	13	35	64	0	270
SALADS								
Fiesta	1 (9.4 oz)	320	16	10	20	44	8	930
Fruit & Cheese Plate	1 (8.6 oz)	400	14	20	50	44	2	560
Vegetable Vinaigrette	1 (10.7 oz)	310	8	15	5	40	10	900
SANDWICHES								
Club Chicken Cheddar Bacon w/ Mayo	1	480	31	18	70	48	2	1180
Club Turkey & Avocado	1	390	26	19	65	33	7	1160
Egg Salad On Multigrain	1	470	19	21	340	53	2	810
Turkey & Swiss w/ Mayo	1	310	26	13	55	26	2	1060
TOPPINGS								
Caramel	1 tbsp	15	0	1	0	2	0	5
Chocolate	1 tsp	5	0	0	0	1	0	0
Flavored Sugar Free Syrup	1 pump	0	0	0	0	0	0	0
Flavored Syrup	1 pump	20	0	0	0	5	0	0
Mocha Syrup	1 pump	25	1	1	0	5	0	0
Sprinkles	1 serv	0	0	0	0	0	0	0

FOOD	PORTION	CALS	PROT	FAT	CHOL	CARB	FIBER	SOD

SUBWAY
ADD-ONS AND SALAD DRESSINGS

FOOD	PORTION	CALS	PROT	FAT	CHOL	CARB	FIBER	SOD
American Cheese	1 serv (0.4 oz)	40	2	4	10	1	0	200
Bacon Strips	2	45	3	4	10	0	0	190
Banana Pepper Slices	3	0	0	0	0	0	0	20
Cheddar	1 serv (0.5 oz)	60	4	5	15	0	0	95
Fat Free Italian	1 serv (2 oz)	35	1	0	0	7	0	720
Fat Free Red Wine Vinaigrette	1 serv (0.7 oz)	30	0	0	1	6	0	340
Jalapeno Pepper Slices	3	<5	0	0	0	0	0	70
Mayonnaise	1 tbsp	110	0	12	10	0	0	80
Mayonnaise Light	1 tbsp	50	0	5	5	tr	0	100
Monterey Cheddar Shredded	1 serv (0.5 oz)	50	3	5	15	1	0	90
Mustard Yellow or Deli	2 tsp	5	0	0	0	tr	0	115
Olive Oil Blend	1 tsp	45	0	5	0	0	0	0
Pepperjack Cheese	1 serv (0.5 oz)	50	3	4	15	0	0	140
Provolone	1 serv (0.5 oz)	50	4	4	10	0	0	125
Ranch	1.5 tbsp	120	0	13	11	1	0	210
Ranch	1 serv (2 oz)	320	0	35	29	3	0	560
Red Wine Vinaigrette	1 serv (2 oz)	80	1	1	0	17	0	910
Sauce Chipotle Southwest	1.5 tbsp	100	0	10	8	1	0	220
Sauce Fat Free Honey Mustard	1.5 tbsp	30	0	0	0	7	0	115
Sauce Fat Free Sweet Onion	1.5 tbsp	40	0	0	0	9	0	85
Swiss	1 serv (0.5 oz)	50	4	5	15	0	0	30
Vinegar	1 tsp	0	0	0	0	0	0	0
BREADS								
6 Inch Italian	6 in	200	7	2	0	38	1	470
Hearty Italian	6 in	220	8	2	0	41	2	470
Honey Oat	6 in	250	10	4	0	48	5	380
Italian Herb & Cheese	6 in	250	10	5	10	40	2	670
Italian White	1 mini	140	5	2	0	26	1	320
Monterey Cheddar	6 in	240	10	5	10	39	1	540

FOOD	PORTION	CALS	PROT	FAT	CHOL	CARB	FIBER	SOD
Parmesan Oregano Bread	6 in	220	8	3	0	40	2	620
Wheat	6 in	200	8	3	0	40	4	360
Wheat	1 mini	140	6	2	0	27	2	240
Wrap	1	190	6	5	0	33	1	470
DESSERTS								
Apple Slices	1 pkg	35	0	0	0	9	2	0
Cookie Chocolate Chip	1	210	2	10	15	30	1	150
Cookie Chocolate Chip w/ M&M's	1 (1.6 oz)	210	2	10	10	32	tr	100
Cookie Chocolate Chunk	1	220	2	10	10	30	tr	100
Cookie Double Chocolate Chip	1 (1.6 oz)	210	2	10	15	30	1	170
Cookie Oatmeal Raisin	1	200	3	8	15	30	1	170
Cookie Peanut Butter	1	220	4	12	15	26	1	200
Cookie Sugar	1	220	2	12	15	28	tr	140
Cookie White Chip Macadamia Nut	1	220	2	11	15	29	tr	160
Raisins	1 pkg	150	2	0	0	33	2	0
SALADS								
Ham w/o Dressing & Croutons	1 serv	120	12	3	25	14	4	840
Oven Roasted Chicken Breast w/o Dressing & Croutons	1 serv	140	19	3	50	11	4	390
Roast Beef w/o Dressing & Croutons	1 serv	120	13	3	20	12	4	480
Subway Club w/o Dressing & Croutons	1 serv	150	18	4	35	14	4	870
Sweet Onion Chicken Teriyaki w/o Dressing & Croutons	1 serv	210	20	3	50	26	4	780
Turkey Breast	1 serv	110	12	3	20	13	4	580
Turkey Breast & Ham w/o Dressing & Croutons	1 serv	120	14	3	25	14	4	790
Veggie Delight w/o Dressing & Croutons	1 serv	60	3	1	0	11	4	80
SANDWICHES								
6 Inch Chicken & Bacon Ranch	1	580	36	30	100	47	6	1390
6 Inch Cold Cut Combo	1	410	21	17	60	47	5	1530

FOOD	PORTION	CALS	PROT	FAT	CHOL	CARB	FIBER	SOD
6 Inch Double Stacked Cold Cut Combo	1	550	31	28	110	49	5	2360
6 Inch Double Stacked Italian BMT	1	630	34	35	100	49	5	2850
6 Inch Double Stacked Steak & Cheese	1	540	46	18	105	49	7	1500
6 Inch Double Stacked Subway Club	1	420	39	8	65	50	5	2080
6 Inch Double Stacked Sweet Onion Chicken Teriyaki	1	480	43	7	100	65	6	1820
6 Inch Double Stacked Turkey Breast	1	330	28	5	40	48	5	1500
6 Inch Ham	1	290	18	5	25	47	5	1260
6 Inch Italian BMT	1	450	23	21	55	47	5	1770
6 Inch Meatball Marinara	1	560	24	24	45	63	8	1590
6 Inch Oven Roasted Chicken Breast	1	310	24	5	25	48	6	830
6 Inch Roast Beef	1	290	19	5	20	45	5	900
6 Inch Spicy Italian	1	480	21	25	55	45	5	1660
6 Inch Steak & Cheese	1	400	29	12	60	48	6	1110
6 Inch Subway Club	1	320	24	6	35	47	5	1290
6 Inch Subway Melt	1	380	25	12	45	48	5	1600
6 Inch Sweet Onion Chicken Teriyaki	1	370	26	5	50	59	5	1200
6 Inch Tuna	1	530	22	31	45	44	5	1010
6 Inch Turkey Breast	1	280	18	5	20	46	5	1000
6 Inch Turkey Breast & Ham	1	290	20	5	25	47	5	1210
6 Inch Veggie Delite	1	230	9	3	0	44	5	500
Mini Sub Ham	1	180	11	3	10	30	4	710
Mini Sub Roast Beef	1	190	13	4	15	30	4	600
Mini Sub Tuna w/ Cheese	1	320	13	18	30	30	4	690
Mini Sub Turkey Breast	1	190	12	3	15	30	4	670
Softwich Santa Fe Turkey	1	520	33	10	55	78	5	1910

TACO BELL

FOOD	PORTION	CALS	PROT	FAT	CHOL	CARB	FIBER	SOD
Border Bowl Southwest Steak	1 serv	600	28	24	55	68	9	2120
Border Bowl Zesty Chicken	1 serv	640	22	35	30	60	10	1800

FOOD	PORTION	CALS	PROT	FAT	CHOL	CARB	FIBER	SOD
Border Bowl Zesty Chicken w/o Dressing	1 serv	440	21	15	30	57	10	1540
Burrito 7 Layer	1	490	17	18	25	65	9	1350
Burrito Bean	1	350	13	9	6	54	8	1190
Burrito Chili Cheese	1	370	16	16	40	40	3	1060
Burrito Grilled Stuft Chicken	1	640	34	23	65	73	7	2160
Burrito Supreme Beef	1	420	17	17	40	51	7	1340
Burrito ½ Lb Beef & Potato	1	530	15	23	30	68	6	1720
Burrito ½ Lb Combo Beef	1	440	21	18	45	51	8	1630
Burrito Fiesta Chicken	1	360	18	10	30	47	3	1320
Burrito Fiesta Steak	1	370	14	13	25	49	4	1200
Burrito Stuft Grilled Steak	1	630	30	25	55	72	7	1930
Burrito Supreme Chicken	1	400	20	13	45	49	6	1360
Burrito Supreme Steak	1	390	18	14	40	49	6	1250
Chalupa Baja Beef	1	410	13	27	35	30	4	780
Chalupa Baja Chicken	1	390	17	23	40	29	3	800
Chalupa Baja Steak	1	390	15	24	35	28	3	690
Chalupa Nacho Cheese Beef	1	370	12	22	20	32	3	770
Chalupa Nacho Cheese Chicken	1	360	16	18	25	30	2	790
Chalupa Nacho Cheese Steak	1	340	14	19	20	30	2	680
Chalupa Supreme Beef	1	380	14	20	40	30	3	620
Chalupa Supreme Chicken	1	360	17	20	45	29	2	650
Chalupa Supreme Steak	1	360	15	21	40	28	2	530
Cheesy Fiesta Potatoes	1 serv	290	4	17	15	29	2	830
Cinnamon Twists	1 serv	170	1	7	0	26	1	200
Crunchwrap Supreme	1	560	17	24	35	68	5	1430
Crunchwrap Supreme Spicy Chicken	1	540	19	24	35	67	4	1360
Crunchy Taco	1	170	8	25	10	13	3	350
Crunchy Taco Supreme	1	210	9	10	25	15	3	370
Empanada Caramel Apple	1	290	3	14	5	37	1	300
Enchirito Beef	1	360	18	17	50	34	7	1420
Enchirito Chicken	1	340	22	13	50	33	6	1450
Fresco Border Bowl Zesty Chicken w/o Dressing	1 serv	350	19	8	25	51	10	1600

FOOD	PORTION	CALS	PROT	FAT	CHOL	CARB	FIBER	SOD
Fresco Burrito Bean	1	330	12	7	0	54	9	1200
Fresco Burrito Fiesta Chicken	1	330	16	8	25	48	3	1240
Fresco Burrito Supreme Chicken	1	330	18	8	25	49	7	1360
Fresco Burrito Supreme Steak	1	330	16	8	20	48	7	1250
Fresco Crunchy Taco	1	150	7	8	20	13	3	370
Fresco Soft Taco Grilled Steak	1	160	10	5	20	20	2	550
Fresco Soft Taco Ranchero Chicken	1	170	12	4	25	21	3	730
Fresco Soft Taco Beef	1	180	8	2	20	21	3	650
Gordita Baja Beef	1	340	13	19	35	29	4	780
Gordita Baja Chicken	1	320	17	16	40	28	3	800
Gordita Baja Steak	1	320	15	17	35	27	3	690
Gordita Nacho Cheese Beef	1	300	12	14	25	31	3	770
Gordita Nacho Cheese Chicken	1	280	16	11	25	29	2	800
Gordita Nacho Cheese Steak	1	270	14	12	20	29	2	680
Gordita Supreme Beef	1	310	14	16	40	29	3	620
Gordita Supreme Chicken	1	290	17	12	45	28	2	650
Gordita Supreme Steak	1	290	15	13	40	28	2	530
Guacamole Side	1 serv	70	1	5	0	5	2	180
Mexican Pizza	1	530	20	30	40	46	6	1000
Mexican Rice	1 serv	180	6	7	15	23	1	790
MexiMelt	1 serv	260	15	14	40	22	3	860
Nacho Supreme	1 serv	440	12	26	35	41	7	800
Nachos	1 serv	330	4	21	5	32	2	530
Nachos Bellgrande	1 serv	770	19	44	35	77	12	1280
Pintos 'n Cheese	1 serv	160	9	6	15	19	7	670
Quesadilla Cheese	1	470	19	26	50	39	2	1100
Quesadilla Chicken	1	520	28	28	75	40	3	1420
Quesadilla Steak	1	520	26	28	70	39	3	1300
Salsa Side	1 serv	15	0	0	0	3	0	160
Soft Taco Grande	1	430	19	20	45	43	5	1440
Soft Taco Grilled Steak	1	270	12	16	35	20	2	660

FOOD	PORTION	CALS	PROT	FAT	CHOL	CARB	FIBER	SOD
Soft Taco Ranchero Chicken	1	270	14	14	35	21	2	820
Soft Taco Supreme Beef	1	250	11	13	40	23	3	650
Sour Cream Side	1 serv	80	1	7	25	3	0	30
Taco Double Decker	1	320	14	13	25	38	6	810
Taco Double Decker Supreme	1	370	14	17	40	40	7	820
Taco Spicy Chicken	1	170	10	8	25	20	2	580
Taco Salad Express	1	610	25	32	65	56	14	1420
Taco Salad Fiesta	1	840	30	45	65	80	15	1780
Taco Salad Fiesta Chicken	1	790	37	38	75	77	13	1830
Taco Salad Fiesta Chicken w/o Shell	1	430	30	18	75	38	11	1560
Taco Salad w/o Shell Fiesta	1	470	23	24	65	41	13	1510
Taquitos Grilled Chicken	1 serv	310	18	11	40	37	2	980
Taquitos Steak Grilled	1 serv	310	16	11	35	36	2	870
Tostada	1	240	11	10	15	27	7	730

TACO JOHN'S
DESSERTS

FOOD	PORTION	CALS	PROT	FAT	CHOL	CARB	FIBER	SOD
Choco Taco	1 serv	300	4	15	15	38	1	110
Churro	1 serv	230	2	11	10	31	1	120

MAIN MENU SELECTIONS

FOOD	PORTION	CALS	PROT	FAT	CHOL	CARB	FIBER	SOD
Burrito Chicken & Potato	1	460	18	19	35	54	8	1470
Burrito Meat & Potato	1	490	15	23	30	55	9	1190
Crispy Taco	1 serv	180	9	10	25	13	3	270
Mexican Rice	1 serv	250	5	5	0	45	2	860
Potato Oles Bravo	1 serv	580	9	36	20	55	6	1760
Potato Oles w/ Nacho Cheese	1 serv	550	7	35	10	52	5	2000
Refried Beans	1 serv	400	18	14	15	50	11	1110
Sierra Taco Beef	1	430	17	23	45	38	4	980
Sierra Taco Chicken	1	390	21	17	50	37	3	1350
Texas Chili	1 serv	270	15	12	35	26	4	1400

SALAD DRESSINGS AND TOPPINGS

FOOD	PORTION	CALS	PROT	FAT	CHOL	CARB	FIBER	SOD
Jalapenos	1 serv (2 oz)	15	1	1	0	3	1	950
Sour Cream	1 serv (2 oz)	120	2	12	25	2	0	30
Super Hot Sauce	1 serv (1 oz)	10	1	0	0	2	tr	25

FOOD	PORTION	CALS	PROT	FAT	CHOL	CARB	FIBER	SOD
TACOTIME								
DESSERTS								
Churro Plain	1 (1.5 oz)	205	2	15	20	16	0	1440
Churro w/ Cinnamon & Sugar	1 (2 oz)	245	2	15	20	26	0	1440
Crustos	1 serv	294	6	6	0	58	3	273
Empanada Apple	1 (4 oz)	234	4	7	0	40	2	201
Empanada Cherry	1 (4 oz)	240	4	7	0	41	2	190
Empanada Pumpkin	1 (4 oz)	256	6	8	23	42	2	198
MAIN MENU SELECTIONS								
Burrito Big Juan Seasoned Ground Beef	1 (13 oz)	651	30	28	73	71	12	2658
Burrito Big Juan Shredded Beef	1 (13 oz)	633	33	25	64	67	10	2616
Burrito Big Juan Chicken	1 (13 oz)	594	35	19	78	68	10	2435
Burrito Casita Chicken	1 (12 oz)	494	34	18	85	43	5	2338
Burrito Casita Seasoned Ground Beef	1 (12 oz)	552	29	25	80	46	6	2561
Burrito Casita Shredded Beef	1 (12 oz)	533	31	25	91	42	5	2520
Burrito Chicken & Black Bean	1 (10 oz)	478	30	16	60	51	9	1219
Burrito Chicken BLT	1 (10 oz)	721	41	41	99	44	8	1642
Burrito Chicken Ranchero	1 (10.8 oz)	654	36	32	80	52	7	1341
Burrito Crisp Chicken	1 (5.5 oz)	336	27	10	42	32	2	566
Burrito Crisp Meat	1 (5.8 oz)	450	23	22	49	36	4	893
Burrito Crisp Pinto Bean	1 (6 oz)	394	13	16	12	50	6	2172
Burrito Soft Meat	1 (6.7 oz)	426	23	16	46	43	8	1095
Burrito Soft Pinto Bean	1 (6.7 oz)	377	14	11	15	54	10	2093
Burrito Veggie	1 (11 oz)	534	18	18	25	74	12	2545
Cheddar Fries	1 sm (6 oz)	374	8	26	23	29	3	877
Cheddar Melt	1 (2.8 oz)	250	11	12	31	25	4	472
Mexi-Fries	1 sm (5 oz)	290	3	19	0	29	2	740
Mexi-Rice	1 serv (4 oz)	87	2	1	0	19	0	401
Nachos Grande	1 serv (16.5 oz)	1132	39	57	90	114	11	4085
Refritos w/ Chips	1 serv (7 oz)	304	14	11	23	35	6	3252
Refritos w/o Chips	1 serv (6.7 oz)	285	13	11	23	32	6	3251

FOOD	PORTION	CALS	PROT	FAT	CHOL	CARB	FIBER	SOD
Stuffed Fries	1 sm (5 oz)	321	7	7	14	29	3	705
Taco Crisp Seasoned Ground Beef	1 (4.3 oz)	225	15	12	40	12	2	512
Taco Super Soft Chicken	1 (11 oz)	540	35	18	77	56	10	2354
Taco Super Soft Seasoned Ground Beef	1 (11 oz)	598	30	25	72	59	12	2577
Taco Super Soft Shredded Beef	1 (11 oz)	579	32	25	84	55	10	2535
Taco Value Soft	1 (5.3 oz)	314	18	13	40	28	6	800
Taco ½ Lb Shredded Beef	1 (9 oz)	440	28	18	65	42	7	1218
Taco ½ Lb Soft Chicken	1 (9 oz)	401	30	11	58	43	7	1037
Taco ½ Lb Soft Seasoned Ground Beef	1 (9 oz)	459	25	18	53	46	9	1260
Taco Chips	1 serv (2 oz)	150	3	3	0	27	1	7
SALAD DRESSINGS AND TOPPINGS								
Cheddar Cheese Milk	1 serv (2 oz)	223	14	18	61	1	0	364
Dressing Chipotle Ranch	1 serv (1 oz)	165	1	18	6	1	0	157
Dressing Ranch	1 serv (1 oz)	181	1	20	7	1	–	187
Dressing Thousand Island	1 serv (1 oz)	132	0	12	5	5	0	369
Guacamole	1 serv (1 oz)	50	0	5	0	2	1	125
Salsa Nuevo	1 serv (1 oz)	8	0	0	0	2	0	131
Salsa Verde	1 serv (1 oz)	6	0	0	0	2	0	149
Sour Cream	1 serv (1.5 oz)	85	1	7	28	1	0	14
SALADS								
Taco Chicken	1 reg (9.2 oz)	351	27	15	58	24	2	899
Taco Seasoned Ground Beef	1 reg (7.8 oz)	396	22	23	53	24	4	860
Taco Shredded Beef	1 reg (7.8 oz)	377	25	22	65	21	2	819
Tostada Delight Chicken	1 (10.5 oz)	565	37	29	100	36	4	2221
Tostada Delight Seasoned Ground Beef	1 (10.5 oz)	623	32	36	95	39	6	2444
Tostada Delight Shredded Beef	1 (10.5 oz)	604	35	36	107	35	5	2402
TASTI D-LITE								
Vanilla	1 sm (4 oz)	40	2	tr	7	7	3	25

FOOD	PORTION	CALS	PROT	FAT	CHOL	CARB	FIBER	SOD
TCBY								
FROZEN YOGURT AND SORBET								
Hand Scooped Butter Pecan Perfection	½ cup	110	4	5	10	14	tr	90
Hand Scooped Chocolate Chocolate Swirl	½ cup	120	4	4	15	19	tr	50
Hand Scooped Chocolate Chunk Cookie Dough	½ cup	160	3	6	15	24	0	75
Hand Scooped Cookies & Cream	½ cup	140	3	4	10	22	0	75
Hand Scooped Cotton Candy	½ cup	120	3	4	15	20	0	60
Hand Scooped Mint Chocolate Chunk	½ cup	140	3	5	10	22	0	55
Hand Scooped Mocha Almond	½ cup	150	3	5	10	22	tr	95
Hand Scooped No Sugar Added Chocolate Chocolate Swirl	½ cup	90	4	1	0	23	6	70
Hand Scooped No Sugar Added Vanilla	½ cup	80	4	1	0	19	5	60
Hand Scooped No Sugar Added Vanilla Fudge Brownie	½ cup	100	4	2	10	22	5	80
Hand Scooped Pralines & Cream	½ cup	140	3	5	10	23	0	80
Hand Scooped Psychedelic Sorbet	½ cup	290	0	0	0	75	0	30
Hand Scooped Rainbow Cream	½ cup	120	3	4	15	20	0	60
Hand Scooped Rocky Road	½ cup	220	3	7	5	36	1	25
Hand Scooped Strawberries & Cream	½ cup	120	2	3	10	21	0	50
Hand Scooped Vanilla Chocolate Chunk	½ cup	140	3	5	10	22	0	55
Hand Scooped Vanilla Bean	½ cup	120	3	4	15	19	0	60
Soft Serve Frozen Yogurt All Flavors 96% Fat Free	½ cup	140	4	3	15	23	0	60
Soft Serve Frozen Yogurt All Flavors Nonfat	½ cup	110	4	0	<5	23	0	60

FOOD	PORTION	CALS	PROT	FAT	CHOL	CARB	FIBER	SOD
Soft Serve Frozen Yogurt All Flavors Nonfat No Sugar Added	½ cup	90	4	0	<5	20	0	35
Soft Serve Frozen Yogurt Low Carb	½ cup	110	3	7	25	16	7	60
Soft Serve Sorbet All Flavors Nonfat Nondairy	½ cup	100	0	0	0	24	0	30
SMOOTHIES								
Berrylicious	1 (16 oz)	290	3	3	10	65	3	65
Black 'N' Blueberry	1 (16 oz)	280	3	3	10	63	2	65
Mando Mango	1 (16 oz)	310	3	3	10	70	2	65
Mango Tango	1 (16 oz)	330	2	3	10	76	2	65
Mangolada	1 (16 oz)	340	3	6	10	70	2	100
Pina Paradise	1 (16 oz)	350	3	12	10	58	1	170
Pink Pineapple	1 (16 oz)	340	3	9	10	63	2	135
Straight Up Strawberry	1 (16 oz)	280	3	4	10	44	1	65
Strawberry Bonanza	1 (16 oz)	320	3	4	10	74	2	65
Strawberry Fling	1 (16 oz)	340	3	3	10	78	2	65

TIM HORTONS
BAKED SELECTIONS

FOOD	PORTION	CALS	PROT	FAT	CHOL	CARB	FIBER	SOD
Bagel Blueberry	1	270	10	1	0	55	2	470
Bagel Cinnamon Raisin	1	270	10	1	0	55	3	350
Bagel Everything	1	280	10	2	0	53	3	460
Bagel Flax Seed	1	290	10	5	0	53	4	520
Bagel Onion	1	260	9	2	0	53	3	460
Bagel Plain	1	260	9	2	0	52	2	450
Bagel Poppy Seed	1	270	9	2	0	53	3	440
Bagel Sesame Seed	1	270	9	3	0	53	3	430
Bagel Sun Dried Tomato	1	310	9	4	0	59	2	550
Bagel Twelve Grain	1	330	10	9	0	52	6	580
Cinnamon Roll Frosted	1	470	4	25	0	57	2	380
Cinnamon Roll Glazed	1	420	4	23	0	50	2	360
Cookie Caramel Chocolate Pecan	1	230	3	11	20	32	1	290
Cookie Chocolate Chip	1	230	3	9	20	34	1	260
Cookie Oatmeal Raisin Spice	1	220	3	8	25	35	1	200
Cookie Peanut Butter Chocolate Chunk	1	260	5	15	20	28	2	260

FOOD	PORTION	CALS	PROT	FAT	CHOL	CARB	FIBER	SOD
Cookie Triple Chocolate	1	250	3	13	30	31	2	220
Cookie White Chocolate Macadamia Nut	1	240	3	12	20	31	1	270
Croissant Butter	1	340	7	18	0	38	1	380
Croissant Cheese	1	370	9	20	15	37	0	410
Danish Chocolate	1	430	4	24	10	51	1	220
Danish Maple Pecan	1	380	4	20	20	46	1	230
Danish Cherry Cheese	1	330	5	13	15	46	1	230
Donut Apple Fritter	1	300	4	11	0	49	2	350
Donut Chocolate Dip	1	210	4	9	0	30	1	190
Donut Chocolate Glazed	1	260	4	10	5	39	2	300
Donut Honey Dip	1	210	4	8	0	33	1	190
Donut Maple Dip	1	210	4	8	0	31	1	200
Donut Old Fashion Glazed	1	320	3	19	10	35	1	230
Donut Old Fashion Plain	1	260	3	19	10	20	1	230
Donut Sour Cream Plain	1	270	3	17	10	27	1	230
Donut Walnut Crunch	1	360	4	23	5	35	1	320
Donut Filled Angel Cream	1	310	4	13	0	46	1	220
Donut Filled Blueberry	1	230	4	8	0	36	1	210
Donut Filled Boston Cream	1	250	4	9	0	38	1	260
Donut Filled Canadian Maple	1	260	4	9	0	41	1	260
Donut Filled Strawberry	1	230	4	8	0	36	1	220
Honey Cruller	1	320	1	19	50	37	0	220
Muffin Blueberry	1	330	4	11	15	54	2	580
Muffin Blueberry Bran	1	300	6	10	10	53	5	770
Muffin Carrot Wheat	1	400	6	19	10	55	4	580
Muffin Chocolate Chip	1	430	5	16	15	69	2	580
Muffin Cranberry Blueberry Bran	1	290	5	10	10	51	5	710
Muffin Cranberry Fruit	1	350	4	12	15	59	2	560
Muffin Fruit Explosion	1	360	4	11	15	61	2	550
Muffin Raisin Bran	1	360	6	10	10	65	6	790
Muffin Strawberry Sensation	1	350	4	11	15	61	1	580
Muffin Low Fat Blueberry	1	290	4	3	0	62	2	750
Muffin Low Fat Cranberry	1	290	4	3	0	62	2	750
Tea Biscuit Plain	1	250	5	9	0	35	1	590
Tea Biscuit Raisin	1	290	6	10	0	45	2	590
Timbits Apple Fritter	1	50	1	2	0	9	0	55

FOOD	PORTION	CALS	PROT	FAT	CHOL	CARB	FIBER	SOD
Timbits Chocolate Glazed	1	70	1	3	0	10	0	75
Timbits Honey Dip	1	60	1	2	0	9	0	50
Timbits Old Fashion Plain	1	70	1	5	5	5	0	60
Timbits Filled Banana Cream	1	60	1	2	0	9	0	65
Timbits Filled Lemon	1	60	1	2	0	9	0	50
Timbits Filled Strawberry	1	60	1	2	0	10	0	55
Timbits Filled Strawberry	1	60	1	2	0	10	0	50
BEVERAGES								
Cafe Mocha	1 (10 oz)	160	1	7	0	25	1	160
Cappuccino Iced	1 (12 oz)	300	0	15	50	41	0	85
Coffee Decaffeinated + Sugar & Cream	1 (10 oz)	75	1	4	15	9	0	15
Coffee + Sugar & Cream	1 (10 oz)	75	1	4	15	9	0	15
English Toffee	1 (10 oz)	220	3	6	0	40	0	240
Flavor Shot	1 serv	5	0	0	0	1	0	0
French Vanilla	1 (10 oz)	240	4	7	0	39	0	240
Hot Chocolate	1 (10 oz)	240	2	6	0	45	2	360
Hot Smoothie	1 (10 oz)	260	5	10	5	39	2	200
Iced Cappuccino w/ Milk	1 (12 oz)	180	3	2	5	39	0	45
Tea + Sugar & Milk	1 (10 oz)	50	1	1	5	10	0	20
CREAM CHEESE								
Garden Vegetable	1.5 oz	120	2	11	45	3	1	230
Light Plain	1.5 oz	60	4	5	20	3	0	200
Plain	1.5 oz	130	2	12	50	2	0	180
Strawberry	1.5 oz	120	6	10	40	6	0	160
SANDWICHES								
B.L.T.	1	450	18	18	30	53	2	850
Breakfast Bacon Egg Cheese	1	410	16	25	185	31	1	760
Breakfast Egg Cheese	1	360	13	21	175	30	1	680
Breakfast Sausage Egg Cheese	1	520	19	37	205	30	1	940
Chicken Salad	1	380	21	9	35	55	3	890
Egg Salad	1	390	17	13	245	52	2	780
Ham & Swiss	1	440	28	12	50	56	3	1690
Toasted Chicken Club	1	460	30	7	50	70	2	1170
Turkey Breast	1	390	27	5	10	59	4	1480

FOOD	PORTION	CALS	PROT	FAT	CHOL	CARB	FIBER	SOD
SOUPS								
Beef Stew	1 serv (10 oz)	236	17	8	30	25	3	1208
Chicken Noodle	1 serv (10 oz)	120	5	2	20	18	1	880
Chili	1 serv (10 oz)	300	21	16	50	18	5	920
Country Field Mushroom	1 serv (10 oz)	150	3	3	0	28	1	1080
Cream Of Broccoli	1 serv (10 oz)	160	6	9	20	16	1	820
Hearty Vegetable	1 serv (10 oz)	70	4	0	0	14	3	1060
Minestrone	1 serv (10 oz)	120	4	3	0	24	2	940
Potato Bacon	1 serv (10 oz)	180	3	6	0	30	2	1260
Split Pea w/ Ham	1 serv (10 oz)	150	8	3	5	27	5	970
Turkey Rice	1 serv (10 oz)	120	3	2	0	21	1	1000
Vegetable Beef Barley	1 serv (10 oz)	110	4	2	5	21	2	980
YOGURT								
Low Fat Creamy Vanilla w/ Berries	1 (6 oz)	160	4	3	10	32	2	80
Low Fat Strawberry w/ Berries	1 (6 oz)	150	4	3	10	28	2	75
T.J. CINNAMONS								
Chocolate Twist	1	250	4	12	5	34	2	110
Cinnamon Twist	1	280	3	14	5	33	1	190
Mocha Chill w/ Whipped Cream	1 (12.5 oz)	306	11	7	29	48	1	214
Mocha Chill w/o Whipped Cream	1 (12.5 oz)	264	11	4	17	48	1	214
Original Roll w/o Icing	1	507	10	10	7	73	4	373
Pecan Sticky Bun	1	688	12	22	7	91	5	420
TJ Icing	1 serv (1 oz)	117	1	5	8	18	0	50

FOOD	PORTION	CALS	PROT	FAT	CHOL	CARB	FIBER	SOD
WENDY'S								
BEVERAGES								
Chocolate Milk 1%	8 oz	170	8	3	15	28	0	200
Coca-Cola	1 med (12 oz)	140	0	0	0	37	0	1
Dasani Water	1 bottle	0	0	0	0	0	0	0
Diet Coke	1 med (11 oz)	0	0	0	0	0	0	15
Frosty	1 sm (8 oz)	330	8	8	35	56	0	150
Milk 2%	8 oz	120	8	5	20	13	0	135
Sprite	1 med (12 oz)	130	0	0	0	34	0	30
CHILDREN'S MENU SELECTIONS								
French Fries	1 serv (3.2 oz)	280	3	14	0	37	3	270
Kid's Meal Cheeseburger	1	320	17	13	40	34	1	820
Kid's Meal Ham & Cheese	1 serv	240	14	6	30	32	1	890
Kid's Meal Hamburger	1	270	15	9	30	33	1	600
Kid's Meal Turkey & Cheese	1 serv	250	14	6	25	34	1	910
Kids'Meal Chicken Nuggets	4 pieces	180	8	11	25	10	0	390
SALAD DRESSINGS AND TOPPINGS								
Ancho Chipotle Ranch	1 pkg	110	1	10	15	4	0	330
Blue Cheese	1 pkg	260	2	27	35	3	0	460
Buttery Best Spread	1 pkg	50	0	6	0	0	0	90
Caesar	1 pkg	120	1	13	20	1	0	220
Cheddar Cheese Shredded	2 tbsp	70	4	6	15	1	0	110
Creamy Ranch	1 pkg	230	1	23	15	5	0	450
Creamy Ranch Reduced Fat	1 pkg	100	1	8	15	6	1	450
Crispy Noodles	1 pkg	60	1	2	0	10	0	170
Croutons Homestyle Garlic	1 pkg	70	2	3	0	9	0	125
Dipping Sauce Deli Honey Mustard	1 pkg	170	1	16	15	6	0	220
Dipping Sauce Heartland Ranch	1 pkg	200	0	22	15	1	0	280
Dipping Sauce Spicy Southwest Chipotle	1 pkg	150	1	15	25	5	0	180
Dipping Sauce Sweet & Sour Hawaiian	1 pkg	70	0	0	0	17	0	350
Dipping Sauce Wild Buffalo Ranch	1 pkg	180	0	19	10	2	0	420

FOOD	PORTION	CALS	PROT	FAT	CHOL	CARB	FIBER	SOD
French Fat Free	1 pkg	80	0	0	0	19	0	210
Granola Topping	1 pkg	110	2	5	0	15	1	0
Honey Mustard	1 pkg	280	1	26	25	11	0	370
Honey Mustard Low Fat	1 pkg	110	0	3	0	21	0	340
Hot Chili Seasoning	1 pkg	5	0	0	0	2	0	270
Italian Vinaigrette	1 pkg	140	0	12	0	9	0	400
Ketchup	1 tsp	7	0	0	0	2	0	80
Mayonnaise	1 tsp	30	0	3	5	1	0	60
Mustard	½ tsp	5	0	0	0	0	0	50
Nuggets Sauce Barbeque	1 pkg	45	1	0	0	10	0	170
Nuggets Sauce Honey Mustard	1 pkg	130	0	12	10	6	0	220
Nuggets Sauce Sweet & Sour	1 pkg	50	0	0	0	13	0	120
Oriental Sesame	1 pkg	190	1	11	0	21	0	490
Roasted Almonds	1 pkg	130	5	11	0	4	2	70
Saltines	2	25	0	1	0	4	0	95
Sour Cream Reduced Fat	1 pkg	45	1	4	10	2	0	30
Thousand Island	1 pkg	260	1	25	20	8	0	440
Tortilla Strips	1 pkg	110	2	5	0	13	1	160
SALADS								
Caesar Chicken w/o Dressing & Croutons	1 serv	180	27	5	70	9	4	550
Ceasar Side Salad w/o Dressing & Croutons	1 serv	70	5	5	15	3	2	135
Chicken BLT w/o Dressing & Croutons	1 serv	340	34	18	105	12	4	840
Mandarin Chicken w/o Dressing	1 serv	170	23	2	60	18	3	480
Side Salad w/o Dressing	1	35	1	0	0	8	2	25
Southwest Taco w/o Dressing Tortilla Strip & Sour Cream	1 serv	440	30	22	80	32	9	1100
SANDWICHES AND SIDES								
Baked Potato Plain	1	270	7	0	0	61	7	25
Baked Potato w/ Sour Cream & Chives	1 serv	320	9	4	10	63	7	55
Big Bacon Classic	1	580	35	29	95	46	3	1400
Chicken Nuggets	5 pieces	220	10	14	35	13	0	490
Chili	1 sm (8 oz)	220	17	6	35	23	5	780

FOOD	PORTION	CALS	PROT	FAT	CHOL	CARB	FIBER	SOD
Classic Single w/ Everything	1	420	25	19	65	37	2	900
French Fries	1 med (5 oz)	440	5	21	0	58	5	430
Frescata Black Forest Ham & Swiss	1	480	28	20	65	50	4	1490
Frescata Club	1	440	23	16	50	50	4	1530
Frescata Roasted Turkey & Basil Pesto	1	420	21	16	40	50	4	1530
Frescata Roasted Turkey & Swiss	1	490	26	21	60	52	4	1530
Hamburger	1	280	15	9	30	34	1	600
Homestyle Chicken Strips	3 pieces	410	28	18	60	33	0	1740
Jr. Bacon Cheeseburger	1	370	19	17	50	34	2	750
Jr. BBQ Cheeseburger	1	330	17	13	40	36	1	800
Jr. Cheeseburger	1	320	17	13	40	34	1	820
Jr. Cheeseburger Deluxe	1	360	18	16	45	37	2	880
Mandarin Orange Cup	1 serv	80	1	0	0	19	1	15
Sandwich Crispy Chicken	1	380	18	15	35	43	1	810
Sandwich Spicy Chicken Fillet	1	510	29	19	55	57	2	1480
Sandwich Ultimate Chicken Grill	1	360	31	7	75	44	2	1100
Yogurt Low Fat Strawberry	1 pkg	140	6	2	5	27	0	85

WETZEL'S PRETZELS

Original w/ Butter	1	320	–	4	10	–	2	<500
Original w/o Butter	1	280	–	1	0	–	2	<500

WHATABURGER
BEVERAGES

Barq's Root Beet	1 sm (16 oz)	220	0	0	0	61	0	28
Cherry Coke	1 sm (16 oz)	210	0	0	0	56	0	9
Coca-Cola	1 sm (16 oz)	207	0	0	0	56	0	5
Coffee	1 sm (8 oz)	5	0	0	0	1	0	9
Coffee Decafe	1 sm (8 oz)	5	0	0	0	1	0	21
Diet Coke	1 sm (16 oz)	0	0	0	0	0	0	19
Dr Pepper	1 sm (16 oz)	190	0	0	0	51	0	47

FOOD	PORTION	CALS	PROT	FAT	CHOL	CARB	FIBER	SOD
Fanta Orange	1 sm (16 oz)	210	0	0	0	56	0	0
Fanta Strawberry	1 sm (16 oz)	230	0	0	0	61	0	0
Iced Tea Sweetened	1 (34 oz)	430	0	0	0	114	0	0
Iced Tea Unsweetened	1 sm (19 oz)	0	0	0	0	0	0	0
Lemonade Hi-C Poppin' Pink	1 sm (16 oz)	200	0	0	0	51	0	84
Malt Chocolate	1 sm (16 oz)	670	13	15	59	123	2	297
Malt Strawberry	1 sm (16 oz)	670	12	15	59	123	0	250
Malt Vanilla	1 sm (16 oz)	600	13	17	66	98	0	250
Milk Reduced Fat	8 oz	120	8	5	20	11	0	115
Orange Juice Tropicana	1 (10 oz)	140	3	0	0	33	0	0
Powerade Fruit Punch	1 sm (16 oz)	130	0	0	0	33	0	107
Shake Chocolate	1 sm (16 oz)	630	14	16	62	111	2	281
Shake Strawberry	1 sm (16 oz)	630	13	16	62	111	0	234
Shake Vanilla	1 sm (16 oz)	560	14	17	69	87	0	243
Sprite	1 sm (16 oz)	200	0	0	0	51	0	47
CHILDREN'S MENU SELECTIONS								
Kid's Meal Chicken Strips	1 serv	770	22	51	30	53	2	720
Kid's Meal Justaburger	1 serv	570	19	29	33	60	3	862
DESSERTS								
Apple Pie A La Mode	1 serv	520	10	20	37	75	2	413
Apple Pie Hot	1	230	3	11	0	29	2	285
Cinnamon Roll	1	400	6	7	15	80	2	380
Cookie Chocolate Chunk	1 (2 oz)	230	2	11	35	33	1	150
Cookie White Chocolate Chunk Macadamia	1 (2 oz)	250	3	14	30	30	0	130
Peach Pie Al La Mode	1 serv	570	10	23	37	82	2	253
MAIN MENU SELECTIONS								
Biscuit	1	300	5	17	0	32	1	644
Biscuit Honey Butter Chicken	1	610	14	38	25	51	1	1072
Biscuit Sandwich Bacon Egg & Cheese	1	500	16	32	232	33	1	1231
Biscuit Sandwich Egg & Cheese	1	450	13	28	224	33	1	1028
Biscuit Sandwich Sausage Egg & Cheese	1	690	26	49	247	33	1	1553
Biscuit w/ Bacon	1	355	8	20	8	32	1	847
Biscuit w/ Gravy	1	530	9	36	12	52	1	1823
Biscuit w/ Sausage	1	540	18	37	23	32	1	1169

FOOD	PORTION	CALS	PROT	FAT	CHOL	CARB	FIBER	SOD
Breakfast Platter w/ Bacon	1 serv	730	24	45	460	53	2	1462
Breakfast Platter w/ Sausage	1 serv	930	34	62	475	53	2	1784
Breakfast On A Bun w/ Bacon	1	380	17	22	232	29	1	942
Breakfast On A Bun w/ Sausage	1	570	27	39	247	29	1	1264
Chicken Strip w/ Gravy	4	840	37	54	62	53	0	1858
Chicken Strips	1	200	9	12	15	11	0	359
French Fries	1 sm	260	4	13	0	31	2	26
Gravy White Peppered	1 serv	60	0	5	0	8	0	421
Hashbrown Sticks	4	200	2	12	0	20	1	368
Justaburger	1	329	15	16	33	30	1	862
Onion Rings	1 med	420	5	28	24	36	3	404
Pancakes Plain	1 serv	580	17	8	1	112	5	2170
Pancakes w/ Bacon	1 serv	630	20	12	9	112	5	2373
Pancakes w/ Sausage	1 serv	820	30	20	24	112	5	2695
Sandwich Chicken Strip Honey BBQ	1	1110	45	59	76	102	3	2759
Sandwich Chicken Strip Junior Honey BBQ	1	720	30	41	60	59	1	1904
Sandwich Egg	1	330	14	18	224	29	1	739
Sandwich Grilled Chicken	1	450	33	18	56	45	6	1101
Taquito Sausage & Egg	1	410	17	24	348	27	3	909
Taquito w/ Bacon & Egg	1	370	17	21	344	27	3	932
Taquito w/ Bacon Egg & Cheese	1	420	19	24	356	27	3	1157
Taquito w/ Potato & Egg	1	430	15	23	336	37	3	912
Taquito w/ Potato Egg & Cheese	1	470	17	27	347	37	3	1137
Taquito w/ Sausage Egg & Cheese	1	450	19	28	359	27	3	1134
Texas Toast	1 slice	180	4	8	0	25	1	230
Whataburger	1	640	30	32	65	61	3	1522
Whataburger Double Meat	1	890	47	51	129	61	3	1770
Whataburger Jr.	1	330	15	16	33	32	1	865
Whataburger Triple Meat	1	1140	65	70	192	61	3	2019
Whataburger w/ Bacon & Cheese	1	800	40	45	98	62	3	2257
Whatacatch	1	480	17	30	41	42	2	1013

FOOD	PORTION	CALS	PROT	FAT	CHOL	CARB	FIBER	SOD
Whatacatch Dinner	1 serv	1095	29	92	113	161	8	1661
Whatachick'n	1	530	32	20	46	61	7	1491
SALADS								
Chicken Strips	1 serv	570	21	38	30	34	4	756
Garden Salad	1	60	3	0	0	12	4	56
Grilled Chicken	1 serv	230	23	7	50	19	4	676

WHITE CASTLE
BEVERAGES

FOOD	PORTION	CALS	PROT	FAT	CHOL	CARB	FIBER	SOD
Barq's Red Cream Soda	1 sm (21 oz)	260	0	0	0	69	0	40
Barq's Root Beer	1 sm (21 oz)	250	0	0	0	68	0	55
Coca-Cola	1 sm (21 oz)	220	0	0	0	61	0	10
Coffee Black	1 sm (12 oz)	<5	0	0	0	1	0	0
Crave Cooler Coke	1 sm (21 oz)	150	0	0	0	41	0	15
Diet Coke	1 sm (21 oz)	0	0	0	0	0	0	20
Fanta Orange	1 sm (21 oz)	240	0	0	0	64	0	0
Hi-C Flashing Fruit Punch	1 sm (21 oz)	240	0	0	0	63	0	20
Hot Chocolate	1 sm (12 oz)	220	1	6	0	40	tr	300
Hot Tea	1 sm (12 oz)	0	0	0	0	0	0	0
Ice Tea Unsweetened	1 sm (21 oz)	0	0	0	0	0	0	30
Iced Tea Sweetened w/ Lemon	1 sm (21 oz)	170	0	0	0	46	0	20
Iced Tea Sweetened w/ Lemon	1 sm (16 oz)	170	0	0	0	46	0	20
Lemonade Raspberry	1 sm (21 oz)	290	0	0	0	78	0	5
Pibb Xtra	1 sm (21 oz)	220	0	0	0	59	0	30
Powerade Mountain Blast	1 sm (21 oz)	140	0	0	0	38	0	139
Sprite	1 sm (21 oz)	220	0	0	0	59	0	50
MAIN MENU SELECTIONS								
Cheeseburger	1	170	7	9	15	15	tr	330
Cheeseburger Bacon	1	200	10	11	20	15	tr	480
Cheeseburger Bacon Double	1	370	19	22	45	23	1	880
Cheeseburger Double	1	300	14	17	30	23	1	590
Cheeseburger Jalapeno	1	180	8	10	20	15	tr	380
Cheeseburger Jalapeno Double	1	320	15	19	40	23	1	680
Chicken Rings	6	210	18	23	80	15	0	670
Clam Strips	1 reg	250	8	22	20	5	0	620
Fish Nibblers	1 reg	280	19	16	30	24	5	820

FOOD	PORTION	CALS	PROT	FAT	CHOL	CARB	FIBER	SOD
French Fries	1 reg	310	4	15	0	39	4	250
Mozzarella Cheese Sticks	3	250	10	14	20	22	1	750
Onion Chips	1 reg	480	7	23	0	62	2	670
Sandwich Chicken Breast w/ Cheese	1	200	12	8	25	21	1	720
Sandwich Chicken Ring	1	180	7	8	35	19	tr	380
Sandwich Chicken Ring w/ Cheese	1	200	8	10	40	19	tr	500
Sandwich Fish w/ Cheese	1	180	9	8	25	19	tr	430
White Castle	1	140	6	7	10	14	tr	210
White Castle Double	1	250	11	13	20	22	1	340
SAUCES AND SPREADS								
Dressing Ranch	1 serv (1 oz)	150	0	17	15	0	0	210
Ketchup	1 pkg	10	0	0	0	3	0	100
Lemon Juice	1 pkg	0	0	0	0	0	0	0
Mayonnaise	1 pkg	60	0	7	5	0	0	55
Sauce BBQ	1 serv (1 oz)	35	0	1	0	8	0	400
Sauce Hot	1 pkg	0	0	0	0	0	0	170
Sauce Marinara	1 serv (1 oz)	15	0	0	0	4	0	260
Sauce Seafood	1 serv (1 oz)	30	0	0	0	7	0	330
Sauce Tartar	1 pkg	30	0	3	0	2	0	115
Sauce Zesty Zing	1 serv (1 oz)	110	0	11	15	3	0	190
Sauce Fat Free Honey Mustard	1 serv (1 oz)	50	0	0	0	12	0	140

WINCHELL'S DONUTS

FOOD	PORTION	CALS	PROT	FAT	CHOL	CARB	FIBER	SOD
Chocolate Bar	1	240	4	16	–	29	–	125
Chocolate Round	1	240	4	16	–	29	–	125
Chocolate Twist	1	240	4	16	–	29	–	125
Croissant	1	260	5	17	–	28	–	280
Glazed Round	1	230	2	15	–	27	–	120
Glazed Twist	1	230	2	15	–	27	–	120
Iced Chocolate	1	230	2	15	–	28	–	220
Traditional	1	215	2	14	–	26	–	215

ZOUP!
DESSERTS

FOOD	PORTION	CALS	PROT	FAT	CHOL	CARB	FIBER	SOD
Cookie Chocolate Chunk	1	410	4	19	–	57	1	–
Cookie Peanut Butter	1	420	6	21	–	43	1	–
SANDWICHES								
Pesto Three Cheese	1	720	44	42	–	42	2	–

FOOD	PORTION	CALS	PROT	FAT	CHOL	CARB	FIBER	SOD
Tuna Melt	1	600	50	23	–	42	2	–
Wrap American Farm	½	435	13	29	–	30	5	–
Wrap Asian	½	615	28	33	–	54	7	–
Wrap Chicken Caesar	½	505	38	19	–	43	5	–
Wrap Greek	½	485	15	33	–	33	6	–
Wrap Tuna	½	365	28	13	–	35	4	–
SOUPS								
Chicken & Dumplings	1 (8 oz)	130	11	3	–	22	1	–
Chicken Potpie	1 (8 oz)	200	13	8	–	21	3	–
Italian Wedding w/ Turkey Meatballs	1 (8 oz)	120	10	4	–	13	1	–
Jamaican Bay Gumbo	1 (8 oz)	140	12	3	–	20	2	–
Lobster Bisque	1 (8 oz)	260	11	18	–	14	0	–
Pepper Steak	1 (8 oz)	160	11	6	–	19	1	–
Potato Cheddar	1 (8 oz)	210	11	13	–	16	1	–
Sesame Noodle Bowl	1 (8 oz)	80	6	3	–	7	1	–
Shrimp & Crawfish Etouffee	1 (8 oz)	130	10	4	–	17	1	–
Sicilian Pizza	1 (8 oz)	150	6	7	–	18	2	–
Spicy Crab & Rice	1 (8 oz)	110	7	2	–	21	1	–
Turkey Chili	1 (8 oz)	120	11	2	–	19	3	–
Wild Mushroom Barley	1 (8 oz)	108	3	3	–	18	2	–